PICTURE

MedE@sy™

Editor-in-Chief

Vaibhav Bharat DNB/MS (General Surgery)
Director, MedE@sy

Authors

Aditi Bharat MD (Anesthesia)
TATA Memorial Hospital
Mumbai, Maharashtra

Gaurav Bharat MD (Pathology)
PathKind Labs

Sapna Bharat DNB (Obs)
Consultant Gynecologist
Cloudnine Hospital
Mumbai, Maharashtra

Associate Authors

Amogh Tiwari MD (Pathology)
People's Medical College
Bhopal, Madhya Pradesh

Vivek Dudeja MS (ENT) DNB, MNAMS
Consultant ENT Surgeon
Hisar, Haryana

Akanksha Jain MD (Community Medicine)
Assistant Professor
Government Medical College
Vidisha, Madhya Pradesh

CBS
Dedicated to Education

CBS Publishers & Distributors Pvt Ltd

• New Delhi • Bengaluru • Chennai • Kochi • Kolkata • Mumbai
• Hyderabad • Nagpur • Patna • Pune • Vijayawada

DISCLAIMER

The content presented in this book is copyrighted to the authors of MedE@sy and is based upon the topics, which have been most frequently asked in Pre PG Medical entrance examinations throughout the world. We don't claim the material presented in this book is exactly same, duplicated or reproduced from any examination conducted by any Board or Authority, statutory or non statutory in India or outside India. We declare that this book is neither sponsored nor related to any board or authority of Government (statutory or non statutory) and neither it contains any proprietary material of any board or authority of Government (statutory or non statutory). The conceptualization of images in this book is purely the work of our authors, however medical science is a generic knowledge and creating similar material by authors is not uncommon. Any resemblance to them is purely a coincidence and by chance. Pictures and color plates presented in the book are copyrighted material of authors of MedE@sy, if not specified otherwise.

Copying and reproducing any of the material of this book in any form completely or partially is prohibited under copyright act and is binding by law.

ISBN: 978-93-89941-93-7

Copyright © Authors and Publishers

First Edition: 2020

All rights reserved. No part of this book may be reproduced or transmitted in any form or by any means, electronic or mechanical, including photocopying, recording, or any information storage and retrieval system without permission, in writing, from the authors and the publishers.

Published by **Satish Kumar Jain** and produced by **Varun Jain** for

CBS Publishers & Distributors Pvt Ltd
4819/XI Prahlad Street, 24 Ansari Road, Daryaganj, New Delhi 110 002, India.
Ph: +91-11-23289259, 23266861, 23266867   Website: www.cbspd.com
Fax: 011-23243014
e-mail: delhi@cbspd.com; cbspubs@airtelmail.in

Corporate Office: 204 FIE, Industrial Area, Patparganj, Delhi 110 092
Ph: +91-11-4934 4934   Fax: 4934 4935
e-mail: feedback@cbspd.com; bhupesharora@cbspd.com

Branches

- **Bengaluru:** Seema House 2975, 17th Cross, K.R. Road, Banasankari 2nd Stage, Bengaluru 560 070, Karnataka
  Ph: +91-80-26771678/79   Fax: +91-80-26771680   e-mail: bangalore@cbspd.com
- **Chennai:** 7, Subbaraya Street, Shenoy Nagar, Chennai 600 030, Tamil Nadu
  Ph: +91-44-26680620, 26681266   Fax: +91-44-42032115   e-mail: chennai@cbspd.com
- **Kochi:** 68/1534, 35, 36-Power House Road, Opp. KSEB, Cochin-682018, Kochi, Kerala
  Ph: +91-484-4059061-65   Fax: +91-484-4059065   e-mail: kochi@cbspd.com
- **Kolkata:** 6/B, Ground Floor, Rameswar Shaw Road, Kolkata-700 014, West Bengal
  Ph: +91-33-22891126, 22891127, 22891128   e-mail: kolkata@cbspd.com
- **Mumbai:** 83-C, Dr E Moses Road, Worli, Mumbai-400018, Maharashtra
  Ph: +91-22-24902340/41   Fax: +91-22-24902342   e-mail: mumbai@cbspd.com

Representatives

- **Hyderabad**   +91-9885175004
- **Pune**   +91-9623451994
- **Patna**   +91-9334159340
- **Vijayawada**   +91-9000660880

Printed At : Goyal Offset Works (P) Limited

PICTURE MEDEASY REVIEW BOARD

Subject	Authors and Reviewers
Anatomy	Dr Aprajita Awasthi
Biochemistry	Dr Ashutosh Saxena
Microbiology	Dr Swati Gupta
Parasitology	Dr Swati Gupta
Pathology	Dr Gaurav Bharat
Histology	Dr Aprajita Awasthi
Forensic Medicine	Dr Shashank Sharma
Preventive & Social Medicine	Dr Akanksha Jain
ENT	Dr Vivek Dudeja, Dr Abhay Kumar Singh
Ophthalmology	Dr Vineet Sehgal
Medicine	Dr Manoj Gupta
Pediatrics	Dr Nikhil Lohiya, Dr Ruby Singh
Obstetrics & Gynecology	Dr Sapna Bharat
Surgery	Dr Vaibhav Bharat, Dr Mayank Porwal
Orthopedics	Dr Anurag Tiwari
Osteology	Dr Aprajita Awasthi
Dermatology	Dr Ishad Aggarwal
Radiodiagnosis	Dr Shweta Khanna Aggarwal, Dr Vaibhav Bharat
Anesthesia	Dr Aditi Bharat, Dr Harshvardhan Bharadwaj

From the Publisher's Desk

Dear Readers,

I extend my warm welcome and convey my heartfelt thanks for appreciating the CBS Exam Books for another successful year. It has been an amazing journey so far and I am highly grateful for your support and cooperation to help us achieve various milestones in this whole span of time. The mission with which we started in the year 2015 was to bring nothing but the best of everything to our target audience and today I can proudly say that we have maintained that standard and are committed to continue the same in future as well.

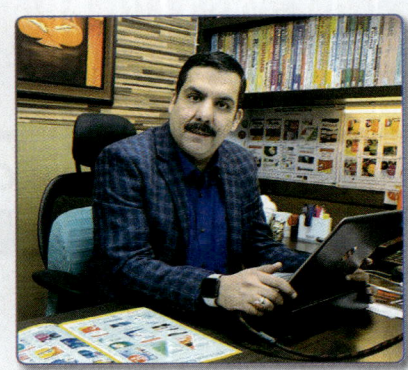

Every single title under the banner of CBS Exam Books has been developed and nurtured like an infant. The authors and our entire team work day and night to bring the best in everything for you. Be it content, presentation, social media contests and offers, we strive to meet your expectations with every passing year. Your trust has motivated us to maintain and upgrade ourselves during this period. I am extremely thankful to all our authors who are the real pillars of the complete series of CBS Exam Books. The contributions of our esteemed authors have laid the foundations of CBS Exam Books.

At this juncture, I can recall these lines by Drake,

"Sometimes it's the journey that teaches you a lot about your destination".

We have grown and changed with the passage of time to upgrade our ways of providing our readers with maximum benefits and help them manage their time and efforts in effective manner. Previous year was the year of great achievements. Let me show you a glimpse of our successful journey:

- Most of the titles of CBS Exam Books received wide acceptance and recognition by the readers of proving their usefulness and supremacy. To mention a few, SARP Anatomy, CRISP, Surgery Sixer, Complete Review of Pathology, Conceptual Review of Pharmacology, SOCH, Forensic Medicine, Complete Review of Medicine, Conceptual Review of PSM, MICRONS, My PGMEE Notes, AIIMS MedEasy, and PRIMEs. With your constant support and our consistent efforts, I am sure that we will together witness an exponential acceptance of all CBS Exam Books in coming future as well.
- The presence of CBS Exam Books has broadened through our various social media platforms. We have received great appreciation for our regular Facebook activities such as online test series, giveaways, scientific content for knowledge enhancement, authors' live sessions, and various contests, like Bid 2 Win, Fastest Finger First, Book Fair and Facebook Community Awards. Join us on all these platforms to avail and enjoy our exciting offers and benefits.

A book is incomplete if it does not have the right readers. We value you and your feedback. Please share your feedback and suggestions directly with me at bhupesharora@cbspd.com. We promise to deliver in our books, what you desire to see.

I would like to sum up with these eternal lines of Robert Frost:

Woods are lovely dark and deep,
But I have promises to keep.
And miles to go before I sleep,
And miles to go before I sleep!
Wishing you success in all your endeavors!

Bhupesh Arora
Vice President – Publishing & Marketing
(PGMEE and Nursing Division)
Email: bhupesharora@cbspd.com
Mobile: (+91) 9555590180

Preface

At the outset, we would like to thank all our readers, who have time and again shown faith in our endeavors. It is always encouraging if your work is appreciated and we are grateful for this overwhelming response. With the success of AIIMS MedE@sy, it gives us immense pleasure to present the picture/video-based book, Picture MedEasy.

The most popular part of our AIIMS MedE@sy book was COLOR PLATES. This inspired us to design this exclusively dedicated Picture Based book for our readers. This books contains a very comprehensive book of images arranged according to subjects, topics and subtopics. The book also covers related images and their theory part alongside for better understanding of the subject and potential future image based questions.

We have done our level best to come up with right answers, but 'To err is Human', and we are humans too. However, we constantly keep in touch with our readers through our website www.medeasyindia.com, and our Facebook fan page https://www.facebook.com/MedEasyindia/ to keep them updated with any correction, change or improvement in our book. We are also operating subject-wise groups by the name of MedE@sy followed by respective subject name.

We heartily invite any suggestions, corrections or discussions of PG Medical entrance MCQs on our mail id infomedeasyindia@gmail.com

Thanks!

Authors/Editors
AIIMS MedE@sy

MEDEASY ONLINE RESOURCE

Visit our dedicated webportal for errata, free downloads and feedback
http://www.medeasyindia.com/
Join our Facebook Page for Updates and Notifications
Join Subject-wise MedE@sy Groups for Discussions
https://www.facebook.com/MedEasyindia/

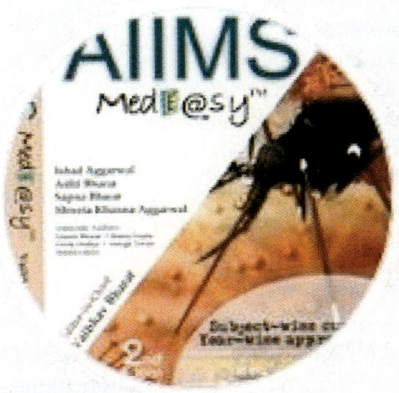

MedEasy Review
@MedEasyindia

 4.9 out of 5 · Based on the opinion of 13 people

Community   See all

- Invite your friends to like this Page
- 88,424 people like this
- 88,211 people follow this
- DrBinayak Bibek Das and 125 other friends like this or have checked in

Dedication and Acknowledgements

We would like to take this opportunity to dedicate this work and to thank people who directly contributed to this book or indirectly inspired us.

Almighty, Our Parents and Grandparents

- Saurabh Bharat (MPCD, NYFA)
- Anuj Shrivastava
- Harshvardhan Bharadwaj (SRMC)
- Saket Kumar (SRMC)
- Pankul Mangla (SRMC)
- Vaibhav Chachra (SRMC, SMC, Ghaziabad)
- Mayank Goel (SRMC, ISB, Hyderabad)
- Raghu Prakash (SRMC, CNMC, LHMC)
- Varun Gupta (SRMC, ASCOMS, Gangaram)
- Vipan Bhandari (SRMC)
- Siaram Sharan Kushwah (SRMC)
- Ashish Kumar Gupta (KIMS, Hubli)
- Rohit Katre (GRMC, MAMC)
- Prashant Bharadwaj (SRMC, LLRM)
- Abhay Kumar Singh (SRMC, VMMC)
- Nirupam Sharan (SRMC, Patel Chest Institute)
- Naval Asija (SRMC, NIHFW)
- Parimal Tara (SRMC)
- Pradeep Kumar (SRMC)
- Md Faizer Nazer (SRMC, RPGMC, MAMC)
- Jamaluddin Ahmed Siddique (SRMC)
- Mankeshwar Kumar (SRMC)
- Brajesh Kumar (SRMC, AMC)
- Deepak Ranjan (SRMC, AMC)
- Diwakar Kumar (SRMC, INS Ashvini)
- Harsha Guduru (SRMC)
- Ranjeet Jha (SRMC)
- Swanay Mondal (SRMC)
- Sandip Singh (SRMC)
- Vinish Agarwal (KMC, GRMC, HIHT)
- Mayank Porwal (GRMC, Gwalior)
- Vikram Singh Rathore (GRMC)
- Aprajita Pandey (GRMC)
- Savyasanchi Tiwari (RDGMC)
- Triloki Nath Soni (RDGMC, People's Bhopal)
- Jorawar Singh Bhatia (RDGMC)
- Vikas Mathur
- Hardik Seth
- N Kulshreshta (Director M&HS, DSP)
- A K Sahay (MCh DNB Plastic Surgery DSP)
- Rohit Shyam Singhal (BHU)
- Ravitej Golive (DSP)
- Noor Ain Khan (DSP)
- Zahid Zahiri (DSP)
- Parthasarthi Buniya (DSP)
- Ashvini Natu (RCSM, TMH, Mumbai)
- Rasika Thosar (RCSM, TMH, Mumbai)
- Tineesh Mathew (TMH, Mumbai)
- Deepika Menon (TMH, Mumbai)
- Renuka Purohit (TMH, Mumbai)
- Anupama Zade (TMH, Mumbai)
- Rishi Shankar (TMH, Mumbai)
- Sanika Patil (TMH, Mumbai)
- Kirti Salunke (TMH, Mumbai)
- Shreyas Bhor (TMH, Mumbai)
- Raghvendra Gowda (TMH, Mumbai)
- Prashant Kumar Yadav (TMH, Mumbai)
- Amit Yadav (TMH, Mumbai)
- Meera Metha (TMH, Mumbai)
- Ritesh Patil (TMH, Mumbai)
- Satish Sarode (TMH, Mumbai)
- Sharada Datar (RCSM)
- Anuradha Dhawal (RCSM)
- Hrishikesh Wagholikar (RCSM, GMC, Miraj)
- Freni Shah (RCSM)
- Priyanka Iyangar (RCSM)
- Chhanvar Lal Mali (RCSM)
- Chinmay Inamdar (RCSM)
- Md Sadat Wasim (IPGIMER)
- Nikhat Ara (CNCI, Kolkata)
- Ankush Sharma (RDGMC)
- Rakesh Soni (RDGMC)
- Nandeep Kushwah (RDGMC)
- Surjeet Shukla (RDGMC)
- Ruby Singh (RDGMC, SAIMS, Indore)
- Malvika Tripathi (RDGMC)
- Jyotsna Khatri (RDGMC)
- Shubha Jaggi (RDGMC)
- Aditi Damle (RDGMC)
- Shravan Patidar (RDGMC, SAIMS)

We appreciate the support of **Mr Satish Kumar Jain** (Chairman CBS Publishers) and **Mr Varun Jain** (Managing Director, CBS Publishers) for their unconditional support in publication of this book. We are overwhelmed by the initiative and support of **Mr Bhupesh Arora**, Vice President – Publishing & Marketing PGMEE and Nursing Division of CBS Publishers and Distributors.

We sincerely thank the entire CBS team for bringing out the book with utmost care and attractive presentation. We thank Dr Mrinalini Bakshi (Editorial Head & Content Strategist) for her editorial support and Ms Nitasha Arora (Production Head & Content Strategist), Dr Anju Dhir (Project Manager & Senior Scientific Coordinator), Mr Shivendu Bhushan Pandey (Senior Editor), Mr Ashutosh Pathak (Senior Proof Reader) and all the production team members, Mr Chaman Lal, Mr Prakash Gaur, Mr Phool Kumar, Mr Bunty Kashyap, Mr Chander Mani, Ms Tahira Parveen, Ms Babita Verma, Ms Manorama Gupta, Mr Raju Sharma, Mr Manoj Chaudhary, Mr Vikram Chaudhary, Mr Manoj Malakar and Mr Rahul Negi for devoting laborious hours in designing and typesetting of the book.

Preface v
Dedication and Acknowledgements vi
Video-based Topics .... xiii - xx

Subjects	Page No.	Number of Plates
Anatomy	1–40	31
Biochemistry	41–48	4
Microbiology	49–68	23
Parasitology	69–98	19
Pathology	99–144	55
Histology	145–164	11
Forensic Medicine	165–186	14
Preventive & Social Medicine	187–202	12
ENT	203–224	27
Ophthalmology	225–254	36
Medicine	255–264	9
Pediatrics	265–274	9
Obstetrics & Gynecology	275–296	22
Surgery	297–328	59
Orthopedics	329–356	31
Osteology	357–368	7
Dermatology	369–410	45
Radiodiagnosis & Radiotherapy	411–452	56
Anesthesia	453–468	16
		Total Plates = 486

Subject-wise cum Topic-wise Color Plates Content List

For quick glance over desired topic/plate, this list has been prepared under each subject, respectively

VIDEO-BASED TOPICS

- Video 1: Allen's Test ... xv
- Video 2: Strongyloides ... xv
- Video 3: Breast Examination ... xvii
- Video 4: Different Seizure Patterns ... xvii
- Video 5: Silverman Scoring ... xviii
- Video 6: Roos Test ... xix
- Video 7: Gower's Sign ... xix
- Video 8: Laparoscopic Falope Ring Applicator ... xix
- Video 9: Fistulogram ... xx
- Video 10: Hysterosalpingography (HSG) ... xx
- Video 11: T Tube Cholangiography ... xx

ANATOMY

- Plate 1: Pharyngeal Pouches and Clefts ... 3
- Plate 2: Notochord & Neurulation ... 4
- Plate 3: 5-week Embryo ... 5
- Plate 4: Dermatomes in Umbilical Region ... 6
- Plate 5: Inferior Surface of Brain ... 8
- Plate 6: Coronal & Transverse Section of Brain ... 9
- Plate 7: Cerebrum: Sections and Functional Areas ... 11
- Plate 8: Base of Skull ... 13
- Plate 9: Structure of Brainstem ... 14
- Plate 10: Arterial Supply to Brain ... 16
- Plate 11: Cavernous Sinus ... 17
- Plate 12: Cross And Sagittal Section of Neck ... 18
- Plate 13: Muscles of Mastication ... 19
- Plate 14: Structures in Neck ... 21
- Plate 15: Intrinsic Muscles of Larynx ... 21
- Plate 16: Clavipectoral Fascia ... 22
- Plate 17: Cross Section of Axilla ... 23
- Plate 18: Muscles of The Chest Wall ... 24
- Plate 19: Ductal Anatomy of The Breast ... 25
- Plate 20: Linea Alba and Inguinal Ligament ... 25
- Plate 21: Muscles of The Forearm ... 26
- Plate 22: Muscles of the Hand ... 29
- Plate 23: Innervation of the Hand ... 31
- Plate 24: Epiploic Foramen ... 31
- Plate 25: Calot's and Hepatobiliary Triangle ... 32
- Plate 26: Coronal & Parasagittal section of Ischiorectal Fossa ... 33
- Plate 27: Gluteal Region Dissection ... 35
- Plate 28: Surface Anatomy of Heart ... 35
- Plate 29: Extraocular and Intraocular Muscles ... 36
- Plate 30: Retroperitoneum Dissection ... 37
- Plate 31: Cadaveric Dissection of Anterior Surface of Heart ... 38

BIOCHEMISTRY

- Plate 1: James Dewey Watson and Francis Harry Compton Crick ... 43
- Plate 2: DNA Structure ... 43
- Plate 3: Urine Analysis ... 44
- Plate 4: Insulin Synthesis and Structure of Human Proinsulin ... 47

MICROBIOLOGY

- Plate 1: Louis Pasteur ... 51
- Plate 2: Sir Ronald Ross ... 51
- Plate 3: Robert Heinrich Herman Koch ... 51
- Plate 4: Antonie Van Leeuwenhoek ... 51
- Plate 5: Charles Louis Alphonse Laveran ... 52
- Plate 6: Sir Alexander Fleming ... 52
- Plate 7: Gram and Acid Fast Microrganisms ... 52
- Plate 8: Microscopy in Genital Ulcer Smear ... 54
- Plate 9: Spirochetes ... 55
- Plate 10: Actinomyces ... 56
- Plate 11: KOH Mount ... 57
- Plate 12: Sporothrix Schenckii ... 57
- Plate 13: Chromoblastomycosis ... 58
- Plate 14: Different Species of Opportunistic Fungi ... 59
- Plate 15: Histoplasma Capsulatum ... 61
- Plate 16: Cytomegalovirus ... 61
- Plate 17: Swarming of Proteus on Blood Agar ... 61
- Plate 18: Haemophilus Influenzae ... 61
- Plate 19: Elek Test for Corynebacterium Diphtheriae ... 62
- Plate 20: Meningococcal Septicemia ... 62
- Plate 21: N 95 Mask for H1N1 ... 63
- Plate 22: Immunoglobulins ... 66
- Plate 23: HBsAg Rapid Card ... 67

PARASITOLOGY

- Plate 1: Entamoeba Histolytica ... 71
- Plate 2: Free Living Amoeba ... 74
- Plate 3: Balantidium Coli (Ciliate) ... 76
- Plate 4: Giardia duodenalis ... 77
- Plate 5: Toxoplasma Gondii (Ciliate) ... 78
- Plate 6: Plasmodium Vivax ... 80
- Plate 7: Plasmodium Malariae ... 80
- Plate 8: Plasmodium Falciparum ... 81
- Plate 9: Plasmodium Ovale ... 81
- Plate 10: Life Cycle of Malaria Parasite (Plasmodium) ... 82
- Plate 11: Leishmania ... 84
- Plate 12: Microfilariae of Medical Importance ... 85
- Plate 13: Fasciola Hepatica (Sheep Liver Fluke) ... 87
- Plate 14: Paragonimus ... 89
- Plate 15: Strongyloides ... 90
- Plate 16: Hymenolepis Nana ... 92
- Plate 17: Trichuris Trichiura ... 94
- Plate 18: Eggs of Nematodes ... 95
- Plate 19: Cryptosporidium Parvum ... 96

PATHOLOGY

- Plate 1: Vacutainer System ... 101
- Plate 2: Urinary Crystals ... 102
- Plate 3: Urinary Casts ... 104
- Plate 4: Pathognomonic Changes in Kidney Damage ... 106

Plate 5: Cells of Peripheral Smear 107
Plate 6: Human RBC with Fluorescent Microscopy 108
Plate 7: Pathologic Red Cells in Blood Smear 108
Plate 8: Hemolytic Disorders 111
Plate 9: Blood Picture Megaloblastic Anemia 112
Plate 10: Blood Picture of Iron Deficiency Anemia 112
Plate 11: Blood Picture of Aplastic Anemia 112
Plate 12: Warm and Cold AIHA 113
Plate 13: Acute Myeloid Leukemia (AML) 113
Plate 14: Chronic Myeloid Leukemia (CML) 113
Plate 15: Acute Lymphoid Leukemia (ALL) 114
Plate 16: Chronic Lymphoid Leukemia (CLL) 114
Plate 17: Michaelis–Gutmann Bodies 115
Plate 18: Pelger-Huët Anomaly 115
Plate 19: Dohle Bodies 115
Plate 20: May-Hegglin Inclusion 116
Plate 21: Plasma Cell Neoplasms 116
Plate 22: Burkitt's Lymphoma 117
Plate 23: Hodgkins Lymphoma 117
Plate 24: Infectious Mononucleosis 119
Plate 25: Gaucher Disease 119
Plate 26: Microscopic Features of Myocardial Infarction .. 119
Plate 27: Rheumatic Heart Disease & Endocarditis 120
Plate 28: Types of Cardiomyopathy 122
Plate 29: Barrett Esophagus and Carcinoma of Esophagus ... 125
Plate 30: Intestinal Polyps 126
Plate 31: Nutmeg Liver; Liver with Chronic Passive
Congestion and Hemorrhagic Necrosis 128
Plate 32: Hemochromatosis 129
Plate 33: Giardia Histopathology 129
Plate 34: Whipple's Disease 130
Plate 35: Crohn's Disease 130
Plate 36: Salivary Gland Tumors 130
Plate 37: Papillary Carcinomas of Thyroid 131
Plate 38: Follicular Carcinomas of Thyroid 132
Plate 39: Medullary Carcinoma of Thyroid 132
Plate 40: Anaplastic Thyroid Carcinoma 132
Plate 41: Breast Tissue Biopsy 134
Plate 42: Malignant Hypertension and
Accelerated Nephrosclerosis 135
Plate 43: Types of Glomerulonephritis 136
Plate 44: Pyelonephritis 138
Plate 45: Renal Amyloidosis 139
Plate 46: Kimmelstiel Wilson Lesion in Diabetic Nephropathy ... 139
Plate 47: Reticulin Stain 140
Plate 48: Chronic Inflammatory Demyelinating
Polyradiculoneuropathy (CIDP) 140
Plate 49: Infection of Brain (Histopathology) 141
Plate 50: Schwannoma 142
Plate 51: Transmissible Spongiform Encephalopathies
(Prion Diseases) 143
Plate 52: Fibrosarcomas 143
Plate 53: Fat Embolism 143
Plate 54: Aspiration Pneumonia 144
Plate 55: Blood Bag with Leukoreduction Filter 144

HISTOLOGY

Plate 1: Electron Microscopic Picture of
Golgi Apparatus and Mitochondria 147
Plate 2: Some Important Epithelium Linings 149
Plate 3: Structural Classification of Exocrine Glands 151
Plate 4: Classification of Exocrine Glands on the
Basis of Mechanism of Secretion 153
Plate 5: Types of Cartilages 155
Plate 6: Muscle Cell's Types 156
Plate 7: Gastric Mucosa Histology 157
Plate 8: Lymphatic Organs 159
Plate 9: Histology of Adrenal Gland 162
Plate 10: Primary Visual Cortex 164
Plate 11: Histology of Cerebellum 164

FORENSIC MEDICINE

Plate 1: Types of Abrasion 167
Plate 2: Types of Wound 167
Plate 3: Signs of Asphyxial Death 168
Plate 4: Shotgun Firearm Injuries 170
Plate 5: Early and Late Signs of Death 173
Plate 6: Autopsy Staining of Myocardium 176
Plate 7: Motorcyclist's Fracture 176
Plate 8: Cardiac Poisons – Herbal 178
Plate 9: Spinal Poisons – Herbal 179
Plate 10: Inorganic Irritant Metal Poisoning Symptoms ... 180
Plate 11: Organic Irritants – Vegetable Origin 181
Plate 12: Deliriant Poisons 184
Plate 13: Animal Poisons 185
Plate 14: Somniferous Poisons (Opioids) 186

PREVENTIVE AND SOCIAL MEDICINE

Plate 1: James Lind 189
Plate 2: John Snow 189
Plate 3: Emblems and Logos 189
Plate 4: Biomedical Waste Categories 193
Plate 5: Mosquito Vectors 195
Plate 6: Sand Fly 197
Plate 7: Oriental Rat Flea 197
Plate 8: Pediculosis (Lice) 198
Plate 9: Scabies 199
Plate 10: Vaccine Vial Monitor 199
Plate 11: Sling Psychrometers 201
Plate 12: Kata Thermometer 201

ENT

Plate 1: Middle Ear Cavity 205
Plate 2: Mastoidectomy 205
Plate 3: Internal Ear Structures 206
Plate 4: Tracheostomy Tubes 208
Plate 5: Tracheostomy Procedure 210
Plate 6: Trousseau Tracheal Dilator 212
Plate 7: Head Mirror 213
Plate 8: Bull's Lamp 213
Plate 9: Aural Speculum 213
Plate 10: Tuning Forks 213

Plate 11: Boyle-Davis Mouth Gag	214
Plate 12: Doyen Mouth's Gag	214
Plate 13: Mollison Self-Retaining Hemostatic Mastoid Retractor	214
Plate 14: Nasal Speculum	215
Plate 15: Walsham and Asch Forceps	215
Plate 16: Luc Forceps	216
Plate 17: Instruments Used In Tonsillectomy	216
Plate 18: Rhinoscopy And Laryngoscopy Mirror	217
Plate 19: Signs of Basilar Skull Fracture	217
Plate 20: Laryngomalacia	218
Plate 21: Respiratory Papillomatosis	218
Plate 22: Audiograms	220
Plate 23: Retropharyngeal Abscess X-Ray	221
Plate 24: The Steeple Sign (Wine Bottle Sign)	221
Plate 25: CT Scan PNS	222
Plate 26: Oral Thrush	223
Plate 27: Peritonsillar Abscess (Quinsy)	223

OPHTHALMOLOGY

Plate 1: Vossius Ring	227
Plate 2: Lid Retraction Signs of Grave's Ophthalmopathy	227
Plate 3: Clinical Signs of Trachoma	228
Plate 4: WHO Grading of Trachoma	229
Plate 5: Habb Striae	230
Plate 6: Signs of Acute (Congestive) Angle-Closure Glaucoma	230
Plate 7: Normal Optic Nerve Head	230
Plate 8: Normal Vs Enlarged Optic Nerve	230
Plate 9: Progression of Optic Nerve Cupping in Glaucoma	231
Plate 10: Optic Disc Changes in Glaucoma	232
Plate 11: Grades of Papilloedema	232
Plate 12: Bilateral Papilloedema (Raised ICT)	233
Plate 13: Acute Angle-Closure Glaucoma Sequelae	233
Plate 14: Fungal Keratitis	233
Plate 15: Cytomegalovirus Retinitis	235
Plate 16: Intermediate Uveitis (Pars Planitis)	235
Plate 17: Microvascular Abnormalities	236
Plate 18: Diabetic Retinopathy	236
Plate 19: Hypertensive Retinopathy	238
Plate 20: Vernal Keratoconjunctivitis	239
Plate 21: Testing Corneal Sensations	240
Plate 22: Maddox Rod	240
Plate 23: Ophthalmoscope	241
Plate 24: Histology of Retinal Layers and OCT of Eye	243
Plate 25: Right Superior Oblique Palsy	245
Plate 26: Berlin's Edema or Commotio Retina	245
Plate 27: Granular Dystrophy	246
Plate 28: Salt and Pepper Appearance of Fundus/Retina	248
Plate 29: Necrotizing Retinochoroiditis	248
Plate 30: Corneal Ulcer	249
Plate 31: Tonometer	249
Plate 32: After Cataract	251
Plate 33: Ptosis	251
Plate 34: Pterygium	252
Plate 35: Cranial Nerve Palsy	252
Plate 36: Metallic Foreign Body (Nail) in Eye	254

MEDICINE

Plate 1: Bone Marrow Biopsy Needles	257
Plate 2: Liver Biopsy Needles	258
Plate 3: Knee Jerk	259
Plate 4: Babinski Sign	261
Plate 5: Types of Facial Nerve Palsy	261
Plate 6: Different Types of Faces	261
Plate 7: Named Signs in Medicine	262
Plate 8: Acral Lentiginous Melanoma	263
Plate 9: Massive Splenomegaly	263

PEDIATRICS

late 1: Infantometer	267
Plate 2: Phototherapy Units/System	267
Plate 3: Turner's Syndrome	268
Plate 4: Sprengel Deformity	269
Plate 5: Neural Tube Defects	269
Plate 6: Unilateral Cleft Lip	271
Plate 7: Muscular Dystrophy	272
Plate 8: Reusable Neonatal SPO_2 Wraps Sensor	273
Plate 9: Sirenomelia	274

OBSTETRICS AND GYNECOLOGY

Plate 1: Pap Smear Collecting Devices	277
Plate 2: Episiotomy Scissors	277
Plate 3: Cusco's Speculum	278
Plate 4: Bakri Postpartum Balloon	278
Plate 5: Karman Cannula	278
Plate 6: Myoma Screw	279
Plate 7: Falope Ring Applicator	279
Plate 8: Ventouse	280
Plate 9: New Generation Ventouse	280
Plate 10: Commonly Used Obstetrics Forceps	281
Plate 11: Hegar's Dilator	283
Plate 12: Intrauterine Devices	283
Plate 13: Ovarian Cancers	284
Plate 14: Vaginal Infections	287
Plate 15: Bacterial Vaginosis	288
Plate 16: Polycystic Ovary	289
Plate 17: Endometrioma	290
Plate 18: Placental Variations	290
Plate 19: Hysterosalpingography	292
Plate 20: Early Pregnancy Ultrasound	292
Plate 21: Types of Abortion	293
Plate 22: Gestational Trophoblastic Disease	294

SURGERY

Plate 1: Foley's Catheter	299
Plate 2: Nasogastric Tube (Ryles)	299
Plate 3: Sengstaken–Blakemore Tube	300
Plate 4: Myer's Vein Stripper	301
Plate 5: Kelly's Proctoscope	301
Plate 6: Bard Parker's Handle and Surgical Blades	302
Plate 7: Needle Holding Forceps	302
Plate 8: Dissecting/Thumb Forceps	302
Plate 9: Surgical Scissors	303
Plate 10: Heath's Suture Cutting Scissors	303

Plate 11	Rampley's Swab (Sponge) Holding Forceps	303
Plate 12	Jones/Doyen's/Mayo's Towel Clip	304
Plate 13	Backhaus Towel Clip	304
Plate 14	Spencer Well's Hemostatic Forceps (Artery Forceps)	304
Plate 15	Halsted's Hemostatic Forceps (Mosquito Forceps)	304
Plate 16	Kocher's Forceps	305
Plate 17	Lister's Sinus Forceps	305
Plate 18	Allie's Tissue Forceps	305
Plate 19	Babcock's Tissue Forceps	305
Plate 20	Lane's Tissue Forceps	306
Plate 21	Cheatle's Forceps	306
Plate 22	Langenbeck's Right Angled Retractor	306
Plate 23	Czerney's Retractor	306
Plate 24	Morris Retractor	306
Plate 25	Deaver's Retractor	307
Plate 26	Doyen's Retractor	307
Plate 27	Desjardin's Choledocholithitomy Forceps	307
Plate 28	Suprapubic Cystolithotomy Forceps	307
Plate 29	Doyen Gastrointestinal Occlusion (Noncrushing) Clamp	308
Plate 30	Moynihan's Gastric Occlusion (Noncrushing) Clamp	308
Plate 31	Lane's Twin Gastrojejunostomy Occlusion Clamp	308
Plate 32	Payr's Crushing Clamp	308
Plate 33	Bulldog Vascular Clamp	309
Plate 34	Satinsky Vascular Clamp	309
Plate 35	Humby's Knife	309
Plate 36	Sutures	310
Plate 37	Diathermy	311
Plate 38	Laparoscope and its Parts	312
Plate 39	Intercostal Chest Tube Drain (Tube Thoracostomy)	314
Plate 40	Vacuum Assisted Closure	316
Plate 41	Damage Control Surgery	316
Plate 42	Myocutaneous Flaps	317
Plate 43	Signs of Appendicitis	318
Plate 44	Cullen's and Grey Turner's Sign	318
Plate 45	Incisional Hernia	318
Plate 46	Ranula	319
Plate 47	Thyroglossus Cyst	319
Plate 48	Raynaud's Phenomenon	320
Plate 49	Common Causes of Leg Ulcers	320
Plate 50	Varicocele	321
Plate 51	Balanoposthitis	322
Plate 52	Balanitis Xerotica Obliterans (BXO)	322
Plate 53	Genital Wart/Condyloma Acuminatum	323
Plate 54	Pilonidal Cyst	323
Plate 55	Retroperitoneal Hemorrhage Zones	324
Plate 56	Basal Cell Carcinoma	324
Plate 57	Gallbladder Pathology Specimens	326
Plate 58	Trichobezoars	327
Plate 59	Mondor's Disease	327

ORTHOPEDICS

Plate 1	Hip Prosthesis	331
Plate 2	Sequestrum Holding Forceps	332
Plate 3	Bone Holding Forceps	332
Plate 4	Bone Surgery Instruments	333
Plate 5	Ligament Injuries of Fingers	333
Plate 6	Stenosing Tenosynovitis (Trigger Finger)	335
Plate 7	Ulnar Claw Hand	335
Plate 8	Ankylosing Spondylitis	337
Plate 9	Fracture of Patella	338
Plate 10	Neer Classification of Proximal Humerus Fracture	339
Plate 11	Scaphoid Fracture	340
Plate 12	Colle's Fracture	341
Plate 13	Galeazzi Fracture	341
Plate 14	Monteggia Fracture	342
Plate 15	Supracondylar Fracture of Humerus	342
Plate 16	Cubitus Valgus	344
Plate 17	Hallux Valgus (Bunion)	344
Plate 18	Forefoot Adduction Deformity	345
Plate 19	Slipped Capital Femoral Epiphysis (SCFE)	345
Plate 20	Posterior Dislocation of Hip	346
Plate 21	Developmental Dysplasia of The Hip	347
Plate 22	Congenital Tibial Pseudoarthrosis	348
Plate 23	Cobb's Angle in Scoliosis	348
Plate 24	Vertebral Anomalies	349
Plate 25	Anatomical Snuff Box	350
Plate 26	Popeye Deformity	350
Plate 27	Osteogenesis Imperfecta	351
Plate 28	Splints in Orthopedics	352
Plate 29	Rail External Fixator	354
Plate 30	Anterior Dislocation of Shoulder Joint	354
Plate 31	Posterior Dislocation of Shoulder Joint	355

OSTEOLOGY

Plate 1	Anatomy of Skull	359
Plate 2	Mandible: Superior Anteriolateral View	363
Plate 3	Atlas (CI) Inferior and Superior View	364
Plate 4	Cervical, Thoracic and Lumbar Vertebra	365
Plate 5	Scapula Bone	366
Plate 6	Clavicle	367
Plate 7	Femur	367

DERMATOLOGY

Plate 1	Histology of Skin	371
Plate 2	Birbeck Granules	372
Plate 3	Wood's Lamp	372
Plate 4	Tinea Versicolor	373
Plate 5	Erythrasma	374
Plate 6	Some Important Conditions of the Tongue	374
Plate 7	Alopecia Areata	375
Plate 8	Trichotillomania	377
Plate 9	Psoriasis Vulgaris	377
Plate 10	Impetigo Herpetiformis	378
Plate 11	Lupus Vulgaris	378
Plate 12	Pemphigus Vulgaris (and Variants)	379
Plate 13	Bullous Pemphigoid	382
Plate 14	Lichen Planus	382
Plate 15	Lichen Nitidus	383
Plate 16	Blister Packs of MDT of Leprosy	384
Plate 17	Tuberculoid Leprosy (TT)/ Paucibacillary	385
Plate 18	Lepromatous Leprosy (LL)/ Multibacillary	386
Plate 19	Borderline Borderline Leprosy	386
Plate 20	Intermediate Leprosy	389
Plate 21	Post Kala Azar Dermal Leishmaniasis	389
Plate 22	Skin Lesions in EM, SJS, TEN	390

Plate 23: Dermatophyte	393
Plate 24: Mycetoma	395
Plate 25: Plantar Warts	395
Plate 26: Molluscum Contagiosum	396
Plate 27: Herpes Zoster (Shingles)	397
Plate 28: Hand, Foot and Mouth Disease (HFMD)	398
Plate 29: Atopic Dermatitis	398
Plate 30: Dermographic Urticaria	399
Plate 31: Tuberous Sclerosis (Bourneville's Disease)	400
Plate 32: Unilateral (Segmental) Vitiligo	401
Plate 33: Types of Acne	403
Plate 34: Acne Rosacea	404
Plate 35: Pityriasis Rosea	404
Plate 36: Congenital Melanocytic Nevus	405
Plate 37: Nevus of OTA	405
Plate 38: Cutaneous Manifestations of Chikungunya Fever	406
Plate 39: Necrobiosis Lipoidica	407
Plate 40: Vesiculobullous Hand Eczema (Pompholyx, Dyshidrosis)	407
Plate 41: Gingival Hyperplasia	408
Plate 42: Piebaldism	408
Plate 43: Dermatological Manifestations of Pallegra	408
Plate 44: Plexiform Neurofibroma	409
Plate 45: Chancre	409

RADIODIAGNOSIS

Plate 1: Wilhelm Conrad Rontgen	413
Plate 2: Normal Chest X-Ray PA View	413
Plate 3: Right Pleural Effusion	414
Plate 4: Chest X-Ray Showing Intercostal Tube Placed for Pleural Effusion	414
Plate 5: Left Pneumothorax	414
Plate 6: Hydropneumothorax	415
Plate 7: Radiological Features of Lung Collapse	415
Plate 8: Right Middle Lobe Consolidation	416
Plate 9: Flail Chest	416
Plate 10: Acute Respiratory Distress Syndrome	416
Plate 11: Pneumatocele	417
Plate 12: Bronchiectasis and/or Cystic Fibrosis	417
Plate 13: Chest X-Ray Signs of Pulmonary Venous Hypertension	418
Plate 14: Pericardial Effusion	418
Plate 15: Rib Notching	419
Plate 16: Congenital Anomalies of Heart	419
Plate 17: Intestinal Obstruction	420
Plate 18: Sigmoid Volvulus Plain Radiograph	421
Plate 19: Caecal Volvulus Plain Radiograph	422
Plate 20: Pneumoperitoneum	422
Plate 21: Achalasia Cardia and Carcinoma of Esophagus	423
Plate 22: Pseudopancreatic Cyst	424
Plate 23: Findings of Ileocaecal (IC) Tuberculosis on Barium Examination	424
Plate 24: Hypertrophic Pyloric Stenosis	424

Plate 25: Sliding Hiatus Hernia	425
Plate 26: Rolling/Paraesophageal Hiatus Hernia	425
Plate 27: Lesions of Liver	425
Plate 28: Diverticular Disease	426
Plate 29: Stages of Pancreatitis	427
Plate 30: IVP, MCU, RUG	428
Plate 31: Urethral Abnormailities	429
Plate 32: Renal Cysts	430
Plate 33: Intracranial Hemorrhage	431
Plate 34: Subarachnoid Hemorrhage & Intracranial Hematomas	433
Plate 35: Cerebral Abscess	433
Plate 36: Cerebral Angiography	434
Plate 37: Acute Osteomyelitis	435
Plate 38: Chronic Osteomyelitis	436
Plate 39: Normal Vertebra with Scottish Dog Sign and Spondylolysis	436
Plate 40: Spondylolisthesis	437
Plate 41: Rickets	437
Plate 42: Scurvy	438
Plate 43: Congenital Syphilis	438
Plate 44: Radiograph of the Knees and Ankle Showing Fractures	439
Plate 45: Deformities of Bones	439
Plate 46: Multiple Myeloma	441
Plate 47: Brown Tumor of Hyperparathyroidism	441
Plate 48: Benign Tumors of Bone	442
Plate 49: Benign Aggressive Bone Tumors	444
Plate 50: Malignant Tumors of Bone	446
Plate 51: Wedge Compression Fracture	448
Plate 52: Lung Ultrasound Signs	448
Plate 53: USG Fast Images	450
Plate 54: PCOD and OHSS	450
Plate 55: Zenker's Diverticulum	451
Plate 56: Coarctation of the Aorta	451

ANESTHESIA

Plate 1: William T. G. Morton	455
Plate 2: Bag Mask Ventilation/Ambu Bag	455
Plate 3: Venturi Mask	455
Plate 4: Guedel's Airway	456
Plate 5: Nasopharyngeal Airway	456
Plate 6: Laryngoscope	457
Plate 7: Endotracheal Tube	458
Plate 8: Types of LMA	459
Plate 9: Lumbar Puncture Needle	462
Plate 10: Tuohy Needle	464
Plate 11: Cannula Sizes and Color Codes	464
Plate 12: Central Venous Catheters	464
Plate 13: Total Parenteral Nutrition	465
Plate 14: Swan Ganz Catheter	466
Plate 15: Gas Cylinders Used in Anesthesia	468
Plate 16: Temperature Measurement Probes (Thermometers)	468

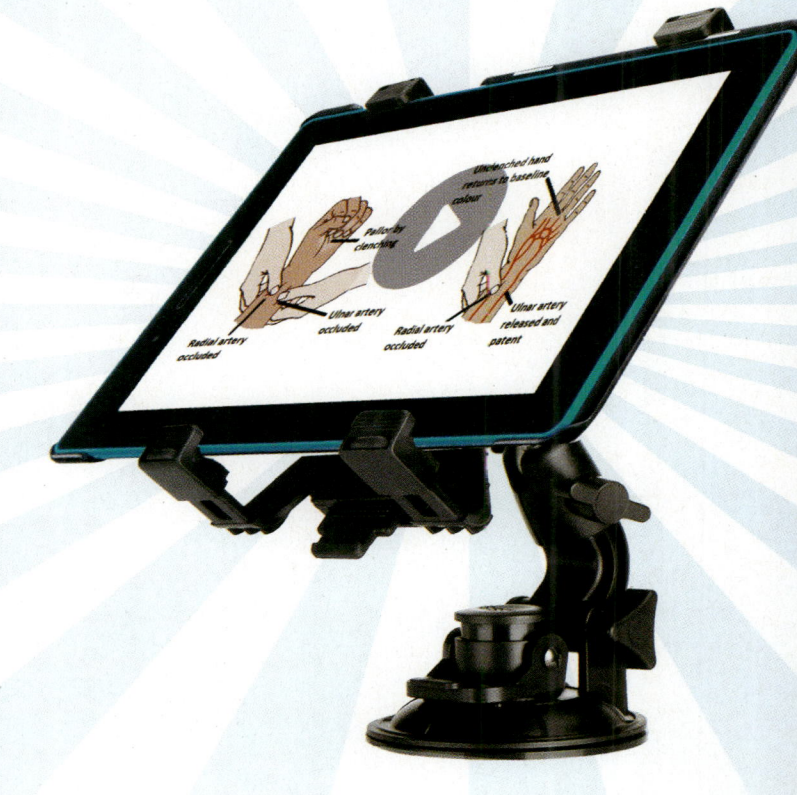

VIDEO-BASED TOPICS

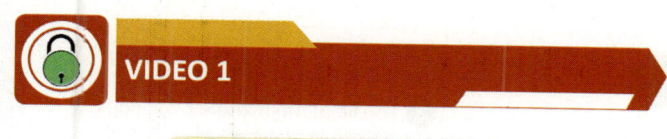

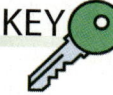 KEY

ALLEN'S TEST

Allen's test, also **Allen test**, is used to test blood supply to the hand, specifically, the patency of the radial and ulnar arteries. It is performed prior to radial arterial blood sampling or cannulation. Allen's test is also performed prior to heart bypass surgery. The radial artery is occasionally used as a conduit for bypass surgery, and its patency lasts longer in comparison to the saphenous veins. Prior to heart bypass surgery, Allen's test is performed to assess the suitability of the radial artery to be used as a conduit

The modified Allen Test

1. The hand is elevated and the patient/person is asked to make a fist for about 30 seconds.
2. Pressure is applied over the ulnar and the radial arteries so as to occlude both of them.
3. Still elevated, the hand is then opened. It should appear blanched (pallor can be observed at the finger nails).
4. Ulnar pressure is released and the color should return in 5-15 seconds.

Inference

Ulnar artery supply to the hand is sufficient and it is safe to cannulate/prick the radial

If color does not return or returns after 5-15 seconds, the test is considered positive and the ulnar artery supply to the hand is not sufficient. The radial artery therefore cannot be safely cannulated.

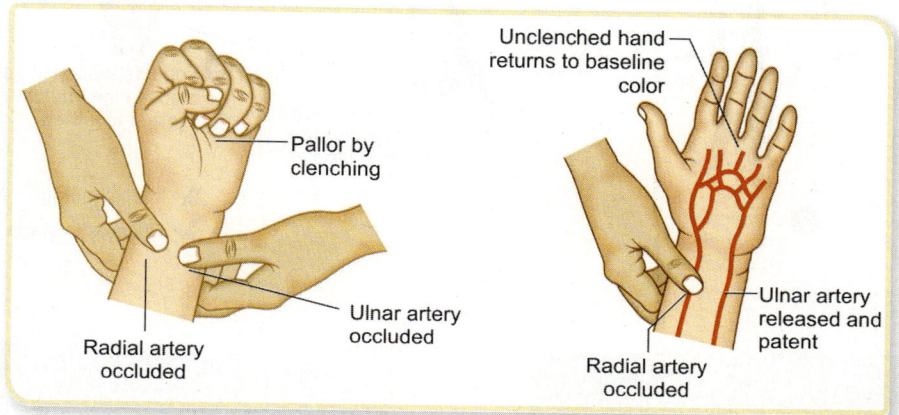

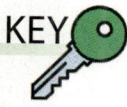 KEY

STRONGYLOIDES

Filariform larvae present in contaminated soil penetrate the human skin, and by various, often random routes, migrate into the small intestine. Historically, it was believed that the L3 larvae migrate via the bloodstream to the lungs, where they are eventually coughed up and swallowed. However, there is also evidence that L3 larvae can migrate directly to the intestine via connective tissues. In the small intestine they moult twice and become adult female worms. The females live threaded in the epithelium of the small intestine and by parthenogenesis produce eggs, which yield rhabditiform larvae. The rhabditiform larvae can either be passed in the stool (see "Free-living cycle" above), or can cause autoinfection. In autoinfection, the rhabditiform larvae become infective filariform larvae, which can penetrate either the intestinal mucosa (internal autoinfection) or the skin of the perianal area (external autoinfection); in either case, the filariform larvae may disseminate throughout the body. To date, occurrence of autoinfection in humans with helminthic infections is recognized only in *Strongyloides stercoralis* and *Capillaria philippinensis* infections. In the case of *Strongyloides*, autoinfection may explain the possibility of persistent infections for many years in persons who have not been in an endemic area and of hyperinfections in immunosuppressed individuals.

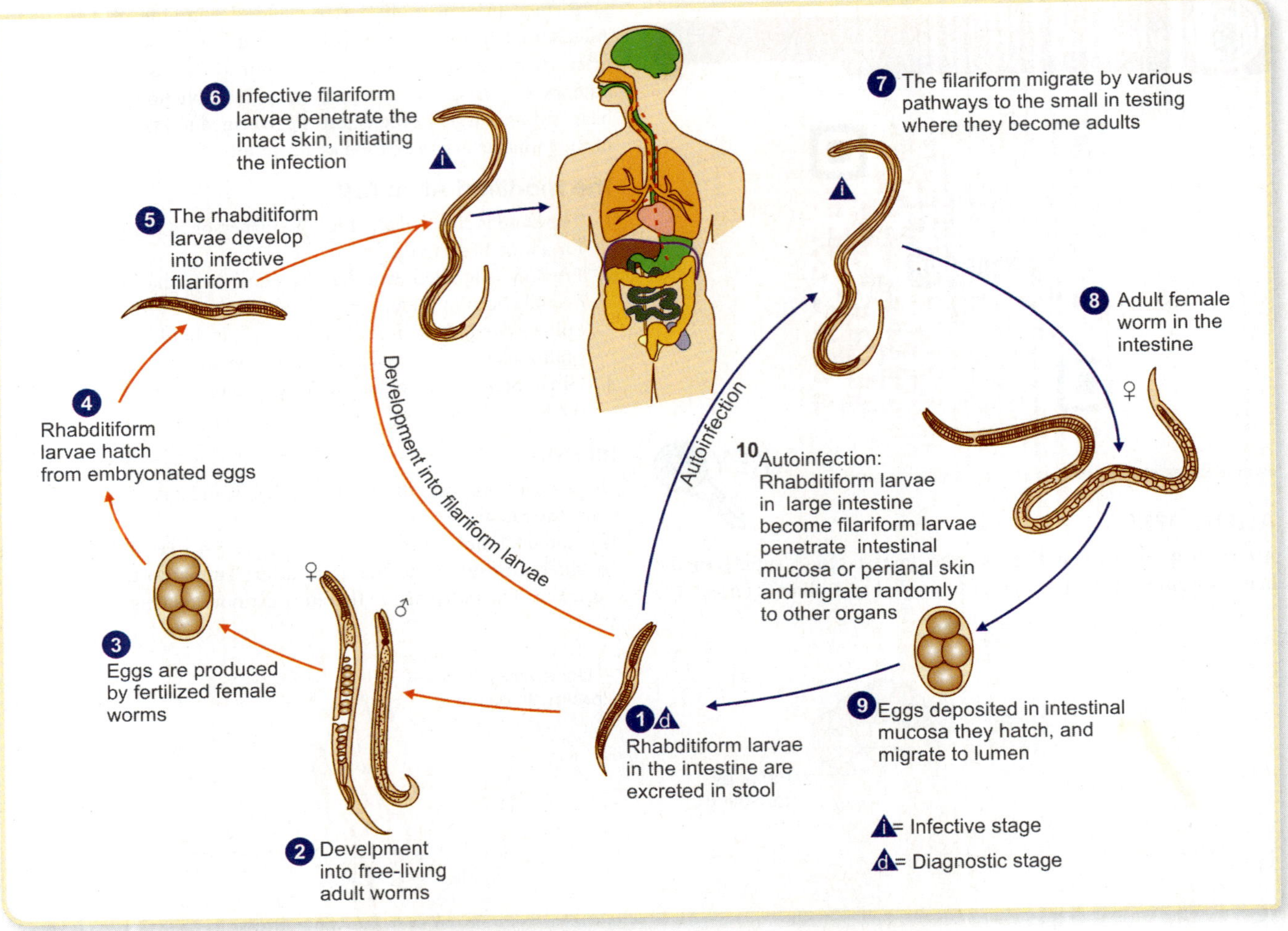

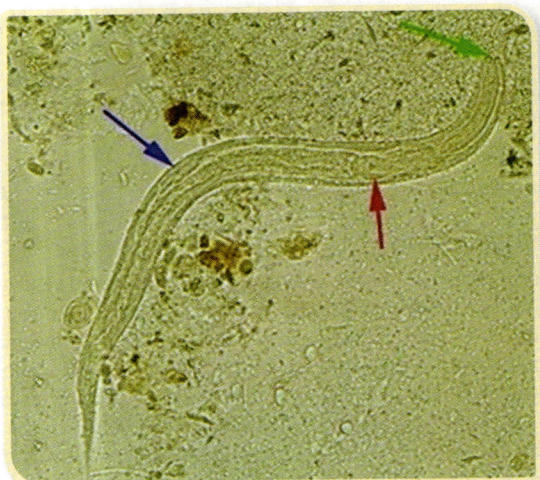

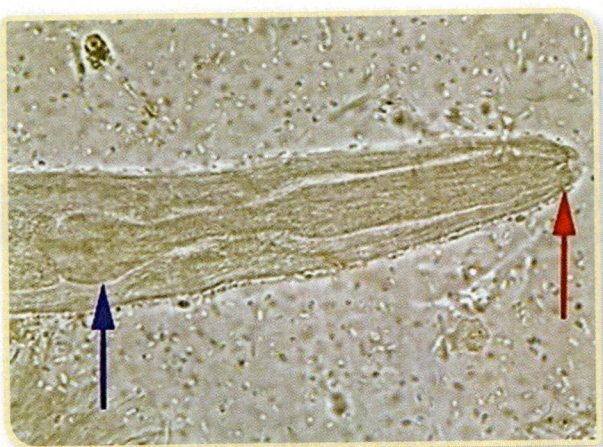

Fig: Strongyloides stercoralis first-stage rhabditiform (L1) larvae: The first-stage rhabditiform larvae (L1) of *Strongyloides stercoralis* are 180-380 μm long, with a short buccal canal, a rhabditoid esophagus and a prominent genital primordium. These L1 larvae are usually found in stool, as the eggs embryonate and hatch in the mucosa of the small intestine of the host. Rhabditiform larva of *S. stercoralis* in an unstained wet mount of stool. Notice the prominent genital primordium (blue arrow), rhabditoid esophagus (red arrow) and short buccal canal (green arrow).

Fig: Close-up of the anterior end of a rhabditiform larva of *S. stercoralis*, showing the short buccal canal (red arrow) and the rhabditoid esophagus (blue arrow). Image taken at 1000x oil magnification.

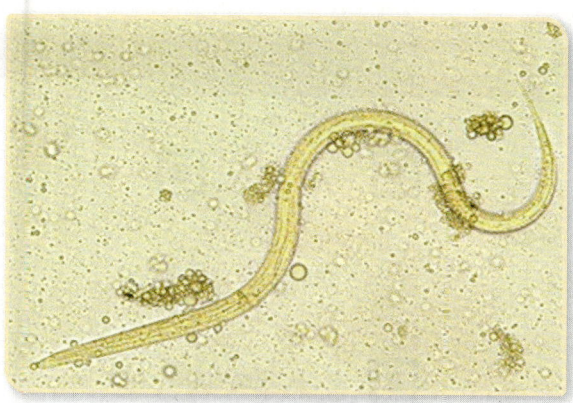

Fig: Strongyloides stercoralis third-stage filariform (L3) larvae: Infective, third-stage filariform larvae (L3) of *Strongyloides stercoralis* are up to 600 μm long. The tail is notched and the esophagus to intestine ratio is 1:1. Infective L3 larvae are found in soil and invade the human host by direct penetration of the skin. They may be found in respiratory specimens during cases of auto nfection.

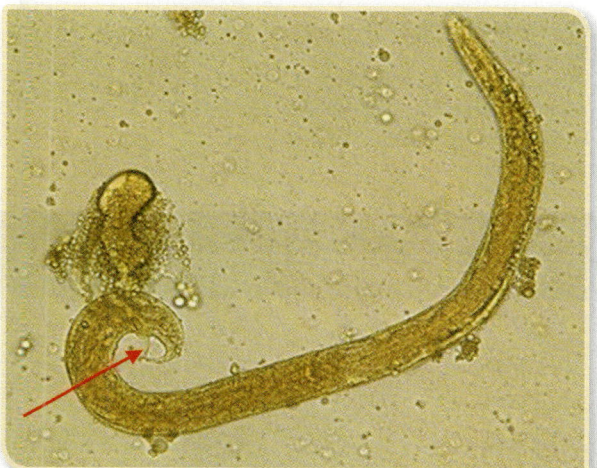

Fig: Strongyloides stercoralis free-living adults: Adults of *Strongyloides stercoralis* may be found in the human host or soil. In the human host, there are no parasitic males, and parasitic females are long, slender and measure 2.0-3.0 mm in length. In the environment, rhabditiform larvae may develop into infective filariform (L3) larvae (direct cycle) or free-living adults that contain both males and females (indirect cycle). Free-living adult males measure up to 750 μm long; free-living females measure up to 1.0 mm long. Free-living adult male *S. stercoralis* is identified by presence of the spicule (red arrow).

 KEY

BREAST EXAMINATION

The breast examination can be done using vertical strip, wedge section, and/or concentric circle detection methods.

1. **Radial spoke or Wedge technique:** The wedge section technique was developed as some women find the circular movement of the hand easier to use during the breast self-examination. In this method, the breast is divided into wedges, moving the palmar pads of the fingers towards the centre of the breast or the nipple. Both breasts are examined wedge by wedge in this manner until completely covered.

2. **Vertical strip method:** With the vertical strip method, the woman should start in the underarm area of the breast, moving the fingers downward slowly until she reaches the area below the breast. The fingers are then moved slightly towards the middle and the process begins again, this time moving the hand upwards, over the breast. This process continues up and down until the whole surface of the breast and underarms is examined. Both breasts should be examined.

3. **Concentric circle method:** In this method, the woman uses a circular motion starting with a small circle around the nipple area to feel the breast. The circle is widened as the woman moves over the surface of the breast. The breast, upper chest and underarm area are fully examined through this circular motion. As with other methods, both breasts should be fully examined.

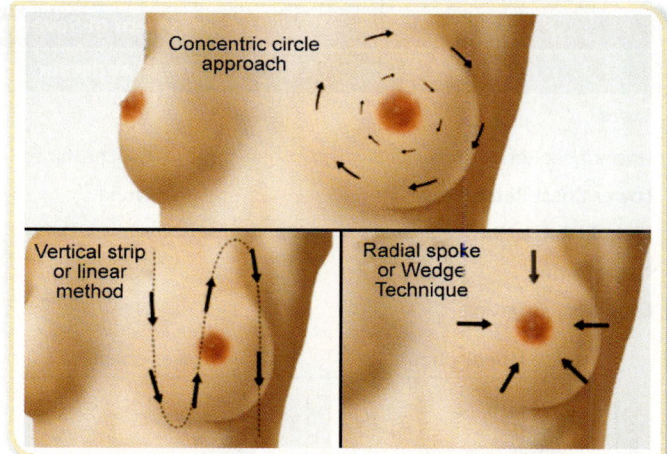

Fig. Different techniques of clinical breast exam

 VIDEO 3

 **VIDEO 4**

The video shows clonic movement of multiple body parts and does not show an extension of limbs hence it is known as Multifocal Clonic seizure.

DIFFERENT SEIZURE PATTERNS

1. **Subtle seizures** do not show any tonic or clonic movement of the limbs. EEG does not show any epileptiform waveforms. Subtle seizures may manifest as eyelid blinking, fluttering or buccal-lingual movement. Subtle seizures lasting for brief duration need not be treated. There may be pedaling or automatic movements because of subcortical neuronal discharges.
2. **Focal Clonic seizures:** Repeated irregular clonic limb movements (1-3 movements/sec) of one limb or both limbs on one side.
3. **Multifocal clonic seizure:** Migratory jerky movements are noted in first limb then another. The migration appear random and does not follow expected pattern of epileptic spread (Jacksonian march)
4. **Myoclonic seizures:** Repeated flexion and extension movements of arms, legs or all limbs.
5. **Tonic seizures** are characterized by extension of extremities and axial muscles. It is usually associated with apnea and upward movement of eyes

SILVERMAN SCORING

Silverman scoring calculation in the given case is:
1. Audible grunt without stethoscope = 2
2. Nasal flare = 2
3. See saw upper chest movement = 2
4. Xiphoid retractions just visible = 1
5. Lower chest retractions just visible = 1

Hence the total score is 8

Assessment of Severity of Respiratory Distress			
Silverman anderson score and its interpretation			
Score	0	1	2
Upper hest Retractions	Synchronized	Lag on inspiration	See-saw movement
Lower Chest Retractions	None	Just visible	Marked
Xiphoid Retractions	None	Just visible	Marked
Nasal Flaring	None	Minimal	Marked
Expiratory Grunting	None	Stethoscope only	Naked eye and ear

	Upper chest	Lower chest	Xiphoid retraction	Nares dilation	Expiratory grunt
Grade 0	Synchronized	No retraction	None	None	None
Grade 1	Lag on Inspiration	Just visible	Just visible	Minimal	Stethoscope only
Grade 2	See saw	Marked	Marked	Marked	Naked ear

Normal babies have a cumulative score close to "0". Severely depressed babies score close to "10"
Score 0-3 = Mild respiratory distress – O_2 by hood
Score 4-6 = Moderate respiratory distress - CPAP
Score > 6 = Impending respiratory failure

Contd...

Downe's Score And Its Interpretation			
RDS Score	0	1	2
Cyanosis	None	Cyanotic in air	Cyanotic in 40% O_2
Retractions	None	Mild	Severe
Grunting	None	Audible with stethoscope	Audible without a stethoscope
Air entry - make baby cry and listen to breath sounds while baby cries	Clear	Delayed or decreased	Barely audible
Respiratory rate	60	60 to 80	80 or apneic episodes

- An RD score of 4 or more for at least 2 hours during the first 8 hours of life denotes clinical RD and requires assessment of the infant by a physician.
- An RD score of 6 or more is an indication for ventilatory assistance.

VIDEO-BASED TOPICS

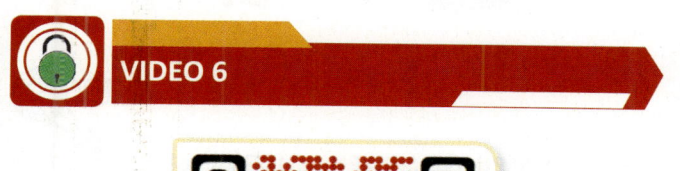

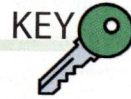

ROOS TEST

Roos Test is diagnostic tool for Thoracic Outlet Syndrome (TOS). It is also knows as the EAST (Elevated Arm Stress Test). In seated position, patient abducts the bilateral shoulders to 90° with the elbow flexed 90°. Patient opens and closes the hands for 3 minutes

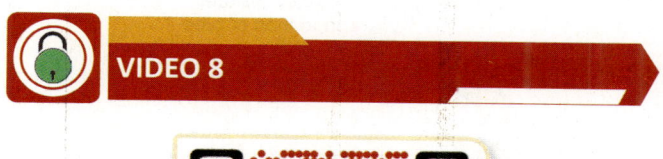

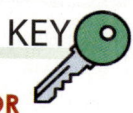

LAPAROSCOPIC FALOPE RING APPLICATOR

The silastic ring is an inert, radio opaque silicone band that is simply applied to a looped section of the fallopian tube with the Silastic Ring Applicator. The Silastic Ring Applicator contains forceps to grasp the fallopian tube 3 to 4 cm from the corneal area. The fallopian tube is gently drawn into the inner cylinder of the instrument, forming a knuckle. The Silastic Ring located on the inner cylinder is released onto the knuckle, occluding the base. This procedure is repeated on the second fallopian tube. Once in place, the Silastic Ring will not slip.

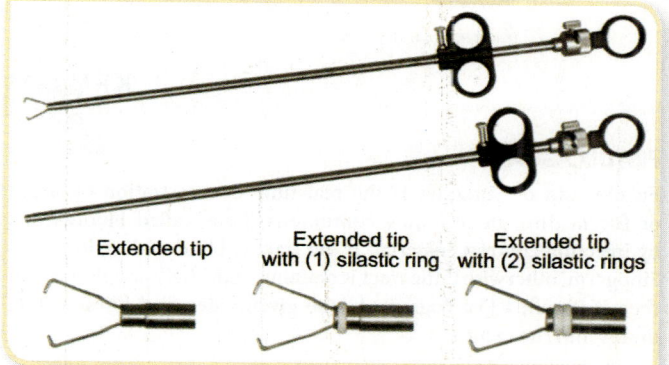

Fig: Falope ring applicators with extended tip

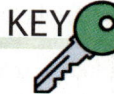

GOWER'S SIGN

Gowers' sign is pathognomonic in patients with Duchenne muscular dystrophy. These patients, when rising, 'climb up' their thighs using their hands in order to overcome the weakness of the pelvic girdle and paravertebral muscles. Gowers' sign is a screening test for muscle weakness, typically seen in Duchenne muscular dystrophy but also seen in numerous other conditions

The Silastic (Falope-yoon) Ring

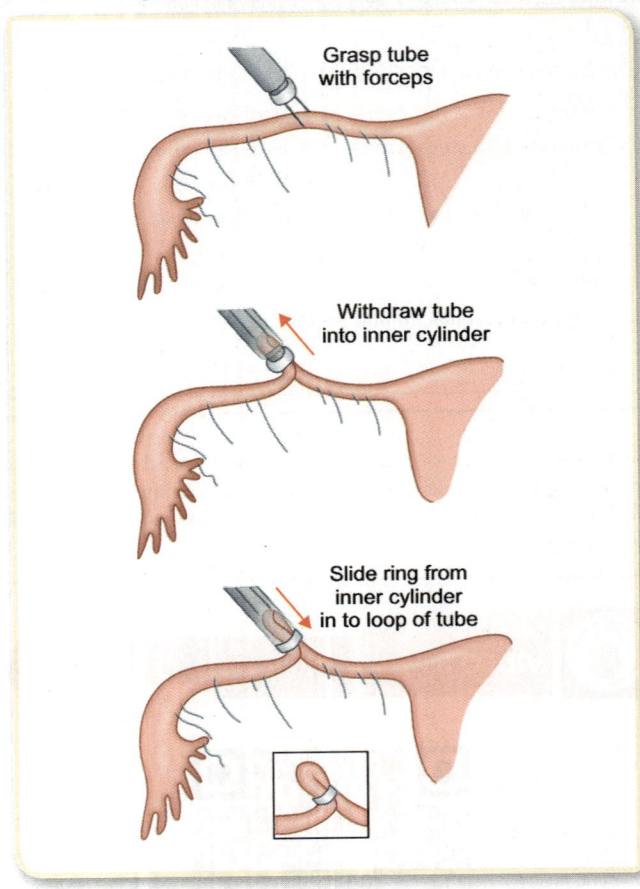

Fig: Falope ring applicator steps illustration

 **VIDEO 10**

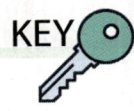 KEY

HYSTEROSALPINGOGRAPHY (HSG)

Hysterosalpingography (HSG) is an X-ray fluoroscopy procedure that is used to evaluate the uterus and fallopian tubes for congenital anomalies and blockage, respectively. There are two contraindications for HSG: pregnancy and active pelvic infection.

The patient is placed supine on the fluoroscopy table in the lithotomy or modified lithotomy position. The perineum is prepared. A **Leech Wilkinson HSG Cannula** or 5-F HSG catheter is positioned in the cervical canal. A scout radiograph of the pelvis is obtained with the catheter in place before contrast material is instilled. Water-soluble contrast material is then slowly instilled, with fluoroscopic images obtained intermittently to evaluate the uterus and fallopian tubes.

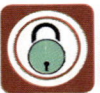 **VIDEO 9**

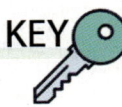 KEY

FISTULOGRAM

Fistulogram or Sinigram is the real time demonstration of sinius or fistula through real time continuous X ray called Fluoroscopy by injecting contrast material. If the tract is blind ending its called Sinogram, otherwise if the tract is opening in the hollow viscus organ then it is called Fistulogram. In the given video and linear fistula drains into the rectum.

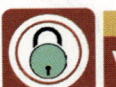 **VIDEO 11**

 KEY

T TUBE CHOLANGIOGRAPHY

A T-tube cholangiogram is a fluoroscopic procedure in which contrast medium is injected through a T-tube into the biliary tree. The T-tube is most commonly inserted during a cholecystectomy operation. Postoperative t-tube cholangiography is performed to exclude a retained bile duct calculus or to assess for any surgical complications such as a bile duct leak.

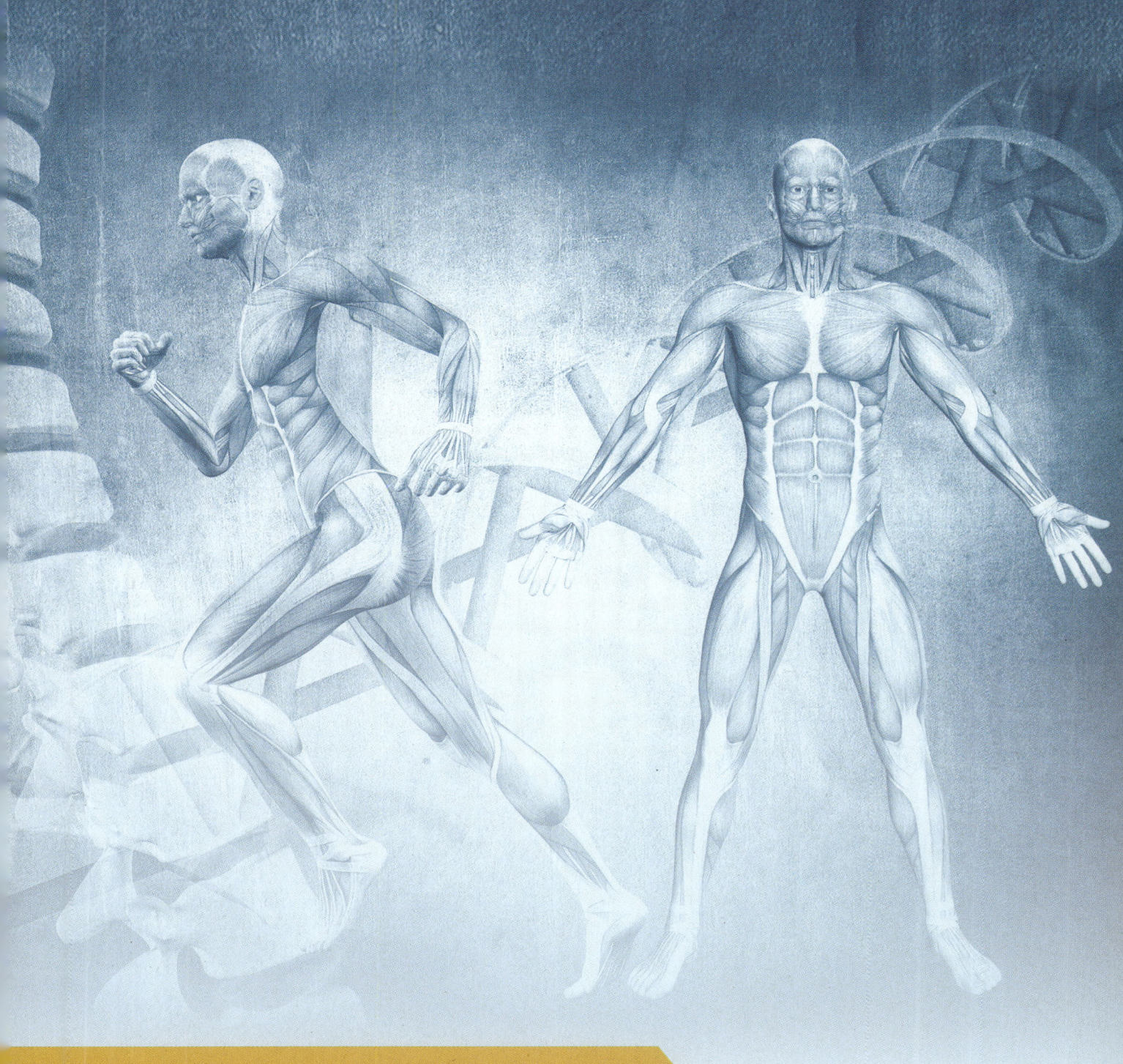

ANATOMY

ANATOMY PLATE 1

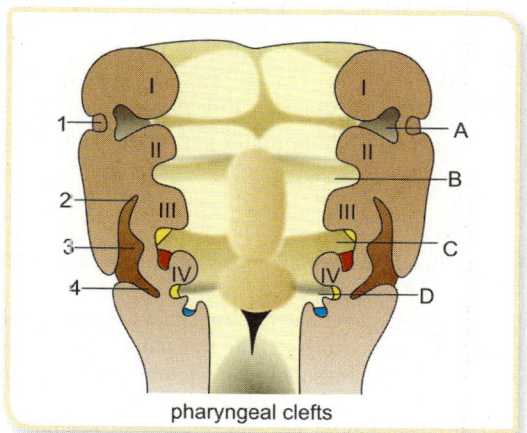

pharyngeal clefts

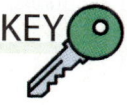

KEY

PHARYNGEAL POUCHES AND CLEFTS

A, B, C, D – Pharyngeal pouches
1, 2, 3, 4 – Pharyngeal clefts

Pharyngeal Arches

There are six pharyngeal arches, but in humans the fifth arch only exists transiently during embryologic growth and development. Since no human structures result from the fifth arch, the arches in humans are I, II, III, IV, and VI. The first three contribute to structures above the larynx, while the last two contribute to the larynx and trachea

Pharyngeal arch	Muscular contributions	Skeletal contributions	Nerve	Artery	Corresponding pouch structures	Corresponding cleft structures
1st (mandibular arch)	Muscles of mastication, Anterior belly of the digastric, Mylohyoid, Tensor tympani, Tensor veli palatini	Maxilla, mandible (only as a model for mandible not actual formation of mandible), Incus and Malleus, Meckel's cartilage, Ant. ligament of malleus, Sphenomandibular ligament	Trigeminal nerve (V2 and V3)	Maxillary artery, external carotid artery	Eustachian tube, Tympanic (Middle ear) cavity, mastoid antrum, and inner layer of the tympanic membrane.	External auditory canal, External auditory meatus
2nd (hyoid arch)	Muscles of facial expression, Buccinator, Platysma, Stapedius, Stylohyoid, Posterior belly of the digastric	Stapes, Styloid process, hyoid (lesser horn and upper part of body), Reichert's cartilage, Stylohyoid ligament	Facial nerve (VII)	Stapedial Artery	Palatine tonsils, Tonsillar fossa	Second, third, and fourth clefts form a cavity lined with ectodermal epithelium, the **cervical sinus**, but with further development, this sinus disappears.
3rd	Stylopharyngeus	Hyoid (greater horn and lower part of body)	Glossopharyngeal nerve (IX)	Common carotid/Internal carotid	Inferior parathyroid, Thymus	
4th	Cricothyroid muscle, all intrinsic muscles of soft palate including levator veli palatini	Thyroid cartilage, epiglottic cartilage	Vagus nerve (X) Superior laryngeal nerve	Right 4th aortic arch: subclavian artery Left 4th aortic arch: aortic arch	Superior parathyroid, ultimobranchial body (which forms the Para follicular C-Cells of thyroid gland)	

Contd...

Pharyngeal Arches

6th	All intrinsic muscles of larynx except the cricothyroid muscle	Cricoid cartilage, arytenoid cartilages, corniculate cartilage	Vagus nerve (X) Recurrent laryngeal nerve	Right 6th aortic arch: pulmonary artery Left 6th aortic arch: Pulmonary artery and ductus arteriosus	Rudimentary structure, becomes part of the fourth pouch contributing to thyroid C-cells.

Footnote:
- **Ultimobranchial body** is the most caudal endodermal invaginations of the pharynx are the fourth pharyngeal pouch and elements of the transitory fifth pharyngeal pouch
- **Pharyngeal arches cut section:** In addition to mesenchyme derived from paraxial and lateral plate mesoderm, the core of each arch receives substantial numbers of **Neural crest cells**, which migrate into the arches to contribute to skeletal components of the face. Each arch consists of a mesenchymal core derived from mesoderm and neural crest cells and each is lined internally by endoderm and externally by ectoderm
- **Parafollicular C cells** are derived from the Neural crest component of Ultimobranchial body, so if neural crest is provided in the options, it is a better answer

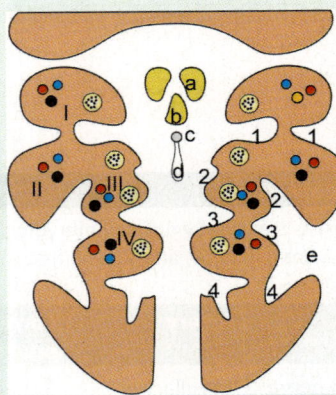

Pattern of the branchial arches
I-IV branchial arches
1-4 branchial pouches (inside)
Pharyngeal grooves (outside)
a. Tuberculum laterale
b. Tuberculum impar
c. Foramen cecum
d. Ductus thyreoglossus
e. Sinus cervicalis

 ANATOMY PLATE 2

 Key

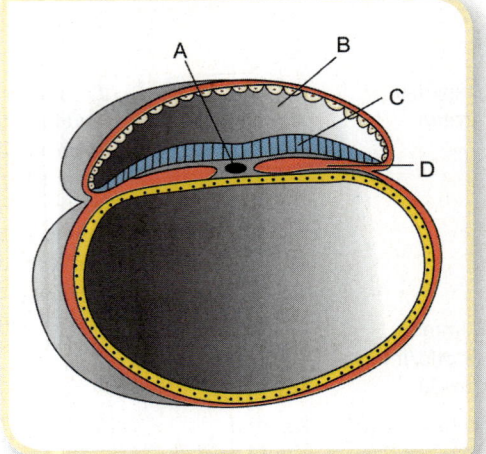

The notochord expands between the developing vertebrae as localized aggregates of cells and matrix that form the nucleus pulposus of the intervertebral disc.

A = Notochord
B = Amniotic cavity
C = Ectoderm
D = Mesoderm

Nucleus pulposus is central gelatinous portion of an intervertebral disc derived from proliferation of notochord cells. Mesenchymal cells between cephalic and caudal parts of the original sclerotome segment do not proliferate but fill the space between two precartilaginous vertebral bodies. In this way, they contribute to formation of the intervertebral disc. Although the notochord regresses entirely in the region of the vertebral bodies, it persists and enlarges in the region of the intervertebral disc. Here it contributes to the Nucleus pulposus, which is later surrounded by circular fibers of the annulus fibrosus. Combined, these two structures form the intervertebral disc.

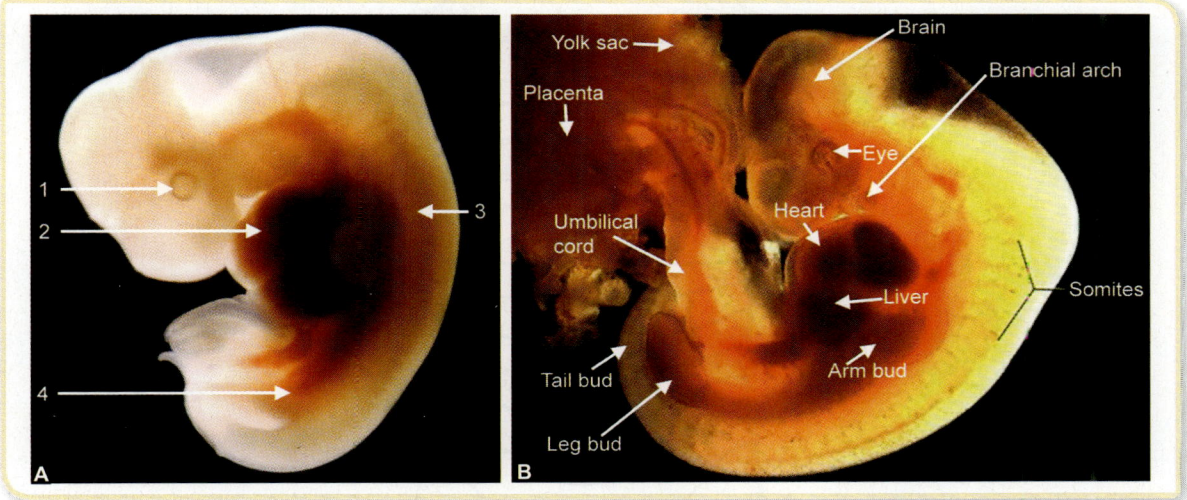

ANATOMY PLATE 3

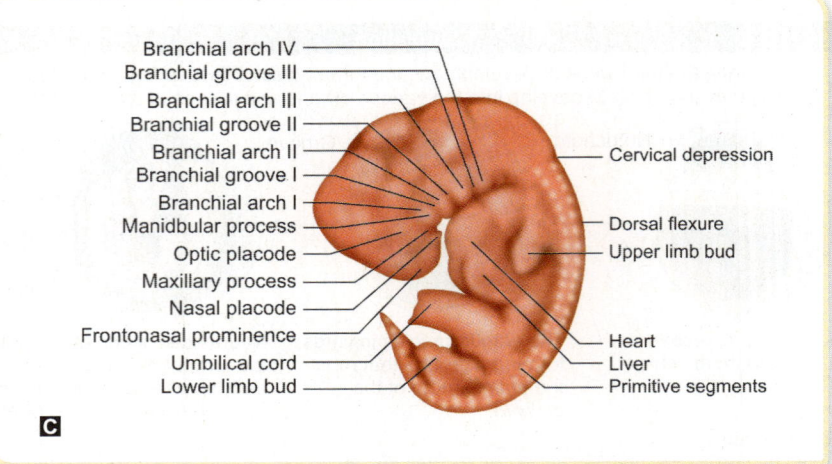

5 – WEEK EMBRYO

A. Major anatomical landmarks of a 5 weeks embryo
   1. Lens pit
   2. Heart prominence[AIIMSPG]
   3. Somites
   4. Limb bud
B. Real embryo at 5 weeks, labelled
C. Illustration of 5 weeks old embryo

 ANATOMY PLATE 4

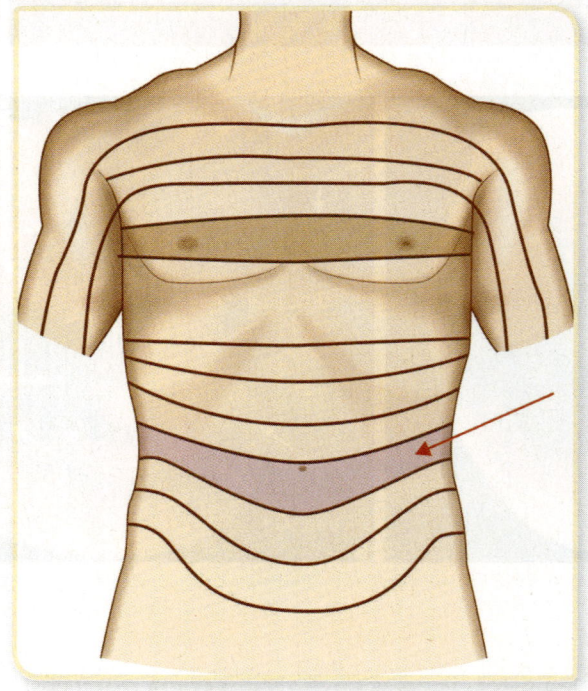

DERMATOME IN UMBILICAL REGION

The area marked is around the umbilicus[NEETPG]. The 10th intercostal nerve supplies the dermatome in the umbilical region.

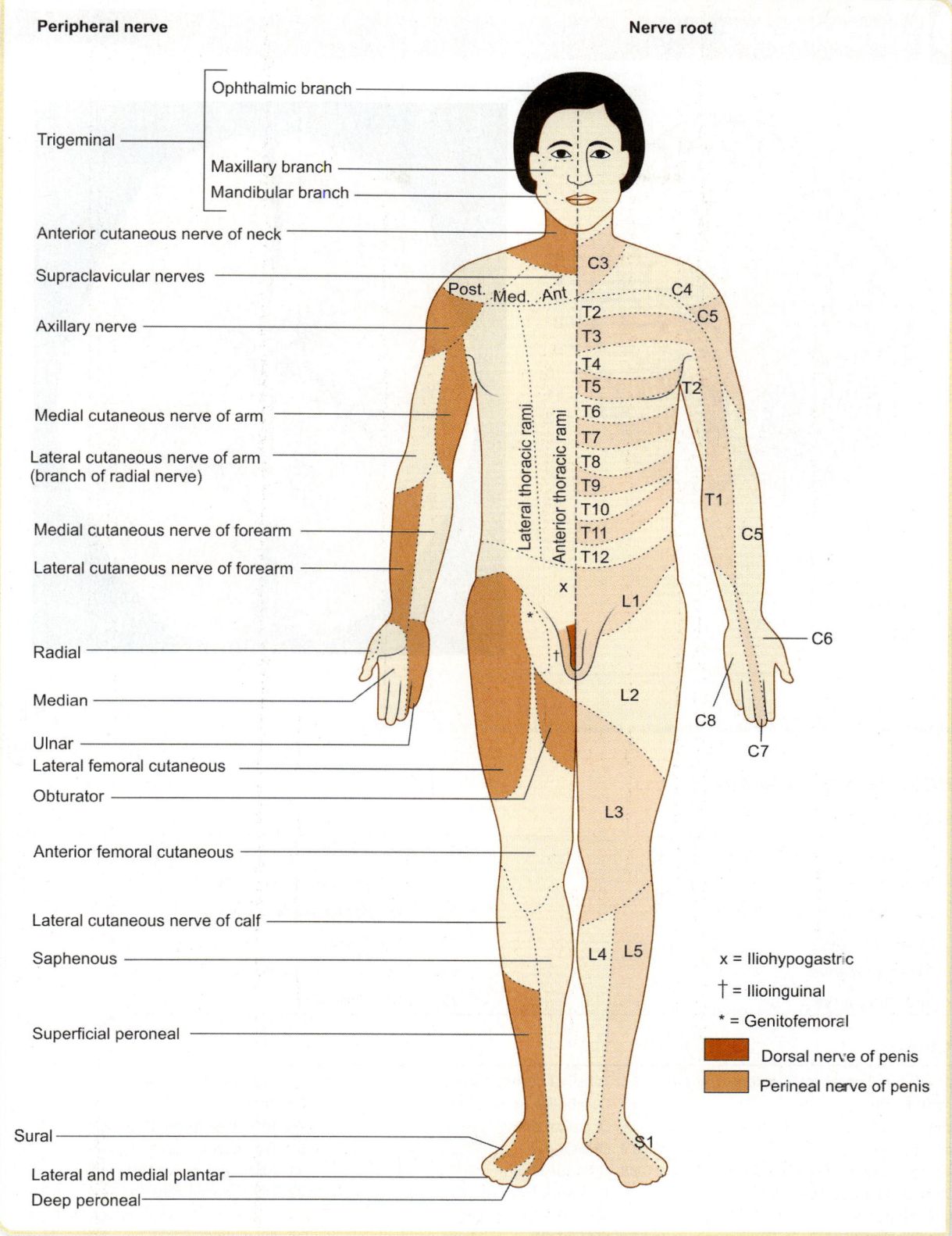

Clinical Importance

- Knowledge of dermatomal supply of various regions helps determining level of regional anesthesia.
- In intrathecal block the level of anaesthesia required is mostly determined by the volume of drug given (along with its baricity as well as patient factors).
- It also helps determine level of insertion of epidural catheter for anesthesia as well as postoperative analgesia.
- Lastly, various nerves are blocked depending upon the dermatome they supply and the respective site of incision during regional blocks.
- Herpes zoster manifests along dermatomes.

ANATOMY PLATE 5

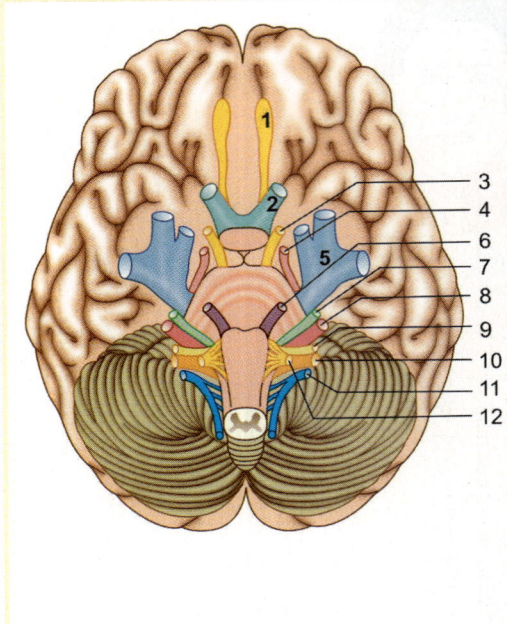
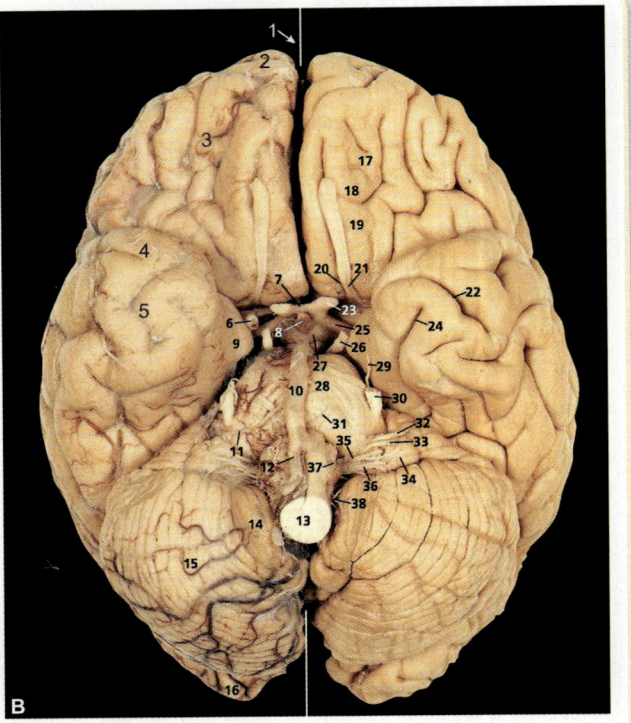
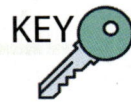

INFERIOR SURFACE OF BRAIN

A. Legends

1.	Olfactory nerve	7.	Facial nerve
2.	Optic nerve	8.	Vestubulocochlear nerve
3.	Oculomotor nerve	9.	Glossopharyngeal nerve
4.	Trochlear nerve	10.	Vagus nerve
5.	Trigeminal nerve	11.	Accessory spinal nerve
6.	Abducens nerve	12.	Hypoglossal nerve

B. Legends

1. Longitudinal cerebral fissure (arrowed)	14. Tonsil of cerebellum	27. Mammillary body
2. Frontal pole	15. Cerebellar hemisphere	28. Pons
3. Inferior surface of frontal pole	16. Occipital pole	29. Trochlear nerve (IV)
4. Temporal pole	17. Orbital gyri	30. Trigeminal nerve (V)
5. Inferior surface of temporal pole	18. Olfactory bulb	31. Abducent nerve (VI)
6. Internal carotid artery	19. Olfactory tract (I)	32. Facial nerve (VII)
7. Optic chiasma	20. Medial olfactory stria	33. Vestibulocochlear nerve (VIII)
8. Infundibulum	21. Lateral olfactory stria	34. Flocculus
9. Parahippocampal gyrus	22. Inferior temporal sulcus	35. Glossopharyngeal nerve (IX)
10. Basilar artery	23. Optic nerve (II)	36. Vagus nerve (X)
11. Labyrinthine artery	24. Collateral sulcus	37. Hypoglossal nerve (XII)
12. Right vertebral artery	25. Optic tract	38. Accessory nerve (XI)
13. Medulla oblongata	26. Oculomotor nerve (III)	

ANATOMY PLATE 6

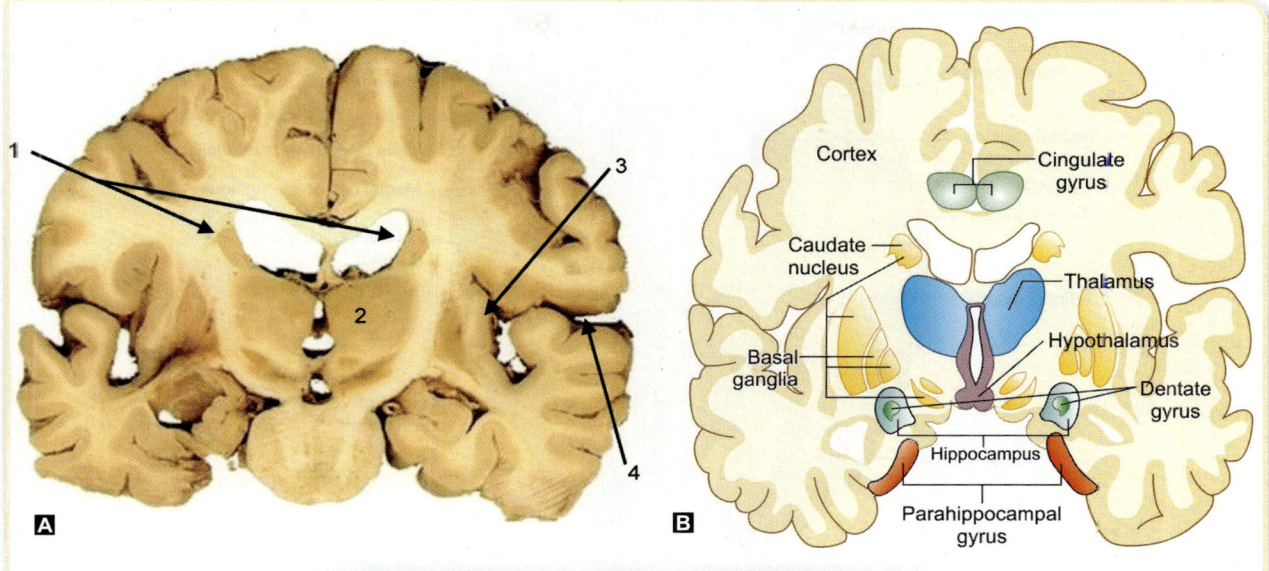
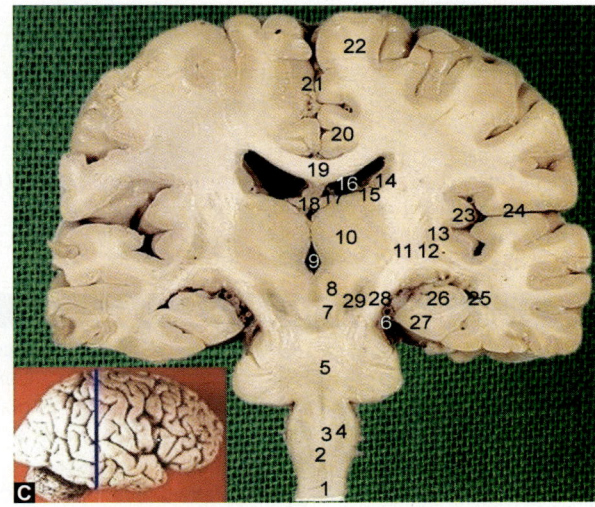
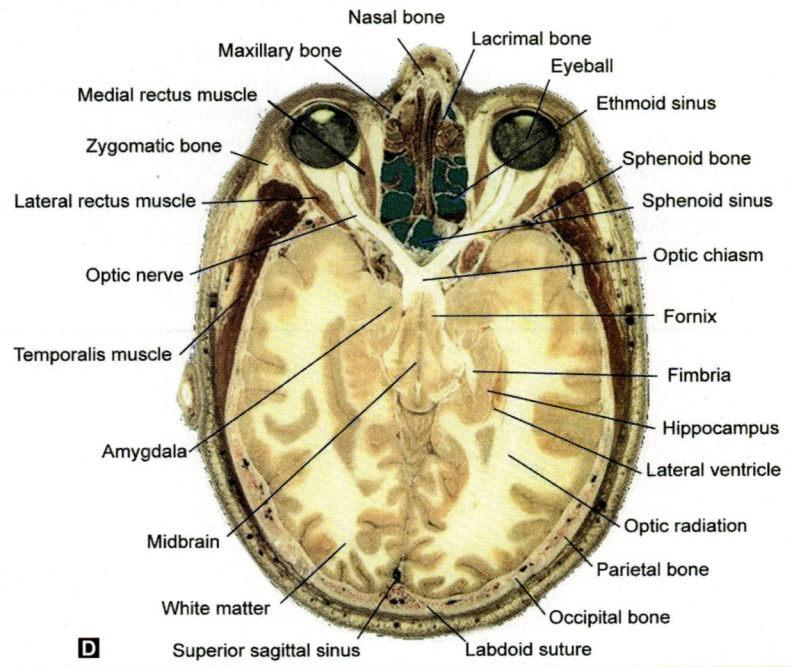

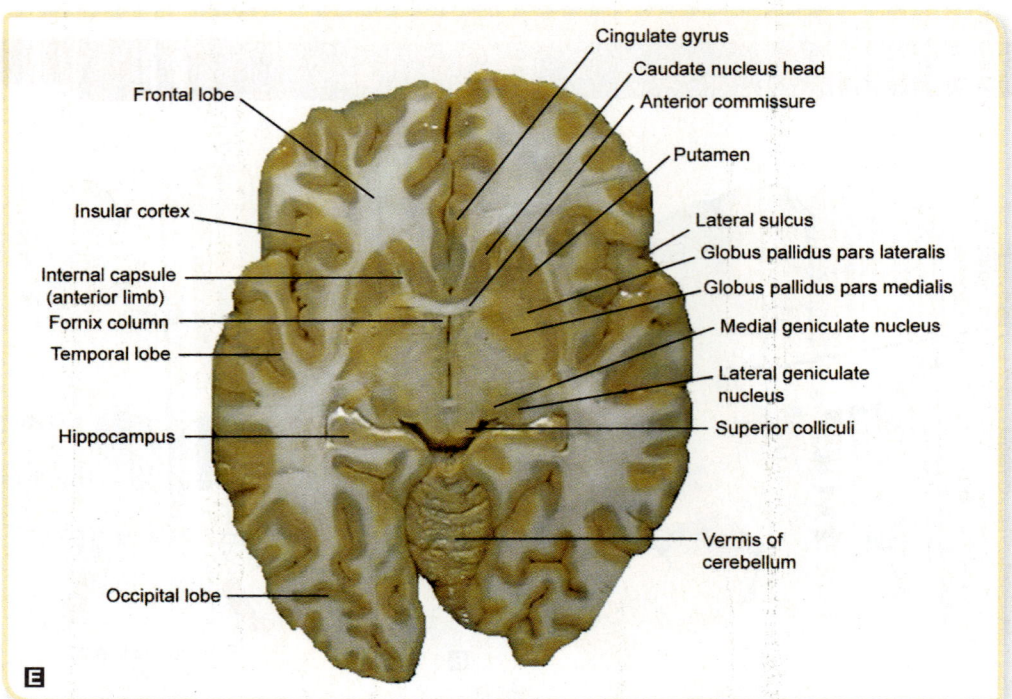

PLATE LEGENDS

A. Coronal section of brain with: Caudate nucleus (marked as arrow 1), Thalamus (marked as 2), Insula (marked as 3), Lateral sulcus (Marked as 4). Note that the Insula is visible on retracting the lateral sulcus.
B. Coronal section anatomy of Limbic system (Representational)
C. Coronal section of Human brain (detailed labelling)

	Human Brain Frontal (Coronal) Section		
1.	Medulla spinalis	16.	Lamina affixa / Ventriculus lateralis, Pars centralis
2.	Decussatio pyramidum	17.	Taenia choroidea / Plexus choroideus ventriculi lateralis
3.	Hilum nuclei olivaris inferioris	18.	Fornix[AIIMSPG, NEETPG], Crus
4.	Nucleus olivaris inferior	19.	Corpus callosum, Truncus
5.	Pons	20.	Gyrus cinguli
6.	Arteria cerebri posterior	21.	Fissura longitudinalis cerebri
7.	Tractus cerebellorubralis	22.	Gyrus frontalis superior
8.	Nucleus ruber	23.	Insula
9.	Ventriculus tertius	24.	Sulcus lateralis
10.	Thalamus	25.	Ventriculus lateralis, Cornu temporale
11.	Capsula interna	26.	Hippocampus
12.	Putamen	27.	Gyrus parahippocampalis
13.	Capsula externa / Claustrum / Capsula extrema	28.	Crus cerebri
14.	Caudate nucleus (Corpus)	29.	Substantia nigra
15.	Stria terminalis et Vena thalamostriata superior		

D. Transverse section of Brain at the level of eyes (Labeled) (Medial rectus muscle [AIIMSPG])
E. Transverse section of Brain at the level of Cerebellum (Labeled)

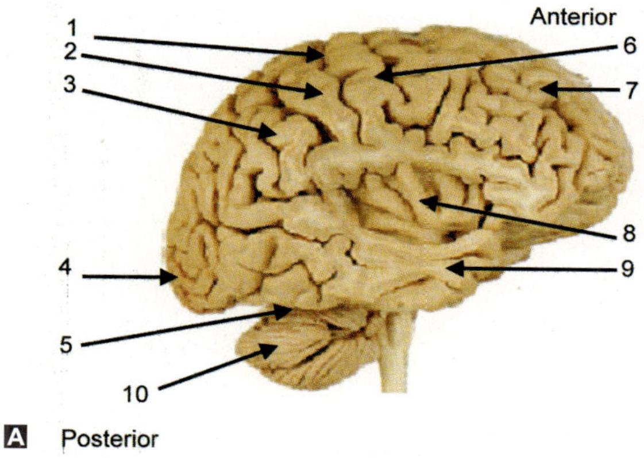

ANATOMY PLATE 7

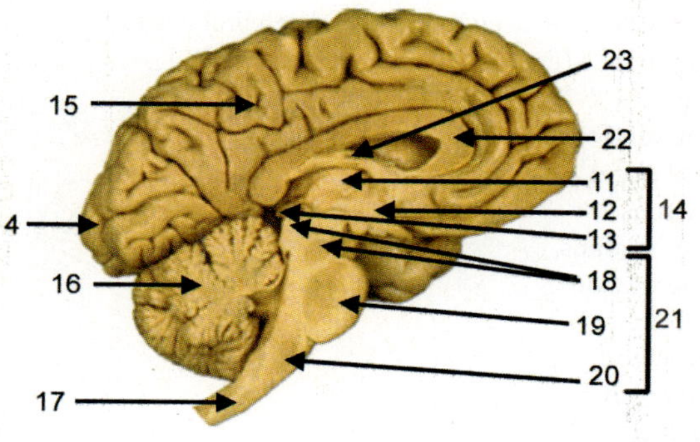

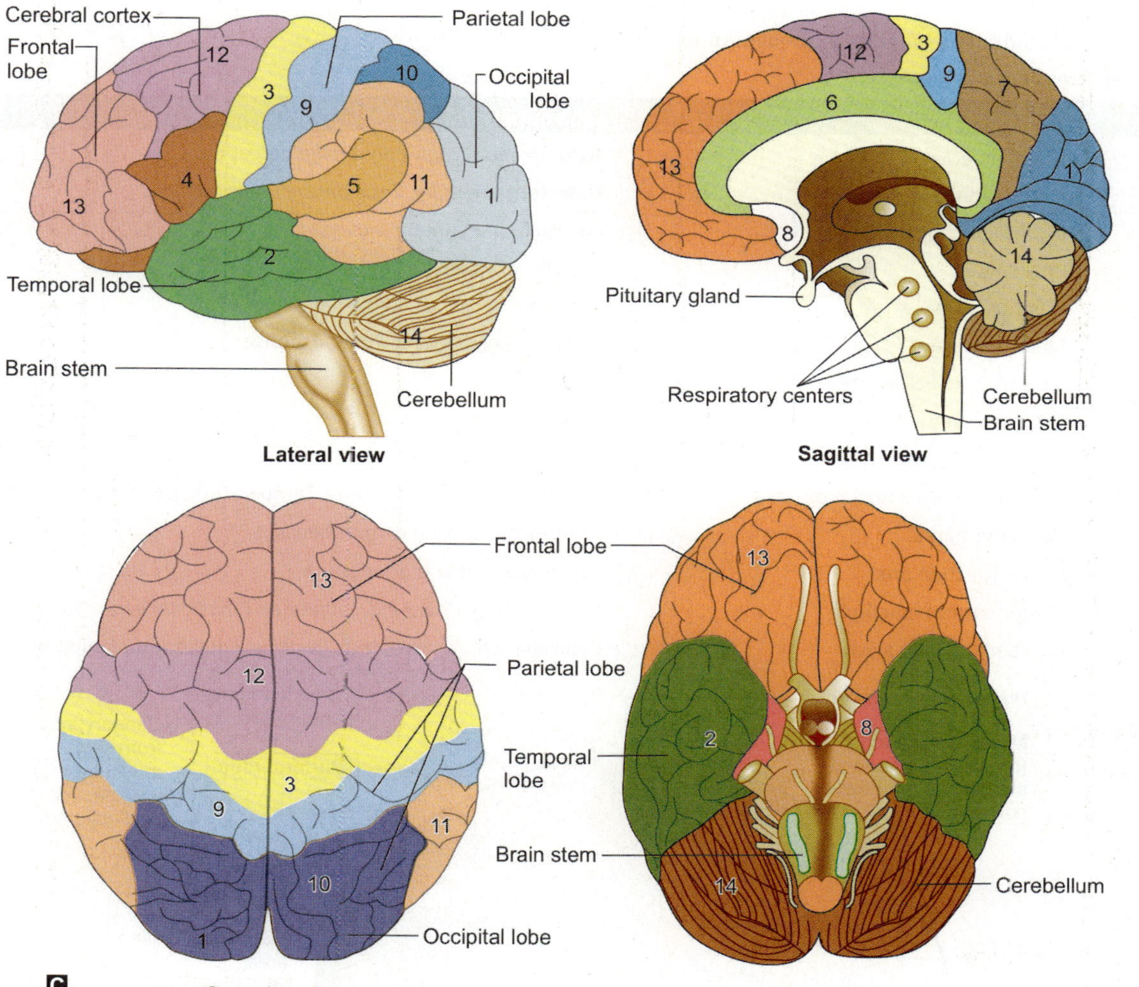

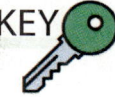

PLATE LEGENDS

A. Right lateral view of Brain with Temporal lobe cut away
1. Central sulcus (shallow groove separating the frontal lobe and parietal lobe)
2. Postcentral gyrus (elevation located just posterior to the central sulcus)

3. Parietal lobe
4. Occipital lobe
5. Transverse fissure (deep groove separating the cerebrum from the cerebellum in the posterior/ inferior part of the brain)
6. Precentral gyrus (elevation located just anterior to the central sulcus)
7. Frontal lobe
8. Insula (inner lobe deep to the lateral cerebral fissure)
9. Temporal lobe (cut)
10. Cerebellum[AIIMSPG, NEETPG]

B. **Sagittal medial section of Brain**
11. Pineal gland
12. Thalamus
13. Hypothalamus
14. Diencephalon
15. Cerebrum
16. Cerebellum
17. Spinal cord
18. Midbrain[AIIMSPG]
19. Pons
20. Medulla oblongata
21. Brainstem
22. Corpus callosum[AIIMSPG]
23. Fornix[AIIMSPG, NEETPG]

(Also know the blood supply of fornix is through Anterior cerebral artery)[AIIMS PG]

C. **Functional areas of cerebral cortex**

Area No.	Area name	Area Function
1.	Visual area	Sight, Image recognition, Image perception
2.	Association area	Short term memory, Equilibrium, Emotion
3.	Motor Function area	Initiation of voluntary muscles
4.	Broca's area	Muscles of speech
5.	Auditory area	Hearing
6.	Emotional area	Pain, Hunger, Flight or Fight response
7.	Sensory association area	
8.	Olfactory area	Smelling
9.	Sensory area	Sensation from muscle and skin
10.	Somatosensory association area	Evaluation of weight, texture, temperature, etc. for object recognition
11.	Wernicke's area	Written and spoken comprehension
12.	Motor function area	Eye movement and orientation
13.	Higher mental function	Concentration, Planning, Judgment, Emotional expression, Creativity
14	Cerebellar motor area	Coordination of movement, Balance, Equilibrium, Inhibition

Note: The above area numbers are arbitrary numbers and do not represent Brodmann area

ANATOMY PLATE 8

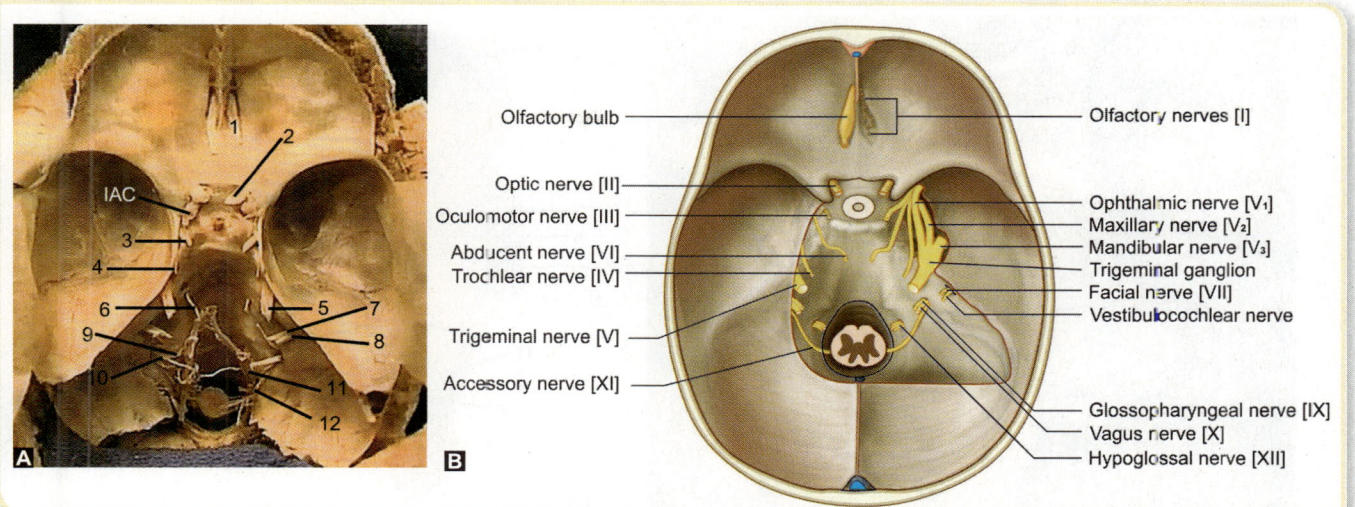

PLATE LEGENDS

A. **Superior view of the base of the skull showing cranial nerves.** The posterior fossa contains the brainstem, cerebellum, and cranial nerves IV-XII.
   1. Olfactory nerve (CN I)
   2. Optic nerve (CN II)
   3. Oculomotor nerve (CN III))^{AIIMSPG} – **Indirectly muscles supplied by/ not supplied by this nerve is asked**
   4. Trochlear nerve (CN IV)
   5. Trigeminal Nerve (CN V)
   6. Abducens nerve (CN VI)^{AIIMSPG}: Abducens nerve located between pons and the clivus in the way to the cavernous sinus.
   7. Facial nerve (CN VII)
   8. Vestibulocochlear nerve (CN VIII)
   9. Glossopharyngeal nerve (CN IX)
   10. Vagus nerve (CN X)
   11. Spinal accessory nerve (CN XI)
   12. Hypoglossal nerve (CN XII)
       IAC = Internal Carotid artery

B. **Superior view of the base of the skull showing cranial nerves (Labeled Illustration)**

ANATOMY PLATE 9

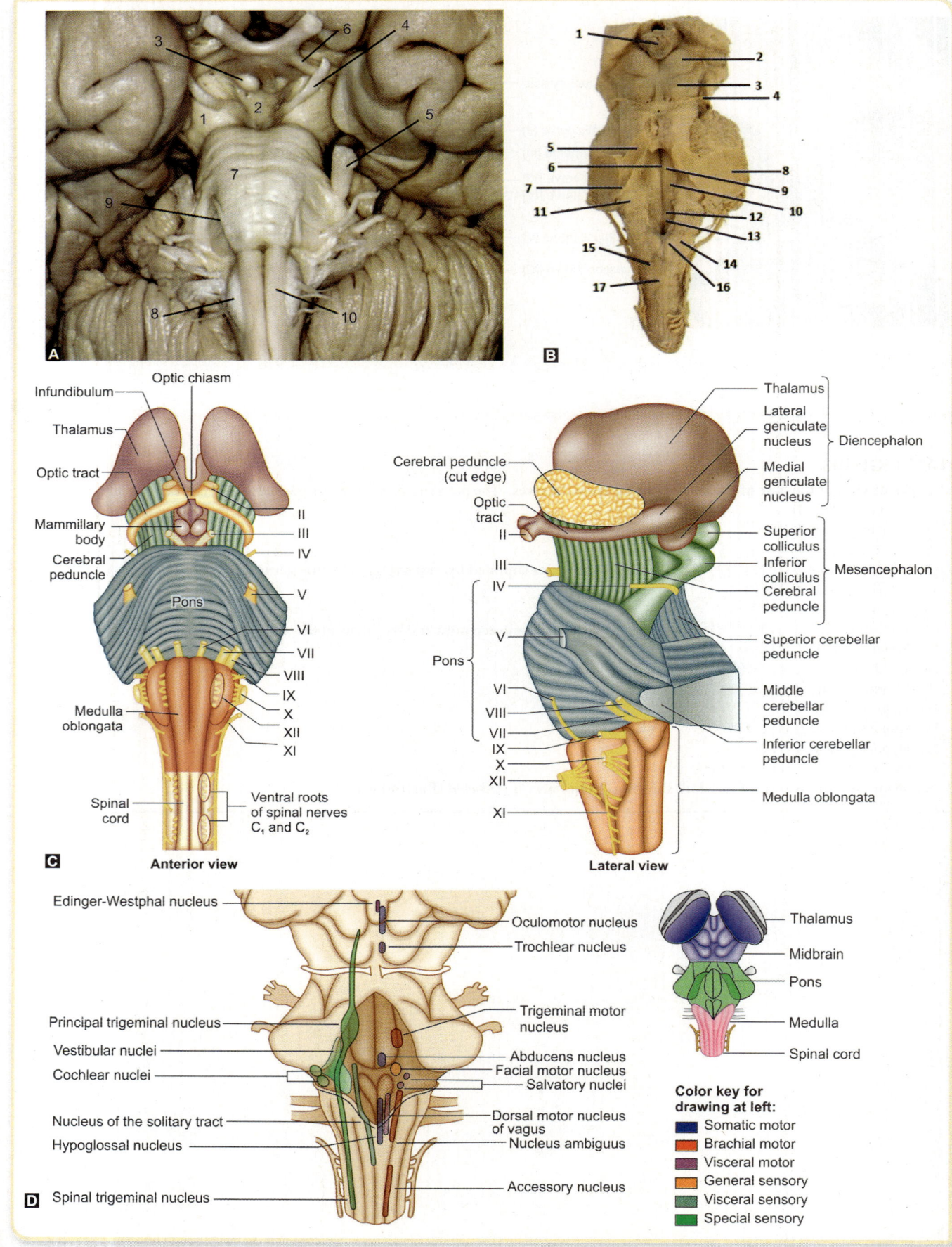

KEY

STRUCTURE OF BRAINSTEM

A. **Ventral View of Brainstem and Basal Forebrain**
   1. Cerebral peduncle
   2. Interpeduncular fossa
   3. Mammillary body
   4. Oculomotor nerve
   5. Trigeminal nerve
   6. Optic tract
   7. Pons
   8. Olive
   9. Trochlear nerve[AIIMSPG, NEETPG]
   10. Medullary Pyramids[AIIMSPG] (Contains Corticospinal tract, damage to which causes contralateral hemiplegia)

B. **Brain stem dissected**
   1. Pineal gland
   2. Superior Colliculus
   3. Inferior Colliculus
   4. Trochlear nerve[AIIMSPG, NEETPG]
   5. Superior cerebellar peduncle
   6. Dorsal median sulcus
   7. Inferior cerebellar peduncle
   8. Middle cerebellar peduncle
   9. Medial eminence
   10. Facial colliculus
   11. Striae medullares
   12. Hypoglossal trigone
   13. Vagal trigone
   14. Cuneate tubercle
   15. Fasciculus cuneatus
   16. Gracilis tubercle
   17. Fasciculus gracilis

C. **Brain stem illustration:** Self explanatory labeling on structures

D. **Brain Stem illustrations:** With emphasis of different nucleus

Structures of Brain Stem

	Ventral surface	Dorsal surface
Midbrain	Cerebral peduncle Interpedincular fossa Occulomotor nerve CN3 Posterior perforated substance created by posterior cerebral and posterior communicating arteries	Superior colliculus (Visual system) Inferior colliculus (Auditory system) **Trochlear nerve CN 4 (Only cranial nerve that exits from dorsal aspect)**[AIIMSPG, NEETPG]
Pons	*Trigeminal nerve CN5* *Abducens nerve CN 6* *Facial nerve CN 7* *Vestibulocochlear nerve CN 8* Ventral cochlear nuclei Facial nucleus	Motor & sensory nucleus of trigeminal Vestibular nuclei Dorsal cochlear nuclei Superficially pontine portion of **Rhomboid fossa** containing Locus ceruleus (Largest collection of norepinephrinergic neurons in CNS) Sulcus limitans Stria medullaris **Facial colliculus** (contains *Abducent nucleus* and internal genu of facial nerve
Medulla	Pyramid (Corticospinal tract)[AIIMS PG] (Causes contralateral hemiplegia) Olive (superior & Inferior olivary nucleus) *Glossopharyngeal nerve CN 9* *Vagus nerve CN 10* *Accessory nerve CN 11* *Hypoglossal nerve CN 12*	Nucleus gracilis Nucleus cuneatus Medullary **Rhomboid fossa** containing **Stria medullaris** Dorsal motor nucleus of vagus CN10 (Vagal trigone) Hypoglossal nucleus CN12 (Hypoglossal trigone) Sulcus limitans Area postrema (Vomiting centre)

Note: Stria medullaris divides rhomboid fossa into pontine and medullary parts

Cerebellar Peduncles

Superior cerebellar peduncle	Middle cerebellar peduncle	Inferior cerebellar peduncle
Cerebellum ↔ midbrain	Cerebellum ↔ pons	Cerebellum ↔ medulla
Fibers that enter cerebellum via superior cerebellar peduncle: 1. Ventral spinocerebellar tract 2. Dentate rubro thalamic tract 3. Trigeminocerebellar tract from the mesencephalic trigeminal nucleus 4. Cerulocerebellar tract from the nucleus ceruleus 5. Tectocerebellar tract from the superior and inferior colliculi	**The fiber systems that enter cerebellum via middle cerebellar peduncle:** 1. Pontocerebellar (corticopontocerebellar) tract from the pontine nuclei 2. Serotonergic fibers from the raphe nuclei	**Fiber systems that enter cerebellum via inferior cerebellar peduncle:** 1. Dorsal spinocerebellar tract 2. Cuneocerebellar tract from the accessory cuneate nuclei 3. Olivocerebellar tract from the inferior olivary nuclei 4. Reticulocerebellar tract from the reticular nuclei of the brain stem 5. Vestibulocerebellar tract (primary afferents from the vestibular end organ and secondary afferents from the vestibular nuclei) 6. Arcuatocerebellar tract from the arcuate nuclei of the medulla 7. Trigeminocerebellar tract from the spinal and main sensory nuclei of the trigeminal nerve

ANATOMY PLATE 10

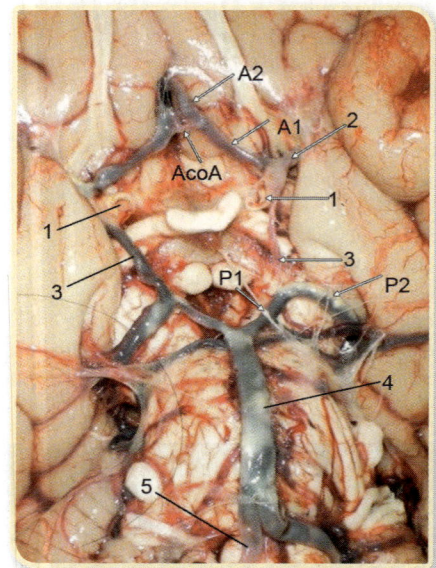

CC BY 4.0 Adapted from De Silva KR, Silva R, Amaratunga D, Gunasekera WS, Jayesekera RW - BMC Neurol (2011) (https://openi.nlm.nih.gov/)

ARTERIAL SUPPLY TO BRAIN

This image shows a normal cerebral arterial circle of Willis
1= Internal carotid artery (cut lumen)
2= Middle cerebral artery
3= Posterior communicating artery
4= Basilar artery
5= Vertebral artery
A1= A1 segment of Anterior cerebral artery
A2= A2 segment of Anterior cerebral artery
P1= P1 segment of posterior cerebral artery
P2= P2 segment of posterior cerebral artery

At 16 weeks' gestation, the anterior, middle and posterior cerebral arteries that contribute to the formation of the **circle of Willis** are well established. The posterior communicating artery originates from the cerebral part of the internal carotid artery and courses caudally to join the posterior cerebral artery (PCA). The part of the PCA medial to this intersection is the P1 segment and the part of the PCA immediately lateral to this junction is the P2 segment. The posterior communicating artery irrigates the hypothalamus and ventral thalamus. An aneurysm of this artery is the second most common aneurysm of the circle of Willis. It commonly results in third-nerve palsy. The posterior cerebral artery is connected to the carotid artery through the posterior communicating artery.

Arterial Supply to Brain		
Artery	**Origin**	**Distribution**
Vertebral	Subclavian artery	Cranial meninges and cerebellum
Posterior inferior cerebellar	Vertebral artery	Posteroinferior aspect of cerebellum
Basilar	Formed by junction of vertebral arteries	Brainstem, cerebellum, and cerebrum
Pontine	Basilar artery	Numerous branches to brainstem
Anterior inferior cerebellar		Inferior aspect of cerebellum
Superior cerebellar		Superior aspect of cerebellum
Internal carotid	Common carotid artery at superior border of thyroid cartilage	Gives branches in cavernous sinus and provides supply to brain
Anterior cerebral	Internal carotid artery	Cerebral hemispheres, except for occipital lobes
Middle cerebral	Continuation of the internal carotid artery distal to anterior cerebral artery	Most of lateral surface of cerebral hemispheres
Posterior cerebral	Terminal branch of basilar artery	Inferior aspect of cerebral hemisphere and occipital lobe
Anterior communicating	Anterior cerebral artery	Cerebral arterial circle
Posterior communicating	Internal carotid artery	

Contd...

Arterial Supply to Brain

Artery	Origin	Distribution

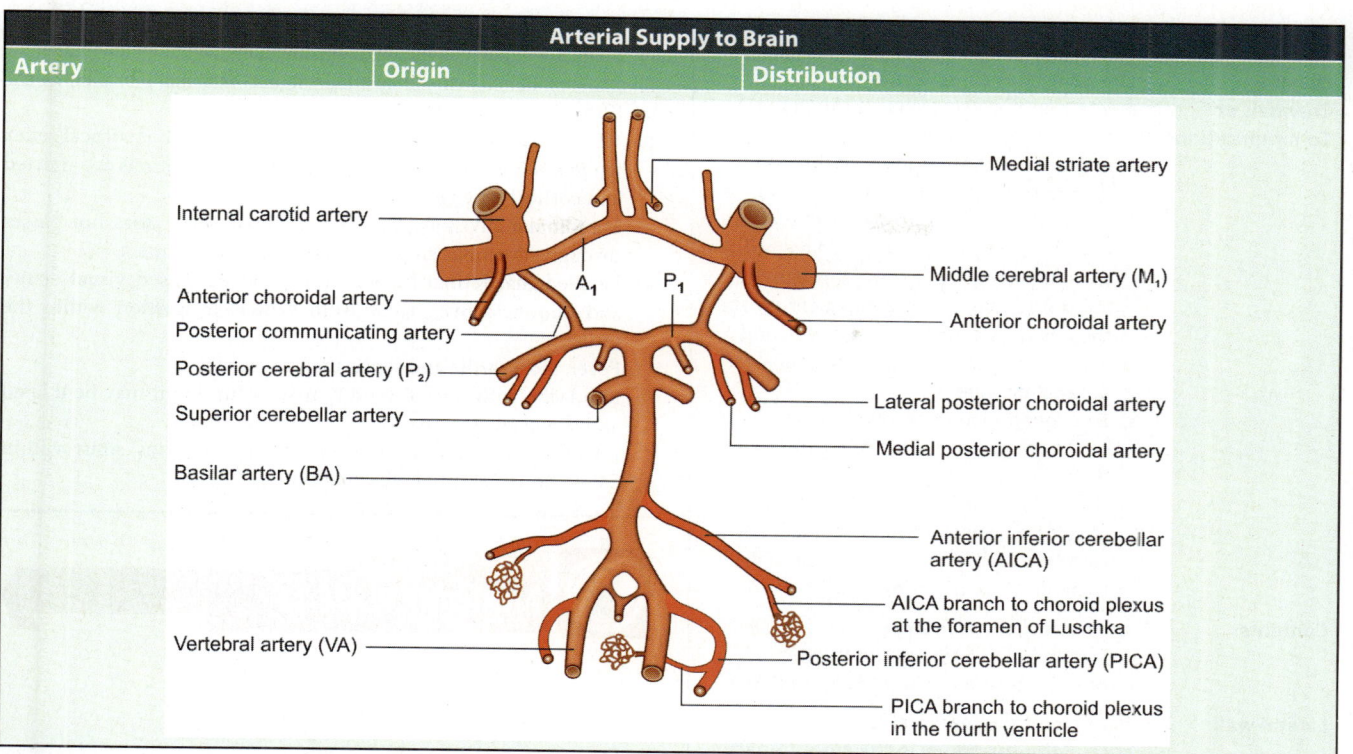

ANATOMY PLATE 11

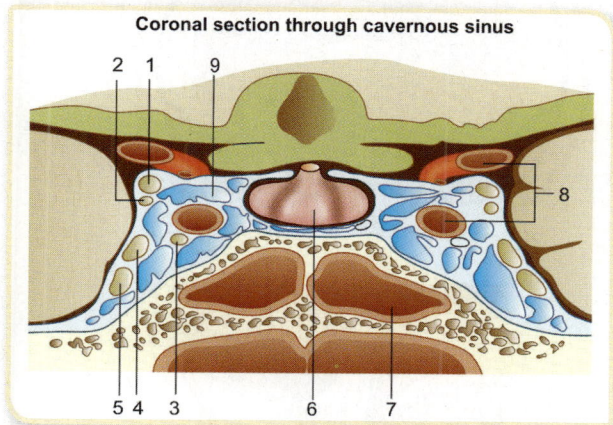

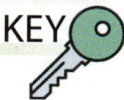
KEY

CAVERNOUS SINUS

1. Occulomotor nerve (III)
2. Trochlear nerve (IV)
3. Abducent nerve (VI)
4. Ophthalmic nerve (V 1)
5. Maxillary nerve (V 2)
6. Pituitary gland
7. Sphenoid sinus
8. Carotid artery
9. Cavernous sinus

Cavernous Sinus

The cavernous sinus is a large venous plexus that lies on both sides of the body of the sphenoid bone. The sinus extends from the superior orbital fissure to the apex of the petrous temporal bone, with an average length of 2 cm and width of 1 cm.

Relationship	**Superiorly:** Optic tract, optic chiasma, olfactory tract, internal carotid artery and anterior perforated substance **Inferiorly:** Foramen lacerum and the junction of the body and greater wing of the sphenoid bone **Medially:** Hypophysis cerebri and sphenoidal air sinus **Laterally:** Temporal lobe with uncus **Anteriorly:** Superior orbital fissure and the apex of the orbit **Posteriorly:** Apex of the petrous temporal and the crus cerebri of the midbrain.
Tributaries or Incoming channels	**From the orbit:** (a) The superior ophthalmic vein; (b) a branch of the inferior ophthalmic vein or sometimes the vein itself; (c) the central vein of the retina may drain either into the superior ophthalmic vein or into the cavernous sinus. **From the brain:** (a) Superficial middle cerebral vein, and (b) inferior cerebral veins from the temporal lobe **From the meninges:** (a) Sphenoparietal sinus (b) the frontal trunk of the middle meningeal vein may drain either into the pterygoid plexus through the foramen ovale or into the sphenoparietal or cavernous sinus

Contd...

Cavernous Sinus	
Draining Channels or Communications	The cavernous sinus drains: a. Into the transverse sinus through the superior petrosal sinus b. Into the internal jugular vein through the inferior petrosal sinus and through a plexus around the internal carotid artery c. Into the pterygoid plexus of veins through the emissary veins passing through the foramen ovale, the foramen lacerum and the emissary sphenoidal foramen, and d. Into the facial vein through the superior ophthalmic vein e. The right and left cavernous sinuses communicate with each other through the anterior and posterior intercavernous sinuses and through the basilar plexus of veins. All these communications are valveless, and blood can flow through them in either direction.
Contents	▫ Internal Carotid artery ▫ Sympathetic chain around the ICA ▫ Abducens nerve (inferiolateral to ICA)
Lateral wall	▫ Uncus of the temporal lobe ▫ **Oculomotor nerve:** In the anterior part of the sinus, it divides into superior and inferior divisions which leave the sinus by passing through the superior orbital fissure ▫ **Trochlear nerve:** In the anterior part of the sinus, it crosses superficial to the oculomotor nerve, and enters the orbit through the superior orbital fissure ▫ **Ophthalmic nerve (V1):** In the anterior part of the sinus, it divides into the lacrimal, frontal and nasociliary nerves ▫ **Maxillary nerve (V2):** It leaves the sinus by passing through the foramen rotundum on its way to the pterygopalatine fossa ▫ **Trigeminal ganglion:** The ganglion and its dural cave project into the posterior part of the lateral wall of the sinus

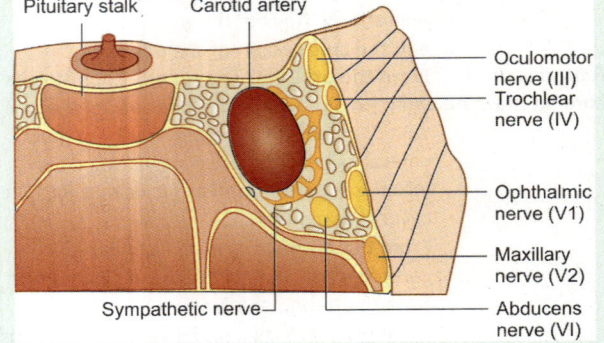

CLINICAL FEATURES OF CAVERNOUS SINUS THROMBOSIS

▫ The most common signs of CST are related to anatomical structures affected within the cavernous sinus, notably cranial nerves III-VI, as well as symptoms resulting from impaired venous drainage from the orbit and eye.
▫ Classic presentations are abrupt onset of unilateral periorbital edema, headache, photophobia, and bulging of the eye (proptosis).
▫ Ptosis, chemosis, cranial nerve palsies (III, IV, V, VI).
▫ Sixth nerve palsy is the most common.
▫ Sensory deficits of the ophthalmic and maxillary branch of the fifth nerve are common.
▫ V1 ophthalmic division of trigeminal is afferent of corneal reflex while CN 7 is the efferent. Hence, corneal sensations are affected and corneal reflex is lost.
▫ Mandibular division (V3) of trigeminal nerve does not passes through cavernous sinus wall hence Jaw jerk is intact.
▫ Papilledema, retinal hemorrhages, and decreased visual acuity and blindness may occur from venous congestion within the retina.
▫ Fever, tachycardia and sepsis may be present.
▫ Headache with nuchal rigidity may occur. Pupil may be dilated and sluggishly reactive.
▫ Infection can spread to contralateral cavernous sinus within 24–48 hours of initial presentation.

 **ANATOMY PLATE 12**

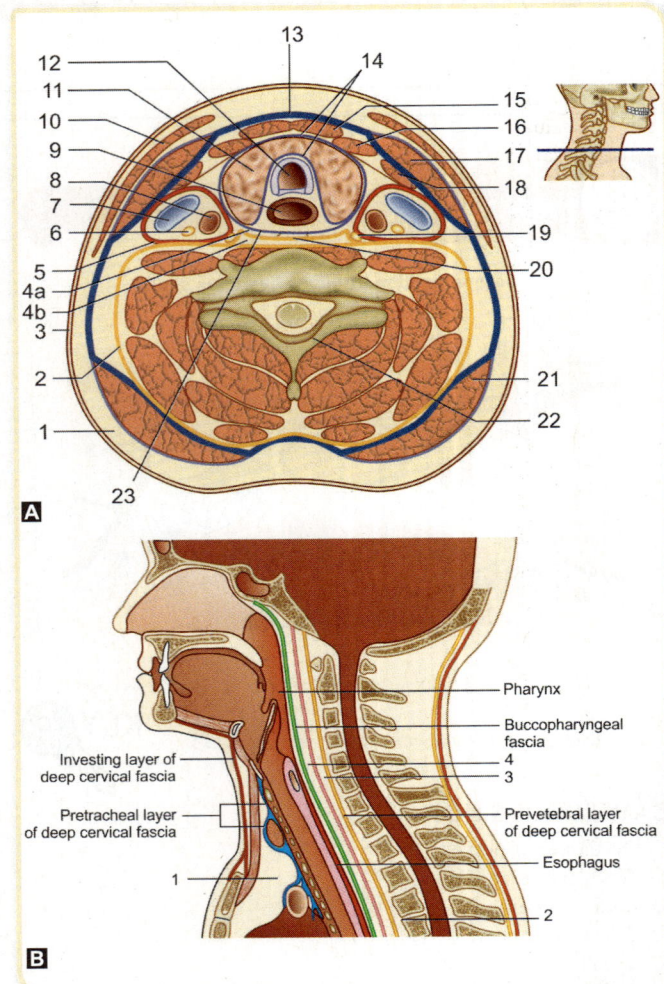

CROSS AND SAGITTAL SECTION OF NECK

A. Cross section of neck
 1. Superficial fascia
 2. Prevertebral fascia

3. Skin
4. **4A. Retropharyngeal space** (Between Buccopharyngeal fascia anteriorly and Alar layer of Prevertebral fascia posteriorly)
   4B. Danger space/Alar space/Space 4 (Grodinsky and Holyoke). Between Alar fascia anteriorly and prevertebral fascia posteriorly and extends from the cranial base above to the level of the diaphragm. Name originates from the risk that an infection in this space can spread directly to the thorax. There exists a midline raphe in this space so some infections of this space appear unilateral.
5. Carotid sheath
6. Vagus nerve
7. Internal Jugular vein
8. Common carotid artery
9. Esophagus
10. Platysma muscle
11. Thyroid gland
12. Trachea
13. Investing (superficial) layer of deep cervical fascia
14. Visceral layer (Skyblue); Pretracheal fascia (Thyroid capsule) Sky blue)
15. Sternohyoid muscle
16. Sternothyroid muscle
17. Sternocleidomastoid muscle
18. Omohyoid muscle
19. Sympathetic trunk
20. Alar fascia (Extension of prevertebral fascia)
21. Trapezius muscle
22. Cervical vertebra
23. Visceral layer (Skyblue) Buccopharyngeal fascia Posteriorly the pretracheal layer gives off Buccopharyngeal fascia.

Carotid Sheath

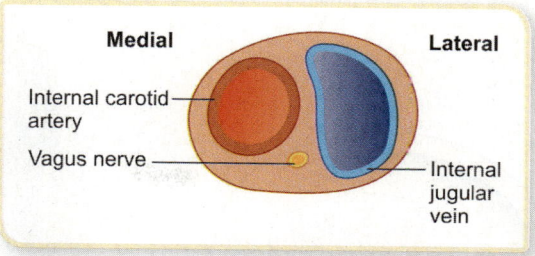

The carotid sheath contains:
1. The common and internal carotid arteries
2. The internal jugular vein (IJV)
3. The vagus nerve (CN X)
4. Some deep cervical lymph nodes
5. The carotid sinus nerve
6. Sympathetic nerve fibers (carotid periarterial plexuses)

B. Sagittal section of Neck:
1. Pretracheal space
2. Prevertebral space
3. **Danger space/ Alar space/ Space 4** (Grodinsky and Holyoke). Between Alar fascia anteriorly and prevertebral fascia posteriorly and extends from the cranial base above to the level of the diaphragm. Name originates from the risk that an infection in this space can spread directly to the thorax. There exists a midline raphe in this space so some infections of this space appear unilateral.
4. **Retropharyngeal space** (Between Buccopharyngeal fascia anteriorly and Alar layer of Prevertebral fascia posteriorly)

 ANATOMY PLATE 13

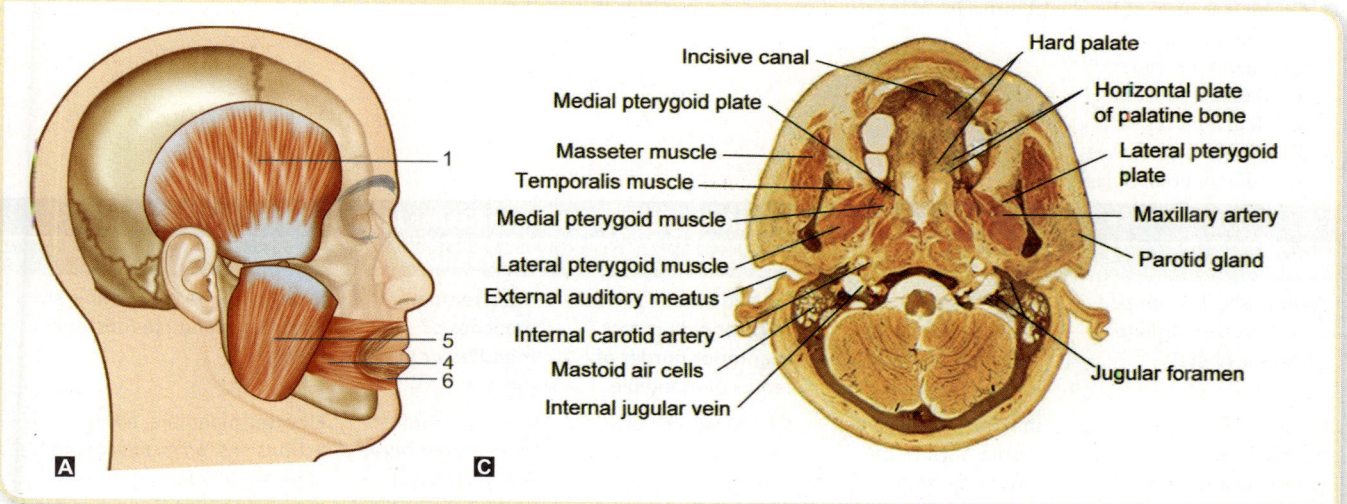

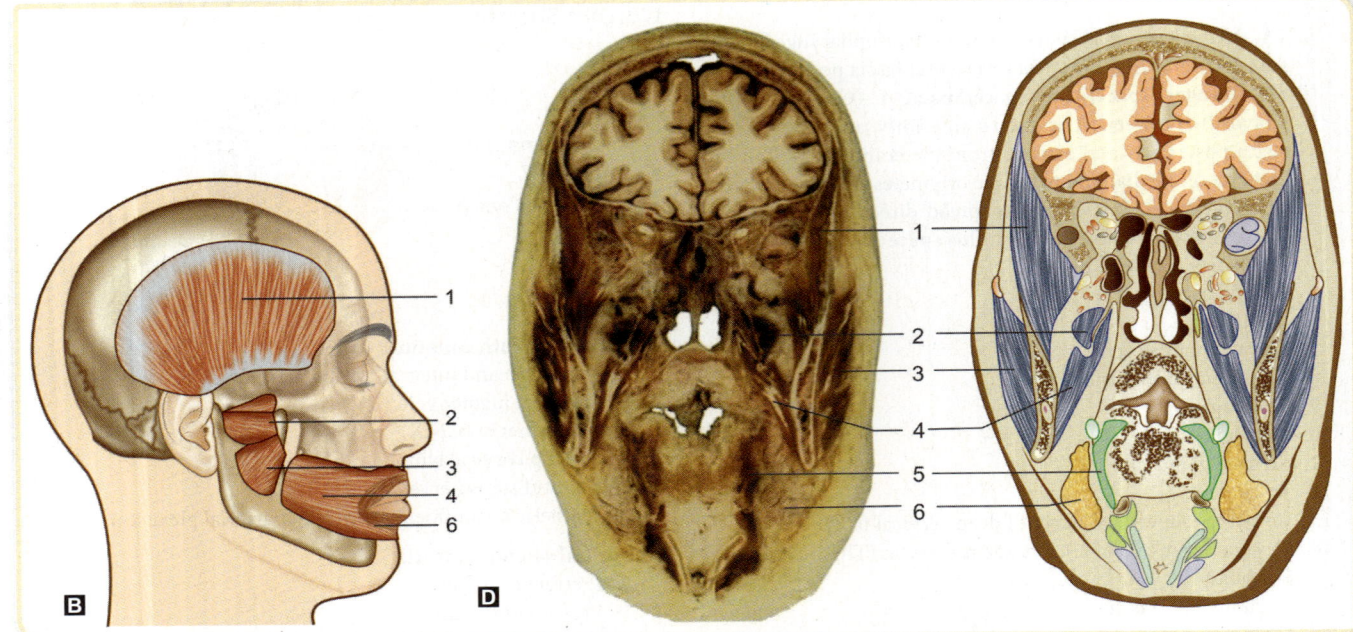
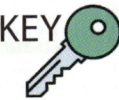

MUSCLES OF MASTICATION

A. Muscles of Mastication Superficial dissection
B. Muscles of Mastication deep dissection
1. Temporalis
2. Lateral pterygoid
3. Medial pterygoid
4. Buccinator
5. Masseter
6. Orbicularis oris

C. Muscles of mastication in transverse/ cross section of Head (Labeled) (Lateral Pterygoid[AIIMSPG])
D. Coronal section of head with muscles of mastication and comparative illustration
1. Temporalis
2. Lateral pterygoid[AIIMSPG]
3. Masseter muscle
4. Medial pterygoid
5. Hypoglossal muscle
6. Submandibular gland

Muscles of Mastication (Acting on Temporomandibular Joint)				
Muscle	**Origin**	**Insertion**	**Innervation**	**Main action**
Temporails (Fan shaped; anterior, intermediate & posterior fibers)	Floor of temporal fossa & deep surface of temporal fascia	Tip and medial surface of coronoid process & anterior border of ramus of mandible	Deep temporal branches of **mandibular nerve** (CN V³)	Elevates mandible (all fibers), Retrudes mandible (posterior fibers)
Masseter (superficial, middle & deep layers) (superficial layer is the largest)	Inferior border & medial surface of zygomatic arch	Lateral surface of ramus of mandible and coronoid process	Anterior trunk of **Mandibular nerve** (CN V³) through masseteric nerve	Elevates mandible, minor actions are: protrudes mandible (superficial fibers), retrudes mandible (deep fibers)
Lateral pterygoid (Upper head & Lower head)	*Superior head:* infratemporal surface and infratemporal crest of greater wing of sphenoid bone *Inferior head:* lateral surface of lateral pterygoid plate	Neck of mandible, articular disc, and capsule of temporomandibular joint	**Mandibular nerve** (CN V³) through lateral pterygoid nerve which enters its deep surface	*Acting bilaterally,* protrude mandible and depress chin; *Acting unilaterally* alternately, they produce side-to-side movements of mandible (pulled medially towards the opposite side)

Contd...

Muscles of Mastication (Acting on Temporomandibular Joint)				
Muscle	Origin	Insertion	Innervation	Main action
Medial pterygoid (small superficial head & major Deep head)	*Deep head:* medial surface of lateral pterygoid plate and pyramidal process of palatine bone *Superficial head:* tuberosity of maxilla	Medial surface of ramus of mandible, inferior to mandibular foramen	**Mandibular nerve** (CN V^3) through medial pterygoid nerve	Acts Synergistically with masseter to elevate mandible, contributes to protrude mandible; *acting unilaterally* produce small grinding movements

\# Unlike the other muscles of mastication, lateral pterygoid is not pennate, nor does it have a significant number of Golgi tendon organs associated with its attachments.

ANATOMY PLATE 14

PLATE LEGENDS
1. Phrenic nerve
2. Scalenus anterior
3. Scalenus medius
4. Transverse cervical artery
5. Brachial plexus
6. Suprascapular artery
7. Thyrocervical trunk originating from the subclavian artery
8. Subclavian vein

ANATOMY PLATE 15

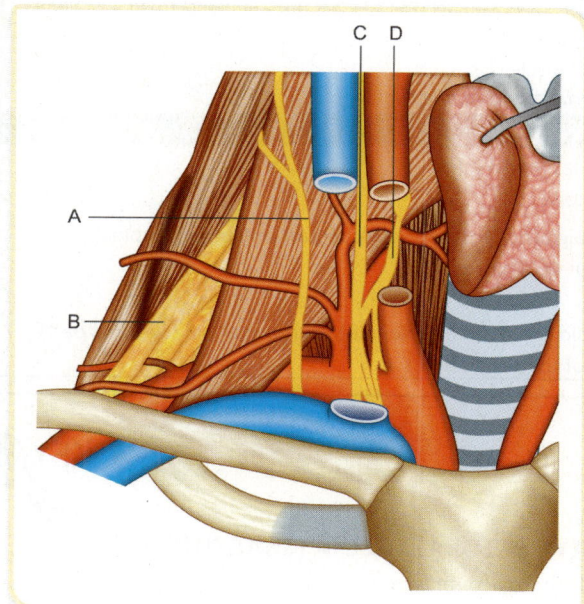

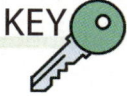

PLATE LEGENDS
A = Phrenic nerve
B = Brachial plexus
C = Vagus nerve
D = Sympathetic trunk

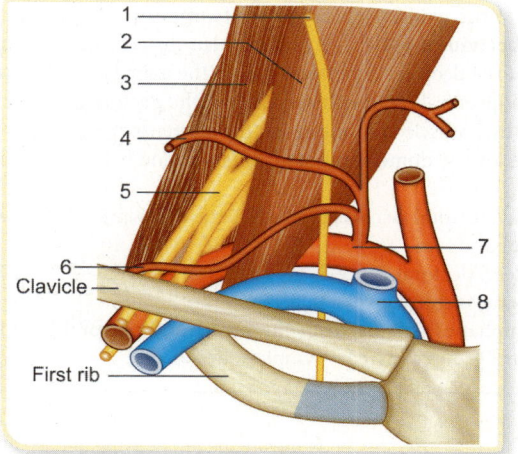

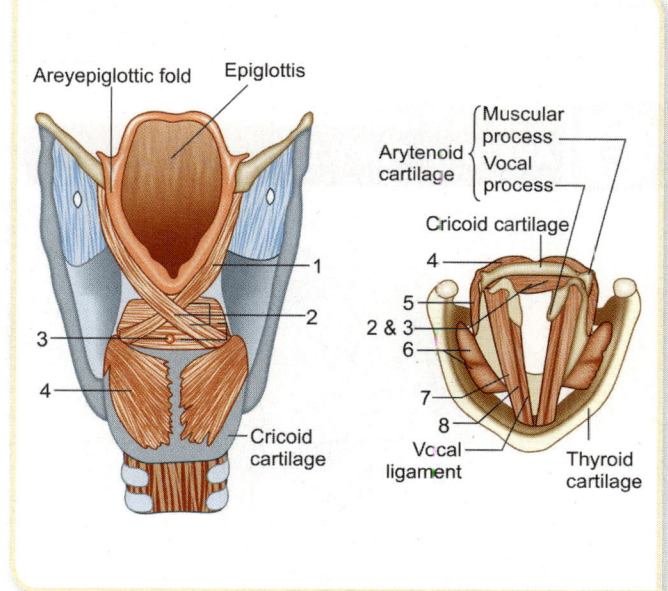

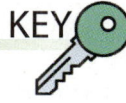

INTRINSIC MUSCLES OF LARYNX (POSTERIOR VIEW & INTERNAL VIEW)
1. Areyepiglottic muscle
2. Oblique Arytenoid muscle
3. Transverse Arytenoid muscle
4. Posterior Cricoarytenoid muscle
5. Lateral Cricoarytenoid muscle
6. Cricothyroid muscle
7. Thyroarytenoid muscle
8. Vocalis muscle

Muscles of Larynx

Muscle	Origin	Insertion	Innervation	Main action (s)
Cricothyroid	Anterolateral part of cricoid cartilage	Inferior margin and inferior horn of thyroid cartilage	External branch of superior laryngeal nerve (CN X)	Tenses vocal fold
Posterior cricoarytenoid	Posterior surface of laminae of cricoid cartilage	Muscular process of arytenoid cartilage	Recurrent laryngeal nerve (CN X)	Abducts vocal fold
Lateral cricoarytenoid	Arch of cricoid cartilage			Adducts vocal fold
Thyroarytenoids[a]	Posterior surface of thyroid cartilage			Relaxes vocal fold
Transverse and oblique arytenoids[b]	One arytenoid cartilage	Opposite arytenoid cartilage		Close inlet of larynx by approximating arytenoid cartilages
Vocalis[c]	Angle between laminae of thyroid cartilage	Vocal ligament, between origin and vocal process of arytenoid cartilage		Alters vocal fold during phonation

[a]Superior fibers of the thyroarytenoid muscle pass into the aryepiglottic fold, and some of them reach the epiglottic cartilage. These fibers constitute the **thyroepiglottic muscle**, which widens the inlet of the larynx.
[b]Some fibers of the oblique arytenoid muscle continue as the aryepiglottic muscle.
[c]This slender muscular slip is derived from inferi*or deeper fibers of the thyroarytenoid musc*le.

Muscles of Larynx FAQ

Intrinsic muscles acting on laryngeal inlet	
Openers of laryngeal inlet	Thyroepiglottic (part of thyroarytenoid)
Closers of laryIngeal inlet	Interarytenoid (oblique part), Aryepiglottic (posterior oblique part of interarytenoids)
Intrinsic muscles acting on vocal cords	
Abductors	Posterior cricoarytenoid
Adductors	Lateral cricoarytenoid, Interarytenoid (transverse arytenoid) Thyroarytenoid (external part)
Tensors	Cricothyroid, Vocalis (internal part of thyroarytenoid)

ANATOMY PLATE 16

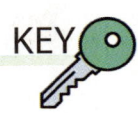

CLAVIPECTORAL FASCIA (SHADED)[AIIMSPG]

1. Thoraco acromian artery
2. Cephalic vein draining in axillary vein
3. Lateral pectoral nerve

Clavipectoral Fascia

- Extent: From clavicle above to axillary fascia below.
- Upper part splits to enclose subclavius muscle while lower part splits to enclose pectoralis minor muscle.
- It helps to pull up axillary fascia.
- Upper thickened part is called the costocoracoidal ligament.

Clavipectoral fascia is a fibrous sheet situated deep to the clavicular portion of the pectoralis major muscle. It extends from the clavicle above to the axillary fascia below. **Its upper part splits to enclose the subclavius muscle.** The posterior lamina is fused to the investing layer of the deep cervical fascia and to the axillary sheath. Inferiorly, the clavipectoral fascia splits to enclose the pectoralis minor muscle. Below this muscle it continues as the suspensory ligament, which is attached to the dome of the axillary fascia, and helps to keep it pulled up.

The clavipectoral fascia is pierced by the following structures:
1. Cephalic vein
2. Lateral pectoral nerve
3. Thoracoacromial vessels
4. Lymphatics passing from the breast and pectoral region to the apical group of axillary lymph nodes.

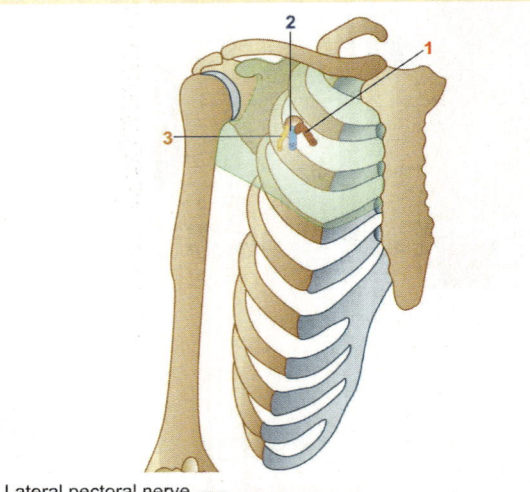
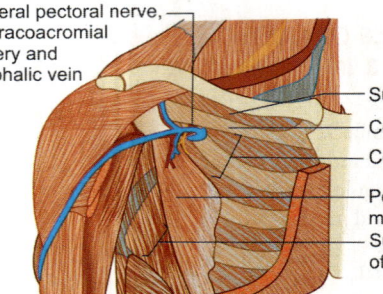
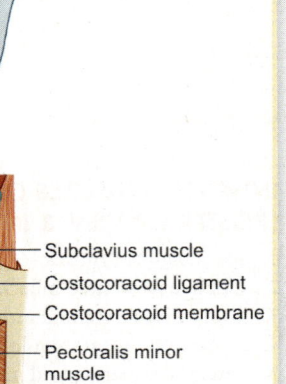

ANATOMY PLATE 17

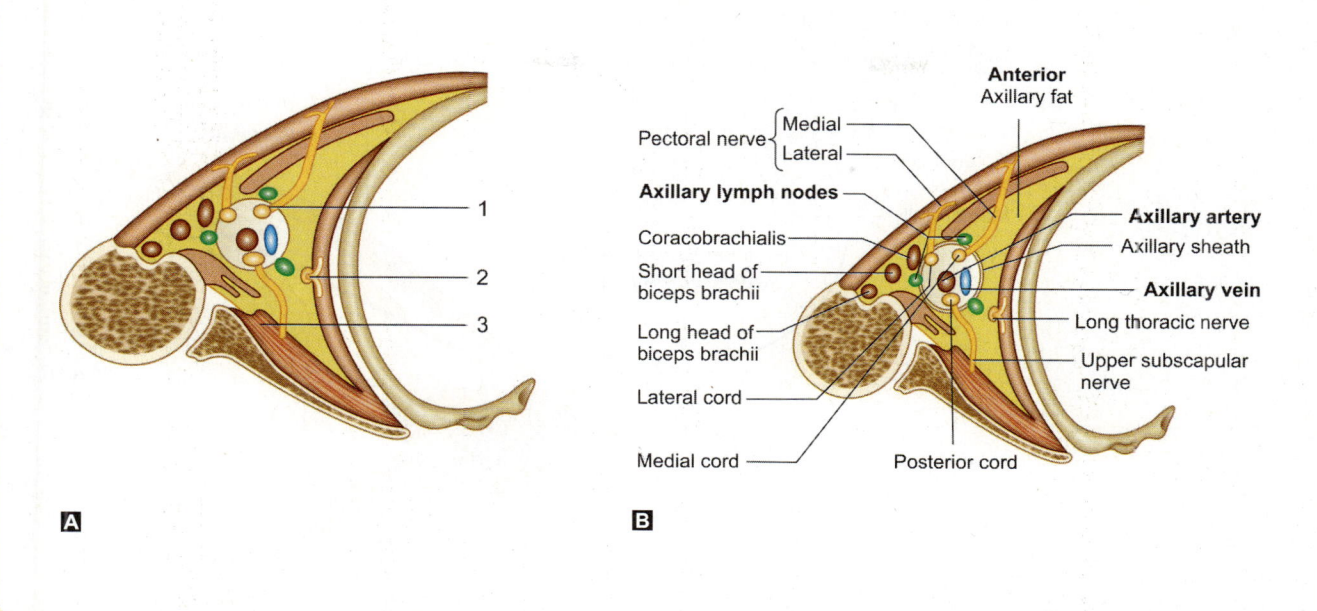

CROSS SECTION OF AXILLA

A. Cross section of Axilla (Unlabeled)[AIIMSPG]
1. Medial cord of brachial plexus (Towards the rib, contrary to lateral cord, which is toward the head of humerus)
2. Long thoracic nerve (supplying the Serratus anterior muscle of the medical wall of axilla)
3. Subscapularis muscle

B. Cross section of Axilla (Labelled)

Axilla
The axilla or armpit is a pyramidal space situated between the upper part of the arm and the chest wall. It resembles a four-sided pyramid, and has (i) an apex, (ii) a base, and (iii) 4 walls—anterior, posterior, medial and lateral. The axilla is disposed obliquely in such a way that the apex is directed upwards and medially towards the root of the neck, and the base is directed downwards.

▫ **Apex:** It is directed upwards and medially towards the root of the neck. It is truncated (not pointed), and corresponds to a triangular interval bounded anteriorly by the clavicle, posteriorly by the superior border of the scapula, and medially by the outer border of the first rib. This passage is called the **cervicoaxillary canal**. The axillary artery and the brachial plexus enter the axilla through this canal.
▫ **Base or floor:** It is directed downwards, and is formed by skin and fasciae
▫ **Anterior wall:** It is formed by the following:
  i. The pectoralis major in front and
  ii. The clavipectoral fascia enclosing the pectoralis minor and the subclavius; all deep to the pectoralis major
▫ **Posterior wall:** It is formed by: (i) Subscapularis above (ii) Teres major and latissimus dorsi below
▫ **Medial wall:** It is formed by: (i) Upper four ribs with their intercostal muscles, (ii) Upper part of the serratus anterior muscle
▫ **Lateral wall:** It is very narrow because the anterior and posterior walls converge on it. It is formed by: (i) Upper part of the shaft of the humerus in the region of the bicipital groove, and (ii) Coracobrachialis and short head of the biceps.

Contd...

Axilla

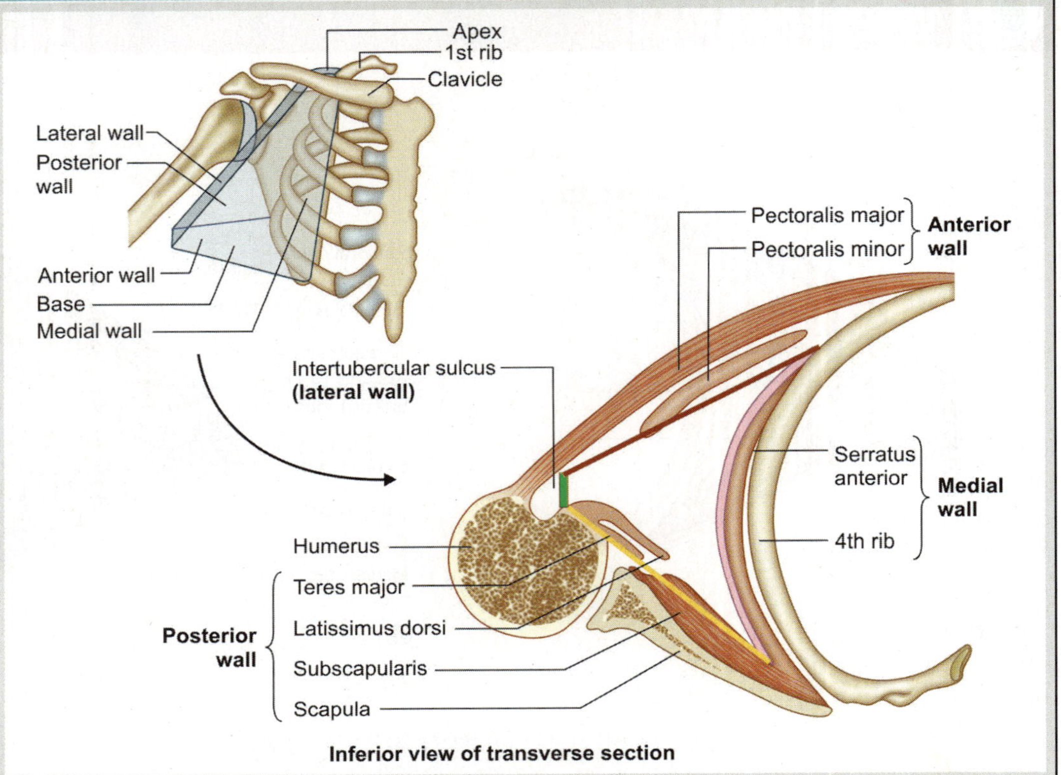

Inferior view of transverse section

Contents in Axilla	1. **Axillary sheath** containing: Axillary artery and its branches, Axillary vein and its tributaries, Brachial plexus (Medial, lateral and posterior cords) 2. Five groups of axillary lymph nodes and the associated lymphatics. 3. The long thoracic and intercostobrachial nerves. 4. Axillary fat and areolar tissue in which the other contents are embedded
Layout in axilla	1. Axillary artery and the brachial plexus of nerves I run from the apex to the base along the lateral wall of the axilla, nearer to the anterior wall than the posterior wall 2. The thoracic branches of the axillary artery lie in contact with the pectoral muscles, the lateral thoracic vessels running along the lower border of the pectoralis minor. 3. The subscapular vessels run along the lower border of the subscapularis. The subscapular nerve and the thoracodorsal nerve (nerve to latissimus dorsi) cross the anterior surface of the muscle. The circumflex scapular vessels wind round the lateral border of the scapula. The axillary nerve and the posterior circumflex humeral vessels pass backwards close to the surgical neck of the humerus.

ANATOMY PLATE 18

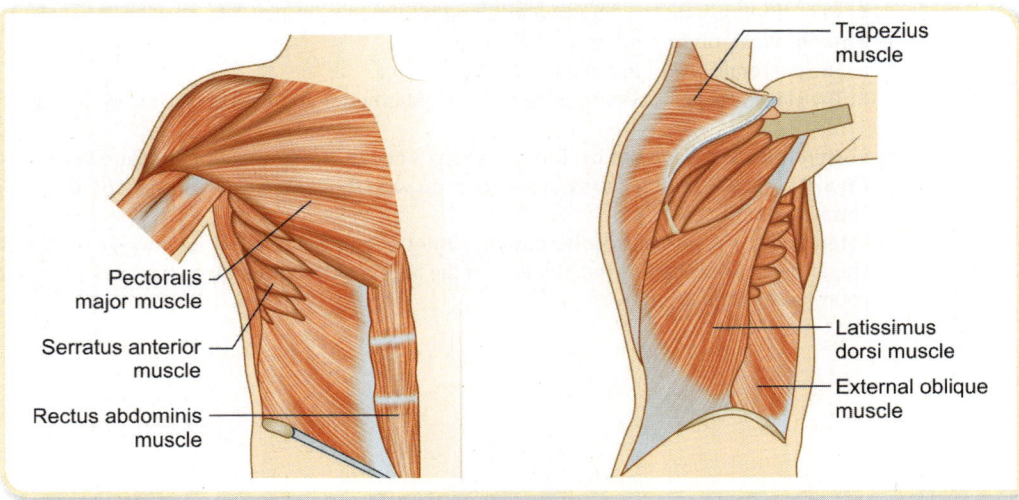

MUSCLES OF THE CHEST WALL (LABELLED)
Pectoralis major[NEETPG]

	Anterior Axioappendicular Muscles			
Muscle	Origin	Insertion	Nerve supply	Action
Pectoralis major	**Clavicular head**: anterior surface of medial half of clavicle **Sternocostal head**: anterior surface of sternum, superior 6 costal cartilages **Abdominal part**: aponeurosis of external oblique muscle	Crest of greater tubercle of intertubercular sulcus (lateral lip of bicipital groove)	Lateral and medial pectoral nerves; clavicular head (C5 and **C6**), sternocostal head (**C7**, **C8**, and T1)	Adducts and medially rotates humerus; draws scapula anteriorly & inferiorly Acting alone: clavicular head flexes humerus & sternocostal head extends it from the flexed position
Pectoralis minor	3rd to 5th ribs near their costal cartilages	Medial border and superior surface of coracoid process of scapula	Medial pectoral nerve (C8 and T1)	Stabilizes scapula by drawing it inferiorly and anteriorly against thoracic wall
Subclavius	Junction of 1st rib and its costal cartilage	Inferior surface of middle third of clavicle	Nerve to subclavius (**C5** and C6)	Anchors and depresses clavicle
Serratus anterior	External surfaces of lateral parts of 1st to 8th–9th ribs	Anterior surface of medial border of scapula	Long thoracic nerve (C5, **C6**, and C7)	Protracts scapula and holds it against thoracic wall; rotates scapula

ANATOMY PLATE 19

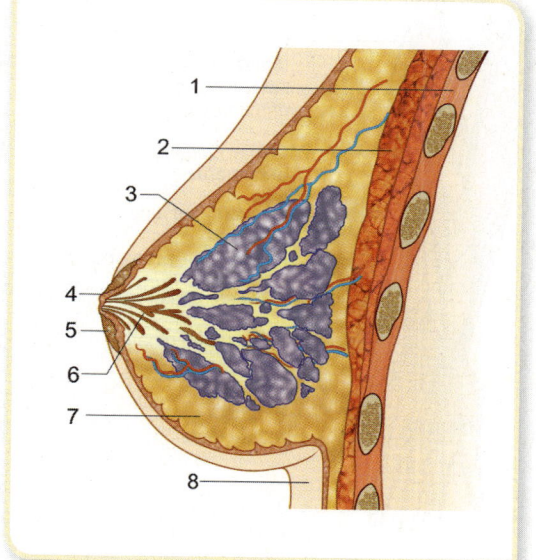

Credit: Patrick J. Lynch, medical illustrator

DUCTAL ANATOMY OF THE BREAST
(1) Chest wall, (2) Pectoral muscles, (3) Lobules, (4) Nipple surface, (5) Areola, (6) Lactiferous duct, (7) Fatty tissue, (8) Skin

ANATOMY PLATE 20

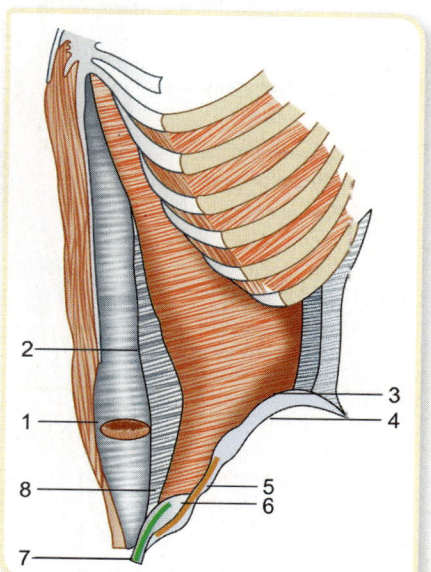

1. **Linea alba:** It is a tendinous raphe extending from xiphoid process to pubic symphysis and pubic crest. It lies between the two recti and is formed by the interlacing and decussating aponeurotic fibers of external oblique, internal oblique and transversus abdominis

2. **Linea Semilunaris:** A few centimeters lateral to the median furrow, the abdominal wall shows a curved vertical groove. Its upper end reaches the costal margin at the tip of I the ninth costal cartilage. Interiorly it reaches the pubic tubercle. This line is called the linea semilunaris. It corresponds to the lateral margin of a muscle called the rectus abdominis
3. **Inner lip of iliac crest:** Iliac crest has internal and external lips and a rough intermediate zone that is narrowest centrally
4. **Outer lip of Iliac crest**
5. **Inguinal ligament:** Extends from the anterior superior iliac spine to the pubic tubercle. It is convex downwards. It is placed at the junction of the anterior abdominal wall with the front of the thigh
6. **Superficial inguinal ring:** It is a hiatus in the aponeurosis of external oblique, just above and lateral to the crest of the pubis. Triangular, with its apex pointing laterally towards the anterior superior iliac spine. The ring is smaller in the female. The base of the triangular opening lies along the crest of the pubis. Its sides are the lateral and medial crura of the opening in the aponeurosis.
7. **Spermatic cord:** present in the male. It can be felt through the skin as it passes downwards near the medial end of the inguinal ligament to enter the scrotum
8. **Conjoint tendon:** is a structure formed from the lower part of the common aponeurosis of the internal abdominal oblique and the transverse abdominal as it inserts into the crest of the pubis and pectineal line immediately behind the superficial inguinal ring. It forms the medial part of the posterior wall of the inguinal canal.

ANATOMY PLATE 21

Anterior superficial view

Posterior superficial view

A

B

C

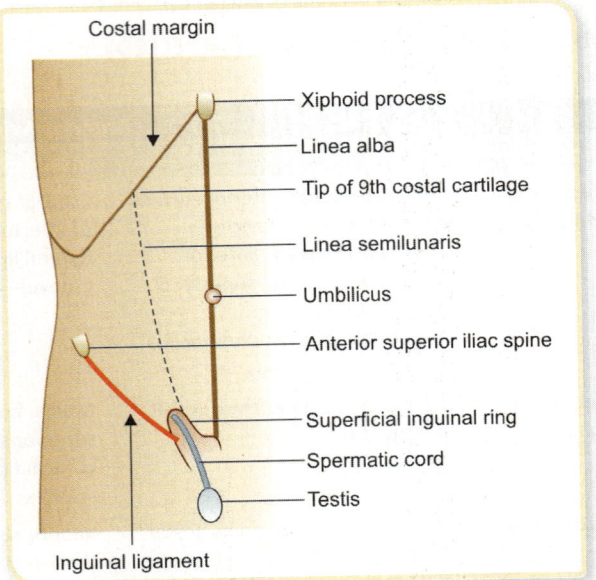

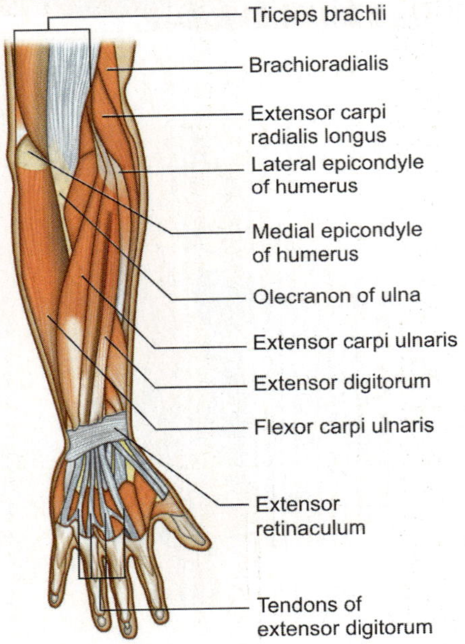

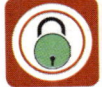

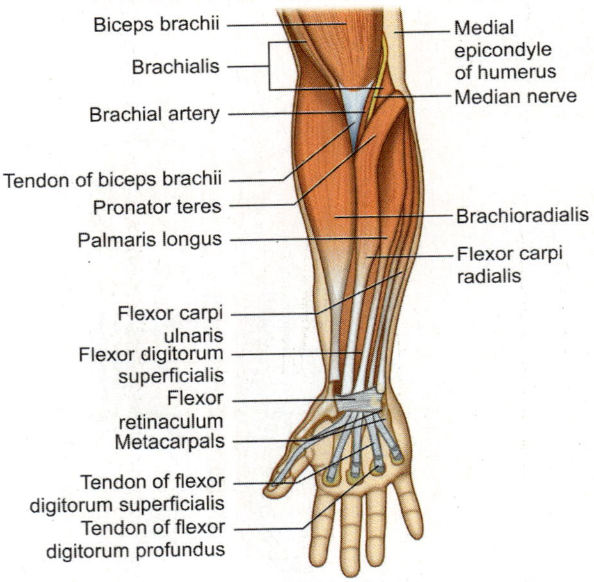

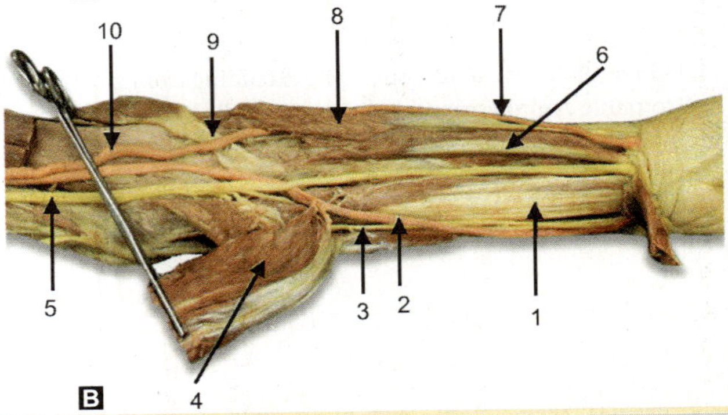

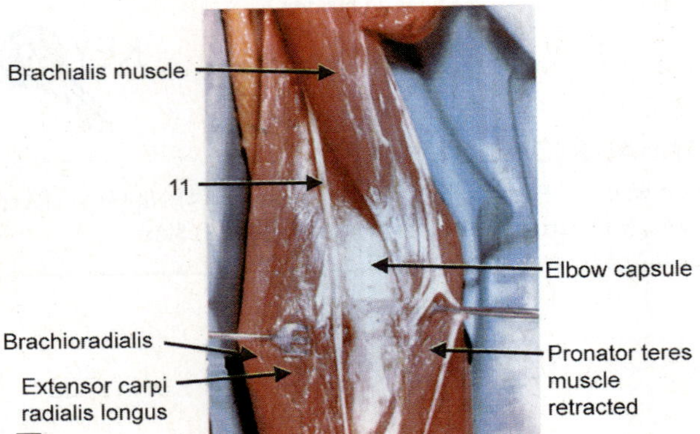

MUSCLES OF THE FOREARM (LABELLED)

A. Muscles of the forearm illustration (Labelled): See Brachioradialis[NEETPG]

B. and C. Forearm dissection
1. Flexor digitorum Profundus
2. Ulnar artery
3. Ulnar nerve[AIIMS PG]
4. Superficial flexor muscles (reflected)
5. Median nerve[AIIMS PG] (Autonomous area of testing median nerve- Tip of index finger dorsal side[AIIMS PG])
6. Flexor pollicis longus
7. Superficial radial artery
8. Brachioradialis[NEET PG]
9. Biceps brachii tendon
10. Superficial radial artery
11. Radial nerve (injury causes wrist drop)[AIIMS PG]

| Muscles of Anterior Compartment of Forearm |||||||
Muscle	Origin	Insertion	Nerve supply	Nerve roots	Action
Superficial (first) layer					
Pronator teres (PT)	*Ulnar head*: Coronoid process of ulna *Humeral head*: Medial epicondyle of humerus	Middle of convexity of lateral surface of radius	Median nerve	C6, **C7**	Pronates and flexes forearm (at elbow)
Flexor carpi radialis (FCR)	Medial epicondyle of humerus	Base of 2nd (3rd) metacarpal	Median nerve	C6, **C7**	Flexes and abducts hand (at wrist)
Palmaris Longus	Medial epicondyle of humerus	Distal half of Flexor retinaculum, palmar aponeurosis	Median nerve	C7, C8	Flexes hand (at wrist) and tenses palmar aponeurosis
Flexor carpi ulnaris (FCU): Humeral head Ulnar head	Olecranon and posterior border (via aponeurosis)	Pisiform, hook of hamate, 5th metacarpal	Ulnar nerve	C7, **C8**	Flexes and adducts hand (at wrist)
Intermediate (second) layer					
Flexor digitorum superficialis (FDS)	*Humero-ulnar head*: Medial epicondyle of humerus and coronoid process of ulna *Radial head*: Oblique line of radius	Shafts (bodies) of middle phalanges of medial four digits	Median nerve	C7, C8, T1	Flexes proximal interphalangeal joints of middle four digits; acting more strongly, it also flexes proximal phalanges at metacarpophalangeal joints
Deep (third) layer					
Flexor digitorum profundus (FDP)	Proximal three quarters of medial and anterior surfaces of ulna and interosseous membrane	Bases of distal phalanges of 2nd, 3rd, 4th, and 5th digits	*Lateral part (to digits 2 and 3):* Median nerve (**C8**, T1) (anterior interosseous branch) *Medial part (to digits 4 and 5):* Ulnar nerve (C8, **T1**)		Flexes distal interphalangeal joints of digits 2, 3, 4, and 5; assists with wrist flexion
Flexor pollicis longus (FPL)	Anterior surface of radius and adjacent interosseous Membrane	Base of distal phalanx of thumb	Anterior interosseous nerve, from median nerve	**C8**, T1	Flexes phalanges of 1st digit (thumb)
Pronator quadratus	Distal quarter of anterior surface of ulna	Distal quarter of anterior surface of radius			Pronates forearm; deep fibers bind radius and ulna together

Contd...

Muscles of Posterior Compartment of Forearm

Origin	Insertion	Nerve supply	Nerve roots	Action
Superficial layer				
Proximal two thirds of lateral supra epicondylar ridge of humerus	Lateral surface of distal end of radius proximal to styloid process	Radial nerve	C5, **C6**, C7	Relatively weak flexion of forearm, maximal when forearm is in midpronated position
Lateral supra-epicondylar ridge of humerus	Dorsal aspect of base of 2nd metacarpal	Radial nerve	C6, C7	Extend and abduct hand at the wrist joint; extensor carpi radialis brevis active during fist clenching
Lateral epicondyle of humerus (common extensor origin)	Dorsal aspect of base of 3rd metacarpal	Deep branch of radial nerve	**C7**, C8	
	Extensor expansions of medial four fingers	Posterior interosseous nerve continuation of deep branch of radial nerve	**C7**, C8	Extends medial four fingers primarily at metacarpophalangeal joints, secondarily at interphalangeal joints
	Extensor expansion of 5th finger			Extends 5th finger primarily at metacarpophalangeal joint, secondarily at interphalangeal joint
Lateral epicondyle of humerus; posterior border of ulna via a shared aponeurosis	Dorsal aspect of base of 5th metacarpal			Extends and adducts hand at wrist joint (also active during fist clenching)
Deep layer				
Lateral epicondyle of humerus; radial collateral and anular ligaments; supinator fossa; crest of ulna	Lateral, posterior, and anterior surfaces of proximal third of radius	Deep branch of radial nerve	C7, **C8**	Supinates forearm; rotates radius to turn palm anteriorly or superiorly (if elbow is flexed)
"Outcropping" muscles of deep layer				
Posterior surface of proximal halves of ulna, radius, and interosseous membrane	Base of 1st metacarpal	Posterior interosseous nerve continuation of deep branch of radial nerve	C7, **C8**	Abducts thumb and extends it at carpometacarpal joint
Posterior surface of middle third of ulna and interosseous membrane	Dorsal aspect of base of distal phalanx of thumb			Extends distal phalanx of thumb at interphalangeal joint; extends metacarpophalangeal and carpometacarpal joints
Posterior surface of distal third of radius and interosseous membrane	Dorsal aspect of base of proximal phalanx of thumb			Extends proximal phalanx of thumb at metacarpophalangeal joint; extends carpometacarpal joint
Posterior surface of distal third of ulna and interosseous membrane	Extensor expansion of 2nd finger			Extends 2nd finger (enabling its independent extension); helps extend hand at wrist

Footnote:
- The posterior compartment of forearm contains the extensor muscles of the forearm and brachioradialis and supinator.
- *Brachioradialis is a flexor of the elbow (despite being supplied by an 'extensor' nerve).*
- All extensor muscles of the forearm are supplied by posterior interosseous nerve C6,7 except
  - Anconeus which is supplied by the radial nerve, C6, 7 and 8
  - Extensor carpi radialis longus which is supplied by the radial nerve C6,7

ANATOMY PLATE 22

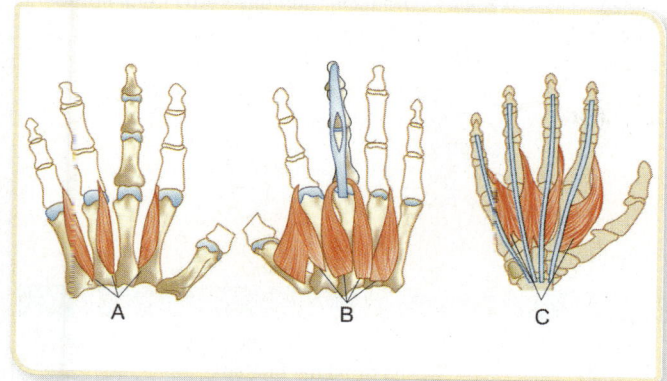

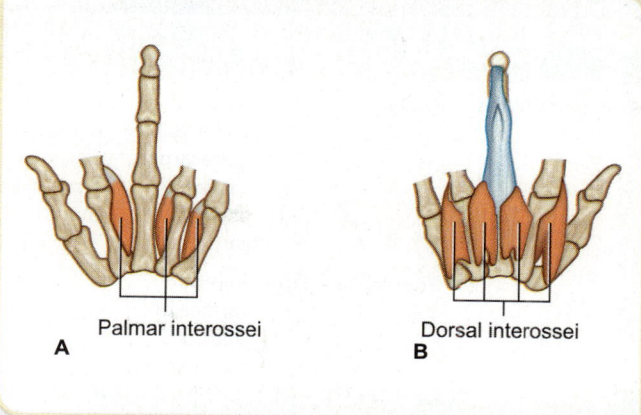

A. Palmar interossei
B. Dorsal interossei

Fig: Intrinsic muscles of the hand are the muscles which have both origin and insertion within the hand

A. Superficial muscles of hand (Palmar view)
B. Superficial muscles of hand (Dorsal view)
C. Deep muscles of hand (Palmar view)
D. Deep muscles of hand (Dorsal view)

KEY

PLATE LEGENDS

A. Palmar interossei
B. Dorsal interossei
C. Lumbricals[NEETPG]

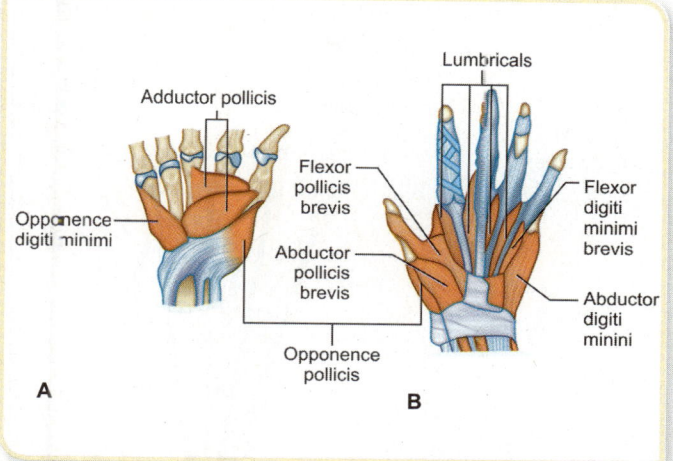

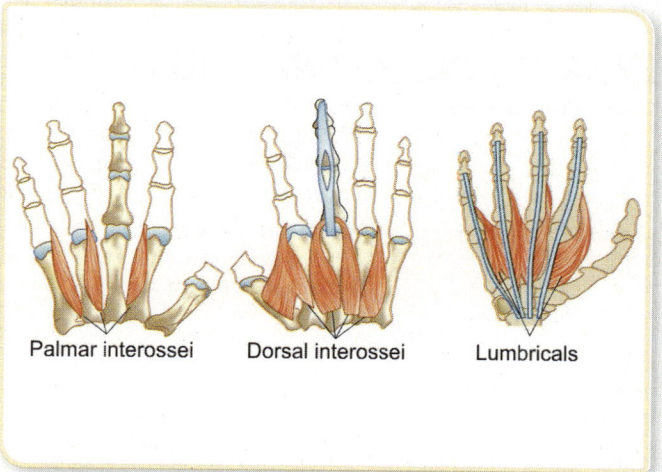

Fig: How to differentiate between Lumbricals and Interossei?

Palmar interossei (3 in number) are all unipennate, Dorsal interossei (4 in number) are all bipinnate while Lumbricals (4 in number) are both Unipnnate and Bipinnate.

Intrinsic Muscles of Hand					
Muscle	Origin	Insertion	Nerve supply	Nerve roots	Action
Thenar muscles					
Opponens Pollicis	Flexor retinaculum and tubercles of scaphoid and trapezium	Lateral side of 1st Metacarpal	Recurrent branch of median nerve	C8, T1	To oppose thumb, it draws 1st metacarpal medially to center of palm and rotates it medially
Abductor pollicis brevis		Lateral side of base of proximal phalanx of thumb			Abducts thumb; helps oppose it
Flexor pollicis brevis (Superficial & Deep head)					Flexes thumb

Contd...

Intrinsic Muscles of Hand

Muscle		Origin	Insertion	Nerve supply	Nerve roots	Action
Adductor Pollicis	Oblique head	Bases of 2nd and 3rd metacarpals, capitate, adjacent carpals	Medial side of base of proximal phalanx of thumb	Deep branch of ulnar nerve	C8, **T1**	Adducts thumb toward lateral border of Palm
	Transverse Head	Anterior surface of shaft of 3rd metacarpal				
Hypothenar muscles						
Abductor digiti Minimi		Pisiform	Medial side of base of proximal phalanx of 5th finger	Deep branch of ulnar nerve	C8, **T1**	Abducts 5th finger; assists in flexion of its proximal phalanx
Flexor digiti minimi brevis		Hook of hamate and flexor retinaculum				Flexes proximal phalanx of 5th finger
Opponens digiti minimi			Medial border of 5th metacarpal			Draws 5th metacarpal anterior and rotates it, bringing 5th finger into opposition with thumb
Short muscles (Lumbricals)						
1 and 2 (Unipinnate)		Lateral two tendons of flexor digitorum profundus (as unipennate muscles)	Lateral sides of extensor expansions of 2nd -5th fingers	Median nerve	C8, **T1**	Flex metacarpophalangeal joints; extend interphalangeal joints of 2nd-5th fingers
3 and 4 (Bipinnate)		Medial three tendons of flexor digitorum profundus (as bipennate muscles)		Deep branch of ulnar nerve	C8, **T1**	
Dorsal interossei, 1-4		Adjacent sides of two metacarpals (as bipennate muscles)	Bases of proximal phalanges; extensor expansions of 2nd-4th fingers			Abduct 2nd-4th fingers from axial line; act with lumbricals in flexing metacarpophalangeal joints and extending interphalangeal joints
Palmar interossei, 1-3		Palmar surfaces of 2nd, 4th, and 5th metacarpals (as unipennate muscles)	Bases of proximal phalanges; extensor expansions of 2nd, 4th, and 5th fingers			Adduct 2nd, 4th, and 5th fingers toward axial line; assist lumbricals in flexing metacarpophalangeal joints and extending interphalangeal joints

ANATOMY PLATE 23

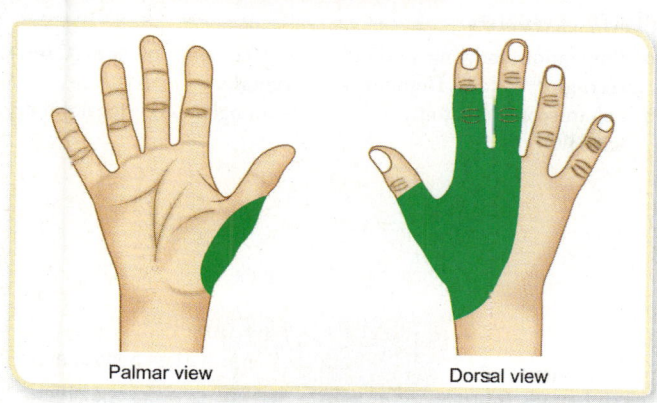

Palmar view | Dorsal view

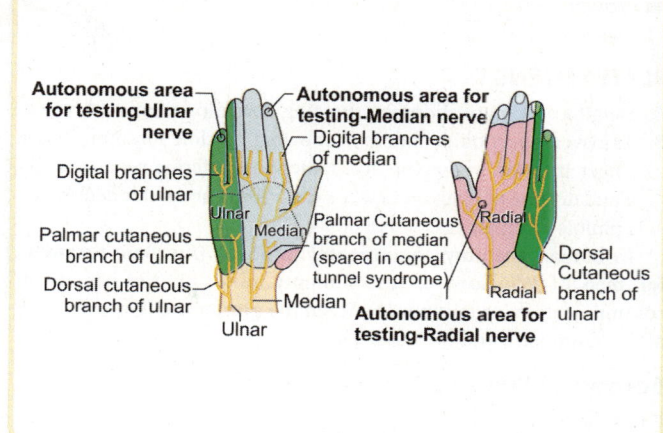

Fig: Cutaneous innervation of dorsal and palmar surface of hand

- Autonomous area of testing median nerve- Tip of index finger dorsal side[AIIMS PG]
- Autonomous area of testing ulnar nerve- Tip of little finger dorsal side
- Autonomous area for testing radial nerve- First interdigital cleft ventral side

PLATE LEGENDS

The area marked in the figure is supplied by the radial nerve. See figure below for distribution of nerve supply in the hand, also note points of testing autonomous innervation of individual nerves.

ANATOMY PLATE 24

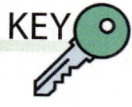

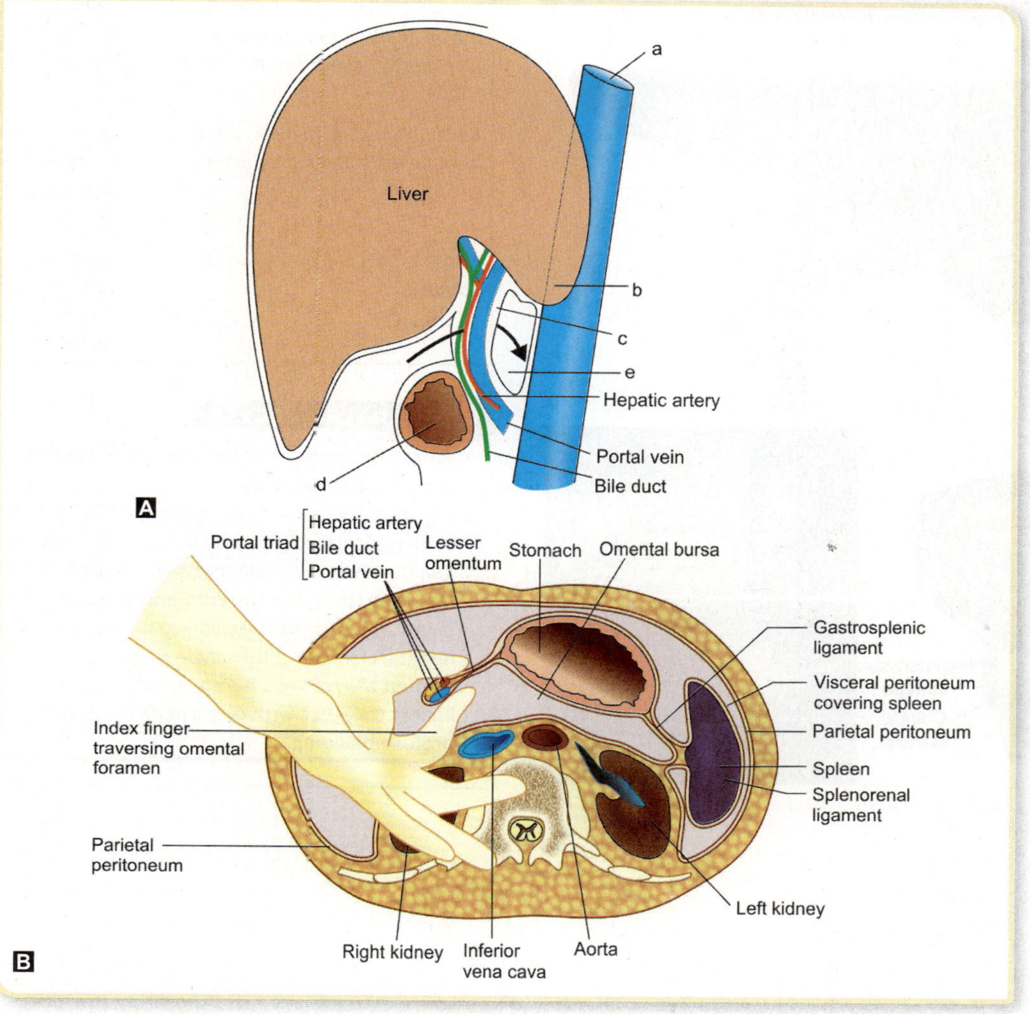

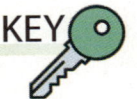

PLATE LEGENDS

A. Saggital section of abdomen showing Epiploic foramen (Arrow)
B. Transverse section of abdomen showing Epicloic foramen (Index finger inserted in epiploic formamen) a= Inferior vena cava, b= Caudate lobe of liver, c= Lesser sac, d= First art of duodenum, e= Epiploic foramen

In human anatomy, the **omental foramen (Epiploic foramen, foramen of Winslow**, or uncommonly aditus) is the passage of communication, or foramen, between the greater sac (general cavity of the abdomen), and the lesser sac.

Borders of Epiploic Foramen

It has the following borders:
1. **Anterior**: the free border of the lesser omentum, known as the hepatoduodenal ligament. This has two layers and within these layers are common bile duct (on the right), portal vein (posteriorly) and hepatic artery (on the left)
2. **Posterior**: IVC and right crus of diaphragm, covered with parietal peritoneum. (They are retroperitoneal). The anterior and posterior walls of the foramen are normally apposed
3. **Superior**: the peritoneum covering the caudate lobe of the liver
4. **Inferior**: the peritoneum covering the commencement of the duodenum (superior or first part of the duodenum)
5. **Left lateral**: Gastrosplenic ligament and Splenorenal ligament.

 ANATOMY PLATE 25

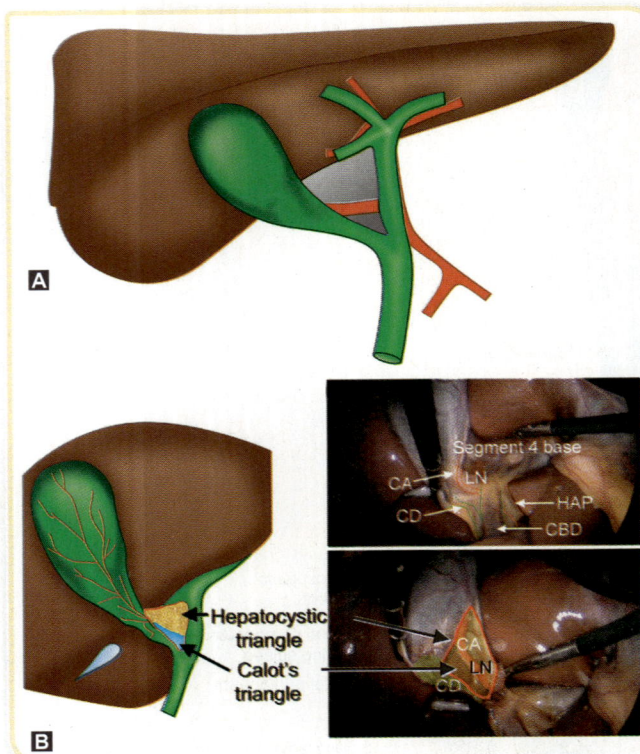

PLATE LEGENDS

A. Illustration showing boundaries and contents of both **Calot's triangle**[NEETPG] **and Hepatobiliary triangle**.
B. Laparoscopic anatomy of Calot's triangle and Hepatobiliary triangle.

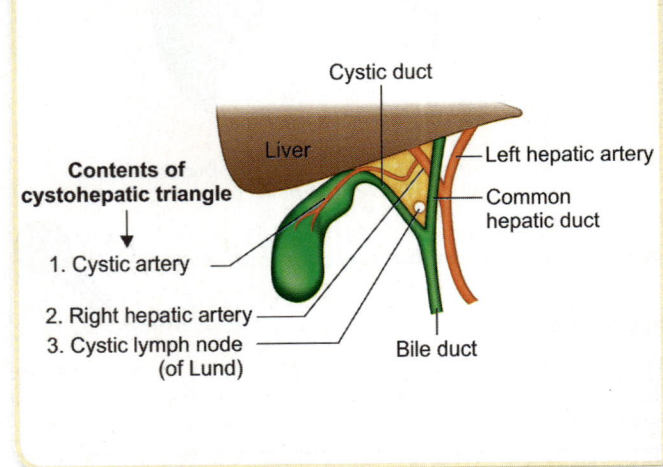

Fig: Hepatobiliary triangle and Calot's triangle

Calot's Triangle	Hepatobiliary Triangle
Originally described by Dr Jean Francois calot in his doctoral thesis in 1891. Later it was also incorrectly called Hepatobiliary triangle.	It is often mistakenly referred to as Calot's triangle (Grey's). AKA Cystohepatic triangle.
Bounded by Cystic duct, Common hepatic duct and Cystic artery	Bounded by Cystic duct, Common hepatic duct and inferior surface of the liver (Segment V)
Cystic artery is a boundary not content	Cystic artery, right hepatic artery and Cystic lymph nodes of Lund are contents.

Clinical Pearls

- When the anatomy of the triangle of Calot is unclear, blind dissection should stop.
- Bleeding adjacent to the triangle of Calot should be controlled by pressure and not by blind clipping or clamping.
- The mistakes in gallbladder surgery frequently happen from failure to recognize the common versions of the extrahepatic biliary system. This takes place particularly when the right hepatic artery in this triangle presents a caterpillar like loop termed **Moynihan's hump**, which may be mistakenly clamped, ligated together with cystic pedicle, and wound leading to profuse bleeding.

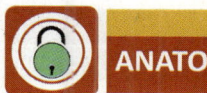

ANATOMY PLATE 26

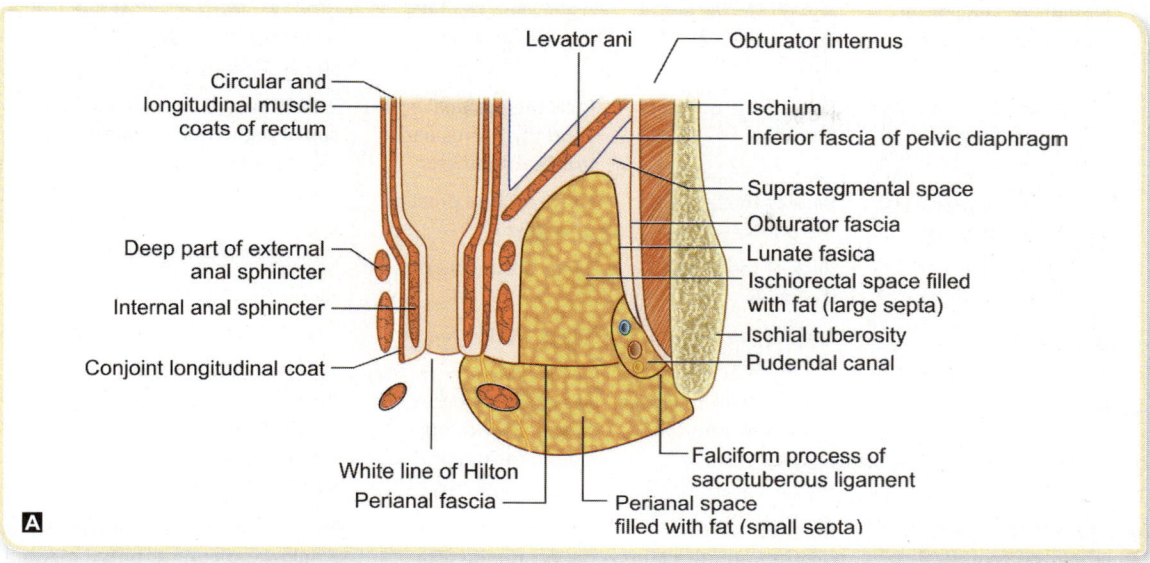

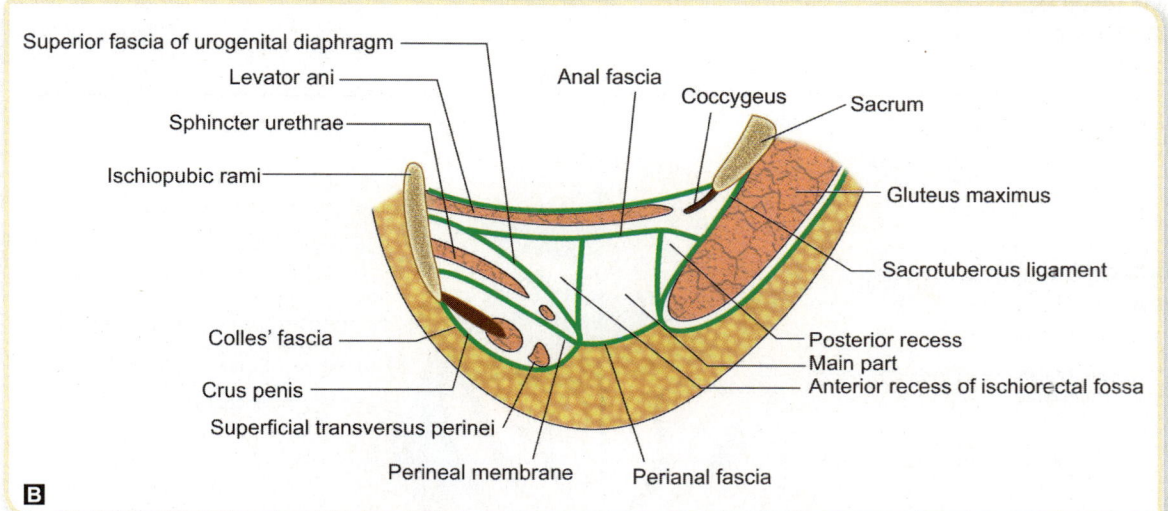

PLATE LEGENDS

A. Coronal section of Ischiorectal fossa (Levator Ani [AIIMSPG])
B. Parasagittal section of Ischiorectal fossa

Muscles of Pelvic Walls and Floor					
	Muscle	Proximal attachment	Distal attachment	Innervation	Main action
Lateral wall	Obturator internus	Pelvic surfaces of ilium and ischium, obturator membrane	Greater trochanter of femur	Nerve to obturator internus (L5, S1, S2)	Rotates thigh laterally; assists in holding head of femur in acetabulum
Posterolateral wall	Piriformis	Pelvic surface of S2–S4 segments, superior margin of greater sciatic notch, sacrotuberous ligament		Anterior rami of S1 and S2	Rotates thigh laterally; abducts thigh; assists in holding head of femur in acetabulum

Contd...

Muscles of Pelvic Walls and Floor

Muscle		Proximal attachment	Distal attachment	Innervation	Main action
Floor or outlet (pelvic diaphragm) — Levator ani	Ischiococcygeus (sometime separately named as coccygeus)	Tip of Ischial spine and obturator fascia	Lateral margins of the coccyx and the fifth sacral segment.	Direct branches of sacral plexus from 3rd & 4th sacral spinal segments	Forms **small part of pelvic diaphragm** that supports pelvic viscera; flexes coccyx
	Pubococcygeus — Puboperinealis (AKA Pubo urethralis)	Back of the body of the pubis	Pulls the perineal body ventrally. Forms part of **urethral sphincter**	2nd & 3rd sacral spinal segments via the **pudendal nerve**	Forms most of **pelvic diaphragm** that helps support pelvic viscera and resists increases in intra abdominal pressure
	Pubococcygeus — Puboprostaticus or pubovaginalis	Back of the body of the pubis	Slings around prostate or vagina		
	Pubococcygeus — Puboanalis	Back of the body of the pubis	Slings around anal canal		
	Pubococcygeus — Puborectalis	Back of the body of the pubis	Slings around rectum		
	Iliococcygeus	Inner surface of Ischial spine and obturator fascia	Sacrum and coccyx but most join with opposite side to form raphe	Direct branches of sacral plexus from 3rd & 4th sacral spinal segments	
Coccygeus (sometimes named as Ischiococcygeus and considered part of Levator ani)		Tip of Ischial spine and obturator fascia	Lateral margins of the coccyx and the fifth sacral segment.	Branches of S4 and S5 spinal nerves	Forms **small part of pelvic diaphragm** that supports pelvic viscera; flexes coccyx

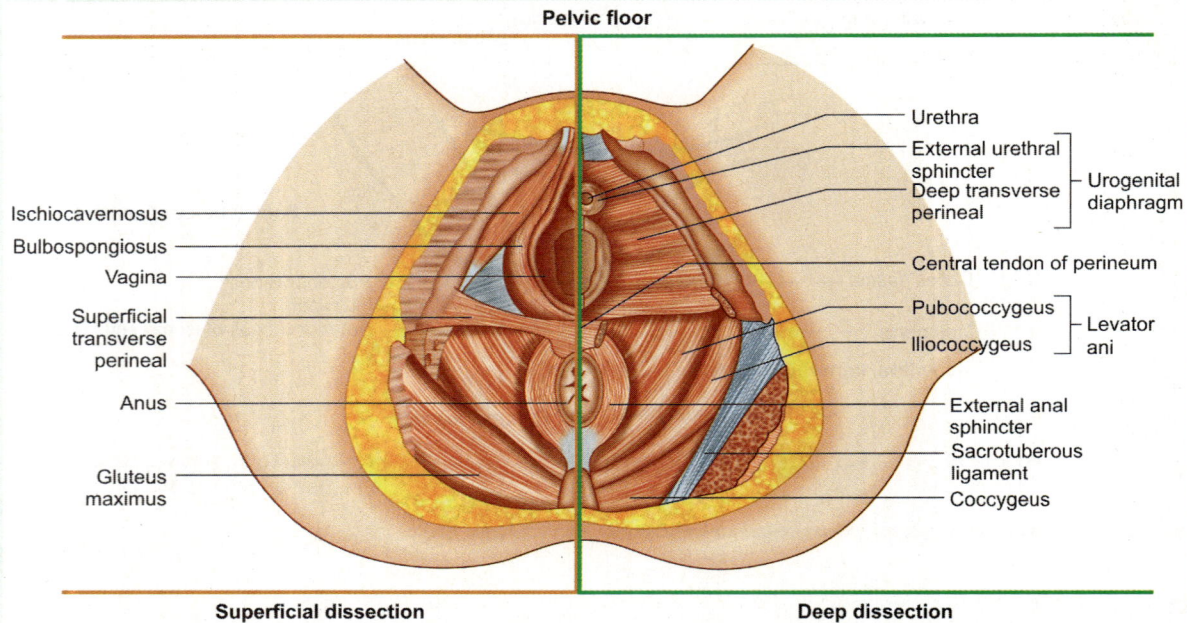

Footnote:
- Whereas the anal sphincters are responsible for the closure of the anal canal to retain gas and liquid stool, the **puborectalis muscle** and the anorectal angle are designed to maintain gross **fecal continence**"
- **Anorectal ring :** This is a muscular ring present at the anorectal junction. It is formed by the fusion of the puborectalis, deep external sphincter and the internal sphincter. It is easily felt by a finger in the anal canal. Surgical division of this ring results in rectal incontinence. The ring is less marked anteriorly where the fibres of the puborectalis are absent. Rectal continence depends solely on the anorectal ring. Damage to the ring results in rectal incontinence. The surgeon has to carefully protect the anorectal ring in operating on the region.

Pelvic Diaphragm
- Forms the **pelvic floor** and **supports all of the pelvic viscera**.
- **Levator ani and coccygeus** form the pelvic diaphragm and delineate the lower limit of the true pelvis.
- The fasciae investing the muscles are continuous with visceral pelvic fascia above, perineal fascia below and obturator fascia laterally.
- Lies posterior and deep to the urogenital diaphragm and medial and deep to the ischiorectal fossa.
- On contraction, **raises the entire pelvic floor.**
- Flexes the anorectal canal during defecation and helps the voluntary control of micturition.
- Helps direct the fetal head toward the birth canal at **parturition.**

Contd...

Muscles of Pelvic Walls and Floor

Muscle	Proximal attachment	Distal attachment	Innervation	Main action
Urogenital Diaphragm				

- The term **"perineal membrane"** replaces the old term **"urogenital diaphragm"**, reflecting the fact that this layer is not a single muscle layer with a double layer of fascia ("diaphragm"), but rather a set of connective tissues that surround the urethra formed by deep transverse perineal muscle, sphincter urethra muscle and transverse perineal ligament.
- Traditionally, a trilaminar UG diaphragm was described as making up the deep perineal pouch. The long-held concept of a flat, essentially two-dimensional UG diaphragm is erroneous (Wendell-Smith, 1995). According to this concept, the UG diaphragm consisted of the **perineal membrane (inferior fascia of UG diaphragm) inferiorly and a superior fascia of the UG diaphragm superiorly,** between which was a flat muscular sheet composed of a disc-like sphincter urethra and the transversely oriented deep transverse perineal muscle.

Structures Piercing Urogenital Diaphragm

In males	In females
▫ Urethra, 2-3 cm behind the inferior border of the symphysis pubis	▫ Urethra, 2-3 cm behind the inferior border of the symphysis pubis
▫ Vessels and nerves to the bulb of the penis	▫ Vagina, centrally
▫ Ducts of the bulbourethral glands, posterolateral to the urethral orifice	▫ Ducts of Bartholin's glands, posterolateral to the urethral orifice
▫ Deep dorsal vessels and dorsal nerves of the penis, behind the pubic arch in the midline	▫ Deep dorsal vessels and dorsal nerves of the clitoris, behind the pubic arch in the midline
▫ Posterior scrotal vessels and nerves, anterior to the transverse perinei.	▫ Posterior labial vessels and nerves, anterior to the transverse perinei

 ANATOMY PLATE 27

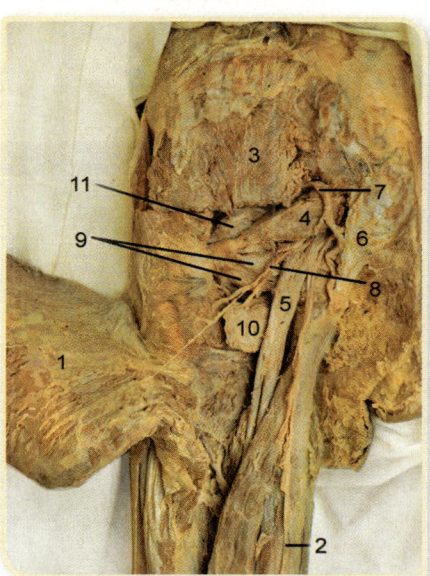

11. Gluteus minimus
12. Tendon of obturator internus (not shown in picture); Explore the area between the two gemelli muscles to positively identify the tendon of the obturator internus muscle.

 **ANATOMY PLATE 28**

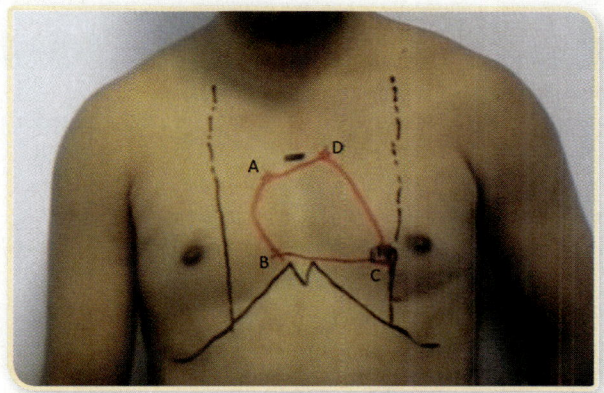

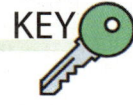 KEY

GLUTEAL REGION DISSECTION

1. Gluteus maximus
2. Posterior femoral cutaneous nerve
3. Gluteus medius^{NEETPG}
4. Piriformis
5. Sciatic nerve
6. Sacro tuberous ligament
7. Superior gluteal neurovascular bundle (superior to piriformis)
8. Inferior gluteal neurovascular bundle (inferior to piriformis)
9. Superior and inferior Gemelli
10. Quadratus femoris

SURFACE ANATOMY OF HEART

Points:
A. Right 3rd costal cartilage
B. Right 6th costal cartilage
C. Cardiac apex
D. Left 2nd costal cartilage

Lines:
A-B: Right heart border- Right atrium
B-C: Inferior or diaphragmatic border- Right and left ventricles
C-D: Left heart border- Left ventricle and left atrium
D-A: Superior border- Right and left atrium and the great vessels

ANATOMY PLATE 29

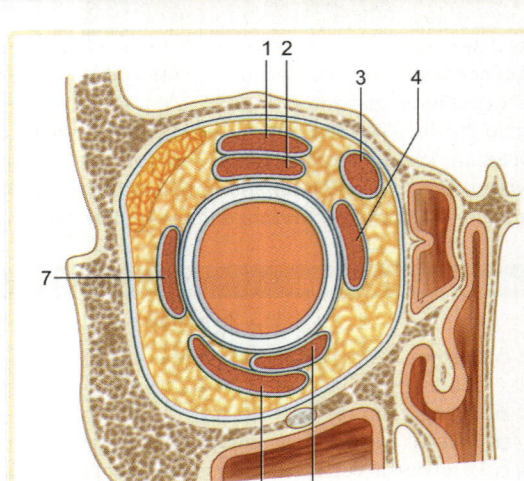
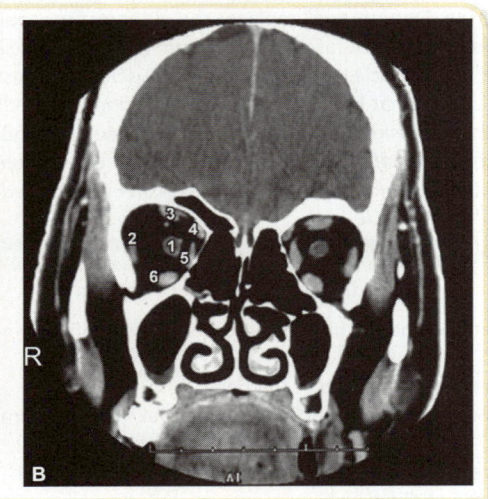

PLATE LEGENDS

A. Coronal section Orbit (Extraocular muscles)
1. Levator palpebrae superioris
2. Superior rectus
3. Superior oblique ᴬᴵᴵᴹˢ ᴾᴳ (Supplied by CN 4- Trochlear nerve)
4. Medial rectus
5. Inferior rectus
6. Inferior oblique
7. Lateral rectus

B. CT anatomy of Intraocular muscles (Coronal section)
1. Optic nerve
2. Lateral rectus
3. Superior rectus
4. Superior oblique ᴬᴵᴵᴹˢ ᴾᴳ (Longest and thinnest Intraocular muscle)
5. Medial rectus
6. Inferior rectus and inferior oblique

				Extraocular Muscles		
Muscle	Innervation	Origin	Insertion	Primary action	Secondary action	Tertiary action
Medial rectus	Oculomotor nerve (inferior branch)	Annulus of Zinn	Eye (anterior, medial surface)	Adduction	None	None
Lateral rectus	Abducens nerve	Annulus of Zinn	Eye (anterior, lateral surface)	Abduction	None	None
Superior rectus	Oculomotor nerve (superior branch)	Annulus of Zinn	Eye (anterior, superior surface)	Elevation	Intorsion	Adduction
Inferior rectus	Oculomotor nerve (inferior branch)	Annulus of Zinn	Eye (anterior, inferior surface)	Depression	Extorsion	Adduction
Superior oblique	Trochlear nerve	Sphenoid bone via the Trochlea	Eye (posterior, superior, lateral surface)	Intorsion	Depression	Abduction
Inferior oblique	Oculomotor nerve (inferior branch)	Maxillary bone	Eye (posterior, inferior, lateral surface)	Extorsion	Elevation	Abduction
Levator palpebrae superioris	Oculomotor nerve	Sphenoid bone	Tarsal plate of upper eyelid	Elevation/retraction of the upper eyelid		

Contd...

Extraocular Muscles

Muscle	Innervation	Origin	Insertion	Primary action	Secondary action	Tertiary action

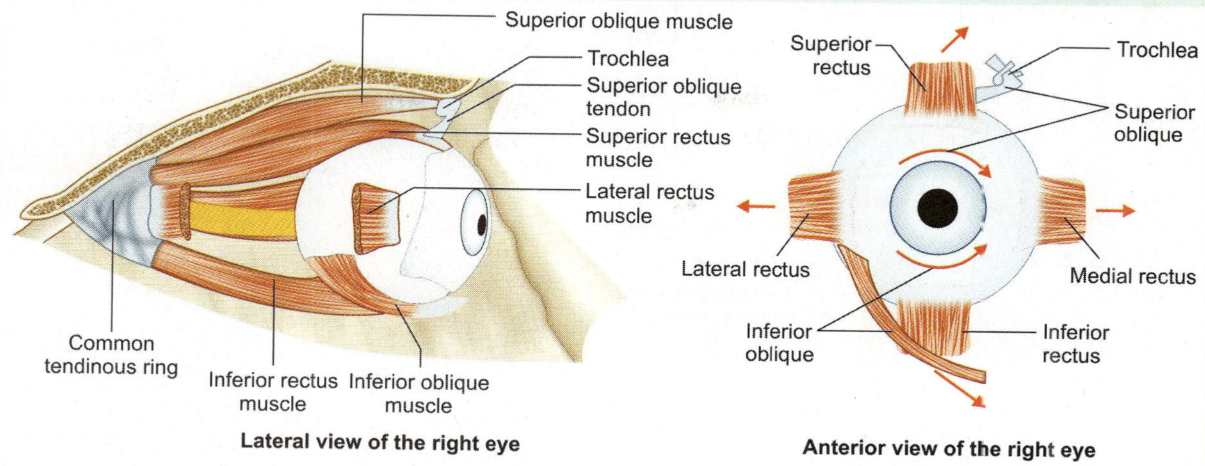

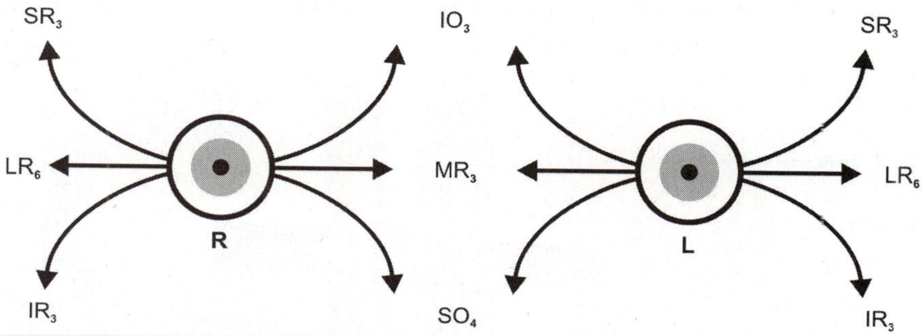

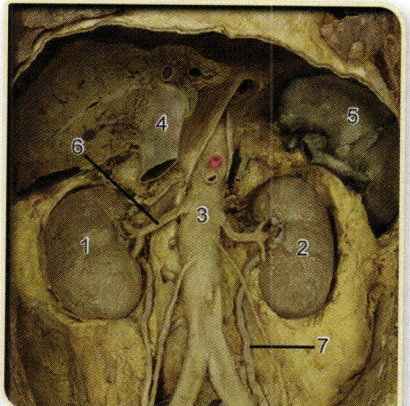

Fig: Schematic demonstration of the actions and cranial nerve innervation (in subscript) of extraocular muscles

Footnote:
- Some books mention only Primary and Secondary action, in which case it will be secondary and Tertiary combined.
- Nerve suply Mnemonic: SO4 LR6 Rest -3 (SO= Superior Oblique, LR = Lateral Rectus)
- Inferior oblique is the only muscle that does not arise from the **Common tendinous ring** (muscular ring) but from the anterior floor of the orbit.

ANATOMY PLATE 30

RETROPERITONEUM DISSECTION

1. Right kidney
2. Left Kidney (Marked arrow on upper pole – Relationship with Gastric area) [AIIMS PG]
3. Abdominal aorta
4. Inferior vena cava
5. Spleen
6. Right renal artery
7. Left Ureter

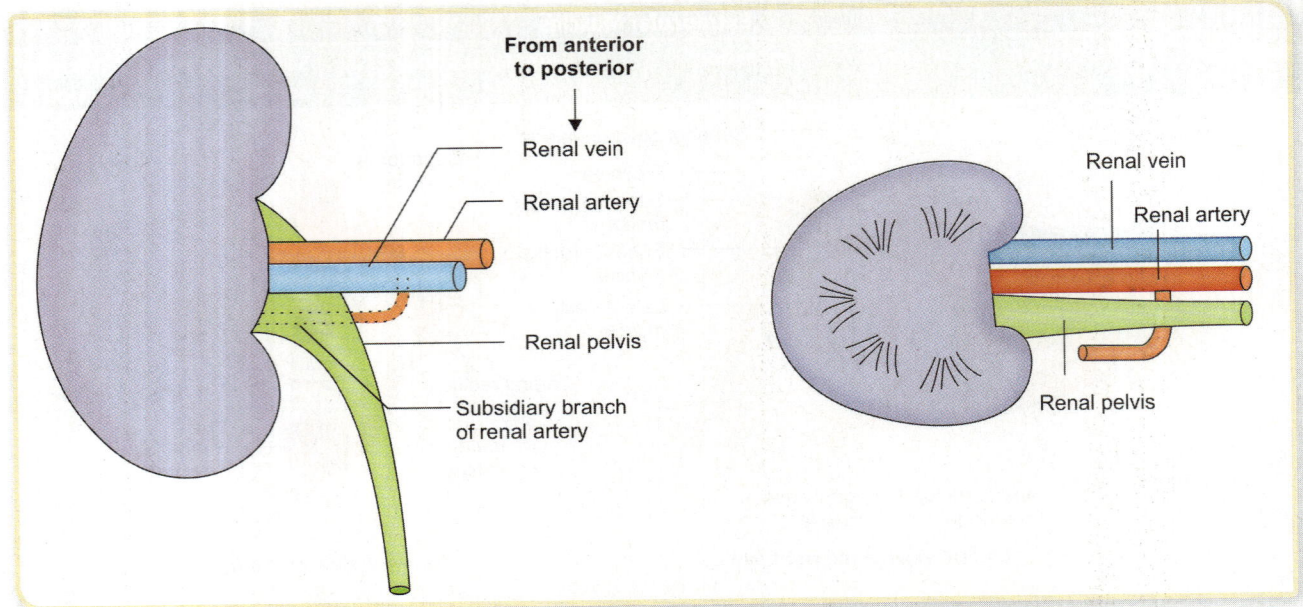

Fig: Renal Hilum relationship: From anterior to posterior; Renal vein → Renal artery → Renal Pelvis

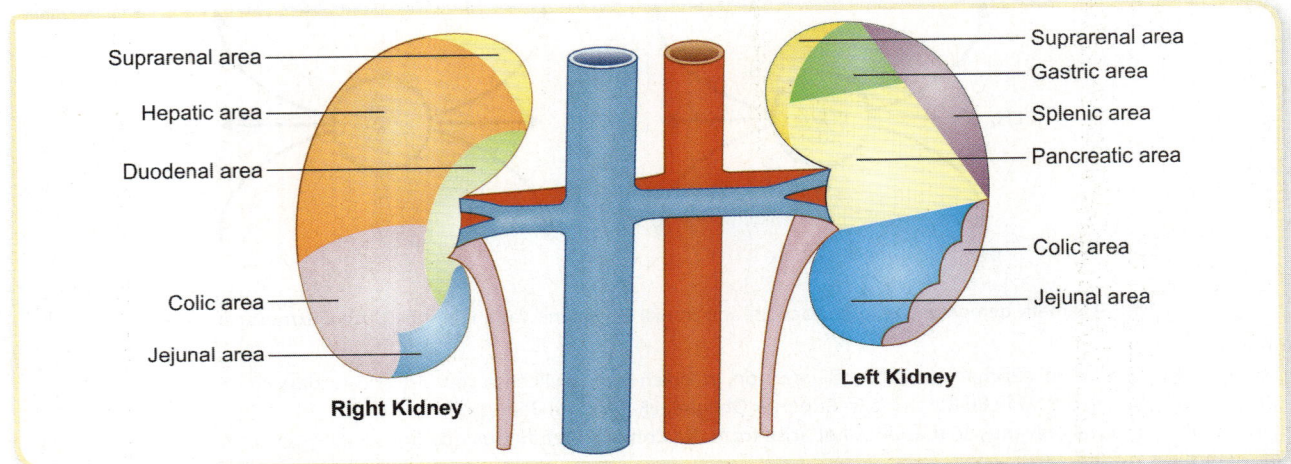

Fig: Illustration of relationship of Kidney

ANATOMY PLATE 31

 **KEY**

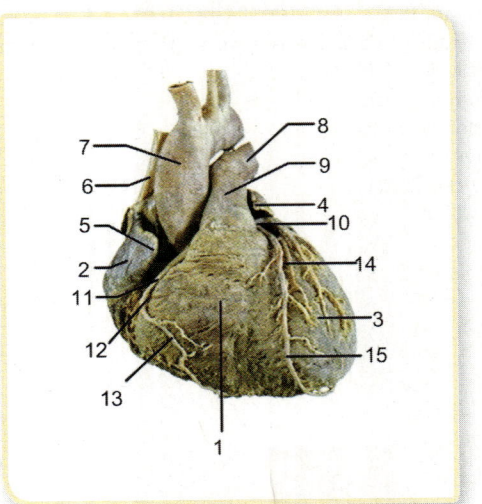

CADAVERIC DISSECTION OF ANTERIOR SURFACE OF HEART

1. Right ventricle [AIIMS PG] (Not supplied by diagonal artery) [AIIMS PG]
2. Right atrium
3. Left Ventricle
4. Auricle of left atrium
5. Auricle of right atrium
6. Superior vena cava
7. Ascending aorta
8. Left pulmonary artery
9. Pulmonary trunk
10. Left coronary artery (LCA)
11. Right coronary artery (RCA)
12. Coronary sulcus
13. Marginal branch of right coronary artery
14. Anterior interventricular sulcus
15. Anterior interventricular branch of LCA

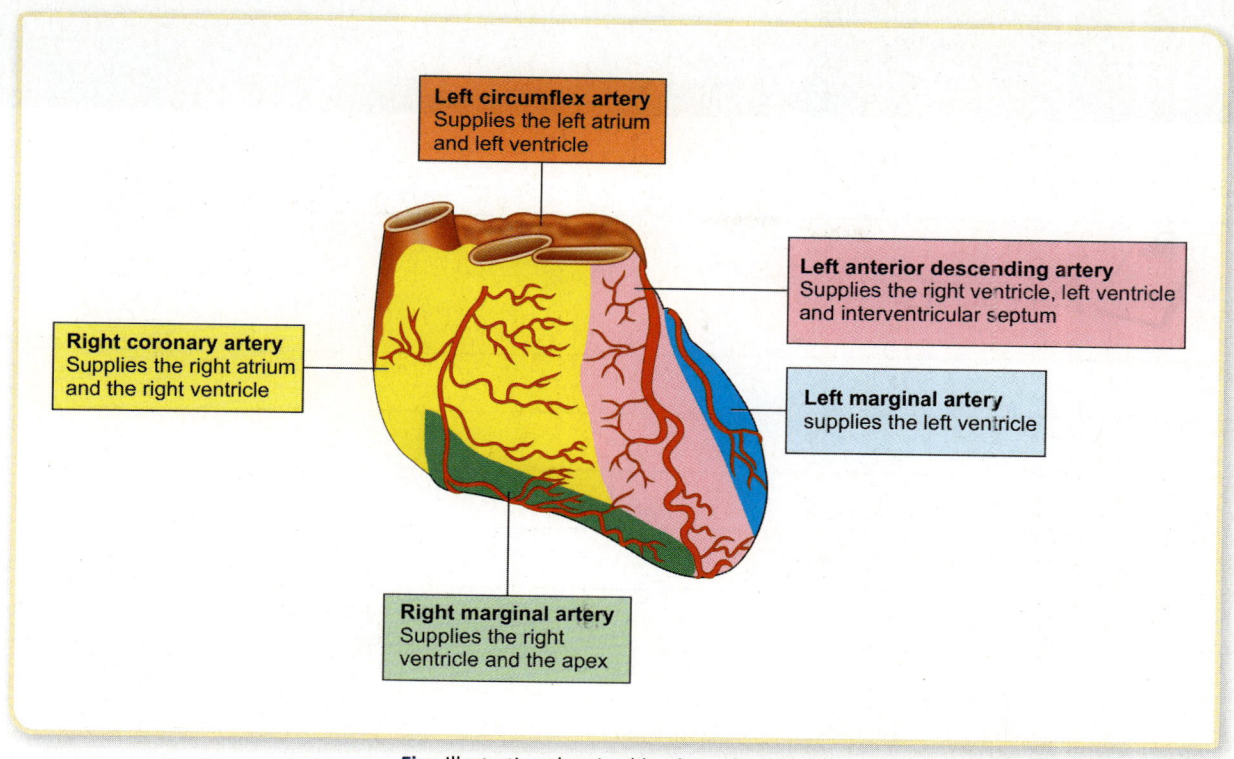

Fig: Illustration showing blood supply of heart

NOTES

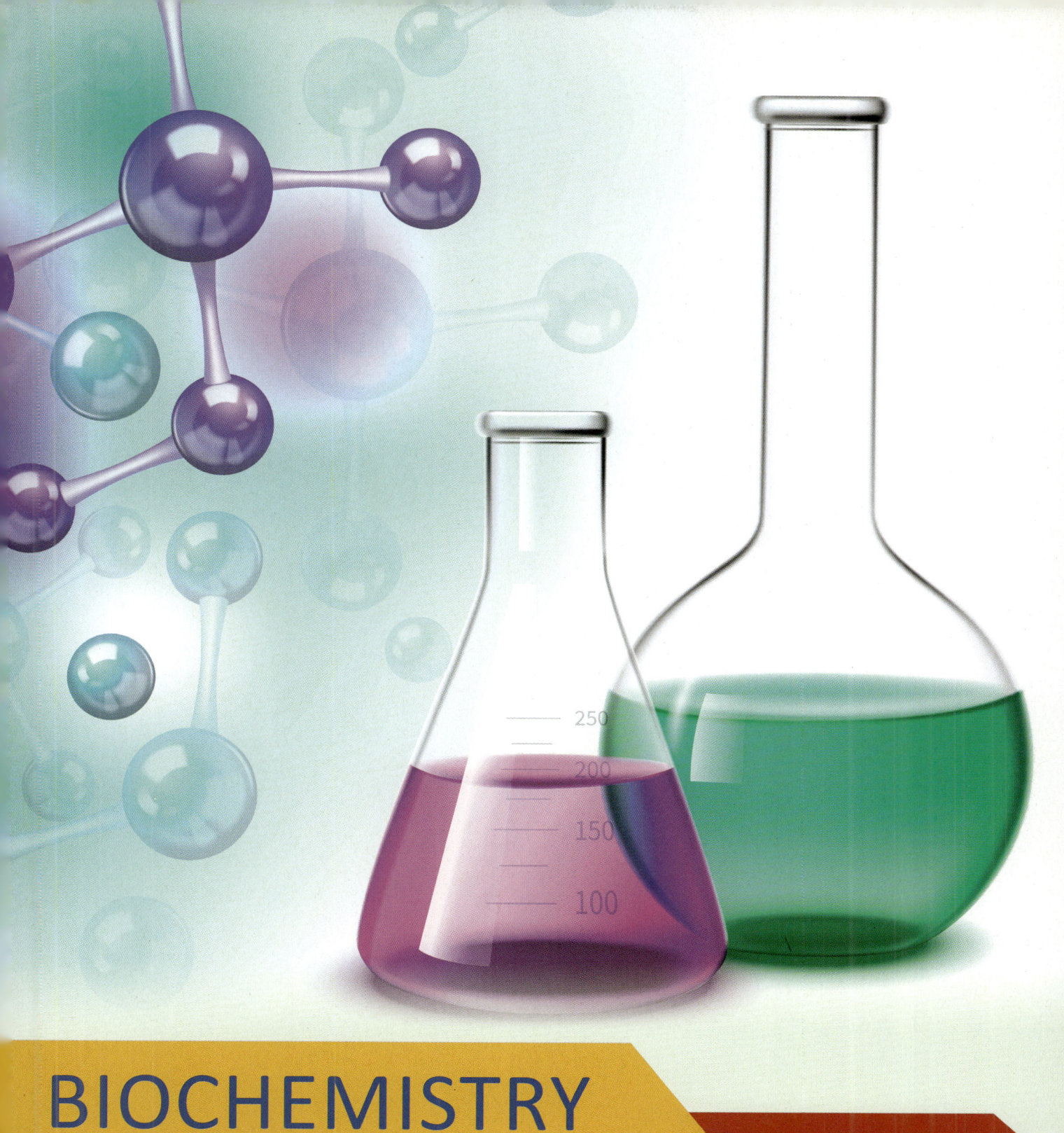

BIOCHEMISTRY

BIOCHEMISTRY PLATE 1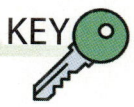

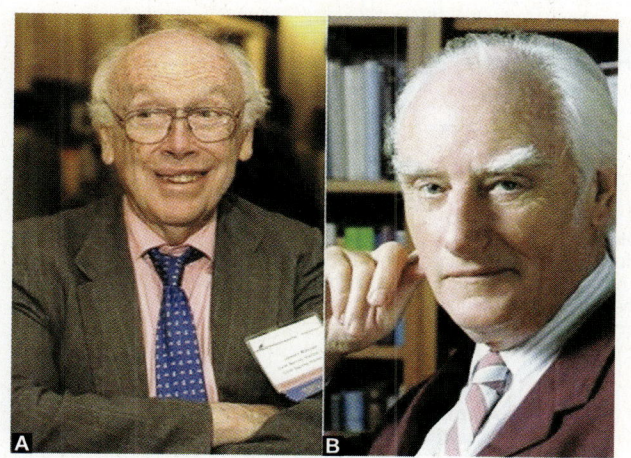

JAMES DEWEY WATSON AND FRANCIS HARRY COMPTON CRICK

A. **James Dewey Watson** was born in Chicago, Ill., on April 6th, 1928. He was awarded The **Nobel Prize in Physiology or Medicine 1962.** Watson wrote "The Double Helix: A Personal Account of the Discovery of the Structure of DNA", which was published in 1968. In 1990, Watson was appointed as the Head of the **Human Genome Project** at the National Institutes of Health, a position he held until April 10, 1992

B. **Francis Harry Compton Crick** was born on June 8, 1916, in Northampton, England. Crick found inspiration in something he read from Erwin Schrödinger— "How can the events of space and time which take place within the ... living organism be accounted for by physics and chemistry?"—and Watson convinced Crick that unlocking the secrets of DNA's structure would both provide the answer to Schrödinger's question and reveal DNA's hereditary role. Using X-ray diffraction studies of DNA, in 1953, Watson and Crick constructed a molecular model representing the known physical and chemical properties of DNA. Watson and Crick published a paper outlining their **DNA double-helical structure** in the scientific journal *Nature* in April 1953.

He was awarded The **Nobel Prize in Physiology or Medicine 1962** with James Watson, Maurice Wilkins. He died on 28 July 2004, San Diego, CA, USA.

BIOCHEMISTRY PLATE 2

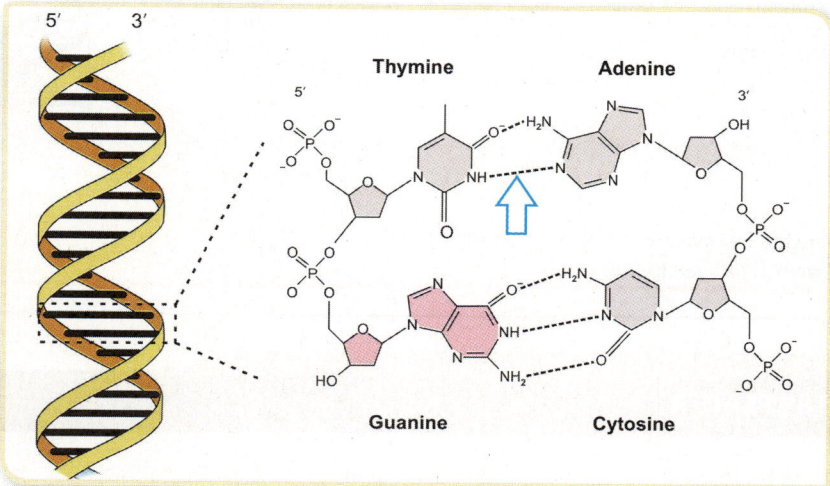

DNA STRUCTURE

In 1953, Watson and Crick postulated a three-dimensional model of DNA structure. It is in the form of a right-handed double helix, the shape of which is maintained by hydrogen bonding between organic bases Nucleic acids (DNA and RNA) are polymers of nucleotides, joined together by phosphodiester linkages between the 5- hydroxyl group of one pentose and the 3- hydroxyl group of the next. There are two types of nucleic acid: RNA and DNA. The nucleotides in RNA contain ribose, and the common pyrimidine bases are uracil and cytosine. In DNA, the nucleotides contain 2-deoxyribose, and the common pyrimidine bases are thymine and cytosine. The primary purines are adenine and guanine in both RNA and DNA.

A nucleotide consists of a nitrogenous base (purine or pyrimidine), a pentose sugar, and one or more phosphate groups. The four types of nitrogen bases are adenine (A), thymine (T), guanine (G) and cytosine (C). The purine and pyrimidine bases of both strands are stacked inside the double helix, with their hydrophobic and nearly planar ring structures very close together and perpendicular to the long axis. The offset pairing of the two strands creates a major groove and minor groove on the surface of the duplex.

Watson and Crick found that the hydrogen-bonded base pairs, G with C and A with T (or U), are those that fit best within the structure, providing a rationale for Chargaff's rule that in any DNA, G = C and A = T. Hydrogen bonds between bases permit a complementary association of two (and occasionally three or four) strands of nucleic acid. *Between cytosine and guanine bases there are three hydrogen bonds. Between adenine and thymine bases there are only two hydrogen bonds*

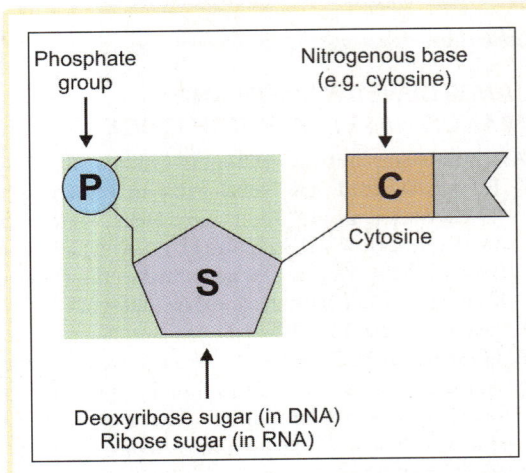
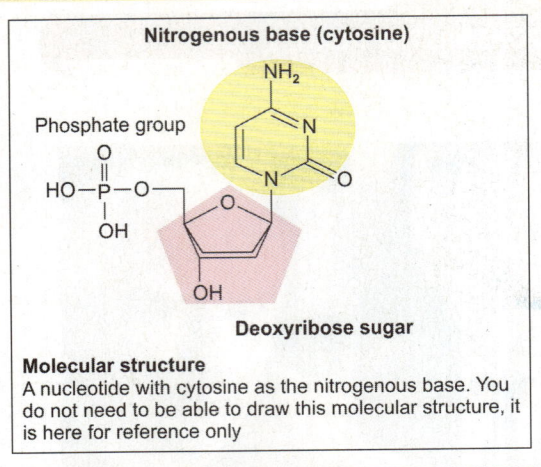
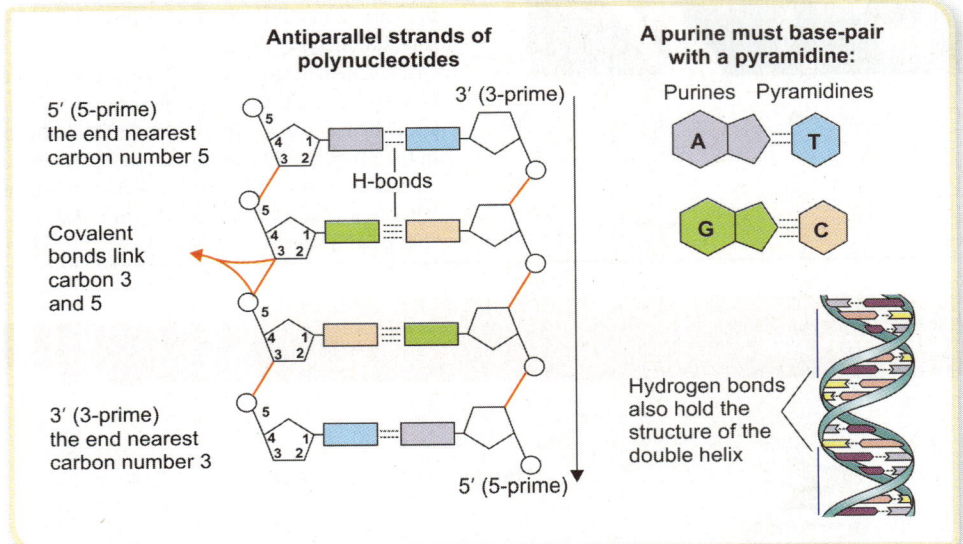

Summary
- Backbone of DNA is connected by covalent 3' 5' Phosphodiester bond
- Bases are connected by weak Hydrogen Bonds

BIOCHEMISTRY PLATE 3

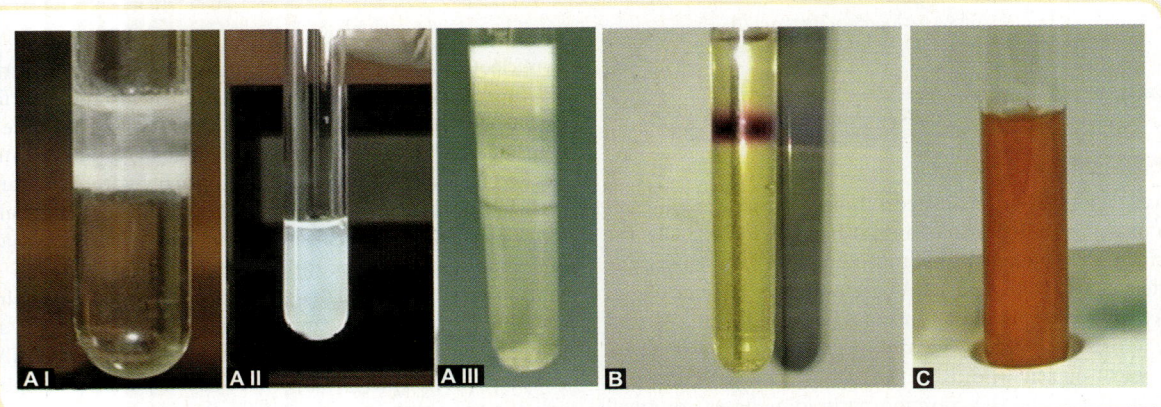

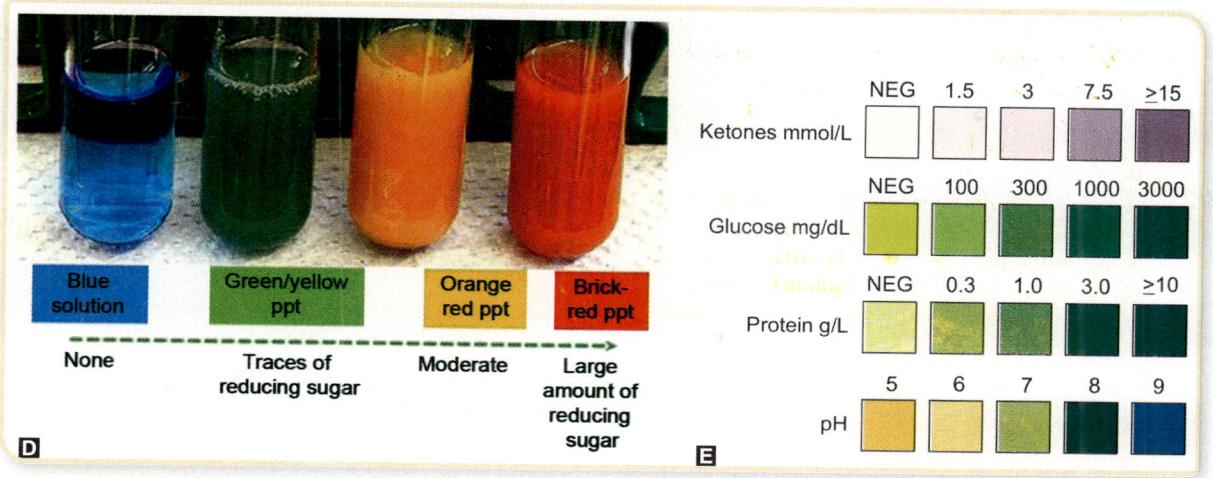

KEY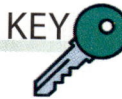

A. URINE PROTEIN TEST

It can be done by several methods.

I. **Heller's Ring Test Reagent:** Concentrated Nitric acid is taken in a test tube and few drops of Urine sample is added to the test tube by sliding down through an angle along the inner side of the test tube. A white ring is formed at the point of contact (white ring of denatured protein) indicating the presence of albumin in the sample

II. **Urine Protein Sulfosalicylic Acid Precipitation Test (SSA)** This technique provides a more quantitative estimate of all the proteins present in the urine, including both albumin and the low molecular weight proteins.

Principle: This test is performed by mixing one part urine supernatant with three parts 30% sulfosalicylic acid. The acidification causes precipitation of protein in the sample (seen as increasing turbidity), which is subjectively graded as trace, 1+, 2+, 3+ or 4+. Unlike the routine urine protein chemistry dipstick pad, the SSA reaction will detect globulin and Bence-Jones proteins, in addition to albumin and essentially detects all urinary proteins (although it is more sensitive to albumin).

Procedure:
1. Pour a small amount of urine into a test tube
2. Add 30% SSA into the tube directly on top of the urine drop by drop
3. Shake tube gently with a quick flick and read for turbidity immediately indicating presence of protein

III. **Heating and acetic acid test:** Proteins are coagulated by heat in acidic urine and do not dissolve on acidification. Whereas, phosphates and carbonates which are also precipitated by heating are dissolved in acid. Heated upper half shows precipitate and lower half is used as control for comparison.

B. TEST FOR KETONE BODIES (ROTHERA'S TEST)

Method

- Take 5 ml of urine in a test tube and saturate it with ammonium sulfate.
- Add a small crystal of sodium nitroprusside. Mix well.
- Slowly run along the side of the test tube liquor ammonia to form a layer.
- Immediate formation of a purple permanganate colored ring at the junction of the two fluids indicates a positive test

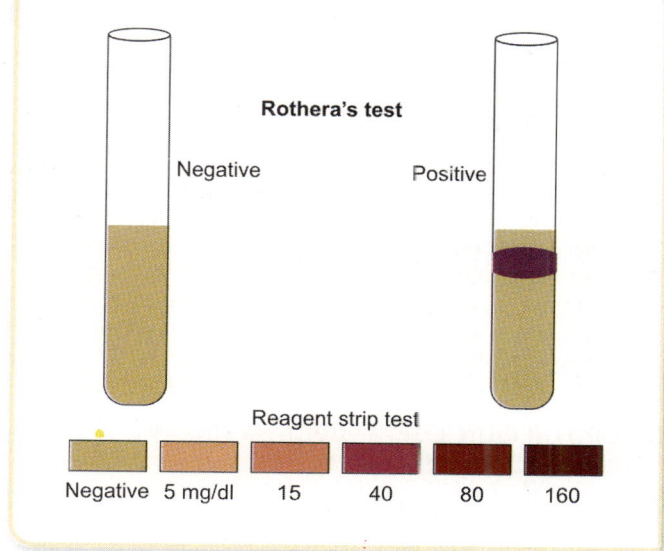

Fig: Rothera's tube test and reagent strip test for ketone bodies in urine. Rothera's test is sensitive to 1-5 mg/dl of acetoacetate and to 10-25 mg/dl of acetone. Reagent strips tests are modifications of nitroprusside test with sensitivity of 5-10 mg/dl of acetoacetate.

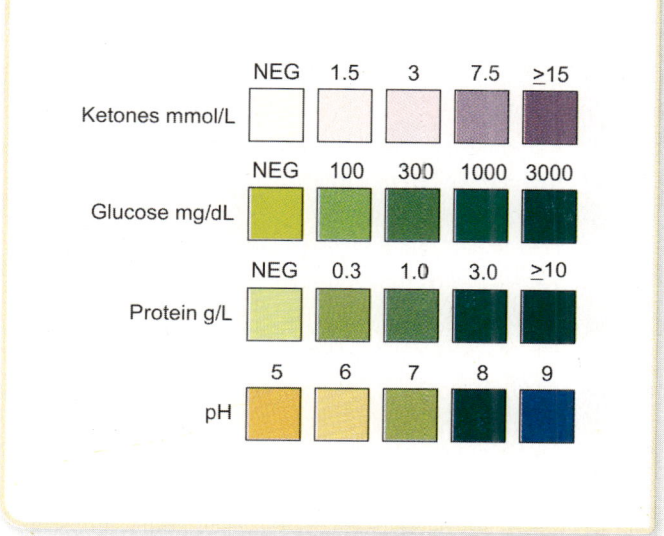

Instructions

Remove one test strip from the vial. Do not touch the test pads with your fingers. Dip the strip in to the urine being tested for 1-2 seconds and remove. After 10 seconds, compare the pH pad to the color chart. After 1 minute, compare the Ketones pad to the color chart, followed by Protein, and Glucose.

Principle: Principles of Rothera's test and reagent strip test for ketone bodies in urine. Ketones are detected as acetoacetic acid and acetone but not β-hydroxybutyric acid. Acetoacetic acid or acetone reacts with nitroprusside in alkaline solution to form a purple-colored complex.

```
                         Rothera's test
Acetoacetate +          Alkaline pH
Sodium nitroprusside    ─────────────→  Purple color

                         Reagent strip test
Acetoacetate +          Alkaline pH
Sodium nitroprusside +  ─────────────→  Purple color
Glycine
```

> **Note**
>
> Ketone bodies in urine = β-hydroxybutyric acid 78%, acetoacetic acid 20%, and acetone 2%. **No method for detection of ketonuria reacts with all the three ketone bodies because β-hydroxybutyric acid is not detected by any of the screening tests.** Rothera's test and Dipstick test (Modified Rothera) and detect acetoacetic acid and acetone (the test is 10-20 times more sensitive to acetoacetic acid than acetone). *Ferric chloride test detects acetoacetic acid only.*

C. TEST FOR GLUCOSE/ REDUCING SUGARS (BENEDICT'S TEST)

- **Reagent:** Benedict's reagent is a chemical reagent named after American chemist Stanley Rossiter Benedict. It is a complex mixture of sodium carbonate, sodium citrate and copper (II) sulfate pentahydrate
- **Principle:** The principle of Benedict's test is that when reducing sugars are heated in the presence of an alkali, they are converted to powerful reducing species known as enediols. Enediols reduce the cupric compounds (Cu^{2+}) present in the Benedict's reagent to cuprous compounds (Cu^+) which are precipitated as insoluble red copper(I) oxide (Cu_2O).

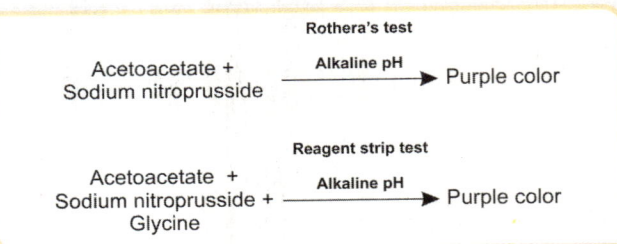

An aldose + Benedict's reagent (blue solution) → Carboxylate anion + Brick-red precipitate

Procedure

- 1 ml of urine sample is placed into a test tube.
- 2 ml (10 drops) of Benedict's reagent ($CuSO_4$) is added in the test tube.
- The solution is then heated in a boiling water bath for 3-5 minutes.
- Observe for color change in the solution of test tubes or precipitate formation.

D. INTERPRETATION OF BENEDICT'S TEST

The color of the obtained precipitate gives an idea about the quantity of sugar present in the solution; hence the test is semi-quantitative.

- Greenish precipitate = 0.1 to 0.5 g% sugar in solution
- Yellow precipitate = 0.5 to 1 g% sugar in solution
- Orange precipitate = 1 to 1.5 g% sugar in solution
- Red precipitate = 1.5 to 2.0 g% sugar in solution
- Brick red means > 2 g% sugar in solution

E. URINE DIPSTICK TESTS

Procedure

- Remove one test strip from the vial. Do not touch the test pads with your fingers.
- Dip the strip in to the urine being tested for 1-2 seconds and remove.
- After 10 seconds, compare the pH pad to the color chart.
- After 1 minute, compare the Ketones pad to the color chart, followed by Protein, and Glucose.

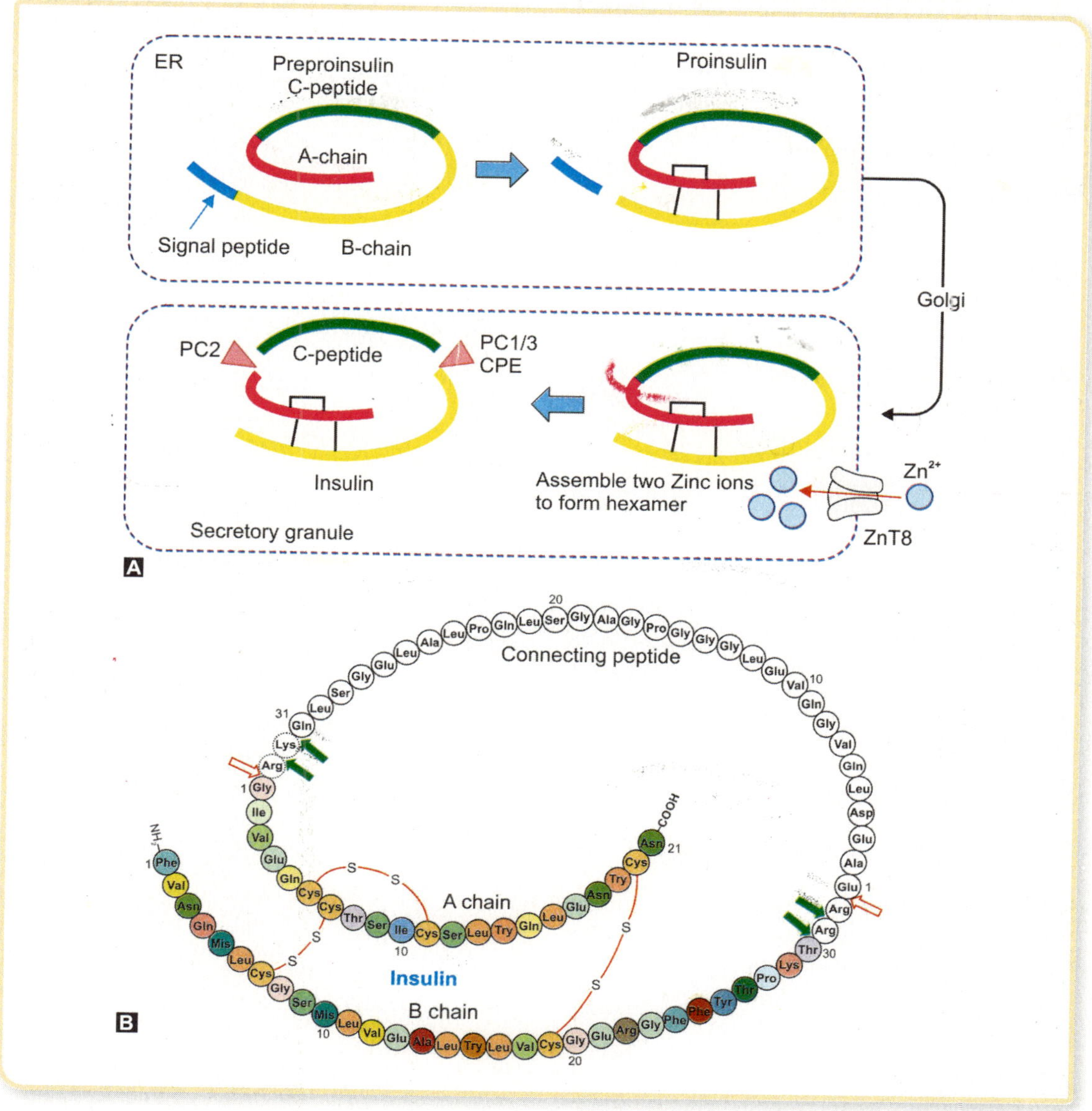

BIOCHEMISTRY PLATE 4

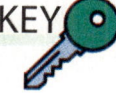

INSULIN SYNTHESIS AND STRUCTURE OF HUMAN PROINSULIN

A. Insulin synthesis: Insulin is synthesized as a preprohormone (molecular weight 11,500). Preproinsulin contains amino terminal sequence that is required in order for the precursor hormone to pass through the endoplasmic reticulum. Upon entering the endoplasmic reticulum the amino terminal sequence is removed proteolytically to form the Proinsulin (9000-MW), which provides the conformation necessary for the proper and efficient formation of the disulfide bridges. Inside the ER, the proinsulin (insulin precursor) folds and two interchain disulfide bridges are formed between cysteines (A7–B7 and A20–B19). The sequence of proinsulin, starting from the amino terminal, is B chain—connecting peptide (C peptide) —A chain. The proinsulin is assembled in the golgi apparatus into two zinc ions containing hexameric proinsulin. Then hexameric proinsulin is converted into the insulin hexamer by excision of the C-peptide by the action of proteolytic enzymes, known as prohormone convertases (PC1/3 and PC2), as well as the exoprotease carboxypeptidase E. Insulin is packed and stored in secretory granules, which accumulate in the cytoplasm until the release is triggered.

B. Structure of human proinsulin: Insulin consists of two polypeptide chains, an A chain (21 amino acid residue) and a B chain (30 amino acid residue). There is one intra A chain with disulfide bridge (CysA6–CysA11) two covalent inter-chain disulfide (SS) bridges (i.e., CysA7–CysB7 and CysA20–CysB19). Insulin and C-peptide molecules are connected at two sites by peptide bonds. An initial cleavage by a trypsin-like enzyme (open arrows) followed by several cleavages by a carboxypeptidase like enzyme (solid arrows) results in the production of the heterodimeric (AB) insulin molecule (coloured) and the C-peptide (white). *A chain shows inter species variation at amino acids A-8, 9, 10 while B chain shows inter species variation at amino acids B-30.*

NOTES

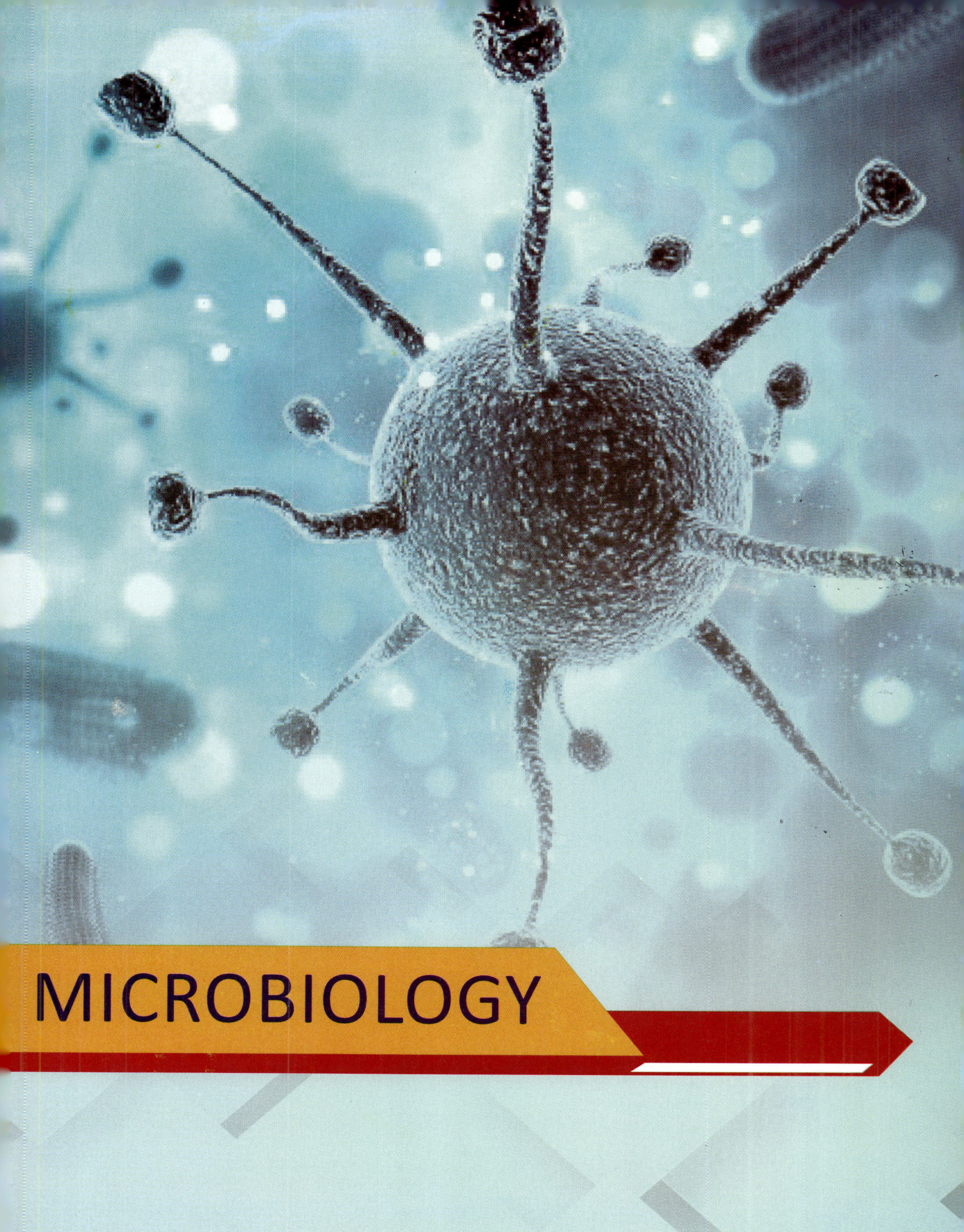

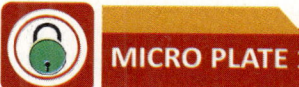
MICRO PLATE 1

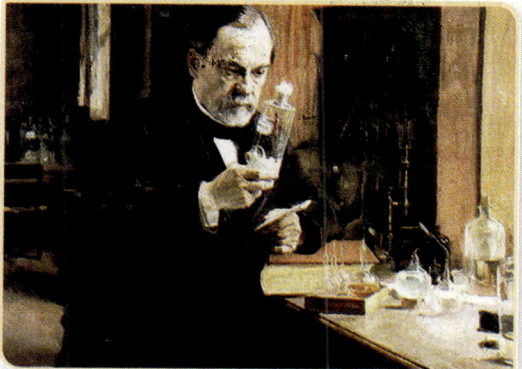

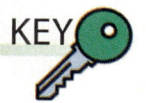

LOUIS PASTEUR

A famous painting of Louis Pasteur is shown in his laboratory in the midst of his experiments. He is holding a jar containing the spinal cord of rabbit infected with rabies which he used to develop a vaccine against rabies.

Painting by Albert Edelfelt

Work of Louis Pasteur
- Germ theory of disease
- Sterilization techniques: Steam sterilizer, hot air oven, autoclave
- Vaccination for anthrax, rabies and cowpox and chicken pox
- Technique of pasteurization

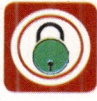
MICRO PLATE 2

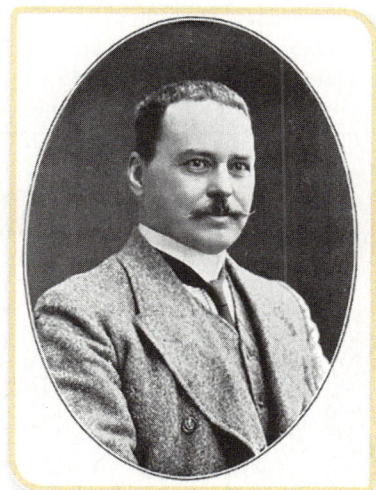

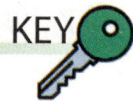

SIR RONALD ROSS

Sir Ronald Ross (13 May 1857 – 16 September 1932) was an India-born British doctor who received the Nobel Prize for Physiology or Medicine in 1902 for his work on malaria. His discovery of the malarial parasite in the gastrointestinal tract of the Anopheles mosquito led to the realization that malaria was transmitted by Anopheles, and laid the foundation for combating the disease.

MICRO PLATE 3

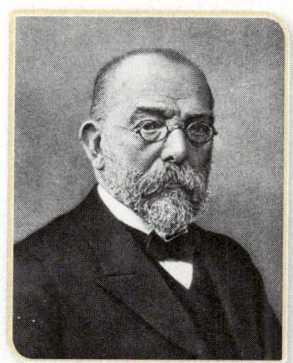

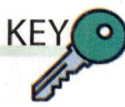

ROBERT HEINRICH HERMAN KOCH

Robert Heinrich Herman Koch (December 11, 1843 – May 27, 1910), considered to be the founder of modern bacteriology, is known for his role in identifying the specific causative agents of tuberculosis, cholera, and anthrax and for giving experimental support for the concept of infectious disease. His research led to the creation of Koch's postulates, a series of four generalized principles linking specific microorganisms to particular diseases which remain today the "gold standard" in medical microbiology. As a result of his ground breaking research on tuberculosis, Koch received the Nobel Prize in Physiology or Medicine in 1905.

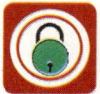
MICRO PLATE 4

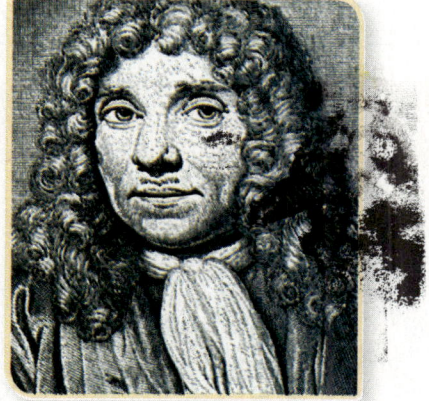

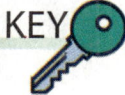

ANTONIE VAN LEEUWENHOEK

Antonie van Leeuwenhoek is known as **"Father of Microbiology"**, and considered to be the first microbiologist. He is best known for his work on the improvement of the microscope and for his contributions toward the establishment of microbiology. Using his handcrafted microscopes, he was the first to observe and describe single-celled organisms, which he originally referred to as *animalcules*, and which we now refer to as microorganisms. He was also the first to record microscopic observations of muscle fibers, bacteria, spermatozoa, and blood flow in capillaries (small blood vessels).

that protozoa were shown to be a cause of disease. He later worked on the trypanosomes, particularly sleeping sickness. For this work and later discoveries of protozoan diseases he was awarded the Nobel Prize for Physiology or Medicine in 1907.

MICRO PLATE 5

MICRO PLATE 6

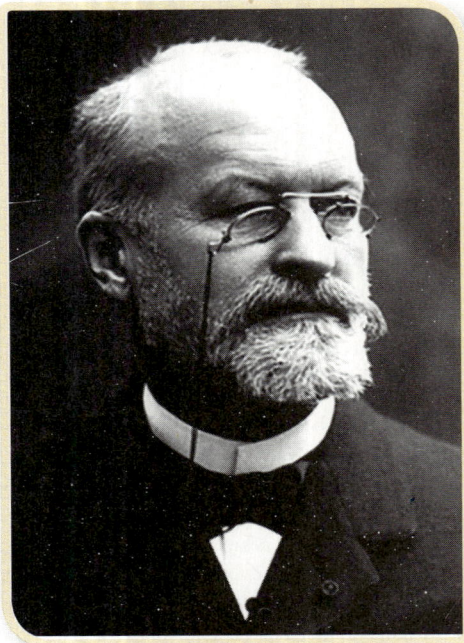

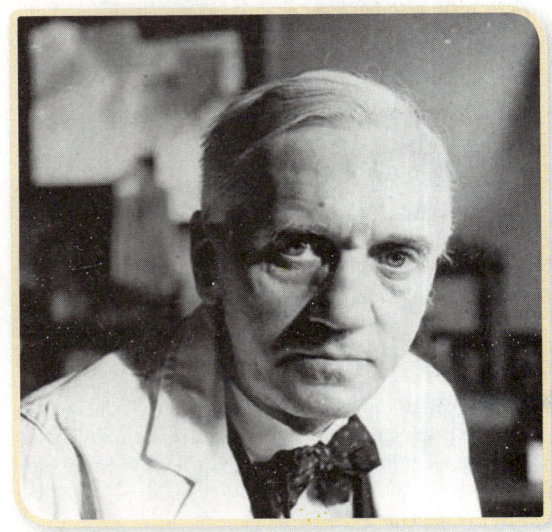

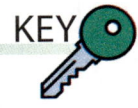
SIR ALEXANDER FLEMING
Sir Alexander Fleming was born at Lochfield near Darvel in Ayrshire, **Scotland on August 6th, 1881.**
In 1928, while working on influenza virus, he observed that mould had developed accidently on a staphylococcus culture plate and that the mould had created a bacteria-free circle around itself. He was inspired to do further experiment and he found that mould culture prevented growth of staphylococci, even when diluted 800 times. He named the active substance as **penicillin** for which he shared the **Nobel Prize in Physiology or Medicine in 1945** with Howard Florey and Ernst Boris Chain. Dr Fleming died on **March 11th in 1955.**

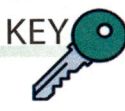
CHARLES LOUIS ALPHONSE LAVERAN
Charles Louis Alphonse Laveran (18 June 1845 – 18 May 1922) was a French physician. In 1880, he discovered that the cause of malaria is a protozoan, after observing the parasites in a blood smear taken from a patient who had just died of malaria. This was the first time

MICRO PLATE 7

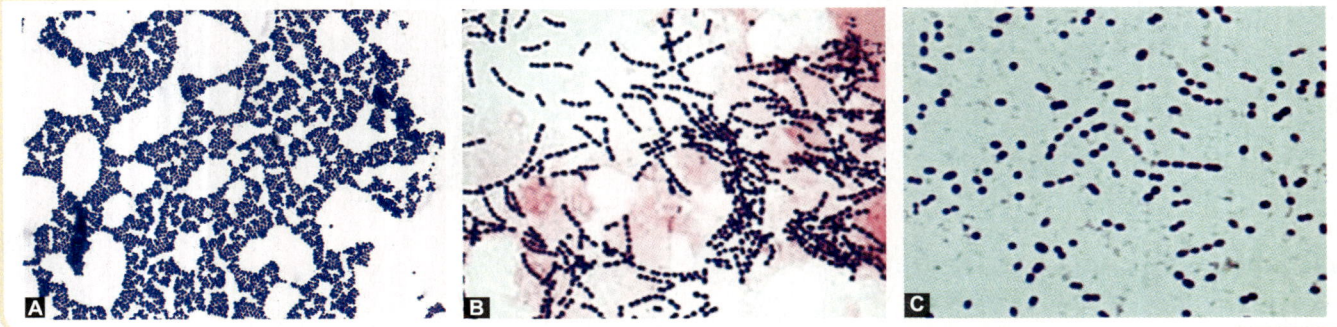

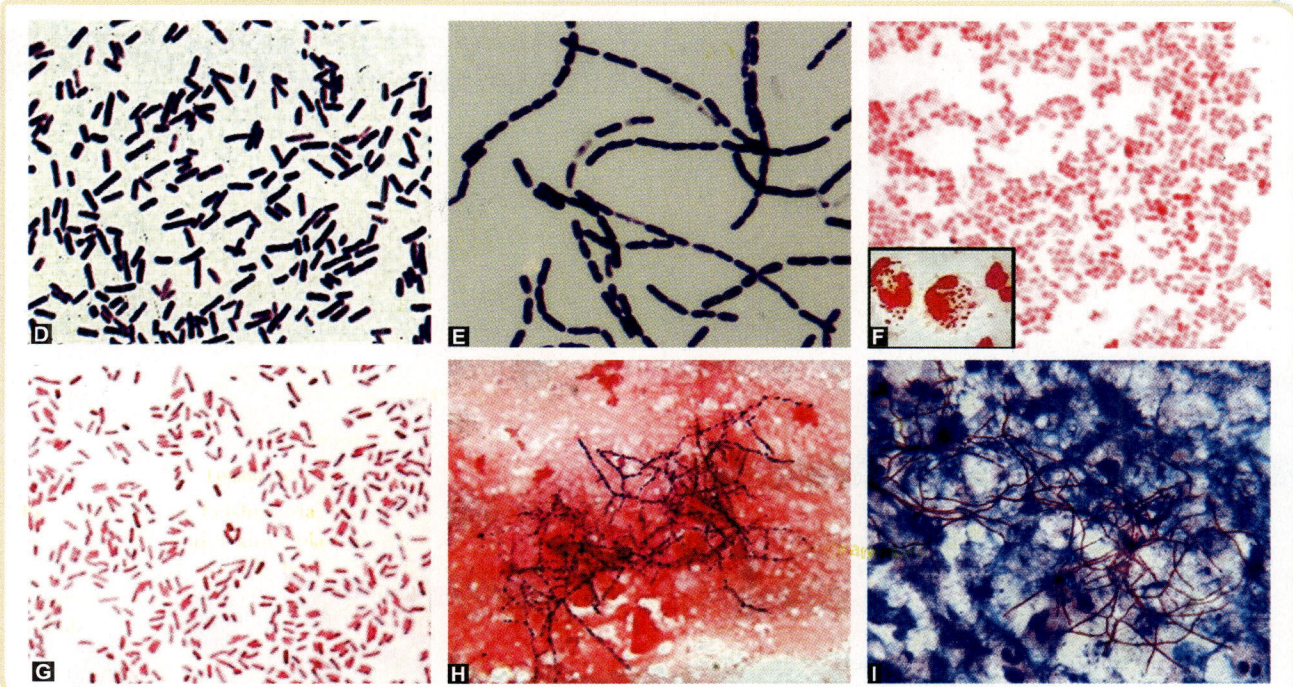

MICROBIOLOGY COLOR PLATES

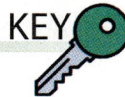 **KEY**

PLATE LEGENDS

A. Gram positive (blue/ purple) cocci (round) in clusters (grape like), e.g. **Staphylococcus**
B. Gram positive cocci in chains, e.g. **Streptococci**
C. Gram positive cocci in group of two (diplococcus/ Lancet shaped), although some very short chains may be seen: **Streptococcus pneumoneae**
D. Gram positive bacillus: **Listeria, Corynebacterium**
E. Gram positive bacillus in chain: **Bacillus species (Anthracis and cereus)**
F. Gram negative cocci (Diplococci), insat shows intracellular Gram-negative diplococci and polymorphonuclear leukocytes in urethral exudate; **Neisseria sp., Moraxella catarrhalis, Acinetobacter, and Brucella.**
G. Gram negative bacillus: **E coli, Pseudomonas, Hemophilus, Klebsiella, Salmonella**
H. **Nocardia Gram Stain;** (Blue in pink background). Showing filamentous, branching gram positive bacilli. (you must know how to differentiate chains from filaments; chains are more beaded and filaments are ore branched)
I. **Nocardia, partially acid-fast staining:** (Pink in blue background). Partial Acid-Fast staining employed: Carbol fuchsin stain (3 min), decolorize with 1% H_2SO_4 (until color no longer comes off ~1 min) and counterstain with methylene blue (30 sec).

Gram and Acid-Fast Staining Methods

Most bacteria are classified as gram-positive or gram-negative according to their response to the Gram staining procedure. This procedure was named for the histologist **Hans Christian Gram**, who developed this differential staining procedure in an attempt to stain bacteria in infected tissues. The Gram stain depends on the ability of certain bacteria (the gram-positive bacteria) to retain a complex of crystal violet (a purple dye) and iodine after a brief wash with alcohol or acetone. Gram-negative bacteria do not retain the dye-iodine complex and become translucent, but they can then be counter stained with safranin (a red dye). **Thus,**

Contd...

Gram and Acid-Fast Staining Methods

gram-positive bacteria look purple under the microscope, and gram-negative bacteria look red. The distinction between these two groups turns out to reflect fundamental differences in their cell envelopes

Gram stain steps
- Fix smear by heat.
- Cover with crystal violet.
- Wash with water. Do not blot.
- Cover with Gram's iodine.
- Wash with water. Do not blot.
- Decolorize for 10–30 seconds with gentle agitation in acetone (30 mL) and alcohol (70 mL).
- Wash with water. Do not blot.
- Cover for 10–30 seconds with safrarin (2.5% solution in 95% alcohol).
- Wash with water and let dry.

School of fish appearance is seen in — *H. ducreyi*
Fish in stream pattern is seen in — *V. cholera*

Ziehl-Neelsen Acid-Fast Stain

- Fix smear by heat.
- Cover with carbol fuchsin, steam gently for 5 minutes over direct flame (or for 20 minutes over a water bath).
- Wash with water.
- Decolorize in acid-alcohol until only a faint pink color remains.
- Wash with water.
- Counterstain for 10–30 seconds with Loeffler's methylene blue.
- Wash with water and let dry.

Kinyoun carbol fuchsin acid-fast stain

1. Formula: 4 g basic fuchsin, 8 g phenol, 20 mL 95% alcohol, 100 mL distilled water.
2. Stain fixed smear for 3 minutes (no heat necessary) and continue as with Ziehl-Neelsen stain.

Acid Fast Organisms/ Structures

| Organisms | All mycobacteria; *M tuberculosis, M leprae,* Atypical mycobacteria |

Contd...

PICTURE MEDEASY

		Actinomycetes including Nocardia (week+) and Rhodococcus **(Except Actinomyces and Streptomyces)**
		Legionella
Oocycts		*Cryptococcus parvum* *Isospora belli* *Cyclospora cayetanensis*
Parasites		Sarcocystis *Taenia saginata* eggs (*Taenia solium* eggs do not stain well, can be used to diff) Hydatid cyst especially hooklets
Others		Bacterial spores Head of sperm

Classification of Bacteria

AEROBES	Bacilli (Rods)	Gram +	Listeria Cornybacterium Bacillus spp
		Gram -	E coli Pseudomonas Haemophilius Klebsiella Bordetella Yersinia Pasteurella Franciscella Brucella Salmonella Proteus Campylobacter Actinobacter
	Cocci	Gram +	Staphylococcus Streptococcus Enterococcus
		Gram -	Neisseria Moraxella
	Filamentous	Gram +	Nocardia
		Gram -	Microthrix parvicella
ANAEROBES	Bacilli (Rods)	Gram +	Clostridia Actinomyces (agar culture) Lactobacillus
		Gram -	Bacteriodes Fusobacterium
	Cocci	Gram +	Streptococcus viridians Peptococcus Peptostreptococcus
		Gram -	Veillonella
	Filamentous	Gram +	Actinomyces (broth culture)
		Gram -	-

MICRO PLATE 8

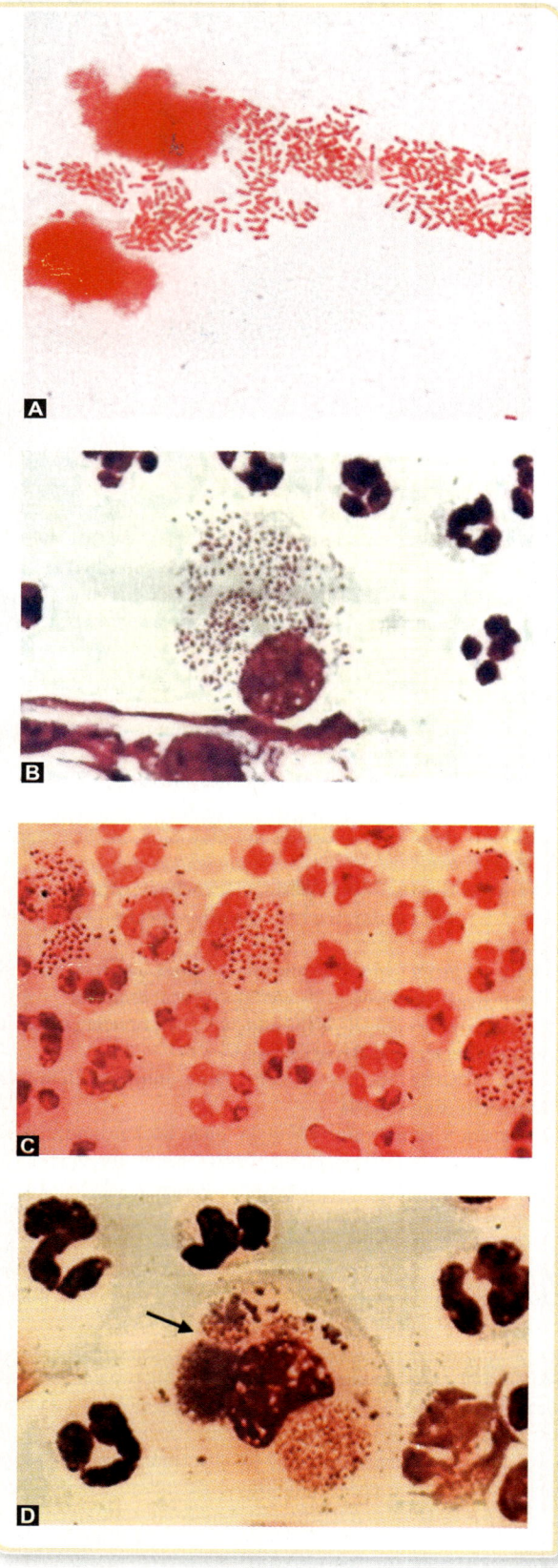

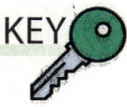

MICROSCOPY

Trick: in genital ulcer smear, check if pathogen is intracellular or extracellular. If intracellular then check the lobes of the nucleus (Monocytes or Neutrophils).

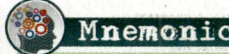

= DUcreyi= Do You Cry= painful ulcer

A. *Haemophilus ducreyi* on gram stain appearance of ulcer shows characteristic "Extracellular schools of fish" appearance.

Haemophilus ducreyi causes chancroid (**soft chancre**), a sexually transmitted disease. Chancroid consists of a ragged ulcer on the genitalia, with marked swelling and tenderness. The regional lymph nodes are enlarged and painful. The disease must be differentiated from syphilis, herpes simplex infection, and lymphogranuloma venereum.

The small gram-negative rods occur in strands in the lesions, usually in association with other pyogenic microorganisms. *H ducreyi* requires X factor but not V factor. It is grown best from scrapings of the ulcer base on chocolate agar containing 1% IsoVitaleX and vancomycin, 3 g/mL, and incubated in 10% CO_2 at 33°C. There is no permanent immunity following chancroid infection. Treatment with intramuscular ceftriaxone, oral trimethoprim-sulfamethoxazole, or oral erythromycin often results in healing in 2 weeks.

B. **Donovanosis** (Granuloma inguinale) causes genital ulceration. The causative organism, Calymmatobacterium granulomatis reclassified as ***Klebsiella granulomatis***. **Donovan body** (safety pin like inclusion bodies inside the monocyte.

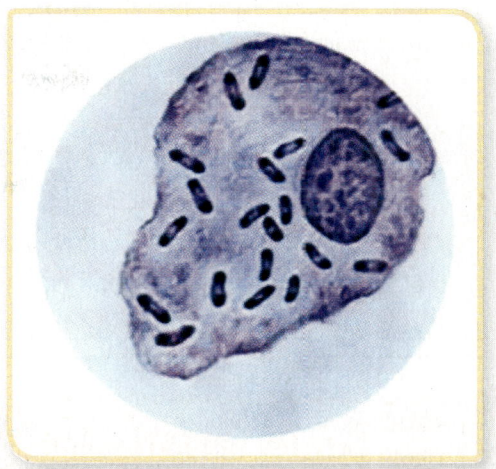

C. Neisseria is an intracellular Gram negative diplococci seen with polymorphonuclear leukocytes (see for multiple lobes of the nucleus) in urethral exudate

D. Chlamydia is gram-negative, obligate intracellular parasite. They grow and reproduce within host cells. Intracytoplasmic basophilic inclusion containing clamps of elementary bodies of Chlamydia -basophilic inclusions.

 MICRO PLATE 9

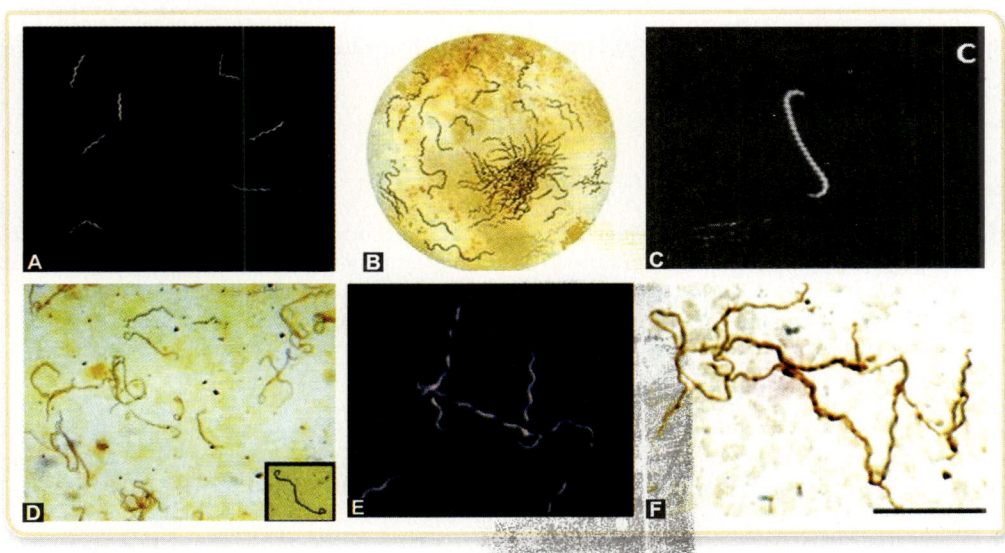

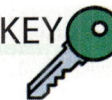

SPIROCHETES

A. *Treponema pallidum* in dark field microscopy
B. *Treponema* in silver impregnation
C. *Leptospira* in dark field microscopy
D. *Leptospira* in Silver impregnation
E. *Borrelia burgdorferi* organisms shown by dark-filed microscopy
F. *Borrelia burgdorferi* organisms shown by dark-filed microscopy; note the large and irregular spirals with pointed ends

Treponema pallidum	Borrelia burgdorferi	Leptospira
T pallidum are **slender spirals** measuring about 0.2 µm in width and 5–15 µm in length. The spiral coils are regularly spaced at a distance of 1 µm from one another. There are about 10 regular spirals. **Ends are smooth.**	B burgdorferi is a spiral organism 20–30 µm long and 0.2–0.3 µm wide. **Large spirals;** The distance between turns varies from 2 to 4 µm. The organisms have variable numbers (7–11) of endoflagella and are highly motile. Both **ends are pointed**. Irregular spirals.	Leptospirae are **tightly coiled (10-18 coils),** thin, flexible spirochetes 5–15 µm long, with very fine spirals 0.1–0.2 µm wide; one end is often bent, forming a **hook** or **umbrella handle.** Secondary spirals give the leptospirae the appearance of **brackets** or the letter **S**.

MICRO PLATE 10

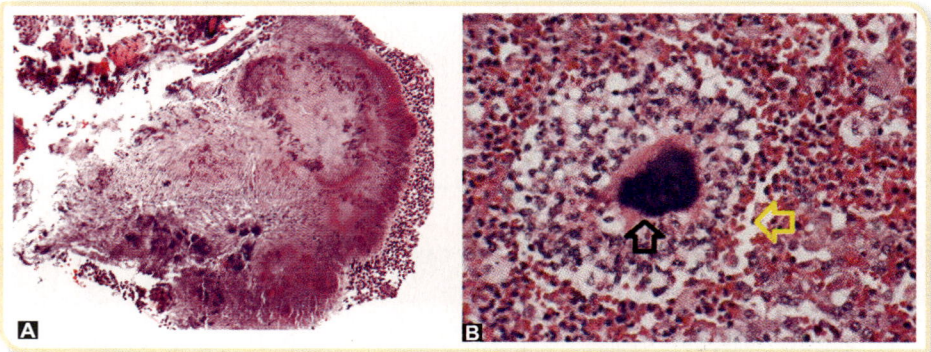

By Nephron - Own work, CC BY-SA 3.0, https://commons.wikimedia.org/w/index.php?curid=18555026

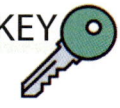 KEY

ACTINOMYCES

A. **Actinomyces H&E stain:** High magnification micrograph of a **sulfur granule** formed by actinomyces in the mandible. Histopathology - For most purposes, recognition is based on the appearances of sulfur granules using the **hematoxylin and eosin (H&E) stain.** These granules actually represent colonies of *A. israelii*, a gram-positive, anaerobic filamentous bacterium.

B. **Actinomyces Grams stain**: Showing tangled mass of branching filaments (black arrow), surrounded by a hypocellular artifactual cleft (yellow arrow) surrounded by neutrophils and macrophages.

 Note

Specific fungal stains such as the methenamine silver and periodic acid Schiff (PAS) stains are useful to ensure that fungi are present, but are seldom helpful for specific diagnosis. Actinomycete filaments also take up silver based stains

	Actinomycosis vs Nocardiasis	
	Actinomycosis	**Nocardia (Aerobic)**
▫ Gram stain	Gram +ve filamentous branching	Gram +ve filamentous branching
▫ Acid fastness	Not	AFB +ve weak (but N. madurai AFB –ve)
▫ Morphology	▫ Non-motile ▫ Non-sporing ▫ Non-capsulated	▫ Non-motile ▫ Non-sporing ▫ Non-capsulated
▫ Infection in	In immunocompitant	In immunocompromised (HIV/AIDS)

Contd...

	Actinomycosis vs Nocardiasis	
Clinical features	□ Oro-cervicofacial (MC type)- woody/lump jaw □ Appendix in GIT □ PID in IUCD users (*A. israelii*)	□ Airborn inhalation –thick sputum □ CXR-Lt. lower lobe nodule with central cavitation.
Microscopy	Spidery colony & Sun-ray appearance- Ray fungus Sulfur granules	Paraffin bait technique
Treatment	Penicillin	TMP-SMX/ Sulfonamides

MICRO PLATE 11

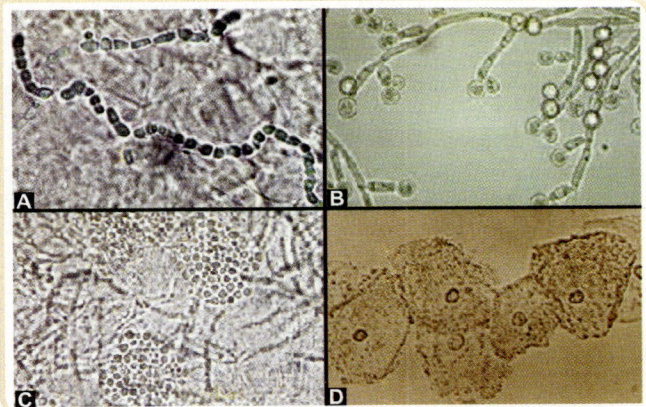

KOH MOUNT

KOH mount used for diagnosis of **superficial fungal infections**. Diagnostic cytology involves various methods like aspiration cytology, imprint smears, skin scraping smear and Tzanck smear. In dermatology, a potassium hydroxide (KOH) mount of a skin scraping is a common procedure performed to demonstrate the evidence of fungal infection in skin, hairs and nails. It can be done on an outpatient basis and the results are available within 1-2 h. In experienced hands, a potassium hydroxide mount is one of the most useful procedures in medical mycology. It has been adjudged more reliable than culture for demonstration of dermatophytes.

KOH MOUNTING

Step 1: Scraping
□ Cleaning by using alcohol or by washing.
□ Scraping is done by a pre flamed scalpel.
□ Scraping should be done from the lesion or the advancing edge in skin.
□ In hairy areas like scalp and beard, scrape along the edges, epilate short hair stubs and crusts.
□ In nail involvement, scrape the affected sites at a considerable depth. Scoop out the deeper keratinous matrix. Nail clippings and avulsed whole nails can also be used.

Step 2: Potassium hydroxide mount
□ The sample is collected on a slide and the collected material is covered with KOH.
□ 10% KOH is used for skin and hair scrapings.
□ 20-30% KOH is used for nail clippings.

Contd...

KOH MOUNTING
□ Heating the sample collected on slide may help in faster clearing of sample.
□ The material is covered with cover slip.

Step 3: Direct microscopic examination
This is a direct microscopic examination of the above specimen to detect fungal spores or hyphae. Initial examination is with low power magnification (x10) and low intensity of light with lowering of the condenser. Later, for a higher magnification (x40), the condenser should be higher for better illumination to study the morphology of the fungus. Fungal spores vary from 2-10 mm in diameter.

Step 4: Interpretation
A. *Dermatophytes:* KOH mount of infected nail material showing typical dermatophyte hyphae breaking up into arthroconidia
B. *Candida:* Pseudo hyphae and budding in candida (yeast)
C. *Tinea Versicolor (Pityriasis Versicolor):* The spores and pseudo hyphae of *Malassezia furfur* (a yeast that can cause tinea versicolor) resemble "spaghetti and meatballs" on a potassium hydroxide slide.
D. *Vaginosis:* Bacterial vaginosis is a common cause of vaginitis in women in the childbearing age who are sexually active. The vaginal fluid obtained on removal of the speculum should be tested for pH and a few drops of 10% potassium hydroxide added to the discharge on a glass slide and sniffed for detection of a fishy odor. Light microscopy of immediate wet mounts can be done to identify *'clue cells'* of *Gardernella*.[AIIMS PG] The ability of G. vaginalis to adhere to vaginal and urinary epithelial cells at a pH of 5 to 6 is thought to contribute to its role in the pathogenesis of BV and urinary tract infections.[AIIMS PG]

MICRO PLATE 12

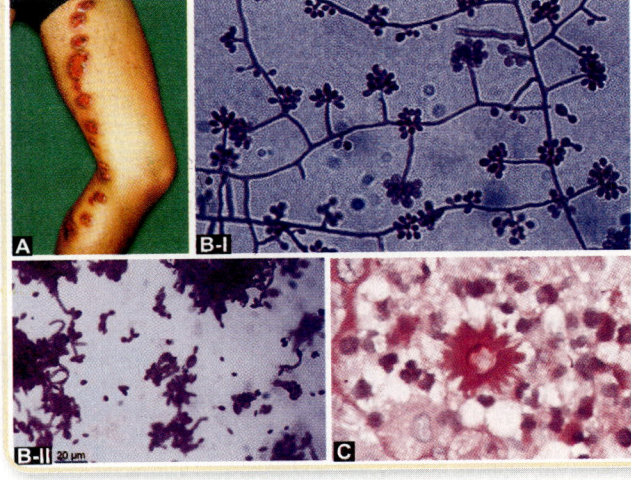

SPOROTHRIX SCHENCKII

Sporothrix schenckii is a thermally *dimorphic fungus* that lives on vegetation. It is associated with a variety of plants—grasses, trees, sphagnum moss, rose bushes, and other horticultural plants. Following traumatic introduction into the skin, *S schenckii* causes sporotrichosis, a chronic granulomatous infection. Multiple subcutaneous nodules and abscesses occur along the lymphatics. The incidence is higher among agricultural workers, and sporotrichosis is considered an occupational risk for forest rangers, horticulturists, and workers in similar occupations. Sporotrichosis (also known as **"rose gardener's disease"**) is a rare infection caused by Sporothrix. This fungus lives throughout the world in soil and on plant matter such as sphagnum moss, rose bushes, and hay. People get sporotrichosis by coming in contact with the fungal spores in the environment.

Types of Sporotrichosis

- **Cutaneous (skin) sporotrichosis** is the most common form of the infection. It usually occurs on a person's hand or the arm after they have been handling contaminated plant matter.
- **Pulmonary (lung) sporotrichosis** is very rare but can happen after someone breathes in fungal spores from the environment.
- **Disseminated sporotrichosis** occurs when the infection spreads to another part of the body, such as the bones, joints, or the central nervous system. This form of sporotrichosis usually affects people who have weakened immune systems, such as people with HIV infection.

PLATE LEGENDS

A. Noduloulcerative lesions (**sporotrichotic chancre**) appear along the lymphatics, proximal to the initial inoculation injury site. It is the most common variety and accounts for 70–80% of the cases of cutaneous sporotrichosis. The extremities are affected most frequently. A noduloulcerative lesion at inoculation site and a string of similar nodules along the proximal lymphatics, with or without transient satellite adenopathy, characterizes this form.

B. **Sporothrix Dimorphism:**
  I. Microscopic morphology of the saprophytic or mould form of Sporothrix schenckii when grown on Sabouraud's dextrose agar at Room temperature (25°C). Conidiophores arise at right angles from the thin septate hyphae and are usually solitary, erect and tapered towards the apex. Conidia are formed in clusters on tiny denticles by sympodial proliferation of the conidiophore, their arrangement often suggestive of a flower.
  II. Microscopic morphology of the saprophytic or mould form of Sporothrix schenckii when grown on Sabouraud's dextrose agar at 37°C with **Cigar Shaped** budding yeast cells.

C. When yeast forms are surrounded by eosinophilic hyaline ray like processes they are referred to as **Sporothrix Asteroid**, usually seen in the center of Granuloma.

MICRO PLATE 13

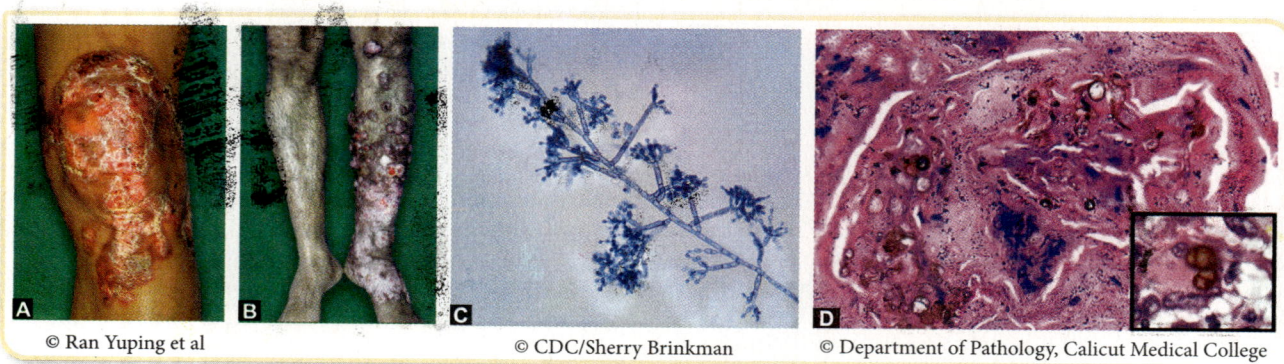

© Ran Yuping et al   © CDC/Sherry Brinkman   © Department of Pathology, Calicut Medical College

CHROMOBLASTOMYCOSIS

A. **Chromoblastomycosis Initial lesion:** The initial erythematous papule grows slowly over months to years, the primary lesion becomes verrucous and wart-like with extension along the draining lymphatics.

B. **Chromoblastomycosis late lesion:** Cauliflower-like nodules with crusting abscesses eventually cover the area. Small ulcerations or "black dots" of hemopurulent material are present on the warty surface. Rarely, elephantiasis may result from secondary infection, obstruction, and fibrosis of lymph channels. Lymphedema is normally observed in the affected limb.

C. **Chromoblastomycosis Microscopy:** Elliptical, brownish conidia from conidiophore. The agents of chromoblastomycosis are identified by their modes of conidiation. The most frequent etiological agents of CBM are- *Fonsecaea pedrosoi, Phialophora verrucosa* and *Cladophialophora carrionii. Rhinocladiella aquaspersa*
   Light microscopy of lactophenol cotton blue preparation of colonies grown on Sabouraud's dextrose agar presenting with Conidiophores suberect, olivaceous brown, apically densely branched

D. **Chromoblastomycosis HPE**[AIIMS PG]**:** Histologic examination shows characteristic pseudoepitheliomatous hyperplasia in the epidermis and a mixed granulomatous inflammatory infiltrate with giant cells containing characteristic dark-brown, round sclerotic body resembling a **"copper penny"** i.e. Dark Brown Pigmented Yeast with reproduction by intracellular wall formation (septation) not budding. The agents of chromoblastomycosis are identified by their modes of conidiation. In tissue, they appear the same, producing spherical brown cells (4–12 µm in diameter) termed muriform or sclerotic bodies that divide by transverse septation.

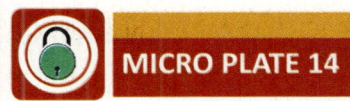
MICRO PLATE 14

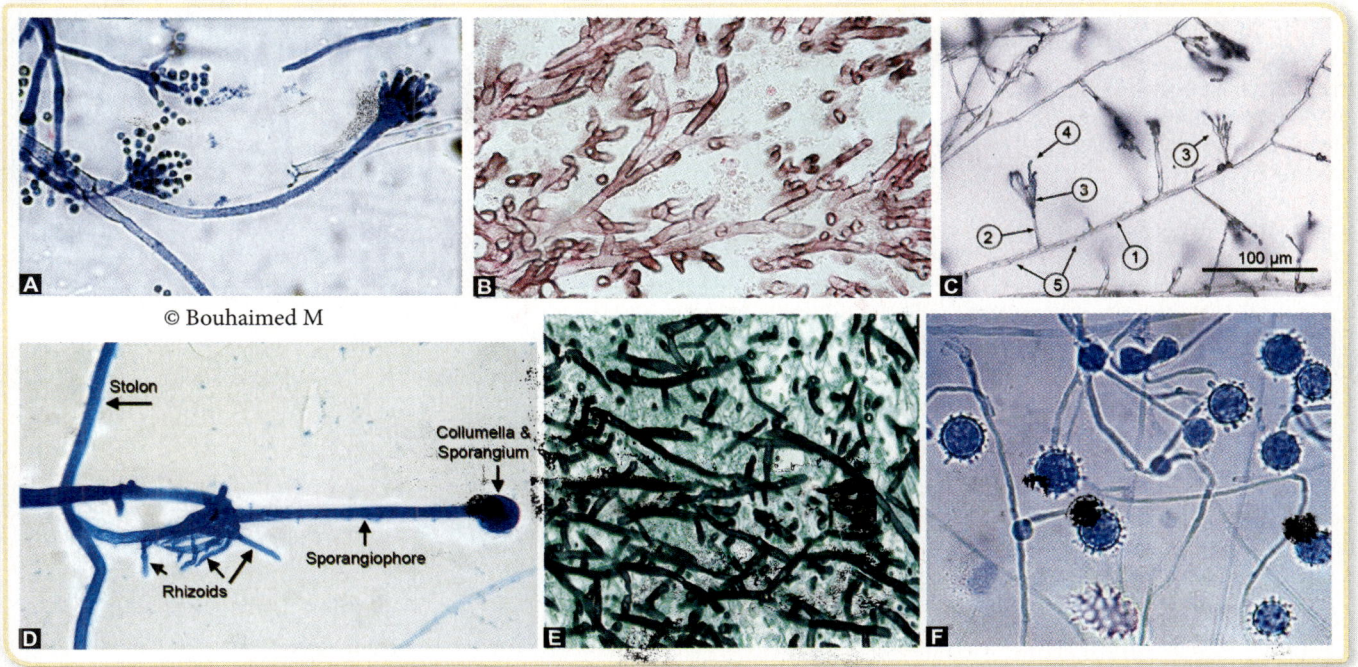

TYPES OF HYPHAE IN DIFFERENT SPECIES

A. **Aspergillus–single hyphae** in Grocott's methenamine silver (GMS) stain showing V-shaped/ Acute angled, 45° septate, branched hyphae and radiating chains of conidia
B. **Aspergillus–multiple hyphae** in Grocott's methenamine silver (GMS) stained tissue section of lung showing narrow width, acute angled branched, septate hyphae
C. **Penicillium–single hyphae** in Grocott's methenamine silver (GMS) stain showing acute angled 25° – 45° septate, branched hyphae. Characteristics are helpful in distinguishing with Aspergillus is clear vacuoles alternating with basophilic zones. Chains of conidia are produced by phialides, which are supported by branched conidiophores. Terminal conidium is oldest. 1. hypha, 2. conidiophore, 3. phialide, 4. conida, 5. septa
D. **Zygomycetes- Rhizopus–single hyphae-** Pauciseptate/Aseptate Ribbon like, Right angled hyphae. Sporangiospores are produced inside a spherical structure, the sporangium. Sporangia are supported by a large apophysate columella atop a long stalk, the sporangiophore. Sporangiophores arise among distinctive, root-like rhizoids.
E. **Zygomycetes- Rhizopus–multiple hyphae-** Pauciseptate/ Aseptate Ribbon like, Right angled hyphae.
F. **Histoplasma** Hyaline septate hyphae. Large single celled Tuberculate macroconidium (with typical thick walls and radial, finger like projections) is a diagnostic structure of *Histoplasma capsulatum*. *Histoplasma capsulatum* exhibits thermal dimorphism growing in living tissue or in culture at 37°C as a budding yeast-like fungus and in soil or culture at temperatures below 30°C as a mould.

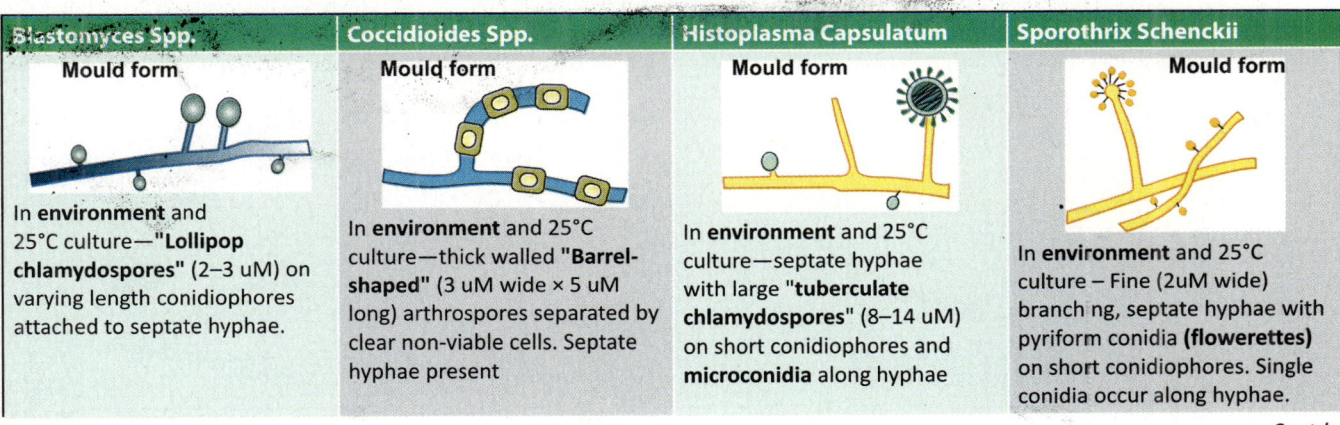

Contd...

Blastomyces Spp.	Coccidioides Spp.	Histoplasma Capsulatum	Sporothrix Schenckii
Yeast form 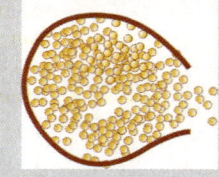 In **tissue** and fungal media at 37°C—**thick walled** yeast (5–20uM) with a **broad base** between mother and daughter cells	**Spherule** 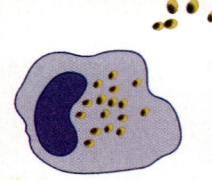 In **tissue** and specialized media at 37°C—immature (20–40uM) and mature **spherule** (50–250uM) containing infectious **endospores**	**Yeast form** Yeast cells in a macrophage In **tissue-intracellular**, small (2–4uM). Culture at 37°C small yeast with a narrow base between mother and daughter cells	**Yeast form** In **tissue – cigar-shaped** (oval and fusiform), small (2uM wide × 3–8uM long) budding yeast. Culture at 37°C —small yeast similar to

Note

Grocott's silver. Both viable and dead hyphae are stained well with this method.

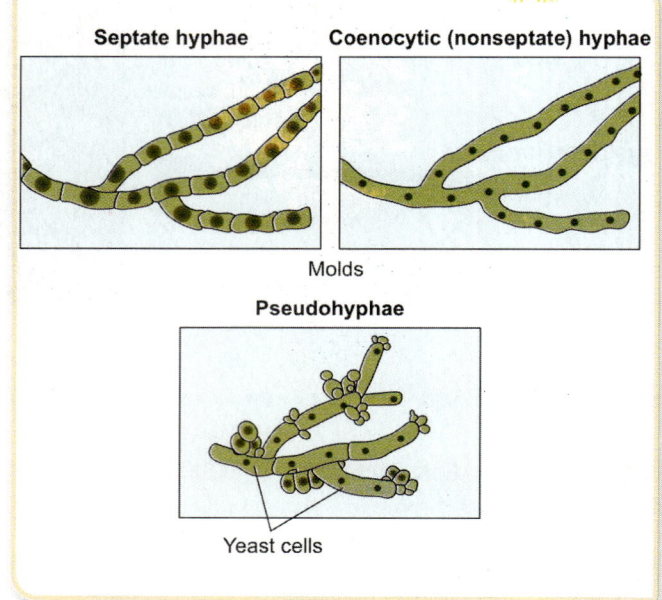

Septate hyphae / Coenocytic (nonseptate) hyphae — Molds

Pseudohyphae — Yeast cells

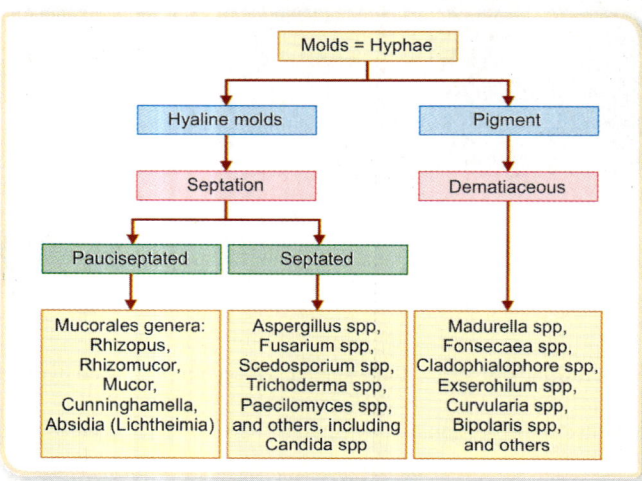

Molds = Hyphae
- Hyaline molds
  - Septation
    - Pauciseptated: Mucorales genera: Rhizopus, Rhizomucor, Mucor, Cunninghamella, Absidia (Lichtheimia)
    - Septated: Aspergillus spp, Fusarium spp, Scedosporium spp, Trichoderma spp, Paecilomyces spp, and others, including Candida spp
- Pigment
  - Dematiaceous: Madurella spp, Fonsecaea spp, Cladophialophore spp, Exserohilum spp, Curvularia spp, Bipolaris spp, and others

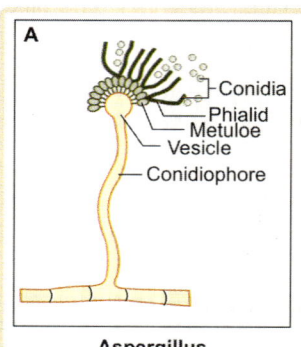

A — Conidia, Phialid, Metuloe, Vesicle, Conidiophore
Aspergillus

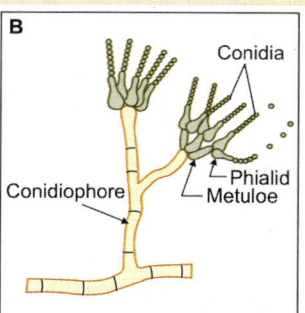

B — Conidia, Phialid, Metuloe, Conidiophore
Penicillium

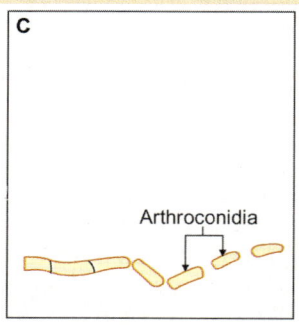

C — Arthroconidia
Geotrichum

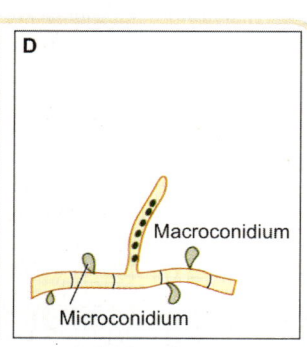

D — Macroconidium, Microconidium
Trichophyton

E — Macroconidium, Microconidium
Microsporum

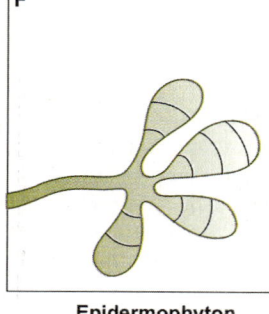

F
Epidermophyton

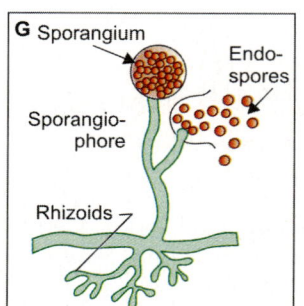

G — Sporangium, Endospores, Sporangiophore, Rhizoids
Rhizopus

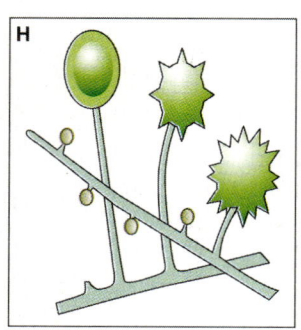

H
Histoplasma

PLATE LEGENDS

A. Aspergillus;
B. Penicillium;
C. Geotrichum;
D. Trichophyton;
E. Microsporum;
F. Epidermophyton;
G. Rhizopus
H. Histoplasma capsulatum

MICRO PLATE 15

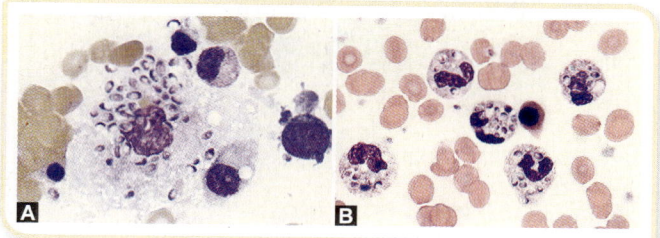

HISTOPLASMA CAPSULATUM

A. **Histoplasma capsulatum:** Wright stain of bone marrow aspirate revealed innumerable oval/ crescent-shaped yeast cells in both intracellular and extracellular distribution, most prominently seen within marrow histiocytes. Also, it is PAS positive and gave a positive Prussian blue reaction.
B. **Histoplasma capsulatum** inside neutrophils in a peripheral blood smear.

MICRO PLATE 16

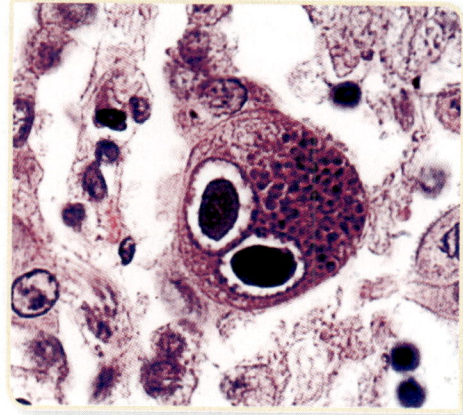

CYTOMEGALOVIRUS

Eosin Hematoxylin stained lung section showing typical owl eye inclusions by CMV. Histologically, the hallmark of CMV infection is the large (mega) cell containing a large centrally situated **intranuclear basophilic inclusion** with peri-inclusion halo and granular multiple basophilic cytoplasmic inclusion, morphologically resembling an '**owl's eye**'.

MICRO PLATE 17

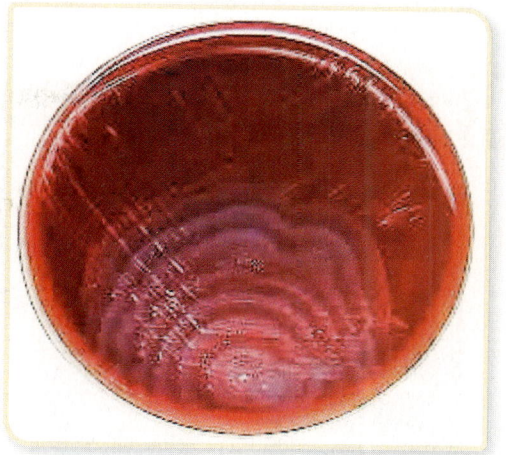

SWARMING OF PROTEUS ON BLOOD AGAR

Swarming of proteus on blood agar: Proteus species move very actively by means of peritrichous flagella, resulting in "swarming" on solid media unless the swarming is inhibited by chemicals, such as phenylethyl alcohol or CLED (cystine-lactose-electrolyte deficient) medium. Swarming does not occur on MacConkey agar on which smooth, colorless colonies are formed.

MICRO PLATE 18

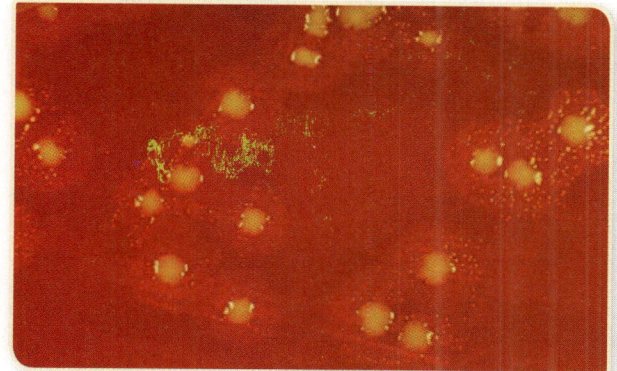

HAEMOPHILUS INFLUENZAE

Haemophilus influenzae colonies on Blood agar showing satellitism around the colonies of staplylococcus.
Satellitism: Although blood agar contains X & V factors, colonies of *H. influenzae* are small due to lake of availability of V factor. Enhancement of growth can be obtained by supplementing medium with NAD or streaking on orgnism, which excretes excess of V factor. After inoculating suspected *H. influenzae* on blood agar plate, *Staph aureus* is streaked across the same plate and incubated overnight at

37° C. In such mixed culture, the colonies of *H. influenzae* are large & well developed around the colonies of staphylococcus, whereas those further away from staphylococcal streak are smaller. This feature is called **"satellitism"** & demonstrates that staphylococci, synthesise V factor in high concentration near the staphylococcal growth.

MICRO PLATE 19

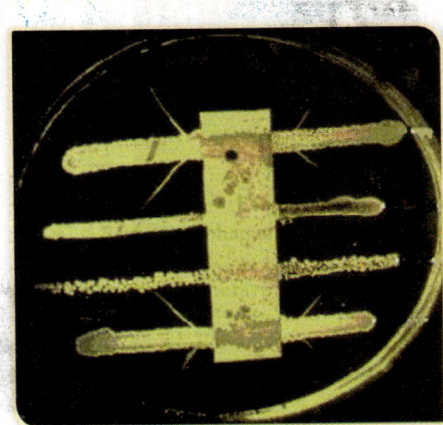

ELEK TEST FOR C. DIPHTHERIAE ENDOTOXINS

All isolates of *C. diphtheriae* should be tested for the production of exotoxin. This has been done historically by an in vitro immunodiffusion assay (**Elek test**), a tissue culture neutralization assay using specific antitoxin.

A filter paper disk containing antitoxin is placed on an agar plate. The cultures to be tested for toxigenicity are spot inoculated 7 to 9 mm away from the disk. After 48 hours of incubation, the antitoxin diffusing from the paper disk has precipitated the toxin diffusing from toxigenic cultures and has resulted in precipitate bands between the disk and the bacterial growth.

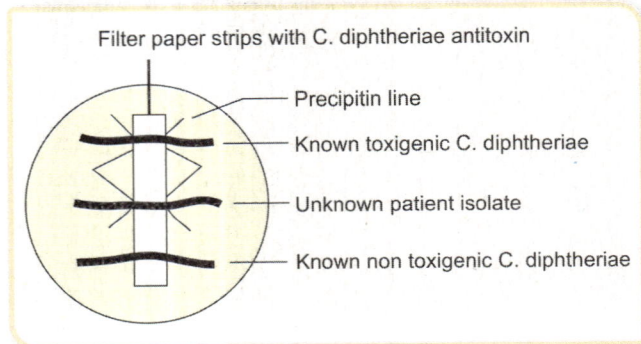

MICRO PLATE 20

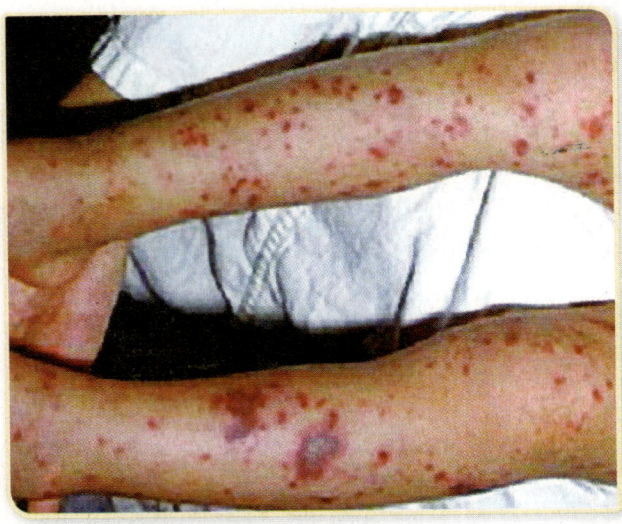

PLATE LEGEND

It's almost impossible to comment without a clinical history. Clinical history of Fever with rash and that of meningitis shall be given with or without the Lumbar puncture CSF analysis.

Nesseria Meningitis

In meningococcal septicemia, a rash is always a very important sign. The rash can appear anywhere on the body. Early skin rash looks like tiny pinpricks (pink, red, or purple). As the infection spreads through the system, the rash becomes more obvious. More bleeding under the skin may cause the spots to turn dark red or deep purple. The rash may resemble large bruises.

In infants and Young Children	In Older Children and Adults
Fever Disinterest in feeding Irritability Extreme tiredness or floppiness Dislike of being handled Vomiting and/or diarrhea Turning away from light Drowsiness Convulsions or twitching Rash of red-purple pinprick spots or larger bruises	Fever Vomiting and/or diarrhea Neck stiffness or aching backache Joint pains and sore muscles General malaise, off food Drowsiness, confusion Rash of red-purple pinprick spots or larger bruises Headache Photophobia (dislike of bright lights).

Glass test: One sign of meningococcal septicemia is that the rash doesn't fade when you apply pressure.

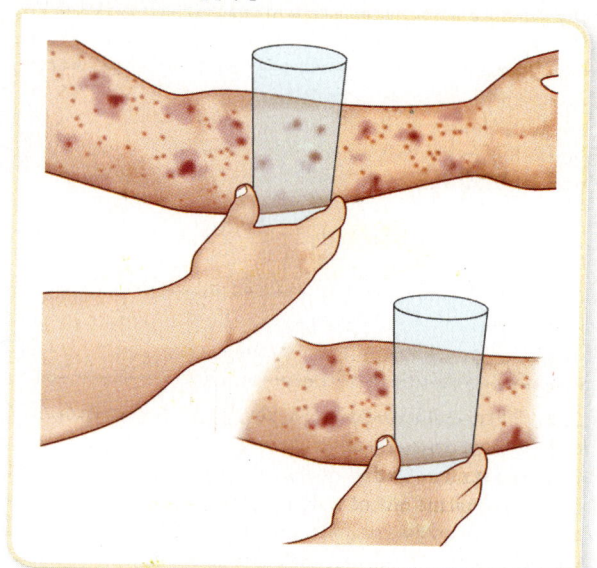

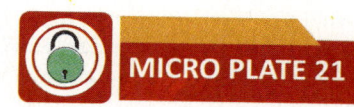
MICRO PLATE 21

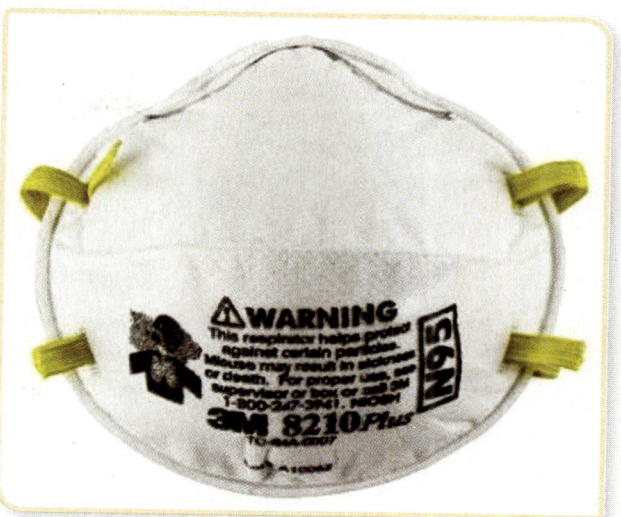

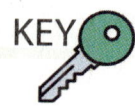
KEY

N 95 MASK FOR H1N1

Influenza A Virus Including Subtype H1N1	
\multicolumn{2}{l}{Influenza A (H1N1) virus is a subtype of influenza A virus and was the most common cause of human influenza (flu) in 2009. Some strains of H1N1 are endemic in humans and cause a small fraction of all influenza-like illness and a small fraction of all seasonal influenza. Other strains of H1N1 are endemic in pigs (swine influenza) and in birds (avian influenza).}
\multicolumn{2}{l}{The virus isolated from patients in the United States was found to be made up of genetic elements from four different flu viruses: 1. North American swine influenza   2. North American avian influenza   3. Human influenza   4. Swine influenza virus.}
Pandemic	On June 11, 2009, the WHO declared an H1N1 pandemic, moving the alert level to phase 6, marking the first global pandemic since the 1968 Hong Kong flu.
Cause of death	A study conducted in coordination with the University of Michigan Health Service published in the December 2009 American Journal of Roentgenology warning that H1N1 flu can cause **pulmonary embolism**, surmised as a leading cause of death in this current pandemic.
Pregnancy	The research team of Andrew Miller MD showed pregnant patients are at increased risk.
Virulence	The virulence of swine flu virus is mild and the mortality rates are very low.
Outbreak	H5N1; Hong Kong H9N2; China H9N2; Hong Kong H7N7; Netherlands 2004/05 H5N1; H7N3; Canada, H10N7; Egypt H5N1 in 13 new countries including India H5N1 in China, Egypt, Indonesia, Nigeria
Drug categories	Two groups of drugs are currently available for the treatment or prophylaxis of influenza infections: 1. **Adamantanes:** The adamantanes (amantadine and rimantadine) are effective only against influenza A and are associated with several toxic effects and with rapid emergence of drug-resistant variants. This potential for the development of resistance especially limits the use of the adamantanes for the treatment of influenza, although the drugs still have a place in planning for prophylaxis during an epidemic.

Contd...

	2. Newer class of neuraminidase inhibitors: The neuraminidase inhibitors (zanamivir and oseltamivir) interfere with the release of progeny influenza virus from infected host cells, a process that prevents infection of new host cells and thereby halts the spread of infection in the respiratory tract. These have activity against both influenza A and B viruses. *A key advantage of the neuraminidase inhibitors, and a major difference from the adamantanes, is that development of resistance is very rare* a. **Zanamivir** is approved for treatment of influenza among children aged ≥7 years. b. **Oseltamivir** is approved for treatment and chemoprophylaxis among persons aged ≥1 year. Recommended treatment and chemoprophylaxis dosages of oseltamivir for children vary by the weight of the child c. **Peramivir,** a newer agent in clinical trials, has also been shown to be a potent and selective inhibitor of influenza A and B neuraminidases. d. **Ribavirin,** a nucleoside analogue has been used in the treatment of human influenza A virus infections, usually administered orally or by aerosolization, and occasionally by the IV route for severe infections or in immunocompromised hosts. A consistent benefit has not been observed in clinical studies, and **currently ribavirin is not considered to be a drug of choice for influenza A infection**
Drug therapy	□ **Oseltamivir,** sold under the trade name Tamiflu and is taken orally in capsules or as a suspension, used to treat and prevent both Influenza virus A and Influenza virus B. □ Oseltamivir is a prodrug (active metabolite, the free carboxylate of oseltamivir) and is the first orally active *neuraminidase inhibitor* serving as a competitive inhibitor towards sialic acid. □ Oseltamivir is approved for use in persons age 1 and over. There is also currently an FDA Emergency Use authorization temporarily allowing the use of Tamiflu in children less than one year old. □ **Treatment dosage:** The usual adult dosage for treatment of influenza is 75 mg twice daily for 5 days, beginning within 2 days of the appearance of symptoms and with decreased doses for children and patients with renal impairment. □ **Prophylaxis dosage:** Standard prophylactic dosage is 75 mg once daily for patients aged 13 and older, which has been shown to be safe and effective for up to six weeks. □ **Co-administration with probenecid:** It has been suggested that co-administration of oseltamivir with probenecid could extend a limited supply of oseltamivir. Probenecid reduces renal excretion of the active metabolite of oseltamivir.
Side effects	□ Common adverse drug reactions (ADRs) associated with oseltamivir therapy (occurring in over 1% of clinical trial participants) include: nausea, vomiting, diarrhea, abdominal pain and headache. □ Rare ADRs include: hepatitis and elevated liver enzymes, rash, allergic reactions including anaphylaxis and Stevens-Johnson syndrome.
Resistance	Mutations conferring resistance are single amino acid residue substitutions (His274Tyr) in the neuraminidase enzyme. As of December 2010, the World Health Organization (WHO) reported 314 samples of 2009 pandemic H1N1 flu tested worldwide have shown resistance to oseltamivir (Tamiflu).

About Zanamavir

- Although zanamivir was the first neuraminidase inhibitor to the market, it had only a few months lead over the second entrant, oseltamivir (Tamiflu), with an oral tablet formulation.
- According to the Centres for Disease Control and Prevention (CDC), no flu, seasonal or pandemic, has shown any signs of resistance to zanamivir.
- Tamiflu, zanamivir's main competitor, is not as effective at treating the influenza viruses as zanamivir, especially in H1N1 Seasonal Flu. In fact, tests showed that 99.6% of the tested strains of seasonal H1N1 flu and 0.5% of 2009 pandemic flu were resistant to Tamiflu while there have been absolutely zero flu samples seasonal or pandemic that shows any resistance to zanamivir.
- Dosing is limited to the inhaled route. This restricts its usage, as treating asthmatics could induce bronchospasm
- Zanamivir has not been known to cause toxic effects.

Use of the Pandemic (H1N1) 2009 Vaccines

- Injectable vaccines contain inactivated (or killed) viruses. These vaccines are given by injection into the upper arm in adults and thigh in infants and younger children. Another type of vaccine is made with live viruses, and it is administered by nasal spray. Both are protective against influenza
- Recommendation is a single dose of vaccine in adults and adolescents from 10 years of age and above. For Immunosuppressed persons two doses of vaccine may be needed.
- In children as over the age of 6 months and younger than 10 years of age recommendations on numbers of dosages may need to be adapted rapidly as new data emerges (WHO).
- Based on currently available information, healthy children 2 through 9 years of age who are receiving live attenuated influenza A (H1N1) 2009 monovalent vaccine should receive two doses of vaccine separated by 28 days.
- Inactivated influenza vaccine can be given at the same time as other injectable, noninfluenza vaccines, but the vaccines should be administered at different injection sites.
- Influenza vaccines only become effective about 14 days after vaccination. Those infected shortly before (1 to 3 days) or shortly after immunization can still get the disease.
- **H1N1 vaccine does not provide protection against seasonal flu.** Therefore, it's advisable to get both a seasonal flu vaccine and the 2009 H1N1 swine flu vaccine at the same time, unless they are both the nasal spray version of the flu vaccine (live vaccine).

Contd...

Microbiology Color Plates

Inactivated, Injectable Influenza Vaccine				
Manufacturer	**Age**	**Dose Presentation**	**Number of doses**	**Route–Site**
PANENZA, the pandemic vaccine procured from Sanofi Pasteur, France	6 through 35 months	0.25 mL—prefilled syringe or from a multi dose vial	2	Intramuscular
	36 months and older	0.5 mL—prefilled syringe or from a multi dose vial	1 or 2	

Live Attenuated Nasal Spray Influenza Vaccine (LAIV)				
Manufacturer	**Age**	**Dose Presentation**	**Number of doses**	**Route–Site**
FluMist by MedImmune (thimerosal-free)	2 through 49 years if healthy and non-pregnant	0.2 mL—Spray ½ of dose into each nostril as indicated on the syringe	1 or 24	Intranasal

Active ingredient of injectable vaccine: (from MOHFW)	1. Split Influenza virus: Inactivated, containing antigen equivalent to: A/California/7/2009 (H1N1) v-like strain (NYMC X-179A)- 15 micrograms per 0.5 ml dose, propagated in eggs. 2. Thiomersal (45 micrograms per 0.5 ml dose) (live nasal vaccine is thimerosal-free). 3. Other ingredients are: Sodium chloride, potassium chloride, disodium phosphate dihydrate, potassium dihydrogen phosphate and water.
Contraindications to vaccine	Inactivated vaccines should not be administered to: 1. People with a history of anaphylaxis (or hypersensitive reactions), or other life-threatening allergic reactions to any of the constituents or trace residues of the vaccine. 2. People with history of a severe reaction to previous influenza vaccination. 3. People who developed Guillain-Barré syndrome (GBS) within 6 weeks of getting an influenza vaccine. 4. Children less than 6 months of age (inactivated influenza vaccine is not approved for this age group). 5. People who have a moderate-to-severe illness with a fever (they should wait until they recover to get vaccinated).
Side effects	1. Most common side effects are headache (muscular pain) and pain at the injection site. 2. These side effects usually disappeared without treatment within 1 to 3 days after onset.
Storage (from MOHFW)	1. Store in a refrigerator (2°C–8°C). Do not freeze. 2. Keep the vial in the carton in order to protect from light. 3. Though the vaccine can be used within 7 days after opening, it is preferred the open vials are used completely
Vaccination preference (TRIAGE)	CDC's Advisory Committee on Immunization Practices (ACIP) recommends that swine flu vaccine should first go to: 1. Healthcare and emergency medical services personnel (1st preference by WHO). 2. Pregnant women (2nd preference). 3. Household contacts and caregivers for children younger than 6 months of age. 4. All children and young adults from 6 months through 24 years of age. 5. Persons aged 25 through 64 years who have health conditions associated with higher risk of medical complications from influenza.
H1N1 Mask: (WHO)	☐ If masks are worn, proper use and disposal is essential to ensure they are potentially effective and to avoid any increase in risk of transmission associated with the incorrect use of masks. ☐ Replace masks with a new clean, dry mask as soon as they become damp/ humid. ☐ When crowded settings or close contact cannot be avoided, the use of N95 mask is recommended. ☐ The pore size for common surgical masks is about 16-51 micron while the size of virus is about 22 nm. N95 mask is 95% efficient at filtering out particles of a size of approximately 0.3 microns and above.

Some models of different masks available

- 3M-8210 — Most common model in the market
- 3M-1860 — Commonly used in healthcare institutions
- 3M-8105 — (Similar to 3M-8210 but for smaller faces)
- 3M-1860S — (Similar to 3M-1860 but for smaller faces)

MICRO PLATE 22

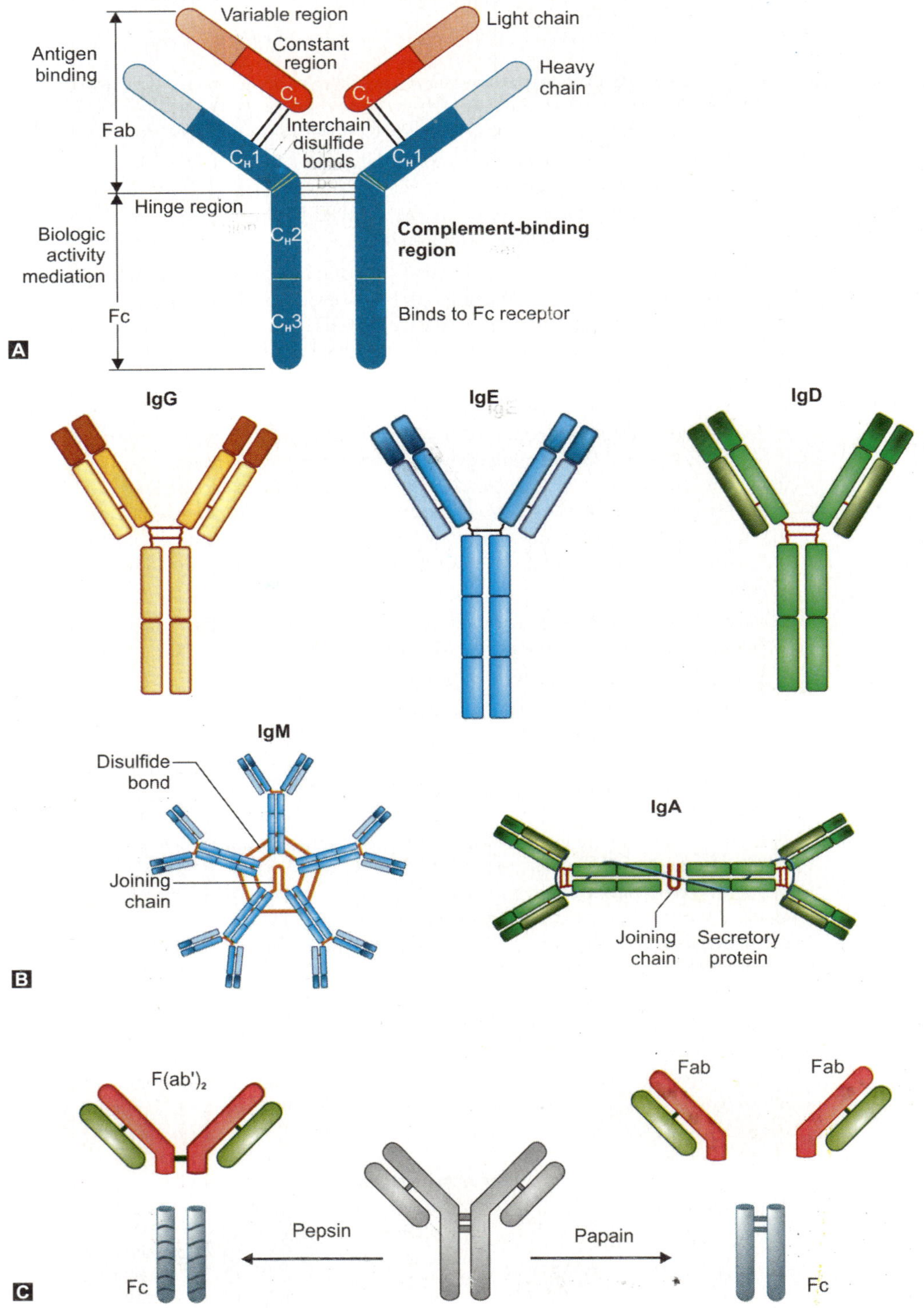

IMMUNOGLOBULINS

A. Basic structure of Immunoglobulin: A glycoprotein, composed of H and L chains, that functions as antibody. All antibodies are immunoglobulins, but not all immunoglobulins have antibody function. An individual antibody molecule always consists of identical H chains and identical L chains. The simplest antibody molecule has a Y shape and consists of minimum four polypeptide chains: minimum of two identical heavy (H) chains (mw 50000) and two identical light (L) chains (mw 25,000). two H chains and two L chains. The four chains are covalently linked by disulfide bonds. L and H chains are subdivided into variable regions and constant regions. The regions are composed of three-dimensionally folded, repeating segments called domains. The structures of these domains have been determined at high resolution by X-ray crystallography. An L chain consists of one variable domain (VL) and one constant domain (CL). Most H chains consist of one variable domain (VH) and three or more constant domains (CH). Each domain is approximately 110 amino acids long. Variable regions are responsible for antigen binding; constant regions are responsible for the biologic functions described below.

B. **Classification of Immunoglobulins:** Light (L) chains are of one of two types, (kappa) or (lambda); classification is made based on amino acid differences in their constant regions. Both types occur in all classes of immunoglobulins (IgG, IgM, IgA, IgE, and IgD), but any one immunoglobulin molecule contains only one type of L chain. The amino terminal portion of each L chain contains part of the antigen-binding site. Heavy (H) chains are distinct for each of the five immunoglobulin classes and are designated (gamma= IgG), (alpha= IgA[NEETPG]), (mu= IgM), (epsilon= IgE) and (delta= IgD).

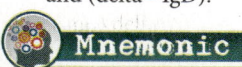

Mnemonic

GAMED (IgG, IgA, IgM, IgE, IgD)

C. If immunoglobulins are treated with a proteolytic enzyme (e.g. papain), peptide bonds in the hinge region are broken. This breakage produces two identical Fab fragments, which carry the antigen-binding sites, and one Fc fragment.

 MICRO PLATE 23

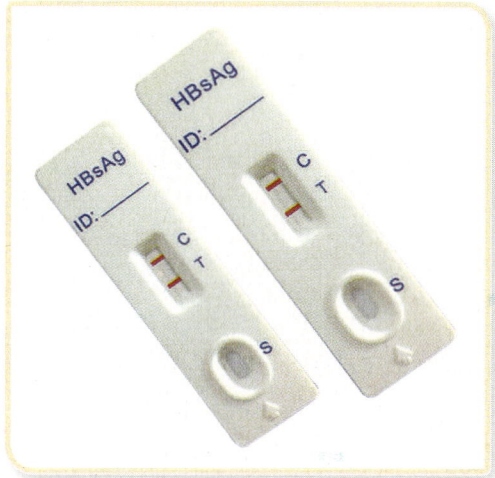

 KEY

HBSAG RAPID CARD[NEETPG]

Infection with the Hepatitis B virus is characterized by the appearance of certain viral markers including Hepatitis B surface Antigen (HBsAg) in the blood. It is recommended that all blood donations are tested for this marker to avoid transmission to recipients.

HBsAg Rapid card is visual, rapid, sensitive and accurate one step immunoassay for the qualitative detection of Hepatitis B surface antigen (HBsAg) in human serum or plasma. If sample contains HBsAg a line will form on the membrane indicating positive result. If antigen is not present no line is formed indicating negative result.

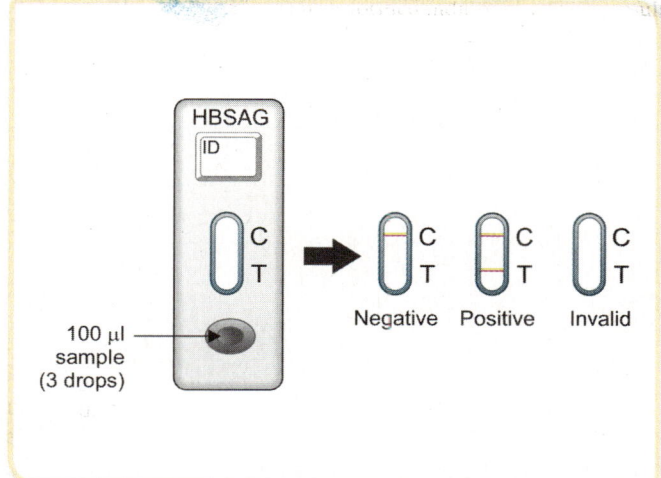

Reagent: The device contains Anti HBsAg particles and Anti HBsAg coated on membrane.

Storage: The kit can be stored in room temperature or refrigerator both (2-30°C).

Limitations: Use is limited to qualitative detection. Negative result is shown when the concentration is below detection limit (20 nanogram/mL).

NOTES

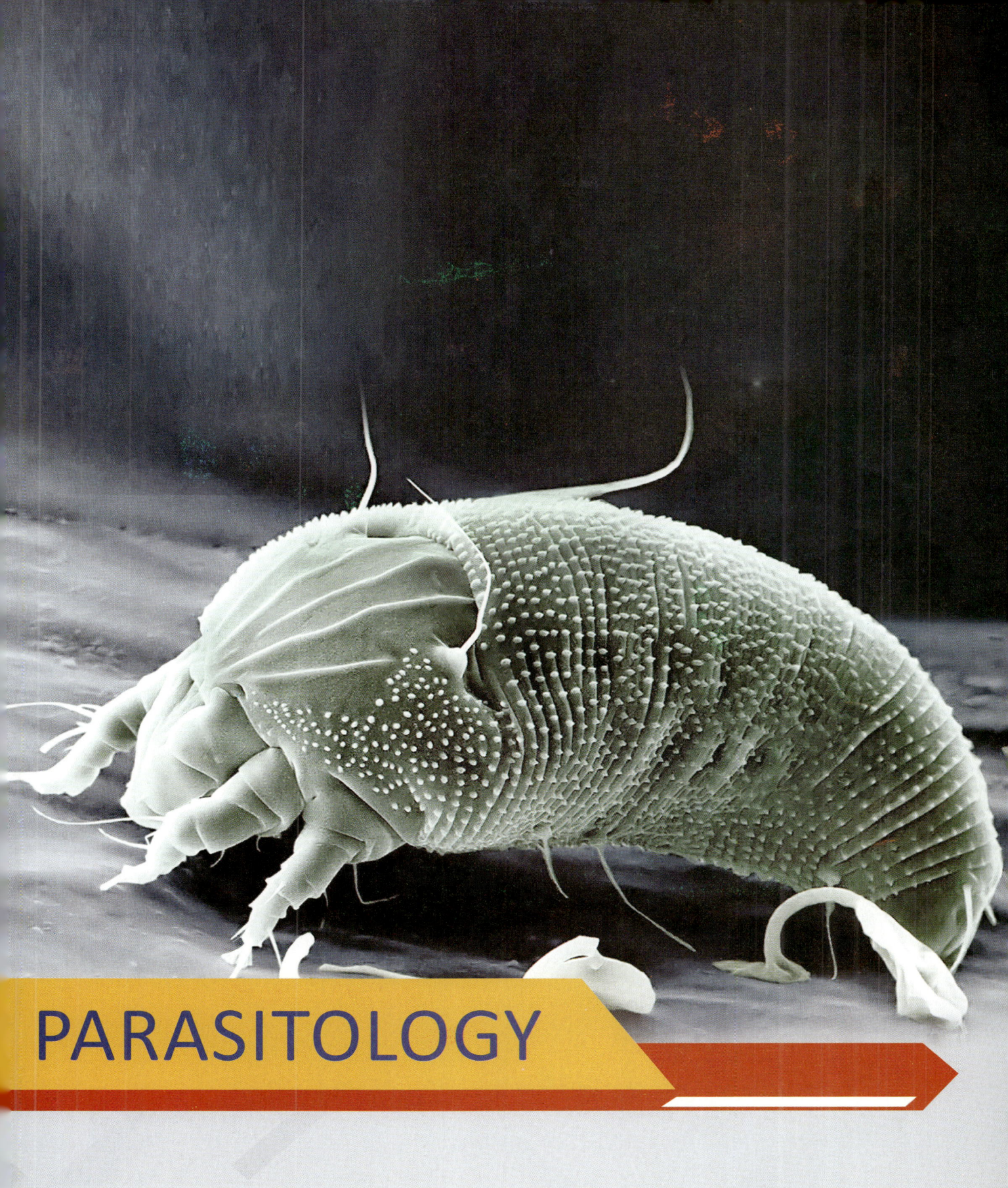

PARASITOLOGY

PARASITOLOGY PLATE 1

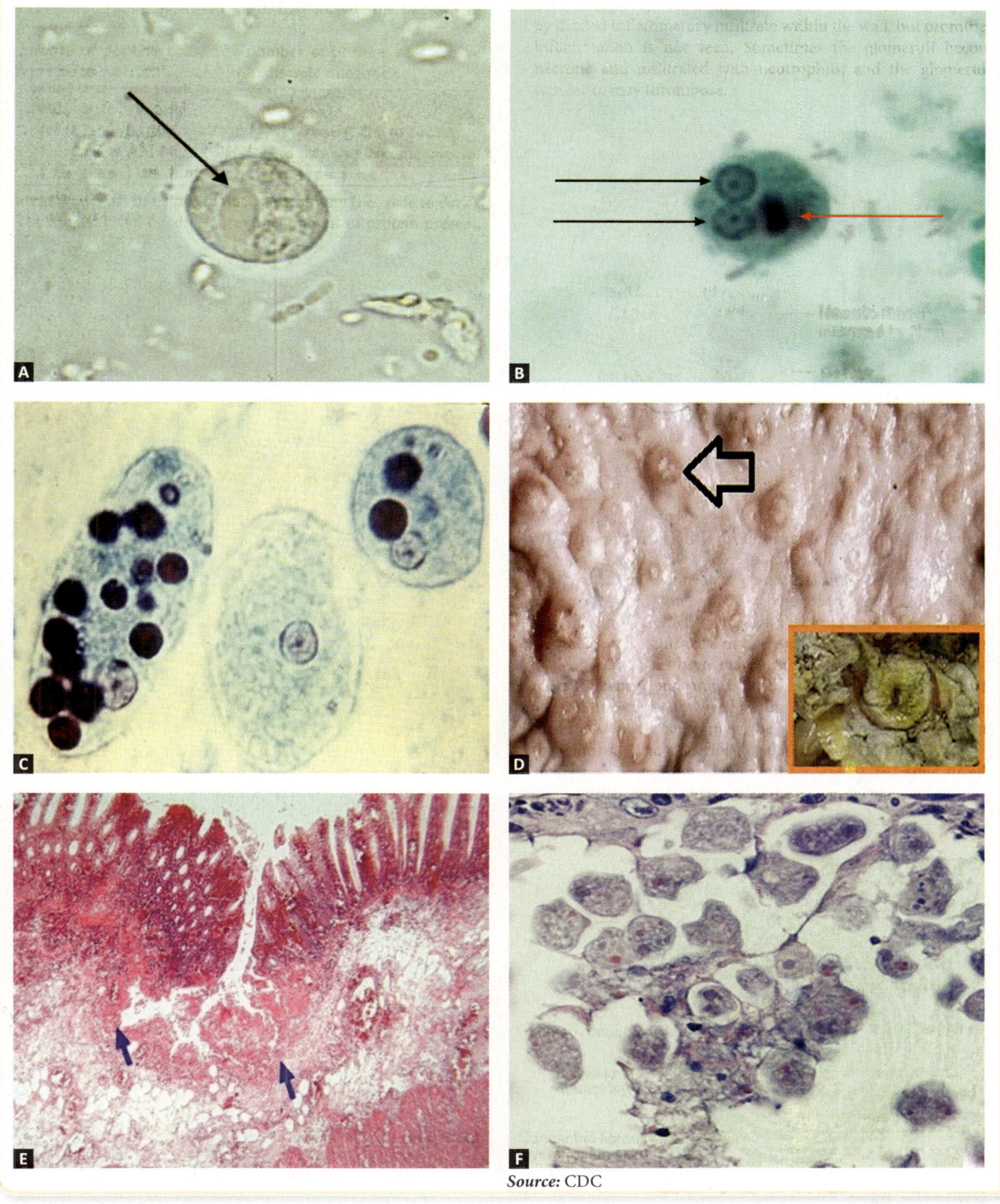

Source: CDC

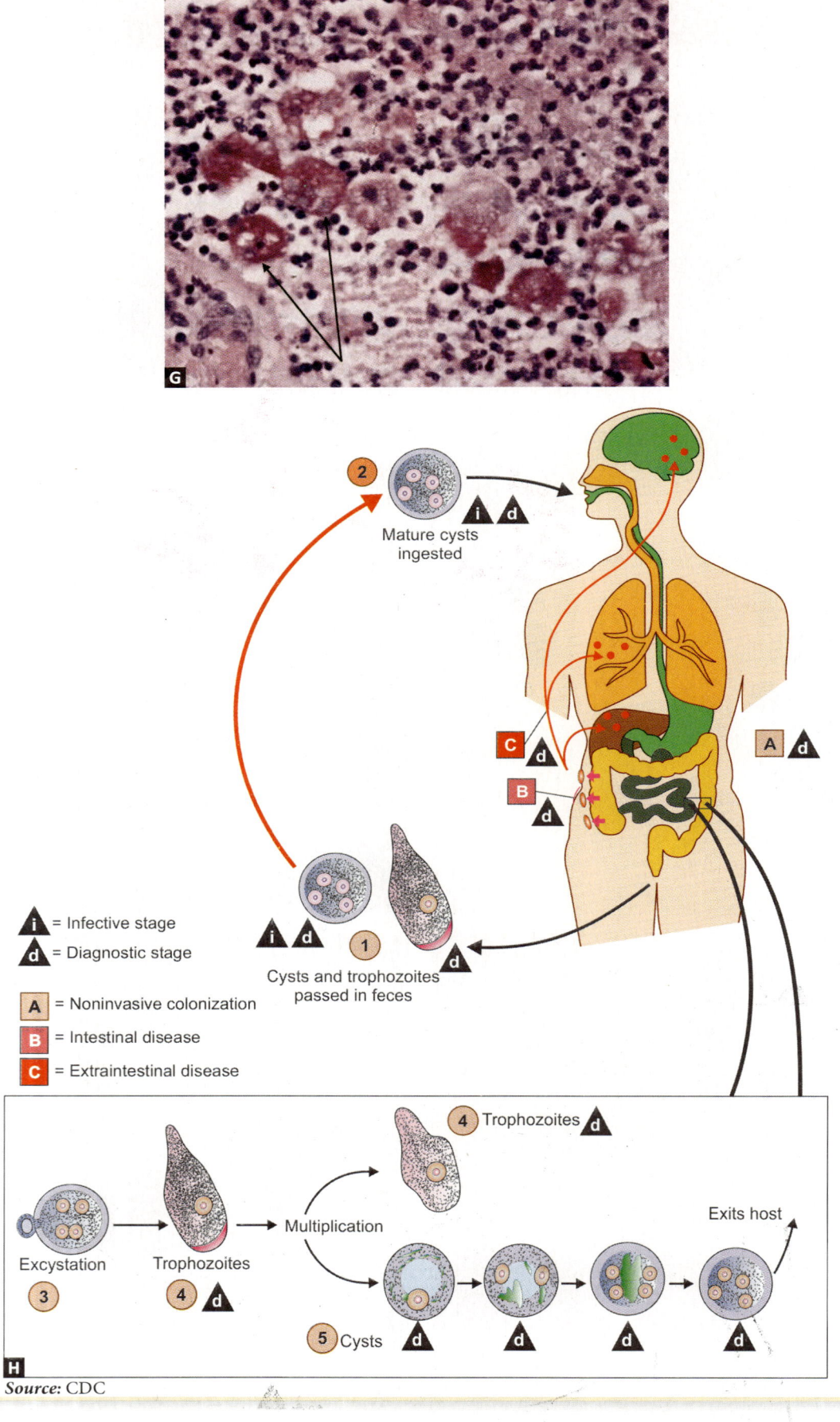

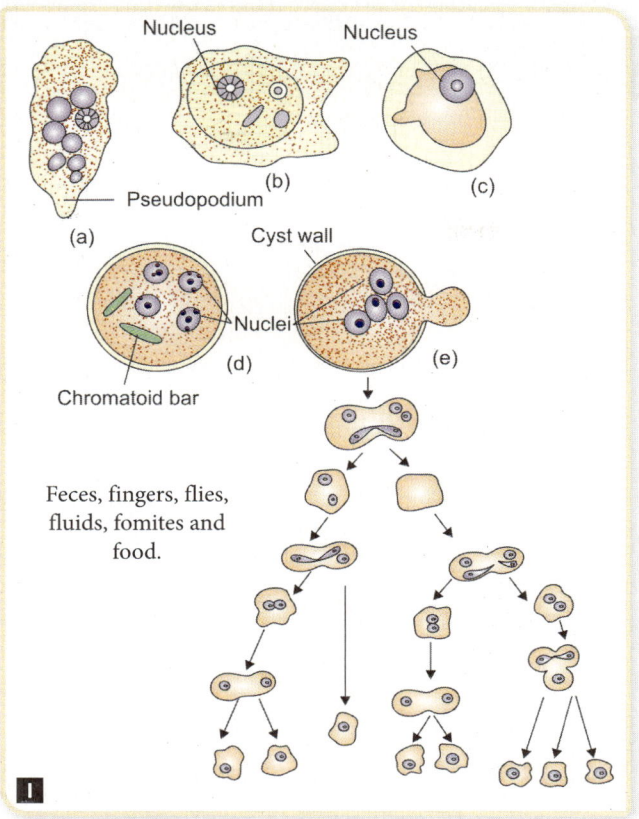

E. **Colonic biopsy specimen in a patient with amoebiasis.** A flask-shaped ulcer with a narrow opening and wide base (arrow) in the colon. Increased chronic inflammatory cells are seen within the lamina propria, and an inflammatory exudate overlies the mucosa.

F. **Colonic biopsy High-magnification** examination of the inflammatory exudate and ulcer base reveals typical trophozoites of *Entamoeba histolytica*. The sizes of trophozoites (arrow) are larger than those of macrophages. They have abundant amorphilic cytoplasm, small nuclei, and erythrophagocytosis (phagocytosis of RBC) in some trophozoites.

G. **Liver biopsy:** Biopsy obtained from the edge of amoebic liver abscess (HE and PAS stained, 20 ×). Notice the presence of trophozoites, hepatocytes, and the large number of inflammatory cells.

Abbreviations: HE - Hematoxylin and eosin; **PAS** - Periodic acid schiff

H. **Life cycle of *E. Histolytica*:** Cysts and trophozoites are passed in feces ❶. Cysts are typically found in formed stool, whereas trophozoites are typically found in diarrheal stool. Infection by *Entamoeba histolytica* occurs by ingestion of mature cysts ❷ in fecally contaminated food, water, or hands. Excystation ❸ occurs in the small intestine and trophozoites ❹ are released, which migrate to the large intestine. The trophozoites multiply by binary fission and produce cysts ❺, and both stages are passed in the feces ❶. Because of the protection conferred by their walls, the cysts can survive days to weeks in the external environment and are responsible for transmission. Trophozoites passed in the stool are rapidly destroyed once outside the body, and if ingested would not survive exposure to the gastric environment. In many cases, the trophozoites remain confined to the intestinal lumen (A: noninvasive infection) of individuals who are asymptomatic carriers, passing cysts in their stool. In some patients the xtraintestinal sites such as the liver, brain, and lungs (C: extraintestinal disease), with resultant pathologic manifestations. It has been established that the invasive and noninvasive forms represent two separate species, respectively *E. histolytica* and *E. dispar*. These two species are morphologically indistinguishable unless *E. histolytica* is observed with ingested red blood cells (erythrophagocystosis). Transmission can also occur through exposure to fecal trophozoites invade the intestinal mucosa (B: intestinal disease), or, through the bloodstream, enter during sexual contact (in which case not only cysts, but also trophozoites could prove infective).

I. **Stages of Life cycle of *E. Histolytica*:** a. Living trophozoite, b. Stained trophozoite, c. Precystic stage, d. Cystic stage: At the tetranucleate stage the cyst is infective to a new host. One tertanucleated cyst transforms to 8 uninucleated cyst, e. Encystment: The excystment is the process by which the cysts are transformed into the trophozoites.

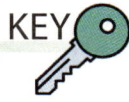
KEY

PLATE LEGENDS

A. **Cyst of *E. histolytica/E. dispar*** in an unstained concentrated wet mount of stool. Notice the chromatoid bodies with blunt, rounded ends (arrow).
B. **Cyst of *E. histolytica/E. dispar* stained with trichrome:** Two nuclei are visible in the focal plane (black arrows), and the cyst contains a chromatoid body with typically blunted ends (red arrow).
C. **Trophozoites of *E. histolytica*** with ingested erythrocytes stained with trichrome. The ingested erythrocytes appear as dark inclusions. The parasites above show nuclei that have the typical small, centrally located karyosome, and thin, uniform peripheral chromatin.
D. **Gross intestinal specimen** with intestinal flask-shaped ulcers observed though rectosigmoidoscopy examination. Arrows indicate small colonic ulcers. Insat shows large flask shaped ulcer of later stages

Protozoan Parasites						
Order	Species	Infective form	Invasive form/host	Diagnosis	Pathogenicity	Remarks
Amoeba — Intestinal	Entamoeba histolytica	-Cyst (1 to 4 nuclei) -Contains glycogen vacuoles & chromatoid bodies	Trophozoite (contains no RBC & Bacteria)	IHA (MC used) ELISA (Best)	Amoebic dysentery liver abscess Flask shaped ulcer	Anchovy sauce pus found in abscess. Aspirates are collected from edge.
Amoeba — Free living	Acanthamoeba spp	Cyst and trophozoite both (soil and water)	Cyst and trophozoite both	Diagnosis of GAE include brain scans, biopsies, or spinal taps.	Acanthamoeba keratitis Granulomatous Amoebic Encephalitis (GAE) and Disseminated infection	Treatment: Miltefosine Most common in individuals who wear contact lenses
Amoeba — Free living	Naegleria fowleri	Trophozoite. Warm fresh water (through nose)	Trophozoite	CSF microscopy	Primary amoebic meningoencephalitis (PAM)	Heat-loving (thermophilic). Acute & fatal Treatment: Miltefosine

Contd...

Protozoan Parasites

Order	Species	Infective form	Invasive form/host	Diagnosis	Pathogenicity	Remarks
Ciliates	Balantidium coli	Cyst	Trophozoites	Trophozoites in stool (V-shaped nucleus)	Abscess & Ulcer	
Mastigophora	Giardia lamblia	Cyst (not killed by chlorination)	Trophozoite pear shaped with tennis racket app.	String test+ Acid fast	Traveler's diarrhea, Non bloody foul-smelling diarrhea	Associated with common variable immunodeficiency
	Trichomonas vaginalis	No cyst stage	Trophozoite pear shaped	Motility in smear	Urethritis, Vaginitis (greenish yellow frothy discharge)	Strawberry cervix on calposcopy, feary red vagina & cervix
Coccidia	Isospora belli	Cyst	Oocyst	Acid fast	Chronic enterocolitis	
	Cryptosporidium	Oocyst	Thick walled cyst	Acid fast	Chronic enterocolitis	
	Toxoplasma gondii	Cyst ingestion in undercooked meat or freshly passed cat's feces	Trophozoites Def. host-Cat Intermediate host-Man	Sabin feldman dye test	Disseminated infection e.g. encephalitis.	Tachyzoites have predilection for parenchymal & RES
Hemosporidia	Plasmodium sp. Babesia	Sporozoite inoculation by mosquito bite	Man is intermediate host		Malaria	
Hemoflagellates	Trypanosoma brucei	Metacyclic trypomastigote	Tse tse fly (Glossina)		Sleeping sickness	Winter bottom sign (due to post cervical lymphadenopathy)
	Trypanosoma cruzi	Infective parasites	Reduvid bug		Chaga's disease	Romana's sign (U/L edema of eye lid)
	Leishmania donovani	Promastigotes Amastigote inside the macrophage	Bite of sandfly (Phlebotomus)	Bone marrow aspirates shows LD bodies	Kalaazar	RES is more severely affected

PARASITOLOGY PLATE 2

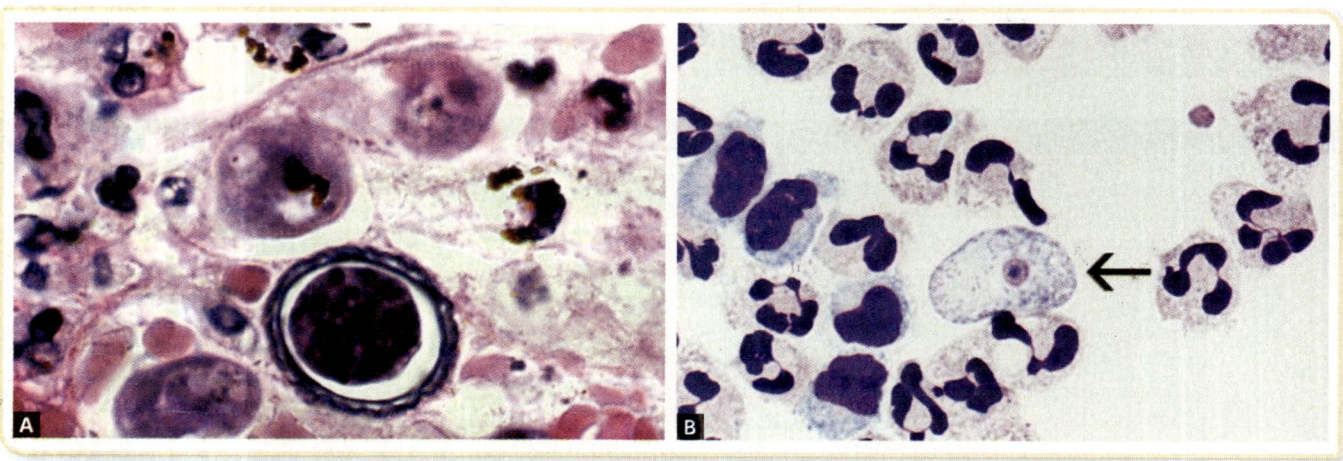

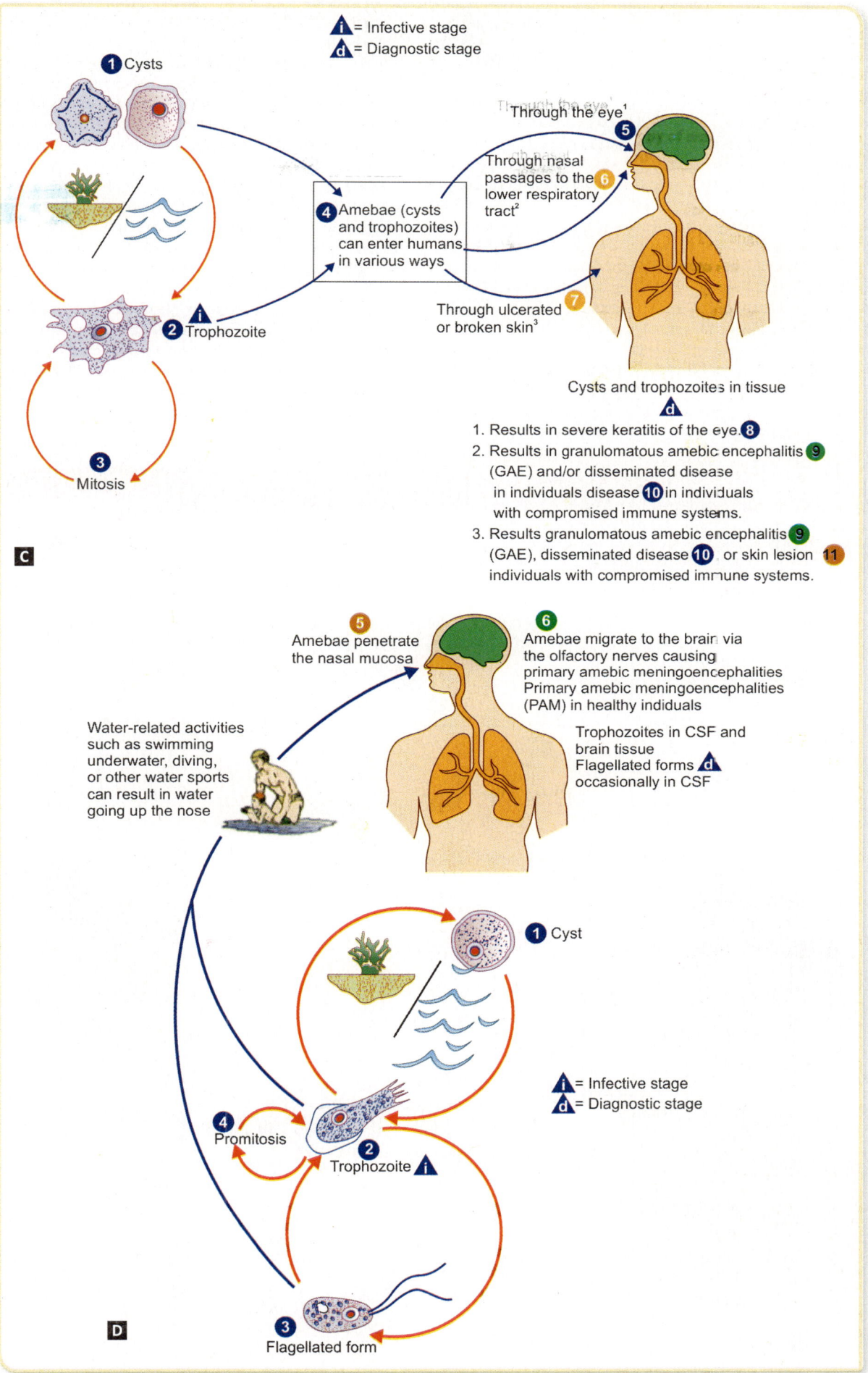

FREE LIVING AMOEBA

A. Acanthamoeba spp cyst: Magnified view of brain tissue within which was a centrally located Acanthamoeba sp. cyst.

B. *Naegleria fowleri* **in CSF:** Naegleria fowleri trophozoite (arrow) is shown in CSF stained with Giemsa stain with polymorphs and few lymphocytes.

C. Acanthamoeba life cycle: Acanthamoeba spp. have been found in soil; fresh, brackish, and sea water; sewage; swimming pools; contact lens equipment; medicinal pools; dental treatment units; dialysis machines; heating, ventilating, and air conditioning systems; mammalian cell cultures; vegetables; human nostrils and throats; and human and animal brain, skin, and lung tissues. Unlike *N. fowleri*, Acanthamoeba has only two stages, cysts ❶ and trophozoites ❷, in its life cycle. No flagellated stage exists as part of the life cycle. The trophozoites replicate by mitosis (nuclear membrane does not remain intact) ❸. The trophozoites are the infective forms, although both cysts and trophozoites gain entry into the body ❹ through various means. Entry can occur through the eye ❺, the nasal passages to the lower respiratory tract ❻, or ulcerated or broken skin ❼. When Acanthamoeba spp. enters the eye it can cause severe keratitis in otherwise healthy individuals, particularly contact lens users ❽. When it enters the respiratory system or through the skin, it can invade the central nervous system by hematogenous dissemination causing granulomatous amebic encephalitis (GAE) ❾ or disseminated disease ❿, or skin lesions ⓫ in individuals with compromised immune systems. Acanthamoeba spp. cysts and trophozoites are found in tissue.

D. *Naegleria fowleri* **life cycle:** Naegleria fowleri has 3 stages in its life cycle: cyst ❶, trophozoite ❷, and flagellate ❸. The only infective stage of the amoeba is the trophozoite. Trophozoites are 10-35 μm long with a granular appearance and a single nucleus. The trophozoites replicate by binary division during which the nuclear membrane remains intact (a process called promitosis) ❹. Trophozoites infect humans or animals by penetrating the nasal tissue ❺ and migrating to the brain ❻ via the olfactory nerves causing primary amebic meningoencephalitis (PAM).

PARASITOLOGY PLATE 3

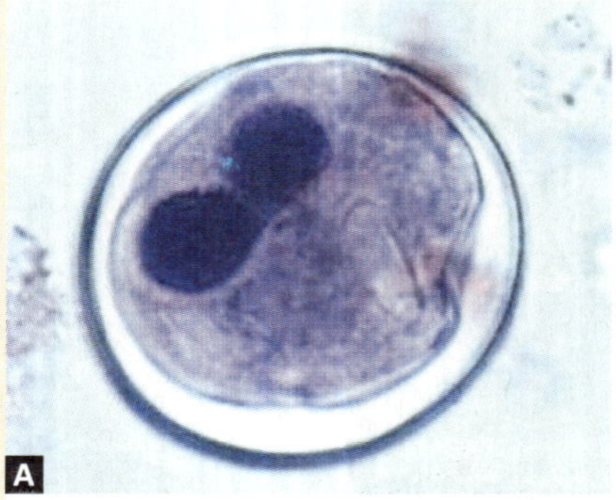

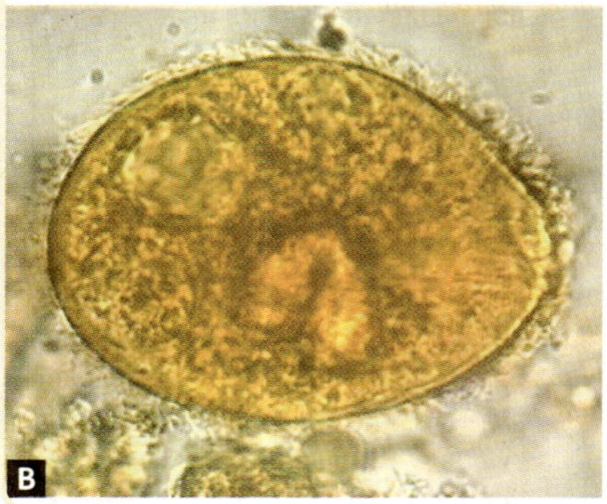

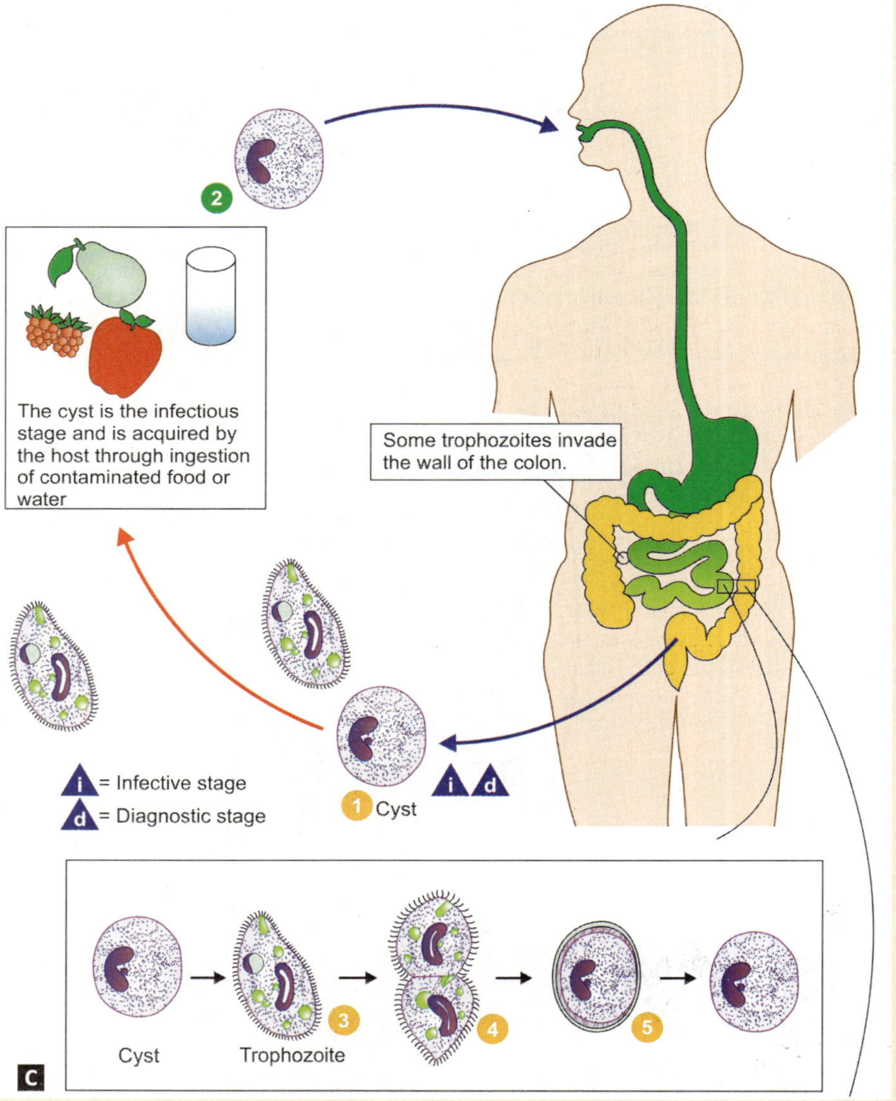

BALANTIDIUM COLI (CILIATE)

A. **B. coli trophozoite cyst**: Only kidney/ bean shaped macronucleus is visible under microscope. It is covered by thick hard cyst wall. Spherical in shape and is the Infective stage.

B. **B. coli trophozoite**: Kidney shaped Macronucleus and spherical micronucleus. No cyst wall but covered by visible cilia. Pointed anterior called cystosome for feeding. Its non infective stage.

C. **Life cycle of *Balantidium coli*:** Cysts are the parasite stage responsible for transmission of balantidiasis ❶. The host most often acquires the cyst through ingestion of contaminated food or water ❷. Following ingestion, excystation occurs in the small intestine, and the trophozoites colonize the large intestine ❸. The trophozoites reside in the lumen of the large intestine of humans and animals, where they replicate by binary fission, during which conjugation may occur ❹. Trophozoites undergo encystation to produce infective cysts ❺. Some trophozoites invade the wall of the colon and multiply. Some return to the lumen and disintegrate. Mature cysts are passed with feces ❶.

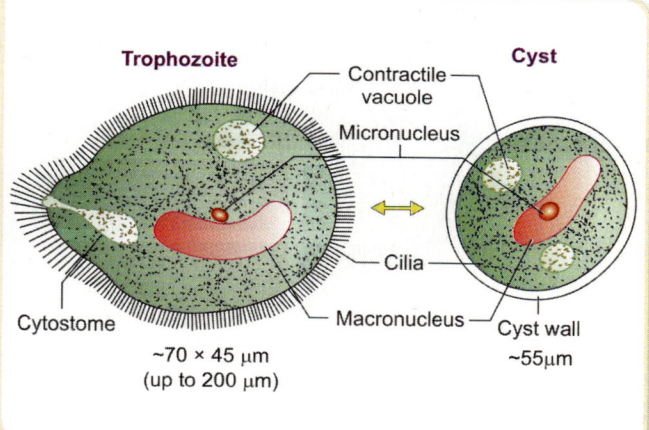

Fig: Balantidium coli

PARASITOLOGY PLATE 4

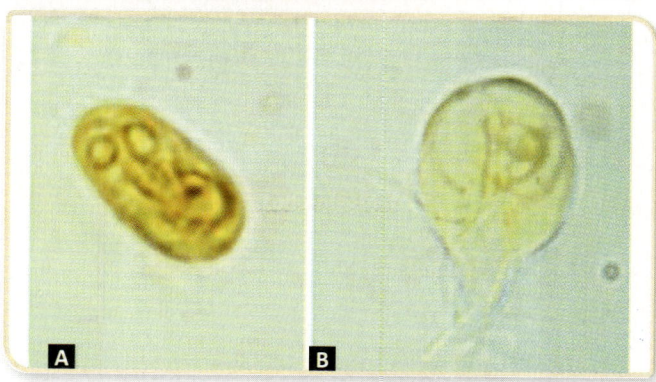

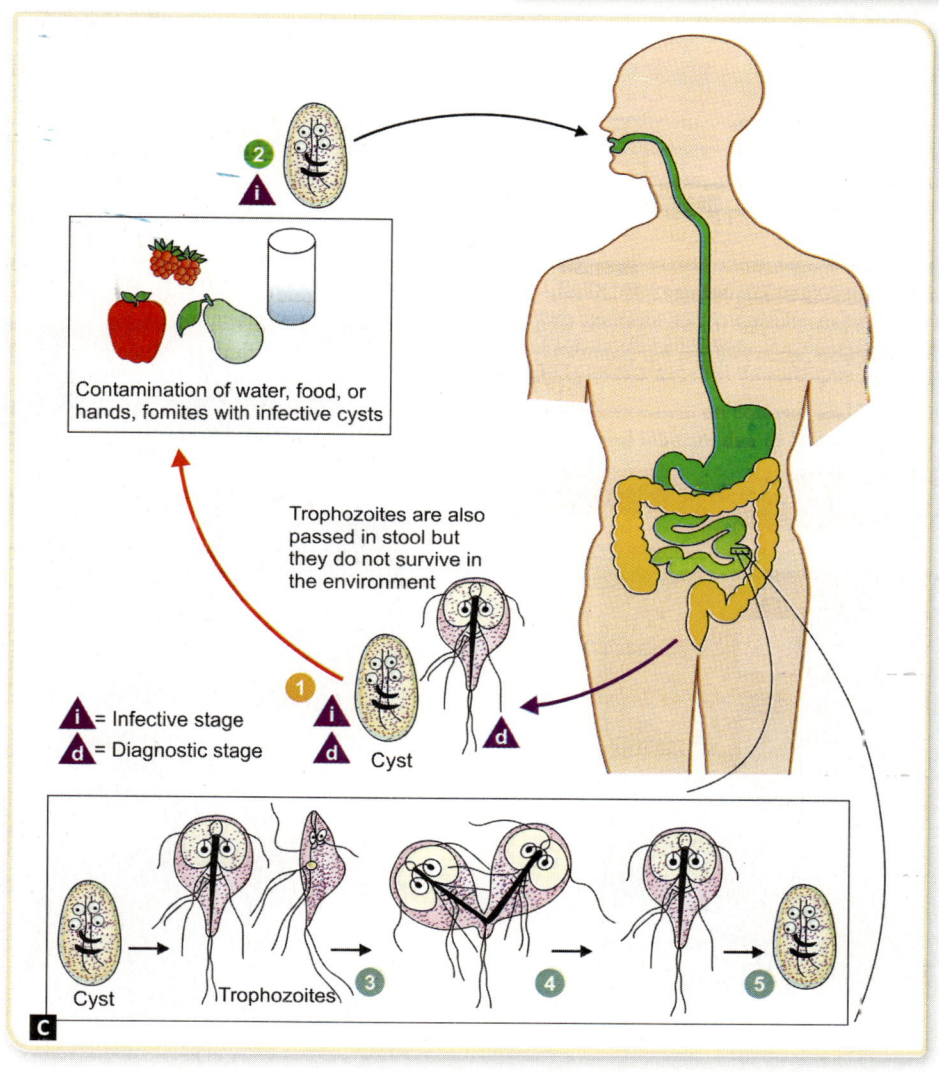

PLATE LEGENDS

A. ***Giardia duodenalis* cysts** are oval to ellipsoid and measure 8-19 μm (average 10-14 μm). Mature cysts have 4 nuclei, while immature cysts have two. Nuclei and fibrils are visible in both iodine-stained wet mounts and trichrome-stained smears.

B. ***Giardia duodenalis* Trophozoite**: Trophozoites are pear-shaped and measure 10-20 micrometers in length. In permanent, stained specimens, 2 large nuclei are usually visible. The sucking disks (used for attaching to the host's mucosal epithelium), median bodies, and flagella may also be seen.

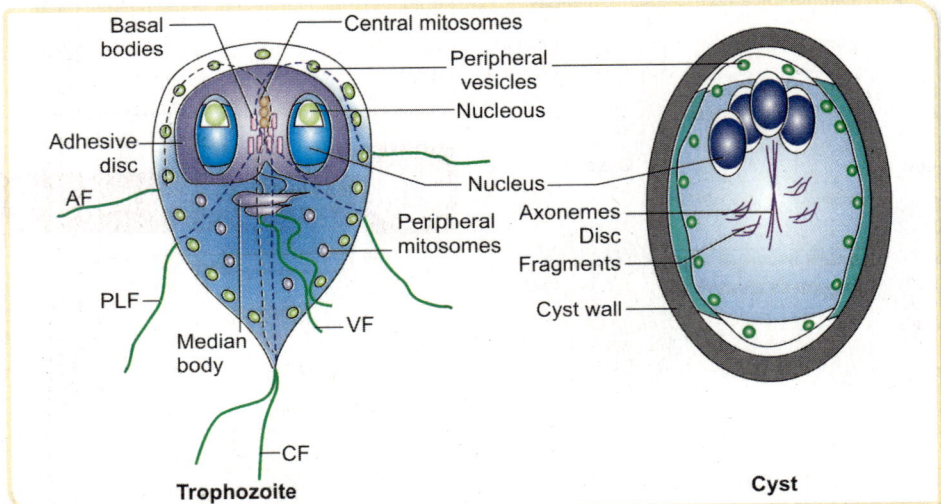

Fig: Giardia

C. Life cycle of giardia: Cysts are resistant forms and are responsible for transmission of giardiasis. Both cysts and trophozoites can be found in the feces (diagnostic stages) ❶. The cysts are hard and can survive several months in cold water. Infection occurs by the ingestion of cysts in contaminated water, food, or by the fecal-oral route (hands or fomites) ❷. In the small intestine, excystation releases trophozoites (each cyst produces two trophozoites) ❸. Trophozoites multiply by longitudinal binary fission, remaining in the lumen of the proximal small bowel where they can be free or attached to the mucosa by a ventral sucking disk ❹. Encystation occurs as the parasites transit toward the colon. The cyst is the stage found most commonly in nondiarrheal feces ❺. Because the cysts are infectious when passed in the stool or shortly afterward, person-to-person transmission is possible. While animals are infected with *Giardia*, their importance as a reservoir is unclear.

PARASITOLOGY PLATE 5

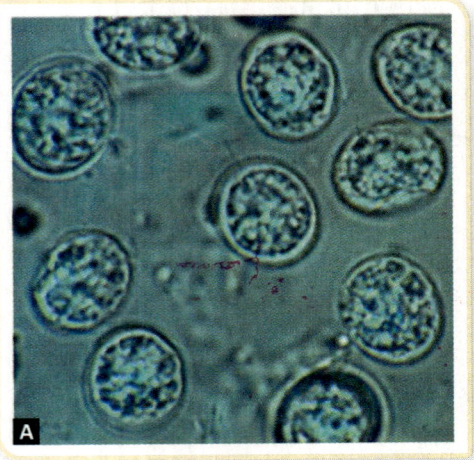

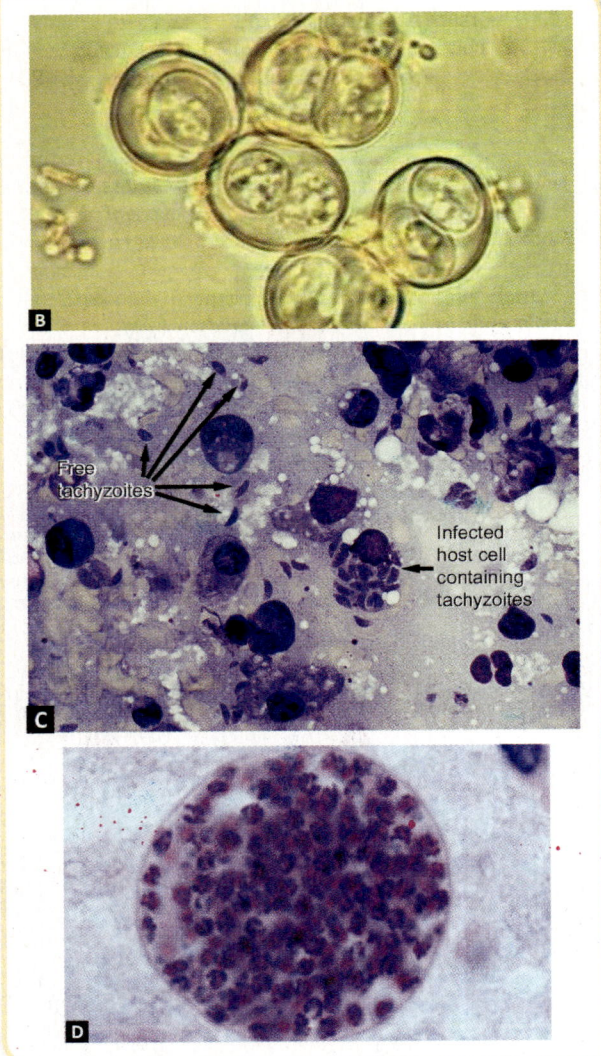

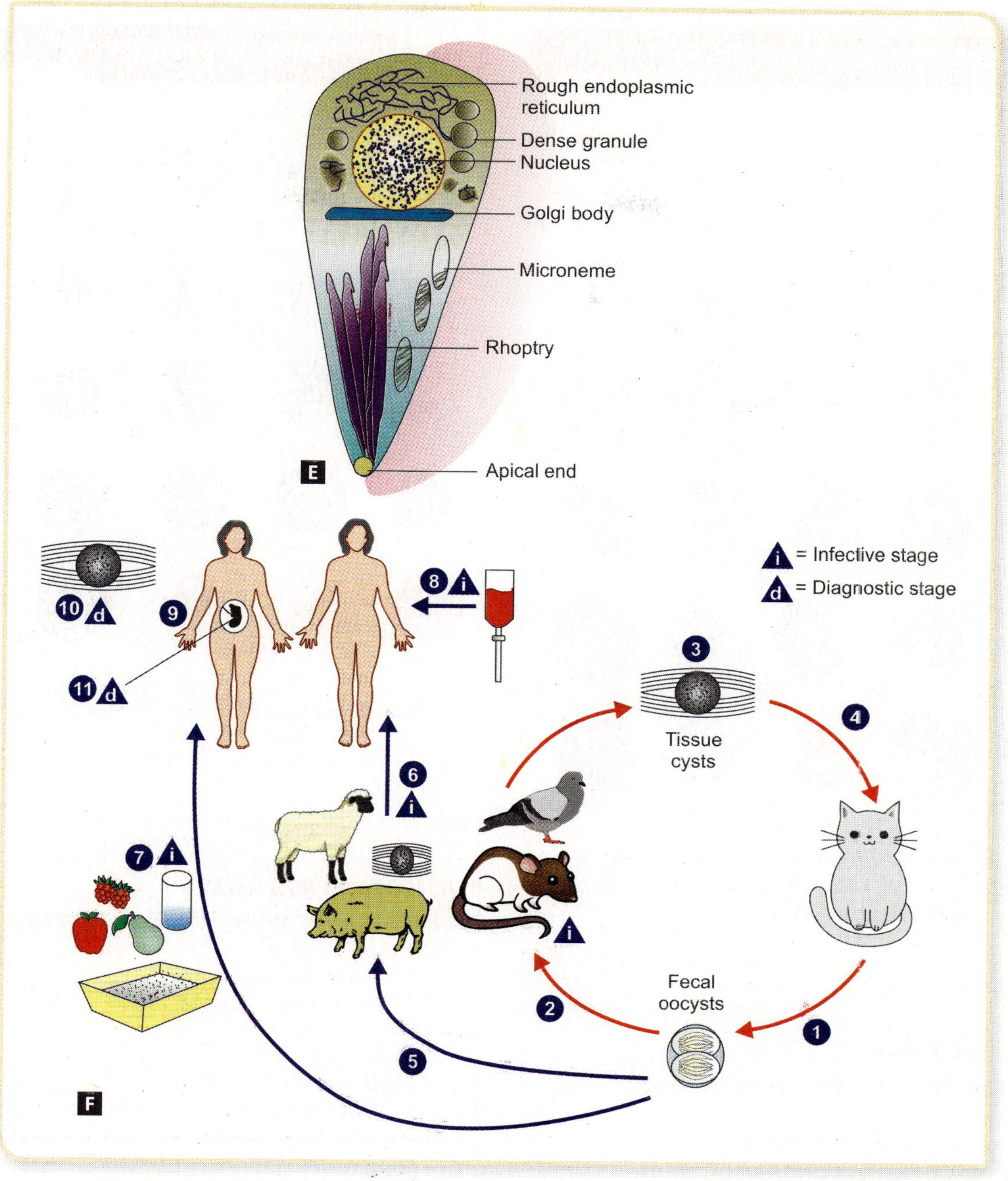

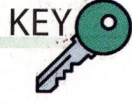

TOXOPLASMA GONDII (CILIATE)

A. ***T. gondii* oocysts unsporulated** in a fecal flotation. Oocysts are unsporulated when excreted in cat feces and usually require 48 to 74 hours to undergo sporulation in the external environment.
B. ***T. gondii* oocysts sporulated** contain two sporocysts, each of which contains four sporozoites.
C. ***T. gondii* tachyzoites** (crescent shaped, 2-3 μm wide by 4-8 μm long) both free tachyzoite and host cell infected with tachyzoites.
D. ***T. gondii* tissue cyst** in a mouse brain, individual bradyzoites can be seen within. Thousands of resting parasites (stained red) are enveloped by a thin parasite cyst wall.
E. *Toxoplasma gondi* tachyzoite diagrammatic representation.
F. ***Toxoplasma gondii* life cycle:** The only known definitive hosts for *Toxoplasma gondii* are cats. Unsporulated oocysts are shed in the cat's feces ❶. Although oocysts are usually only shed for 1-2 weeks, large numbers may be shed. Oocysts take 1-5 days to sporulate in the environment and become infective. Intermediate hosts in nature (including birds and rodents) become infected after ingesting soil, water or plant material contaminated with oocysts ❷. Oocysts transform into tachyzoites shortly after ingestion. These tachyzoites localize in neural and muscle tissue and develop into tissue cyst bradyzoites ❸. Cats become infected after consuming intermediate hosts harboring tissue cysts ❹. Cats may also become infected directly by ingestion of sporulated oocysts. Animals bred for human consumption and wild game may also become infected with tissue cysts after ingestion of sporulated oocysts in the environment ❺. Humans can become infected by any of several routes:

1. Eating uncooked meat of animals harboring tissue cysts ❻
2. Consuming food or water contaminated with cat feces ❼
3. Blood transfusion or organ transplantation ❽
4. Transplacentally from mother to fetus ❾

PARASITOLOGY PLATE 6

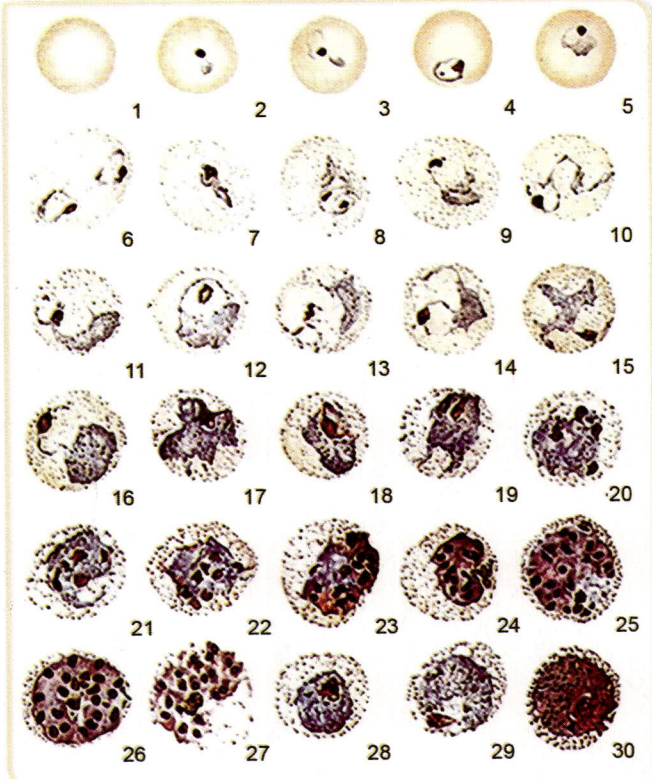

CDC Illustrations from: Coatney GR, Collins WE, Warren M, Contacos PG. The Primate Malarias. U.S. Department of Health, Education and Welfare, Bethesda, 1971

PLASMODIUM VIVAX
Blood Stage Parasites: Thin Blood Smears

Fig. 1: Normal red cell
Figs. 2-6: Young trophozoites (ring stage parasites)
Figs. 7-18: Trophozoites
Figs. 19-27: Schizonts
Figs. 28 and 29: Macrogametocytes (female)
Fig. 30: Microgametocyte (male)

PARASITOLOGY PLATE 7

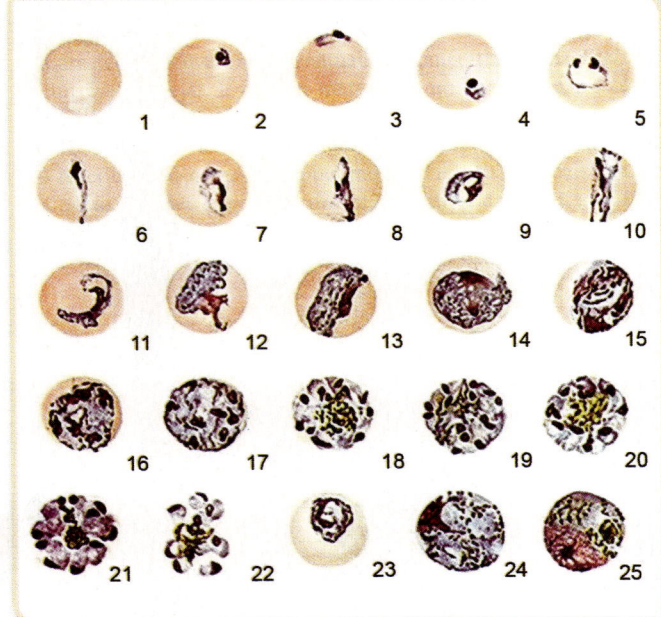

CDC Illustrations from: Coatney GR, Collins WE, Warren M, Contacos PG. The Primate Malarias. U.S. Department of Health, Education and Welfare, Bethesda, 1971

PLASMODIUM MALARIAE
Blood Stage Parasites: Thin Blood Smears

Fig. 1: Normal red cell
Figs. 2-5: Young trophozoites (rings)
Figs. 6-13: Trophozoites
Figs. 14-22: Schizonts
Fig. 23: Developing gametocyte
Fig. 24: Macrogametocyte (female)
Fig. 25: Microgametocyte (male)

PARASITOLOGY PLATE 8

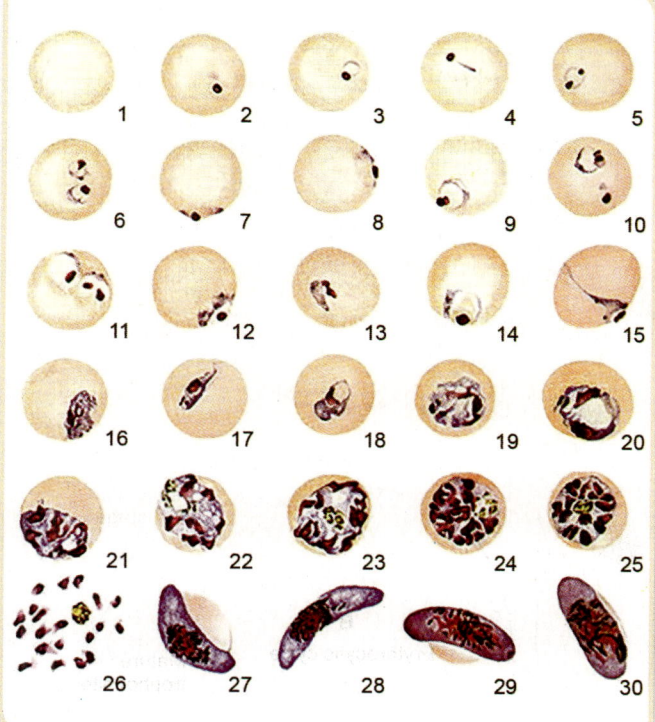

CDC Illustrations from: Coatney GR, Collins WE, Warren M, Contacos PG. The Primate Malarias. U.S. Department of Health, Education and Welfare, Bethesda, 1971

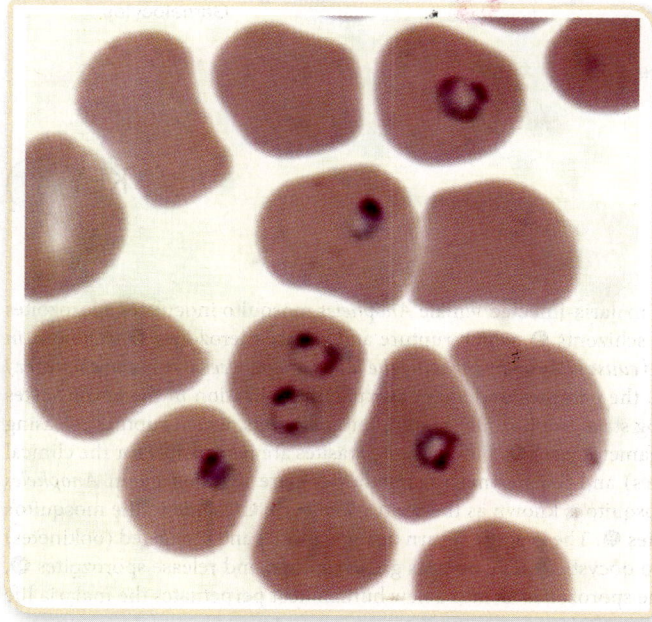

Source: CDC

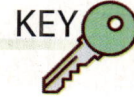 KEY

PLASMODIUM FALCIPARUM
Blood Stage Parasites: Thin Blood Smears (Total 30)

Fig. 1: Normal red cell
Figs. 2-18: Trophozoites (among these, Figs. 2-10 correspond to ring-stage trophozoites; as shown in Fig B^{NEETPG})
Figs. 19-26: Schizonts (Fig. 26 is a ruptured schizont)
Figs. 27, 28: Mature macrogametocytes (female); **Banana shaped**
Figs. 29, 30: Mature microgametocytes (male); **Banana shaped**

PARASITOLOGY PLATE 9

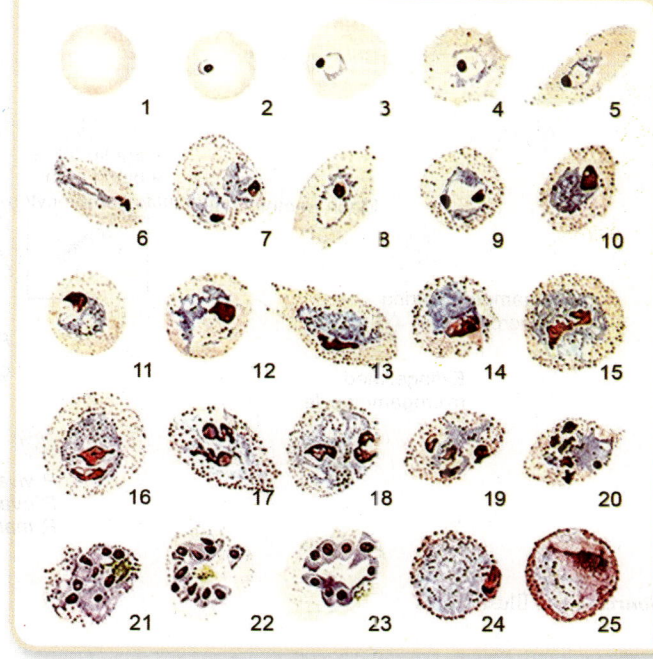

CDC Illustrations from: Coatney GR, Collins WE, Warren M, Contacos PG. The Primate Malarias. U.S. Department of Health, Education and Welfare, Bethesda, 1971

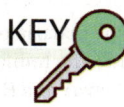 KEY

PLASMODIUM OVALE
Blood Stage Parasites: Thin Blood Smears

Fig. 1: Normal red cell
Figs. 2-5: Young trophozoites (Rings)
Figs. 6-15: Trophozoites
Figs. 16-23: Schizonts
Fig. 24: Macrogametocytes (female)
Fig. 25: Microgametocyte (male)

PARASITOLOGY PLATE 10

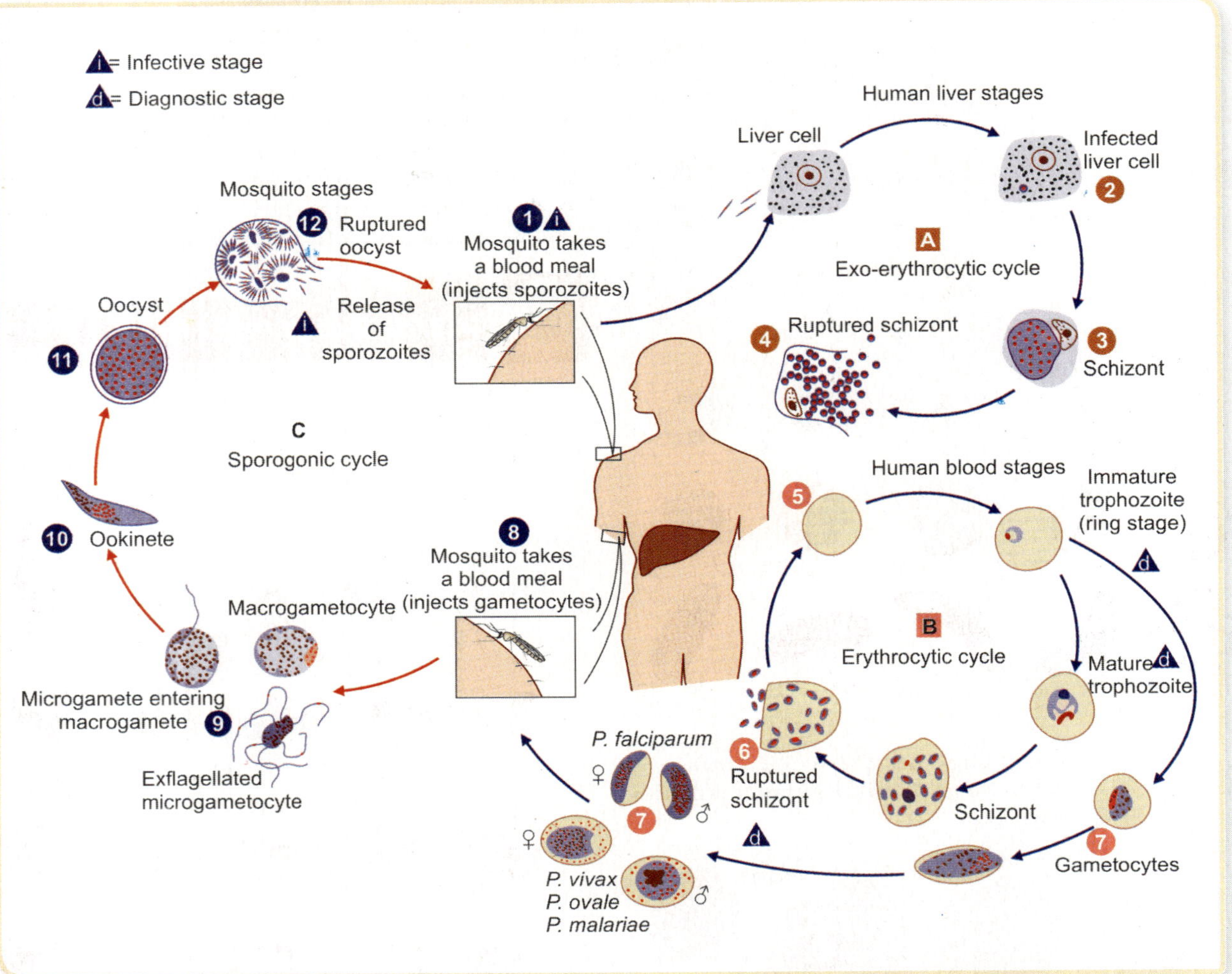

LIFE CYCLE OF MALARIA PARASITE (PLASMODIUM)

The malaria parasite life cycle involves two hosts. During a blood meal, a malaria-infected female *Anopheles* mosquito inoculates sporozoites into the human host ❶. Sporozoites infect liver cells ❷ and mature into schizonts ❸, which rupture and release merozoites ❹. (Of note, in *P. vivax* and *P. ovale* a dormant stage [hypnozoites] can persist in the liver and cause relapses by invading the bloodstream weeks, or even years later.) After this initial replication in the liver (exo-erythrocytic schizogony **A**), the parasites undergoes asexual multiplication in the erythrocytes (erythrocytic schizogony **B**). Merozoites infect red blood cells ❺. The ring stage trophozoites mature into schizonts, which rupture releasing merozoites. Some parasites differentiate into sexual erythrocytic stages (gametocytes) ❼. Blood stage parasites are responsible for the clinical manifestations of the disease. The gametocytes, male (microgametocytes) and female (macrogametocytes), are ingested by an *Anopheles* mosquito during a blood meal ❽. The parasites' multiplication in the mosquito is known as the sporogonic cycle **C**. While in the mosquito's stomach, the microgametes penetrate the macrogametes generating zygotes ❾. The zygotes in turn become motile and elongated (ookinetes) ❿ which invade the midgut wall of the mosquito where they develop into oocysts ⓫. The oocysts grow, rupture, and release sporozoites ⓬, which make their way to the mosquito's salivary glands. Inoculation of the sporozoites ❶ into a new human host perpetuates the malaria life cycle.

Characteristic Features of the Malaria Parasite (Romanowsky-Stained Preparations)

	P vivax (Benign Tertian Malaria)	*P malariae* (Quartan Malaria)	*P falciparum* (Malignant Tertian Malaria)	*P ovale* (Ovale Malaria)
Parasitized red cells	Enlarged, pale. Fine stippling (**Schüffner's dots**). Primarily invades reticulocytes, young red cells.	Not enlarged. No stippling (except with special stains). Primarily invades older red cells.	Not enlarged. Coarse stippling (**Maurer's clefts**). Invades all red cells regardless of age.	Enlarged, pale. **Schüffner's dots** conspicuous. Cells often oval, fimbriated, or crenated.
Level of usual maximum parasitemia	Up to 30,000/µL of blood.	Fewer than 10,000/µL.	May exceed 200,000/µL; commonly 50,000/µL.	Fewer than 10,000/µL.
Ring stage trophozoites	Large rings (1/3–1/2 red cell diameter). Usually one chromatin granule; ring delicate.	Large rings (1/3 red cell diameter). Usually one chromatin granule; ring thick.	Small rings (1/5 red cell diameter). Often two granules; multiple infections common; ring delicate, may adhere to red cells.	Large rings (1/3 red cell diameter). Usually one chromatin granule; ring thick.
Pigment in developing trophozoites	Fine; light brown; scattered.	Coarse; dark brown; scattered clumps; abundant.	Coarse; black; few clumps.	Coarse; dark yellow-brown; scattered.
Older trophozoites	Very pleomorphic.	Occasional band forms.	Compact and rounded.	Compact and rounded.
Mature schizonts (segmenters)	More than 12 merozoites (14–24).	Fewer than 12 large merozoites (6–12). Often in rosette.	Very rare in peripheral blood except in severe cases. When seen, schizonts contain anywhere from 8-24 merozoites (usually > 12). A mature schizont usually fills about 2/3 of the infected RBC.	Fewer than 12 large merozoites (6–12). Often in rosette.
Gametocytes	Round or oval.	Round or oval.	Crescentic or sausage shaped, about 1.5 times the diameter of RBC in length. Sometimes in thin blood smears, the remnants of the host RBC can be seen; this is often referred to as **Laveran's bib**.	Round or oval.
Distribution in peripheral blood	All forms.	All forms.	Only rings and crescents (gametocytes).	All forms.
Length of Sexual Cycle (Mosquito at 27°C)	8–9 days	15–20 days	9–10 days	14 days
Prepatent Period (in Humans) (Preerythrocytic Cycle)	8 days	15–16 days	5–7 days	9 days
Length of Asexual Cycle (in Humans)	48 hours	72 hours	36-48 hours	48 hours

PARASITOLOGY PLATE 11

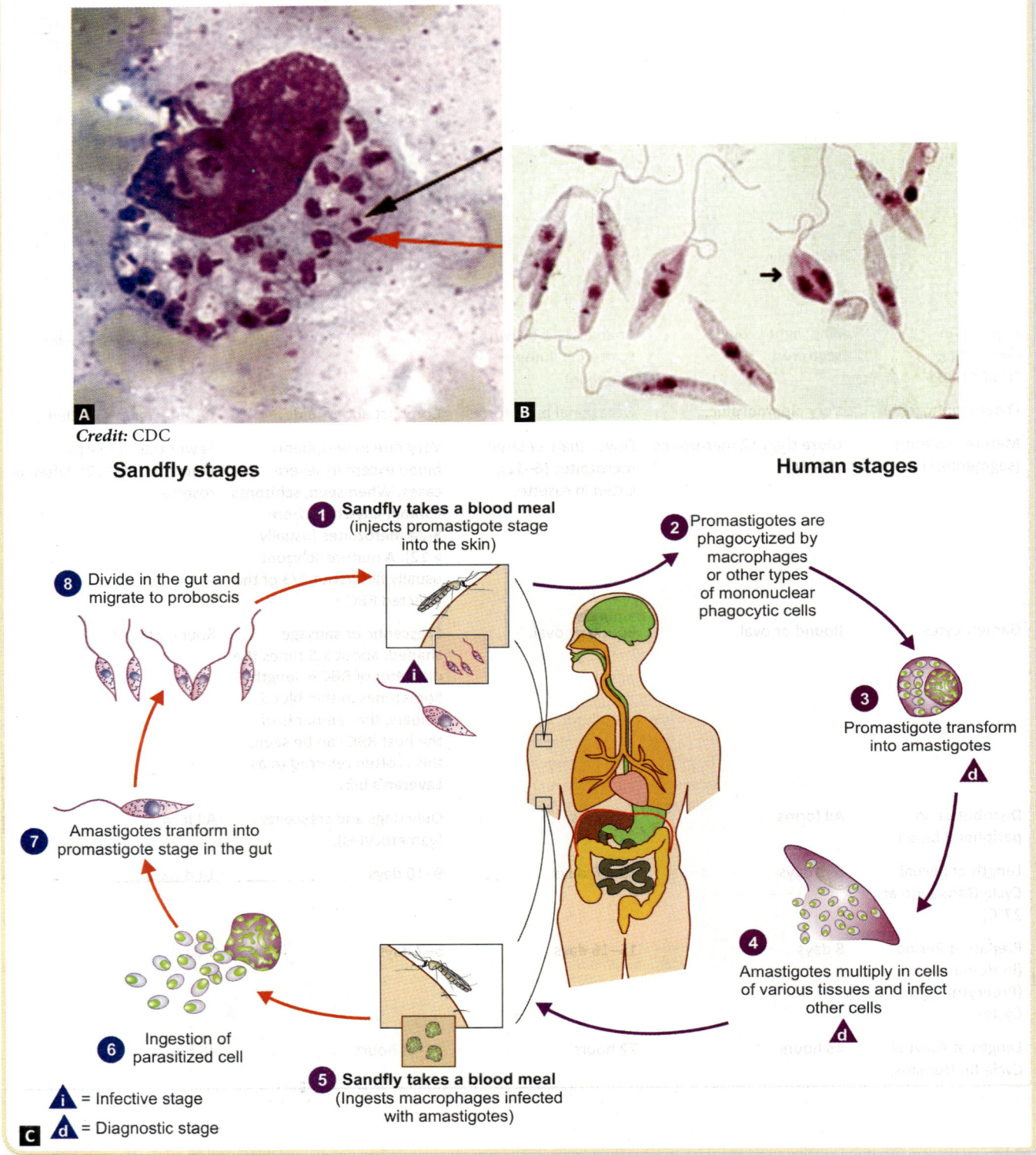

Credit: CDC

PLATE LEGENDS

A. Light-microscopic examination of a stained bone marrow specimen from a patient with visceral leishmaniasis—Showing a macrophage containing multiple Leishmania amastigotes (the tissue stage of the parasite). Note that each amastigote has a nucleus (red arrow) and a rod-shaped kinetoplast (black arrow).

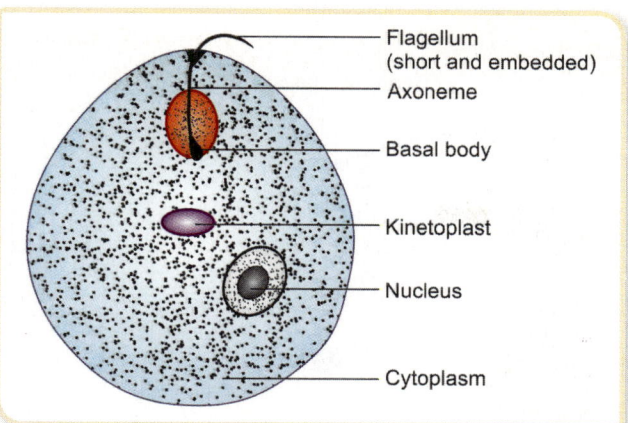

Fig: Leishmania amastigote form

B. Promastigotes of Leishmania: Promastigotes are characterized by a flagellum and a kinetoplast anterior to the nucleus. They are the infective stage to humans. Note the multiplication by longitudinal binary fission (arrow) that occurs naturally in the gut of sandfly vectors.

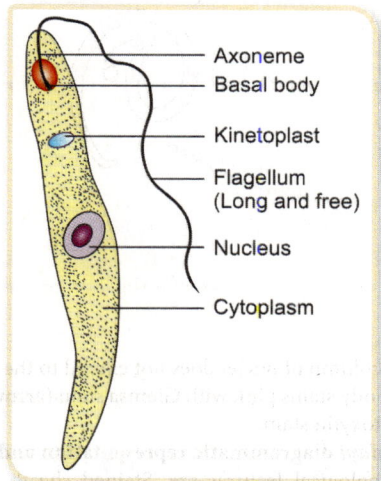

Fig: Leishmania promastigote form

C. Leishmania life cycle: Leishmaniasis is transmitted by the bite of infected female phlebotomine sand flies. The sand flies inject the infective stage (i.e., promastigotes) from their proboscis during blood meals ❶. Promastigotes that reach the puncture wound are phagocytized by macrophages ❷ and other types of mononuclear phagocytic cells. Promastigotes transform in these cells into the tissue stage of the parasite (i.e., amastigotes) ❸, which multiply by simple division and proceed to infect other mononuclear phagocytic cells ❹. Parasite, host, and other factors affect whether the infection becomes symptomatic and whether cutaneous or visceral leishmaniasis results. Sand flies become infected by ingesting infected cells during blood meals (❺, ❻). In sand flies, amastigotes transform into promastigotes, develop in the gut ❼ and migrate to the proboscis ❽

PARASITOLOGY PLATE 12

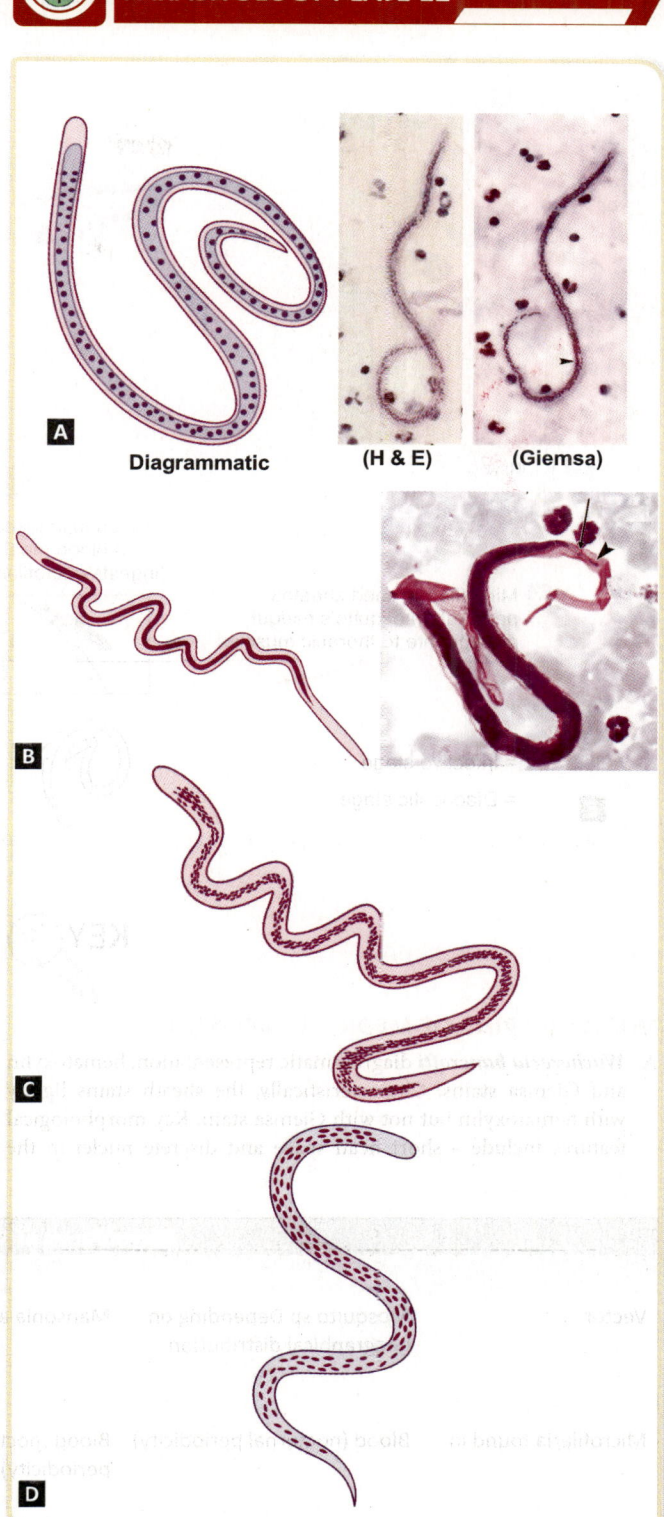

85

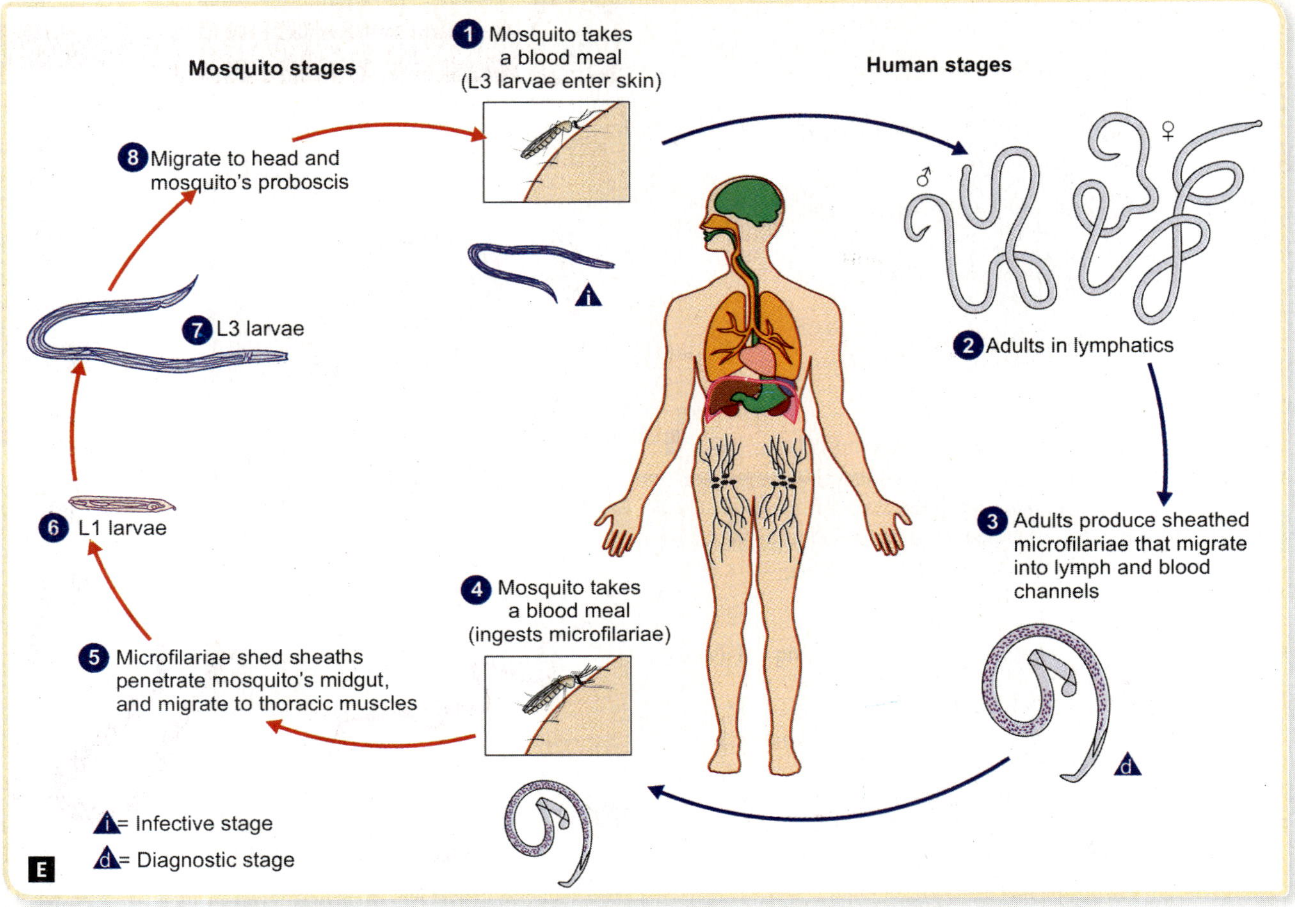

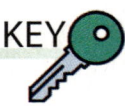

KEY

MICROFILARIAS OF MEDICAL IMPORTANCE

A. **Wuchereria bancrofti** diagrammatic representation, hematoxylin and Giemsa stains. Characteristically, the sheath stains lightly with hematoxylin but not with Giemsa stain. Key morphological features include a short head space and discrete nuclei in the body. The column of nuclei does not extend to the end of the tail. The innerbody stains pink with Giemsa stain (arrowhead) but not with hematoxylin stain.

B. **Brugia malayi** diagrammatic representation and Giemsa stain. Key morphological features are, Stained sheath, long cephalic space, compact nuclei in body, terminal nuclei (arrowhead) and subterminal nuclei (arrow). Life cycle is similar to W. bancrofti

C. **Loa loa** diagrammatic representation

D. **Onchocerca volvulus** diagrammatic representation

	Microfilarias of Medical Importance			
	A. Wuchereria bancrofti	**B. Brugia malayi**	**C. Loa Loa**	**D. Onchocerca volvulus**
Vector	Mosquito sp Depending on geographical distribution	Mansonia and Aedes	Deerflies (also known as mango flies or mangrove flies) of the genus Chrysops	Blackflies of the genus Simulium
Microfilaria found in	Blood (nocturnal periodicity)	Blood (nocturnal periodicity)	Blood (Diurnal)	**Tissue** (skin) (No periodicity, sample can be collected ay time)
Sheath	Present (unstained with hematoxylin, stains pale pink on giemsa)	Present (stains pink red on giemsa, unstained on hematoxylin), loose sheath with kinky curves	Present (stained pink with hematoxylin but unstained on giemsa)	Absent
Head space	Length = width (free of nuclei)	*Twice as long as width* (long head/cephalic space)	Short cephalic/head space	*Long head space*
Body	Smooth/Sweeping graceful curves	Folded in angular fashion	Irregular curves with **corkscrew appearance**	Long body with less curves

Contd...

Microfilarias of Medical Importance				
	A. Wuchereria bancrofti	**B. Brugia malayi**	**C. Loa Loa**	**D. Onchocerca volvulus**
Body Nuclei	Well separated/dispersed yet numerous	Crowded and darkly stained	Coarse and crowded (**single row of nuclei** till the end of tail)	Well-marked, moderately compact nuclei and elongated terminal nuclei.
Interbody (amorphous mass seen in some sp)	**Stained pink with giemsa** but not stained with Hematoxylin	Not easily identified	Not easily identified	Not easily identified
Cytoplasm	Cytoplasm extends beyond the last nuclei	Terminal nuclei	Terminal nuclei (are irregularly spaced)	Cytoplasm extend beyond the last nuclei
Tail	Taper, Anucleate	Tapers, **Subterminal and terminal nuclei** (2 nuclei that appears connected by fine thread)	Taper, Nuclei irregularly spaced to extend to the tip of tail. Tail is sometimes flexed/coiled within the sheath.	Tapers to a sharp point, **typically flexed**, Anucleate

Microfilariae are found in peripheral blood (in blood smear) only at night (nocturnal periodicity), largely at night or during crepuscular hours (subperiodicity), largely during daylight hours (diurnal periodicity), or without clear distinction (nonperiodic).

E. **Life cycle of *W. bancrofti* filariasis:** (With permission from CDC) During a blood meal, an infected mosquito introduces third-stage filarial larvae onto the skin of the human host, where they penetrate into the bite wound ❶. They develop in adults that commonly reside in the lymphatics ❷. Adults produce microfilariae, which are sheathed and have nocturnal periodicity, except the South Pacific microfilariae which have the absence of marked periodicity. The microfilariae migrate into lymph and blood channels moving actively through lymph and blood ❸. A mosquito ingests the microfilariae during a blood meal ❹. After ingestion, the microfilariae lose their sheaths and some of them work their way through the wall of the proventriculus and cardiac portion of the mosquito's midgut and reach the thoracic muscles ❺. There the microfilariae develop into first-stage larvae ❻ and subsequently into third-stage infective larvae ❼. The third-stage infective larvae migrate through the hemocoel to the mosquito's proboscis ❽ and can infect another human when the mosquito takes a blood meal ❶.

PARASITOLOGY PLATE 13

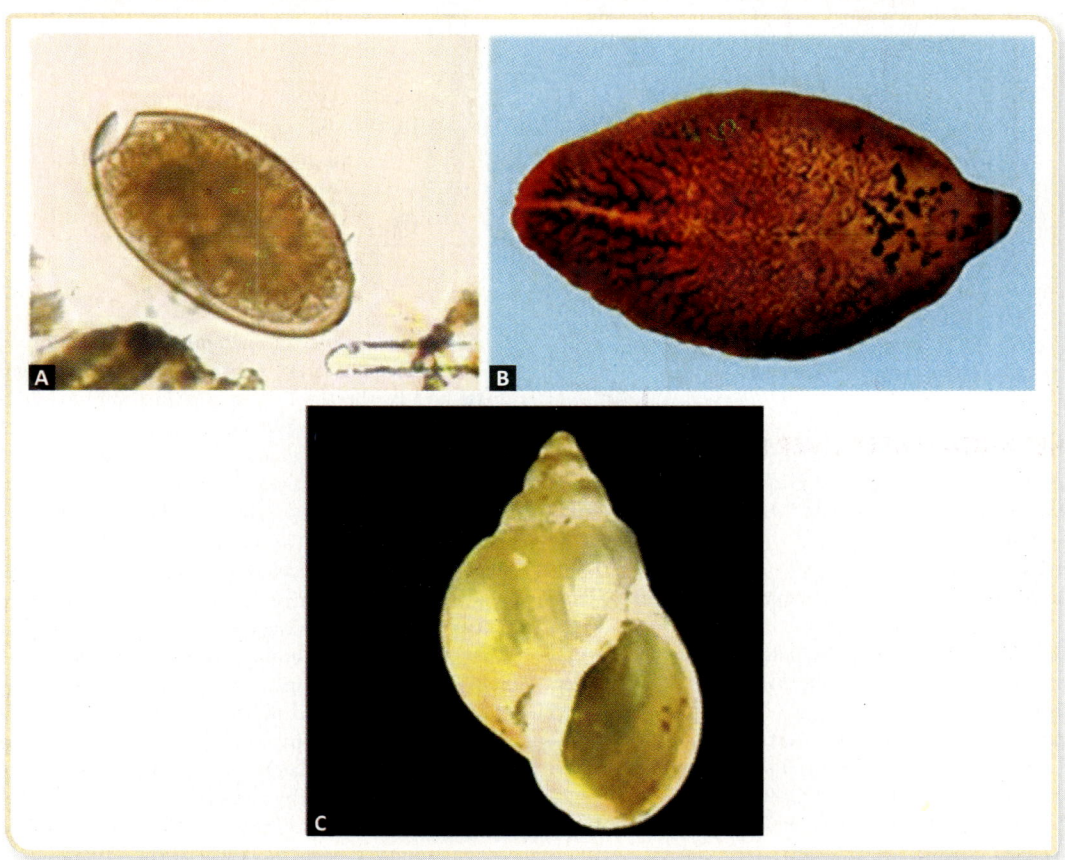

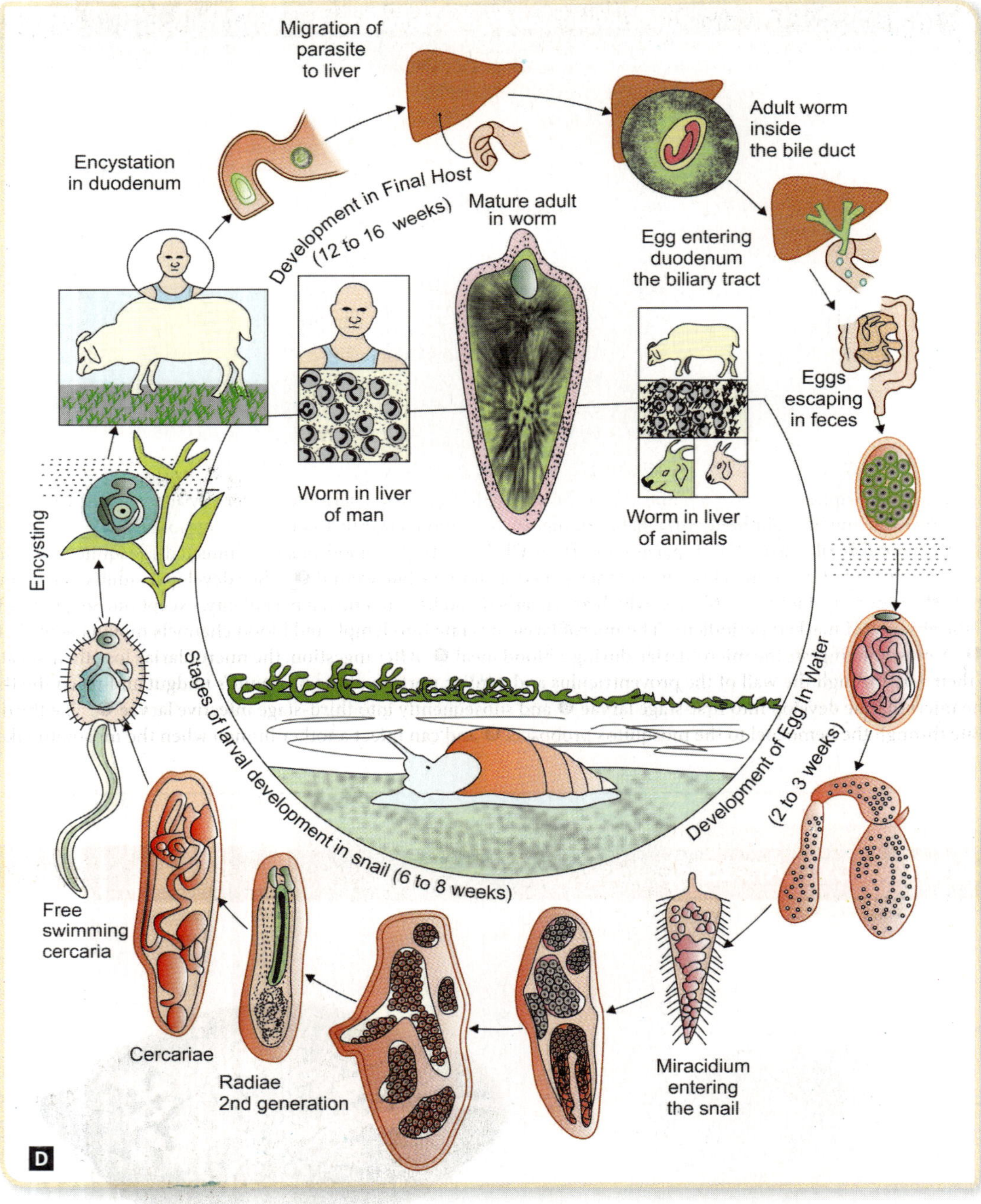

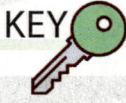

FASCIOLA HEPATICA (SHEEP LIVER FLUKE)

Disease: Fascioliasis is a parasitic infection typically caused by *Fasciola hepatica*, which is also known as "the common liver fluke" or "the sheep liver fluke."
Reservoir host: Sheep, cattle, humans
Mode of transmission: Ingestion of contaminated aquatic plants (watercress)
Progression in Humans: Cysts germinate in duodenum, exit through wall into liver, and proceed to bile ducts, where they mature; eggs enter feces in bile.

A. *Fasciola hepatica* egg in an unstained wet mount (400 × magnification). F. hepatica eggs are broadly ellipsoidal, operculated on one end, and measure 130-150 μm by 60-90 μm.
B. Adult *Fasciola hepatica* fluke stained with carmine (30 mm by 13 mm).
C. *Fossaria bulamoides*, a snail host for *F. hepatica*
D. **Life cycle:** Immature *Fasciola* **eggs** are discharged in the biliary ducts and in the stool. Eggs become embryonated in water, eggs release **miracidia**, which invade a suitable snail intermediate host, including the genera *Galba*, *Fossaria* and *Pseudosuccinea*. In the snail, the parasites undergo several developmental stages (sporocysts, rediae, and cercariae). The **cercariae** are released from the snail and encyst as **metacercariae** on aquatic vegetation or other surfaces. Mammals acquire the infection by eating vegetation containing metacercariae. Humans can become infected by ingesting metacercariae-containing freshwater plants, especially watercress. After ingestion, the metacercariae excyst in the duodenum and migrate through the intestinal wall, the peritoneal cavity, and the liver parenchyma into the biliary ducts, where they develop into adult **flukes**. In humans, maturation from **metacercariae** into **adult flukes** takes approximately 3 to 4 months. The adult flukes (*Fasciola hepatica*: up to 30 mm by 13 mm; *F. gigantica*: up to 75 mm) reside in the large biliary ducts of the mammalian host. *Fasciola hepatica* infect various animal species, mostly herbivores (plant-eating animals).

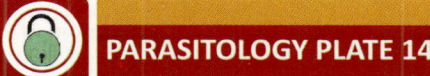

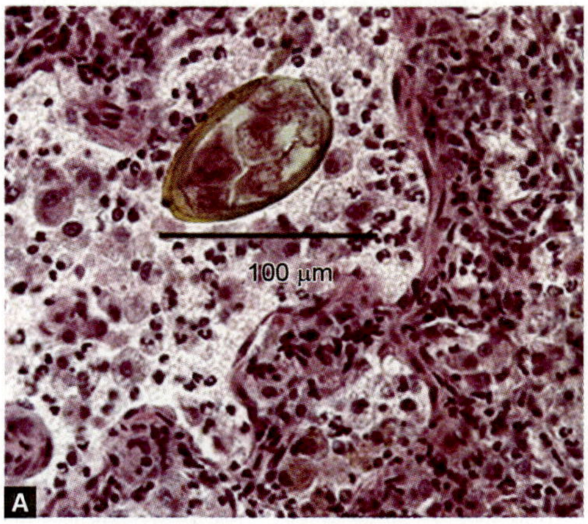

PARASITOLOGY PLATE 14

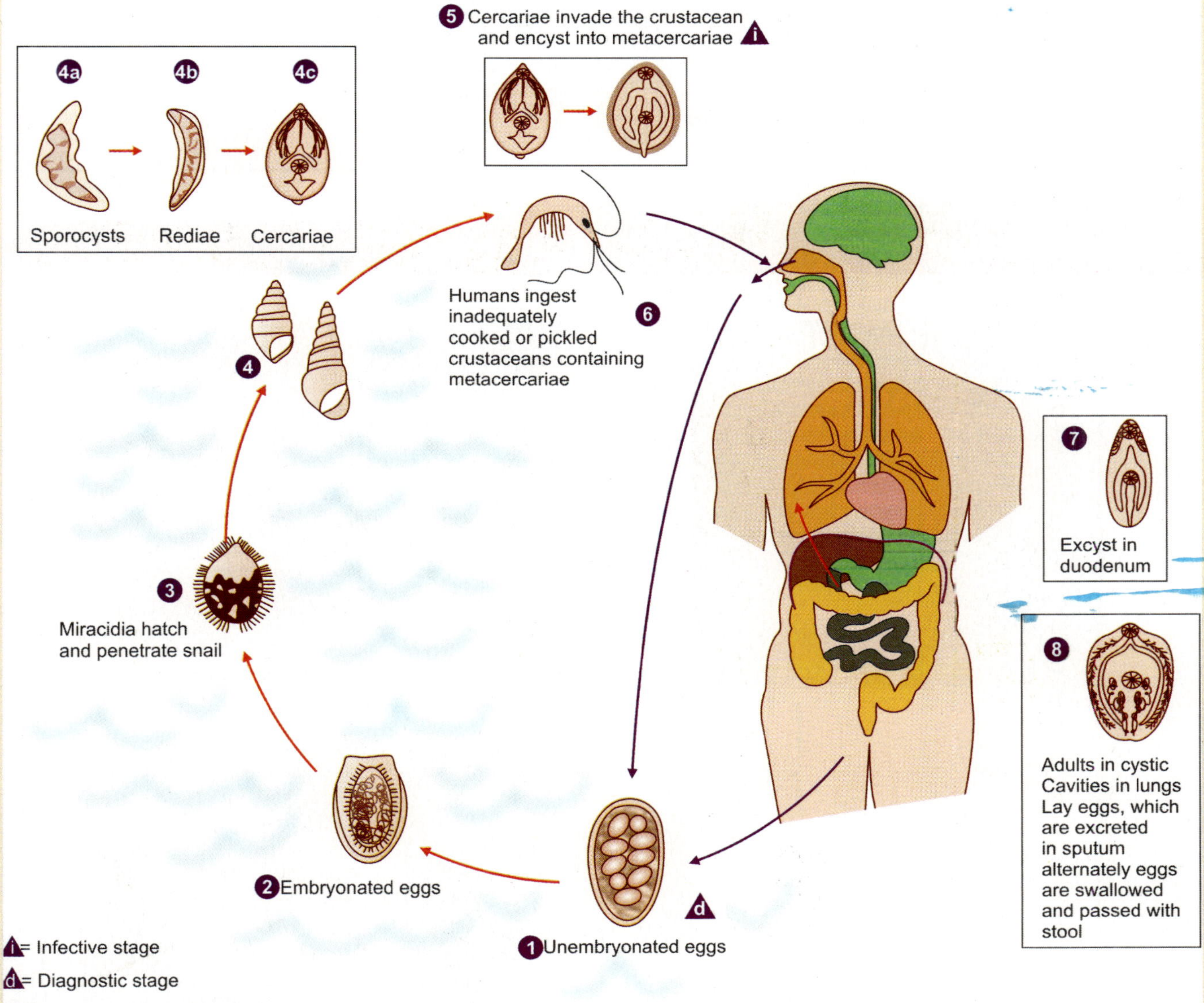

KEY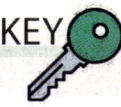

PLATE LEGENDS

A. **Paragonimus Cyst**: The pathologic lesions of paragonimiasis may be due to invasion and migration by the worms and host's immune responses to the invading parasites.
- The basic pathology is the formation of a worm cyst primarily in the **lungs.** Usually located superficially, sometimes deep in the lung parenchyma contained dark red or rusty brown viscous fluid, red blood cells, inflammatory cells, eosinophils, necrotic tissue, Charcot-Leyden crystals, and adult worms and ova.
- The adult worms are usually found at the periphery of the cyst, adhered to the cyst wall. Generally, a cyst contained paired worms, but single or more than two worms of the same or different species may be found.
- The cyst is communicated with bronchioles through which the cystic fluid, including the ova is discharged in the sputum to the exterior environment. If the sputum is swallowed as in case of young children, the ova can be detected in the feces.
- *Histopathologically, the worm cyst is composed of an outer fibro collagenous cyst wall with focal hemosiderin laden macrophages and an inner layer of congested blood vessels, inflammatory cells and normal or distorted ova.*
- The size of the egg, approximately 85 micrometers, which was in the size range for Paragonimus spp. eggs.
- The presence of an **operculum.** This feature eliminates other helminth eggs in the same size range, Trichostrongylus, Ascaris (infertile), and Schistosoma japonicum.
- Location (lung tissue) where the eggs were found.

B. **Life Cycle of Paragonimus:** The eggs are excreted unembryonated in the sputum, or alternately they are swallowed and passed with stool❶. In the external environment, the eggs become embryonated ❷, and miracidia hatch and seek the first intermediate host, a snail, and penetrate its soft tissues ❸. Miracidia go through several developmental stages inside the snail ❹: sporocysts ❹a, rediae ❹b, with the latter giving rise to many cercariae ❹c, which emerge from the snail. The cercariae invade the second intermediate host, a crustacean such as a crab or crayfish, where they encyst and become metacercariae. This is the infective stage for the mammalian host ❺. Human infection with *P. westermani* occurs by eating inadequately cooked or pickled crab or crayfish that harbor metacercariae of the parasite ❻. The metacercariae excyst in the duodenum ❼, penetrate through the intestinal wall into the peritoneal cavity, then through the abdominal wall and diaphragm into the lungs, where they become encapsulated and develop into adults ❽ (7.5 to 12 mm by 4 to 6 mm). The worms can also reach other organs and tissues, such as the brain and striated muscles, respectively. However, when this takes place completion of the life cycles is not achieved, because the eggs laid cannot exit these sites. Time from infection to oviposition is 65 to 90 days.

PARASITOLOGY PLATE 15

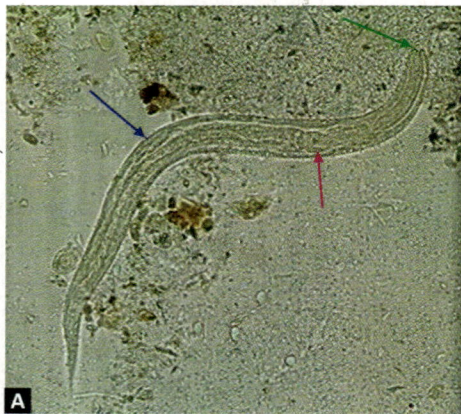

A
Source: CDC

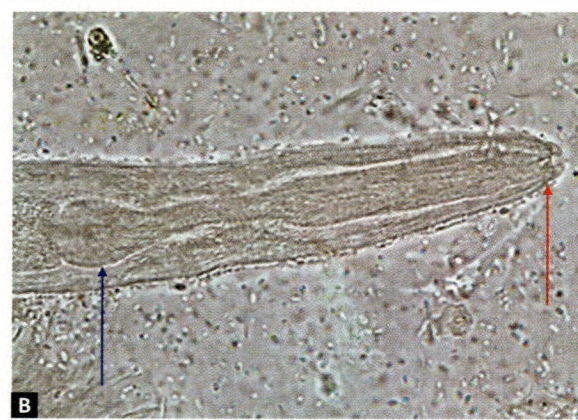

B
Source: CDC

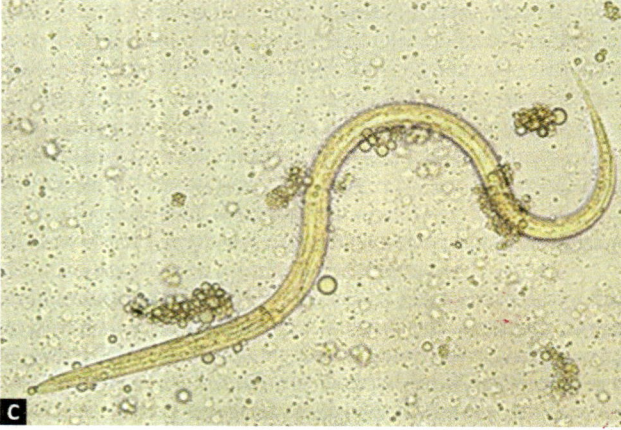

C
Source: CDC

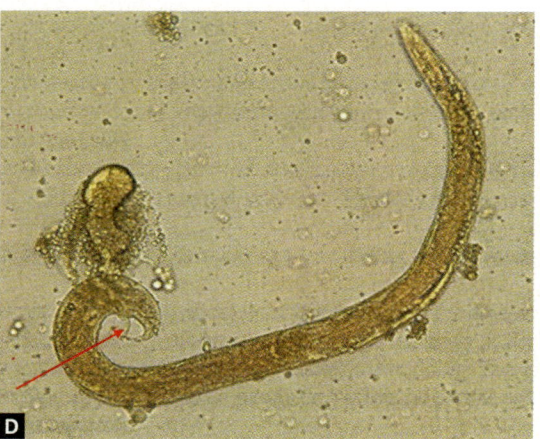

D
Source: CDC

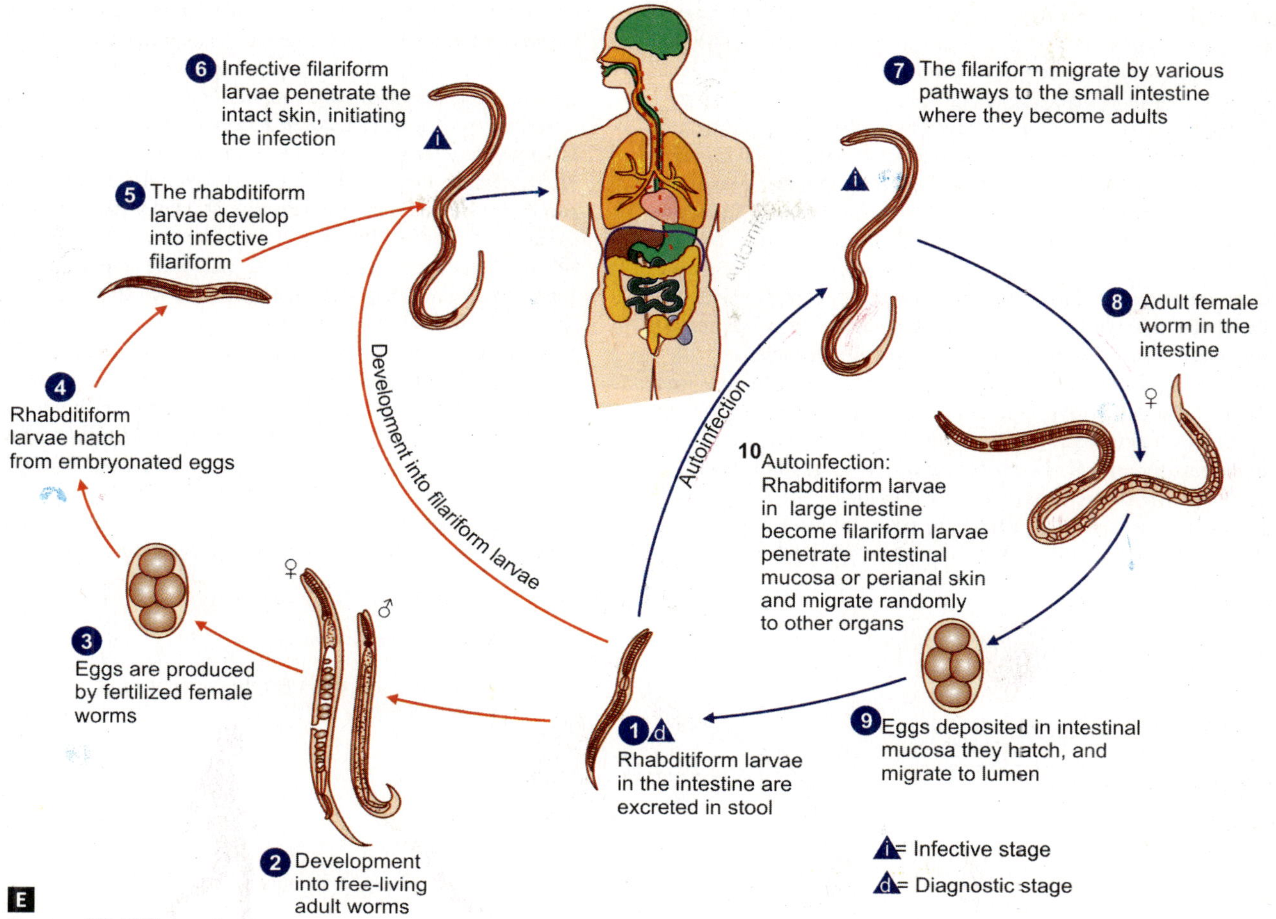

KEY

STRONGYLOIDES

A. Strongyloides stercoralis first-stage rhabditiform (L1) larvae: The first-stage rhabditiform larvae (L1) of Strongyloides stercoralis are 180-380 μm long, with a short buccal canal, a rhabditoid esophagus and a prominent genital primordium. These L1 larvae are usually found in stool, as the eggs embryonate and hatch in the mucosa of the small intestine of the host. Rhabditiform larva of S. stercoralis in an unstained wet mount of stool. Notice the prominent genital primordium (blue arrow), rhabditoid esophagus (red arrow) and short buccal canal (green arrow).

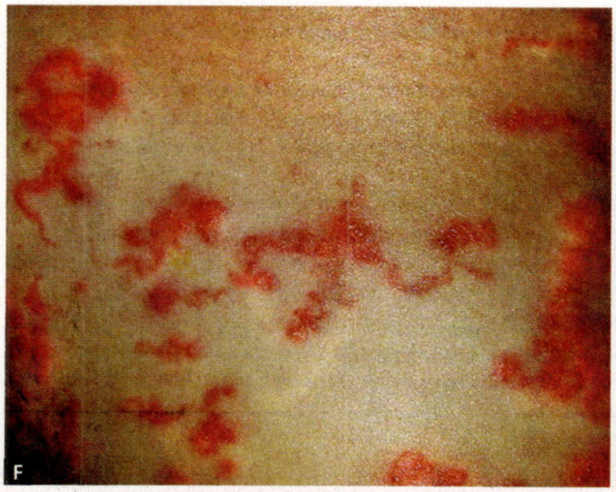

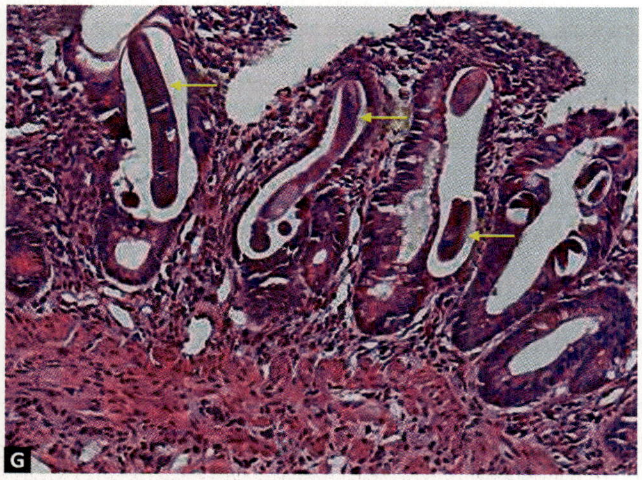

B. Close-up of the anterior end of a rhabditiform larva of S. stercoralis, showing the short buccal canal (red arrow) and the rhabditoid esophagus (blue arrow). (Image is taken at 1000x oil magnification).

C. Strongyloides stercoralis third-stage filariform (L3) larvae: Infective, third-stage filariform larvae (L3) of Strongyloides stercoralis are up to 600 μm long. The tail is notched and the esophagus to intestine ratio is 1:1. Infective L3 larvae are found in soil and invade the human host by direct penetration of the skin. They may be found in respiratory specimens during cases of autoinfection.

D. **Strongyloides stercoralis free-living adults:** Adults of Strongyloides stercoralis may be found in the human host or soil. In the human host there are no parasitic males, and parasitic females are long, slender and measure 2.0-3.0 mm in length. In the environment, rhabditiform larvae may develop into infective filariform (L3) larvae (direct cycle) or free-living adults that contain both males and females (indirect cycle). Free-living adult males measure up to 750 μm long; free-living females measure up to 1.0 mm long. Free-living adult male *S. Stercoralis* is identified by presence of the spicule (red arrow).

E. **Life cycle of strongyloides:** The *Strongyloides* life cycle is more complex than that of most nematodes with its alternation between free-living and parasitic cycles, and its potential for autoinfection and multiplication within the host. Two types of cycles exist:

Free-living cycle: The rhabditiform larvae passed in the stool ❶(see "Parasitic cycle" below) can either become infective filariform larvae (direct development) ❺ or free living adult males and females ❷ that mate and produce eggs ❸ from which rhabditiform larvae hatch ❹. and eventually become infective filariform larvae ❺. The filariform larvae penetrate the human host skin to initiate the parasitic cycle (see below) ❻.

Parasitic cycle: Filariform larvae in contaminated soil penetrate the human skin ❻, and by various, often random routes, migrate into the small intestine ❼. Historically it was believed that the L3 larvae migrate via the bloodstream to the lungs, where they are eventually coughed up and swallowed. However, there is also evidence that L3 larvae can migrate directly to the intestine via connective tissues. In the small intestine they molt twice and become adult female worms ❽. The females live threaded in the epithelium of the small intestine and by parthenogenesis produce eggs ❾, which yield rhabditiform larvae. The rhabditiform larvae can either be passed in the stool ❶ (see "Free-living cycle" above), or can cause autoinfection ❿. In autoinfection, the rhabditiform larvae become infective filariform larvae, which can penetrate either the intestinal mucosa (internal autoinfection) or the skin of the perianal area (external autoinfection); in either case, the filariform larvae may disseminate throughout the body. To date, occurrence of autoinfection in humans with helminthic infections is recognized only in *Strongyloides stercoralis* and *Capillaria philippinensis* infections. In the case of *Strongyloides*, autoinfection may explain the possibility of persistent infections for many years in persons who have not been in an endemic area and of hyperinfections in immunosuppressed individuals.

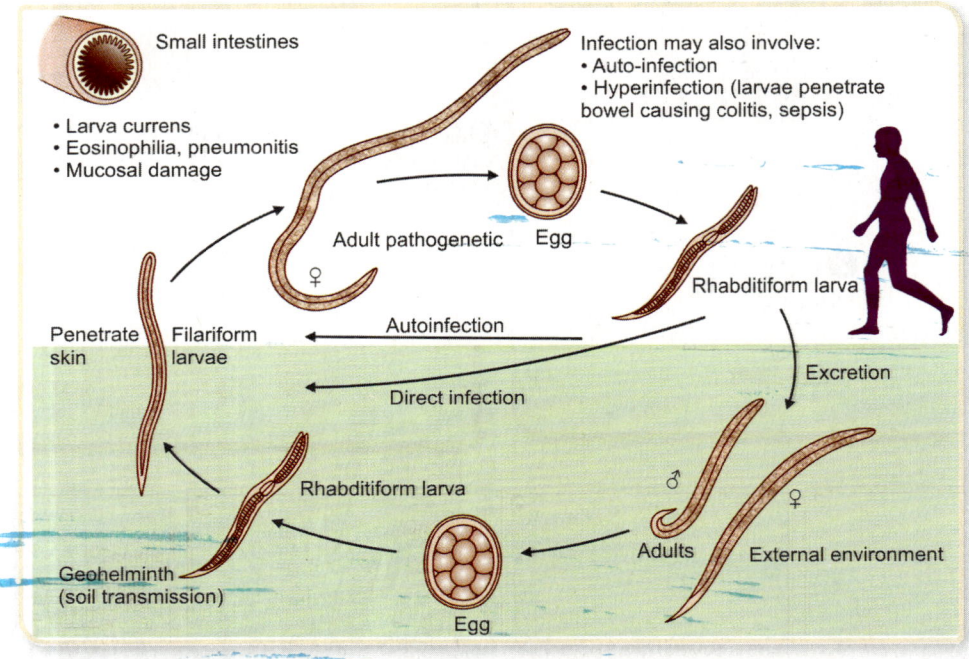

F. Strongyloides larva under the skin (**Cutaneous larva migrans**)^AIIMSPG
Note: Common causes of Cutaneous larva migrans are Ancylostoma, Strongloides, Loa Loa, Fasciola, Paragonimus
G. Duodenal biopsy showing Strongyloides stercoralis larval infection in the mucosal crypts (arrow) (HE).

PARASITOLOGY PLATE 16

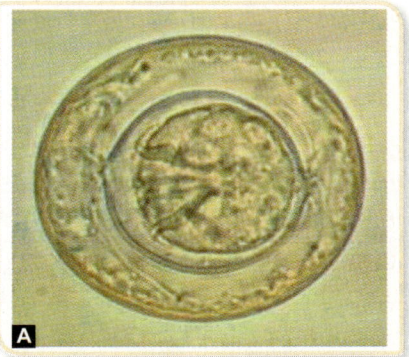

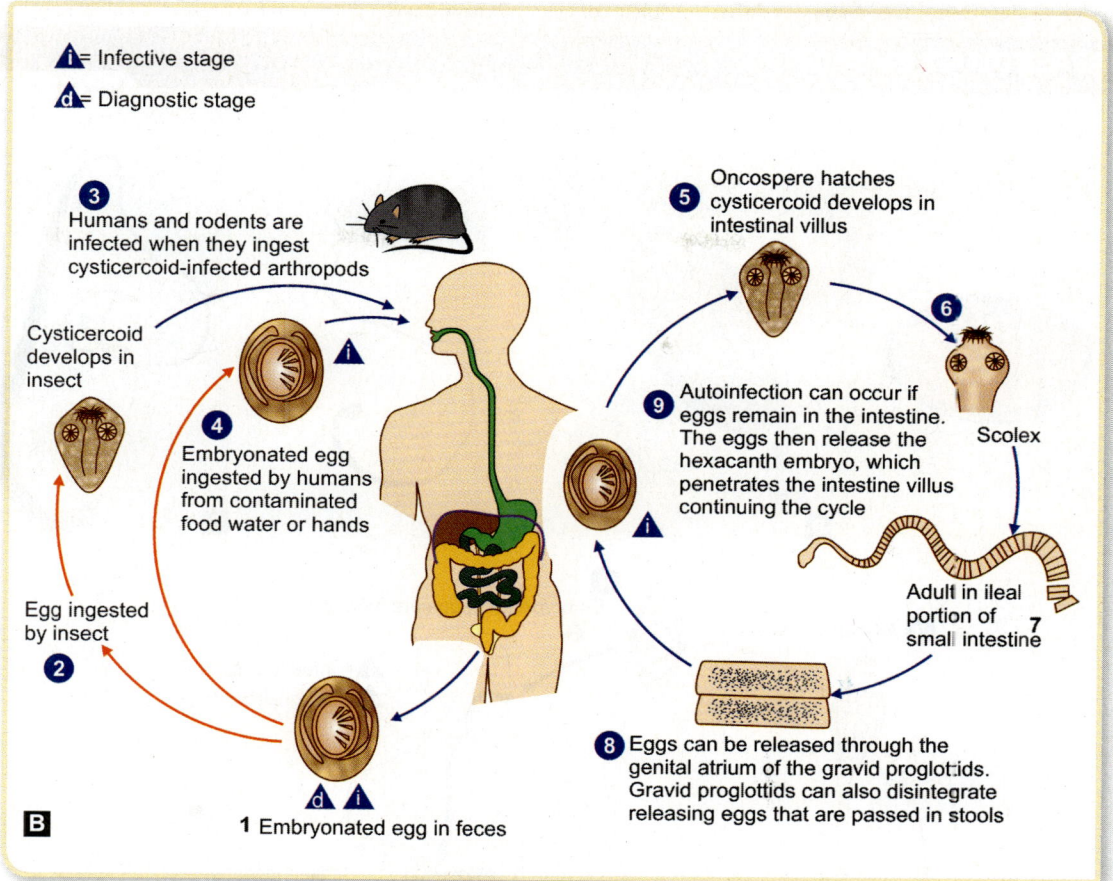

PLATE LEGENDS

A. Egg of *H. nana* in an unstained wet mount. Note the presence of hooks in the oncosphere and polar filaments within the space between the oncosphere and outer shell.

B. Life cycle of H nana: Eggs of *Hymenolepis nana* are immediately infective when passed with the stool and cannot survive more than 10 days in the external environment ❶. When eggs are ingested by an arthropod intermediate host ❷ (various species of beetles and fleas may serve as intermediate hosts), they develop into cysticercoids, which can infect humans or rodents upon ingestion ❸ and develop into adults in the small intestine. A morphologically identical variant, *H. nana* var. *fraterna*, infects rodents and uses arthropods as intermediate hosts. When eggs are ingested ❹ (in contaminated food or water or from hands contaminated with feces), the oncospheres contained in the eggs are released. The oncospheres (hexacanth larvae) penetrate the intestinal villus and develop into cysticercoid larvae ❺. Upon rupture of the villus, the cysticercoids return to the intestinal lumen, evaginate their scoleces ❻, attach to the intestinal mucosa and develop into adults that reside in the ileal portion of the small intestine producing gravid proglottids ❼. Eggs are passed in the stool when released from proglottids through its genital atrium or when proglottids disintegrate in the small intestine ❽. An alternate mode of infection consists of internal autoinfection, where the eggs release their hexacanth embryo, which penetrates the villus continuing the infective cycle without passage through the external environment ❾. The life span of adult worms is 4 to 6 weeks, but internal autoinfection allows the infection to persist for years.

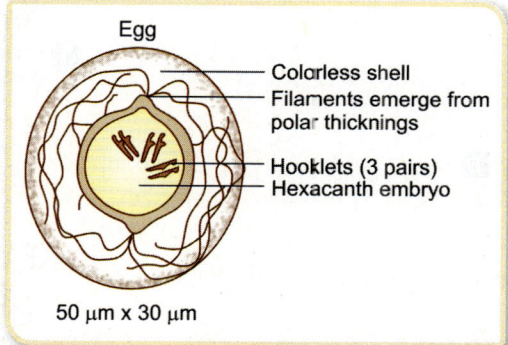

Hymenolepiasis is caused by two cestodes (tapeworm) species, *Hymenolepis nana* (the dwarf tapeworm, adults measuring 15 to 40 mm in length) and *Hymenolepis diminuta* (rat tapeworm, adults measuring 20 to 60 cm in length). *Hymenolepis diminuta* is a cestode of rodents infrequently seen in humans and frequently found in rodents.

PARASITOLOGY PLATE 17

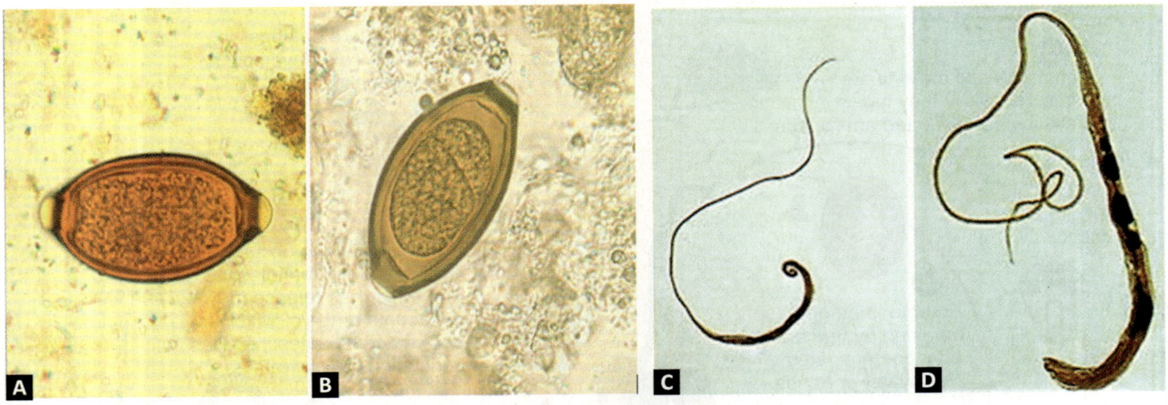

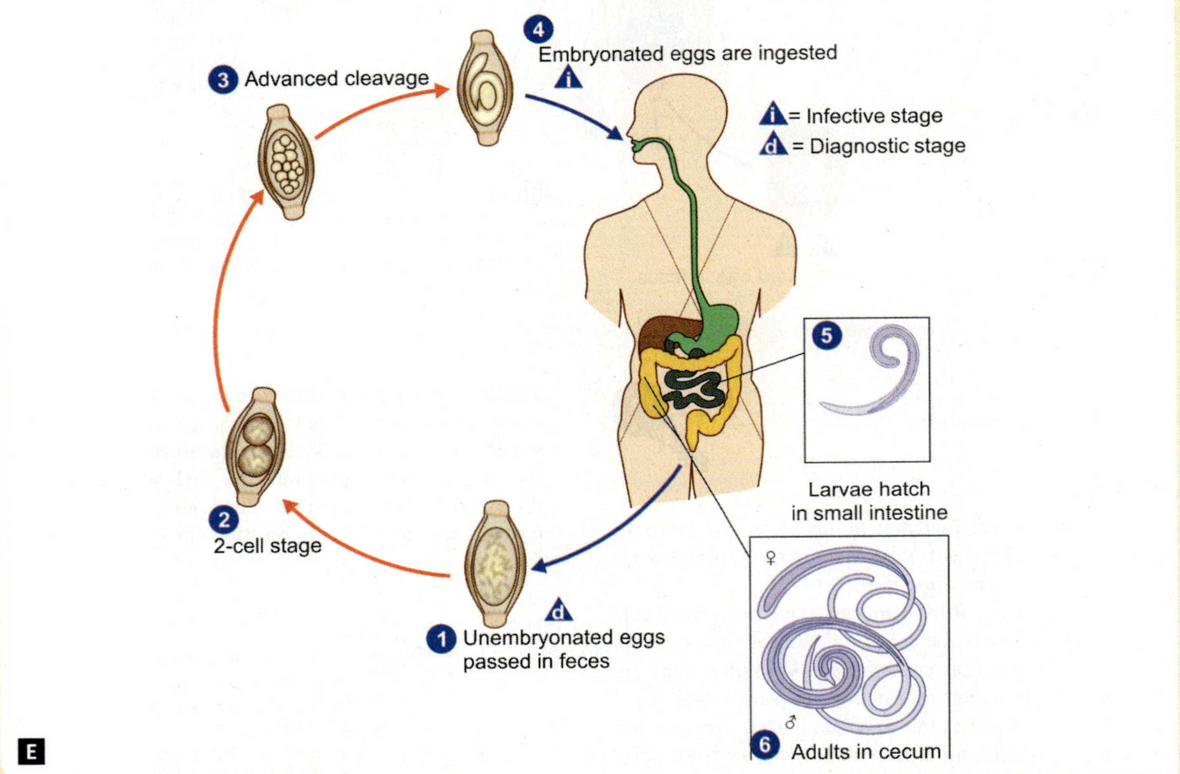

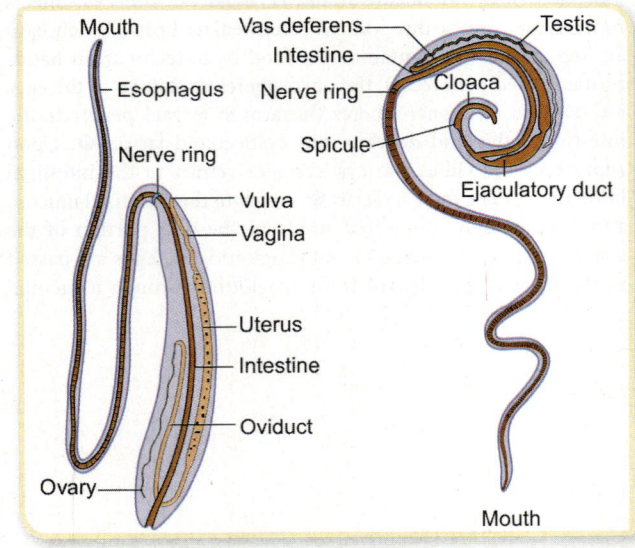

PLATE LEGENDS

The nematode (roundworm) *Trichuris trichiura*, also called the human whipworm.
- **A.** Egg of *T. trichiura*[NEETPG] in an iodine-stained wet mount of stool. Elongated barrel shaped with distinctive bipolar plugs, smooth outer shells
- **B.** Egg of *T. trichiura* in an unstained wet mount of stool
- **C. Adult male trichuris (whipworm):** 4 cm long, characteristic whiplike shape, posterior end is coiled with one protruding spicule
- **D. Adult female trichuris:** 5 cm long, posterior end is not coiled, straight and blunt

E. Life cycle of Trichuris trichura: (With permission from CDC) The unembryonated eggs are passed with the stool ❶. In the soil, the eggs develop into a 2-cell stage ❷, an advanced cleavage stage ❸, and then they embryonate ❹; eggs become infective in 15 to 30 days (minimum 10 days). After ingestion (soil-contaminated hands or food), the eggs hatch in the small intestine, and release larvae ❺ that mature and establish themselves as adults in the colon ❻. The adult worms (approximately 4 cm in length) live in the cecum and ascending colon. The adult worms are fixed in that location, with the anterior portions threaded into the mucosa. The females begin to oviposit 60 to 70 days after infection. Female worms in the cecum shed between 3,000 and 20,000 eggs per day. The life span of the adults is about 1 year.

PARASITOLOGY PLATE 18

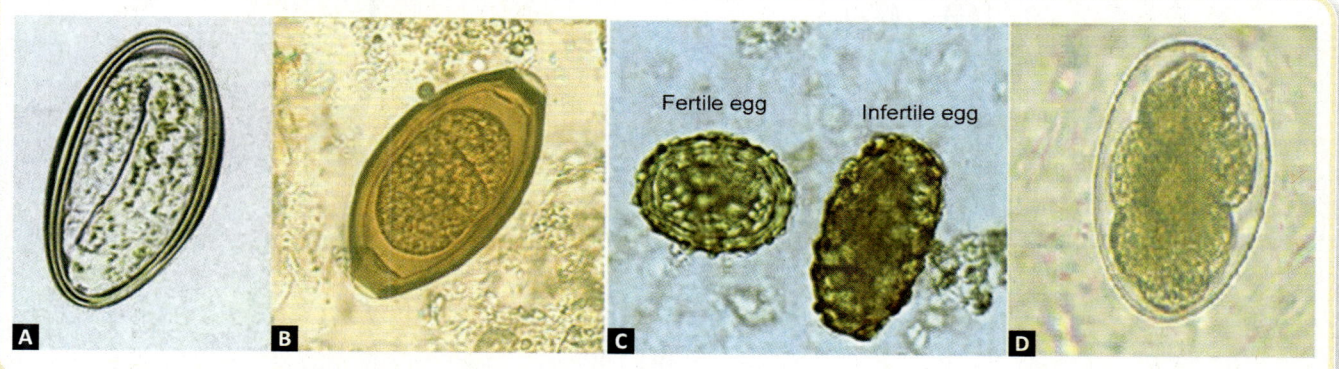

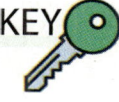

NEMATODES EGG

A. *Enterobius vermicularis* egg: Elongate-oval and slightly flattened on one side. They are usually partially-embryonated when shed. Enterobiasis can be diagnosed by applying cellulose tape to the anus of a suspected patient, especially in the morning before the patient's first bowel movement. Eggs will adhere to the tape and can be seen microscopically.

B. *Trichuris trichura* egg (unstained wet mount): Elongated barrel shaped with distinctive bipolar plugs, smooth outer shells. The eggs are unembryonated when passed in stool

C. *Ascaris lumbricoides* egg: Both fertilized and unfertilized Ascaris lumbricoides eggs are passed in the stool of the infected host.
- **Fertilized eggs** are rounded and have a thick shell with an external mammilated layer that is often stained brown by bile. Fertile eggs range from 45 to 75 μm in length.
- **Unfertilized eggs** are elongated and larger than fertile eggs (up to 90 μm in length). Their shell is thinner and their mammillated layer is more variable, either with large protuberances or practically none. Unfertile eggs contain mainly a mass of refractile granules.

D. *Ancylostoma duodenale* or *Necator americanus* egg. (outside circles represent RBC): The eggs of Ancylostoma and Necator cannot be differentiated microscopically. The eggs are thin-shelled, colorless and measure 60-75 μm by 35-40 μm.

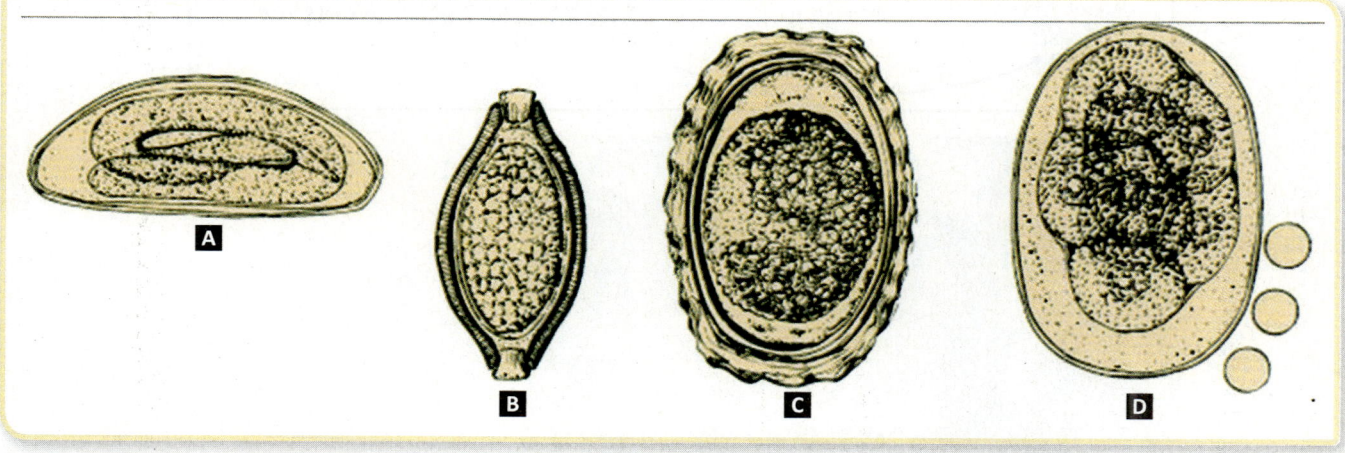

Fig: A. Enterobius vermicularis egg. **B.** Trichuris trichura egg. **C.** Ascaris lumbricoides egg. **D.** Ancylostoma duodenale or Necator americanus egg. (Circles represent RBC)

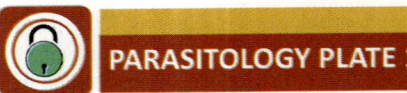

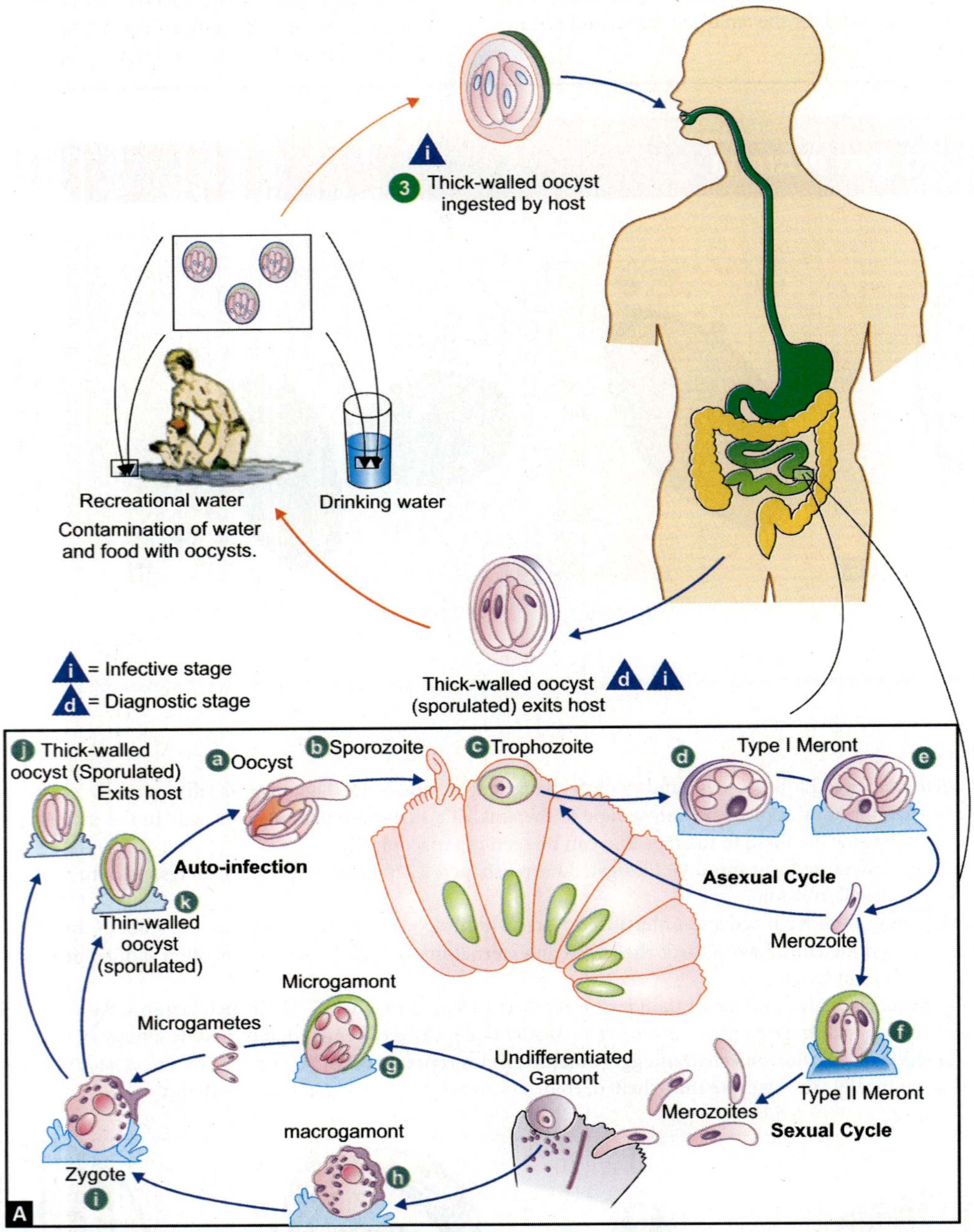

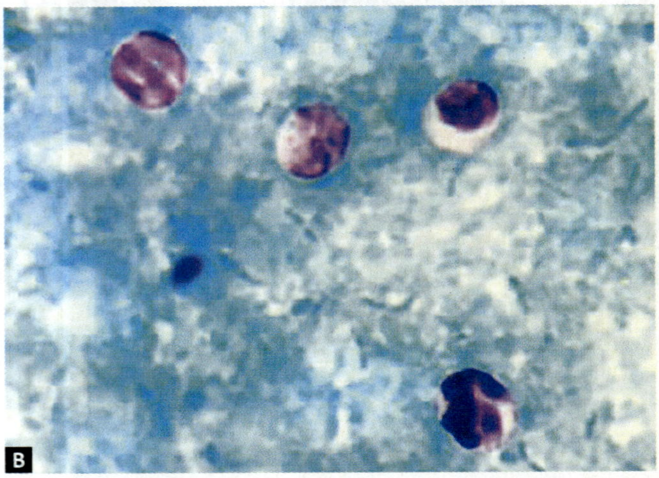

PLATE LEGENDS

Cryptosporidiosis is a Coccidian disease caused by Cryptosporidium that causes watery diarrhea. Although Crypto can affect all people immunocompromised status is likely to produce more serious illness.

- **A. Life cycle of *Cryptosporidium parvum*:** Sporulated oocysts, containing 4 sporozoites, are excreted by the infected host through feces and possibly other routes such as respiratory secretions ❶. Transmission of *Cryptosporidium parvum* and *C. hominis* occurs mainly through contact with contaminated water (e.g., drinking or recreational water). Occasionally food sources, such as chicken salad, may serve as vehicles for transmission. Many outbreaks in the United States have occurred in waterparks, community swimming pools, and day care centers. Zoonotic and anthroponotic transmission of *C. parvum* and anthroponotic transmission of *C. hominis* occur through exposure to infected animals or exposure to water contaminated by feces of infected animals ❷. Following ingestion (and possibly inhalation) by a suitable host ❸, excystation ⓐ occurs. The sporozoites are released and parasitize epithelial cells (ⓑ, ⓒ) of the gastrointestinal tract or other tissues such as the respiratory tract. In these cells, the parasites undergo asexual multiplication (schizogony or merogony) (ⓓ, ⓔ, ⓕ) and then sexual multiplication (gametogony) producing microgamonts (male) (ⓖ) and macrogamonts (female) (ⓗ). Upon fertilization of the macrogamonts by the microgametes (ⓘ), oocysts (ⓙ, ⓚ) develop that sporulate in the infected host. Two different types of oocysts are produced, the thick-walled, which is commonly excreted from the host (ⓙ), and the thin-walled oocyst (ⓚ) which is primarily involved in autoinfection. Oocysts are infective upon excretion, thus permitting direct and immediate fecal-oral transmission.
- **B. Cryptosporidium oocysts in a modified acid-fast stain**[AIIMS PG]. Diagnosis of cryptosporidiosis is made by examination of stool samples. Most often, stool specimens are examined microscopically using different techniques (e.g., acid-fast staining, direct fluorescent antibody [DFA], and/or enzyme immunoassays for detection of Cryptosporidium sp. antigens).

Notes

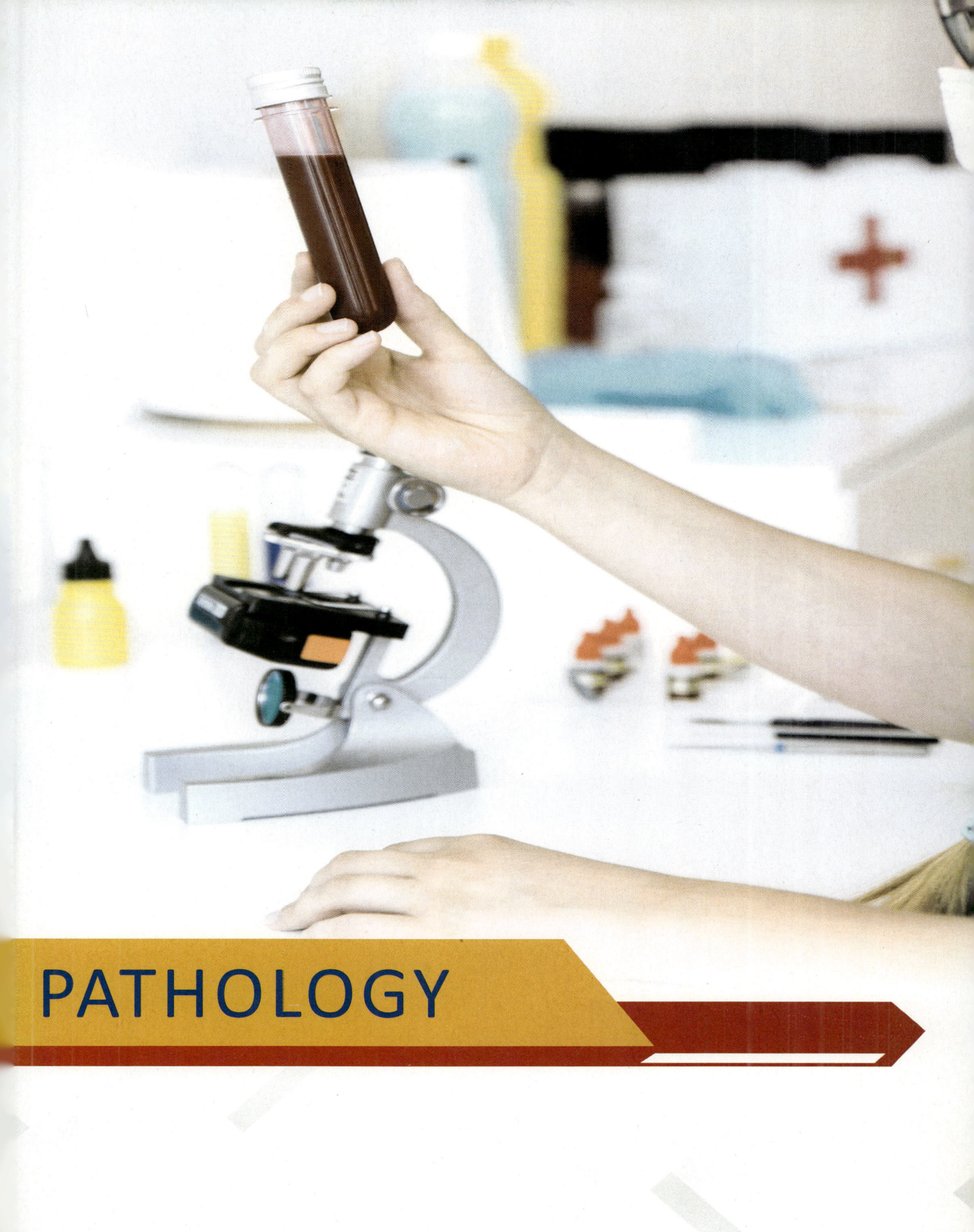
PATHOLOGY

PATHO PLATE 1

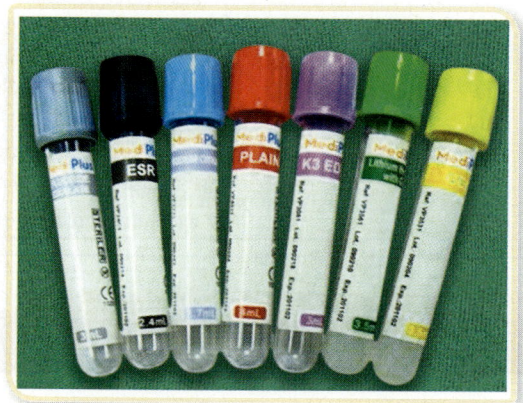

KEY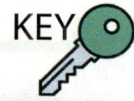

Blood Collection System (Vacutainer System)					
	Color code	Additive	Blood draw	Mixing	Clinical use
Serum blood collection tubes	Yellow / Golden (4)	Plain, No additive, Serum Separator Tube (SST) contains clot activator with gel separator at the bottom to separate blood from serum on centrifugation	4 ml 6 ml	5 times	Serum biochemistry, Dug monitoring, Serum immunology
	Red (3)	Plain, No additive, clot activator (Blood clots and serum is separated by centrifugation)	4 ml 4 ml 6 ml	5 times for plastic tubes, no mixing for glass tubes	Serum biochemistry, Dug monitoring, Serum immunology Blood bank profiles
Whole blood collection tubes	Lavender (6)	EDTA Liquid (Form calcium salts to remove calcium)	2 ml	8-10 times	Hematology (FBC), Blood Bank (Cross Match); gently invert bottle after filling to prevent clotting and platelet clumping
	Pink (7)	EDTA	2 ml	8-10 times	Blood grouping, cross matching, Direct Coomb's test, Antenatal grouping
	Black (2)	Sodium citrate ESR	2 ml	8-10 times gently	Erythrocyte sedimentation rates
Plasma blood collection tubes	Grey (8)	Sodium Fluoride + potassium oxalate (Antiglycolytic agent preserves glucose upto 5 days)	2 ml	8-10 times	For Glucose levels (Blood sugar)
	Light blue (1)	Buffered Sodium Citrate 3.2% (Form calcium salts to remove calcium) studies (9 volume of blood added to 1 volume of 10^9 mmol/L sodium citrate soL)	2 ml	3-4 times	Coagulation test (INR), Full draw required
	Green (5)	Plasma Separating Tube (PST) with Lithium Heparin (Anticoagulates with lithium heparin; Plasma is separated with PST gel at the bottom of the tube)	2 ml	8 10 times	Cytogenetics (chromosome studies), carboxy Hb, MethHb

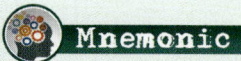

Order of draw (Brackets): Blood culture packs (Read Sterile for Mnemonic), Followed by Light **b**lue, **B**lack, **R**ed, **Y**ellow, **G**reen, **L**avender, **P**ink, **G**rey
(**S**tupid **B**oys bravely **r**ead, **y**et **g**et **l**ow & **p**oor **G**rades)

Contd...

Anticoagulants used for blood and their uses	
Sodium fluoride	Estimation of glucose since it inhibits enolase
Double oxalate	Used where vol of RBC is preserved like ESR, PCV
Sodium citrate	Coagulation studies and ESR by westergren's method
EDTA	EDTA is the preferred anticoagulant for blood counts because it produces complete anticoagulation with minimal morphologic and physical effects on cells
Heparin	Heparin is often used for red cell testing, osmotic fragility testing, and functional or immunologic analysis of leukocytes
ESR	All except coagulation studies

PATHO PLATE 2

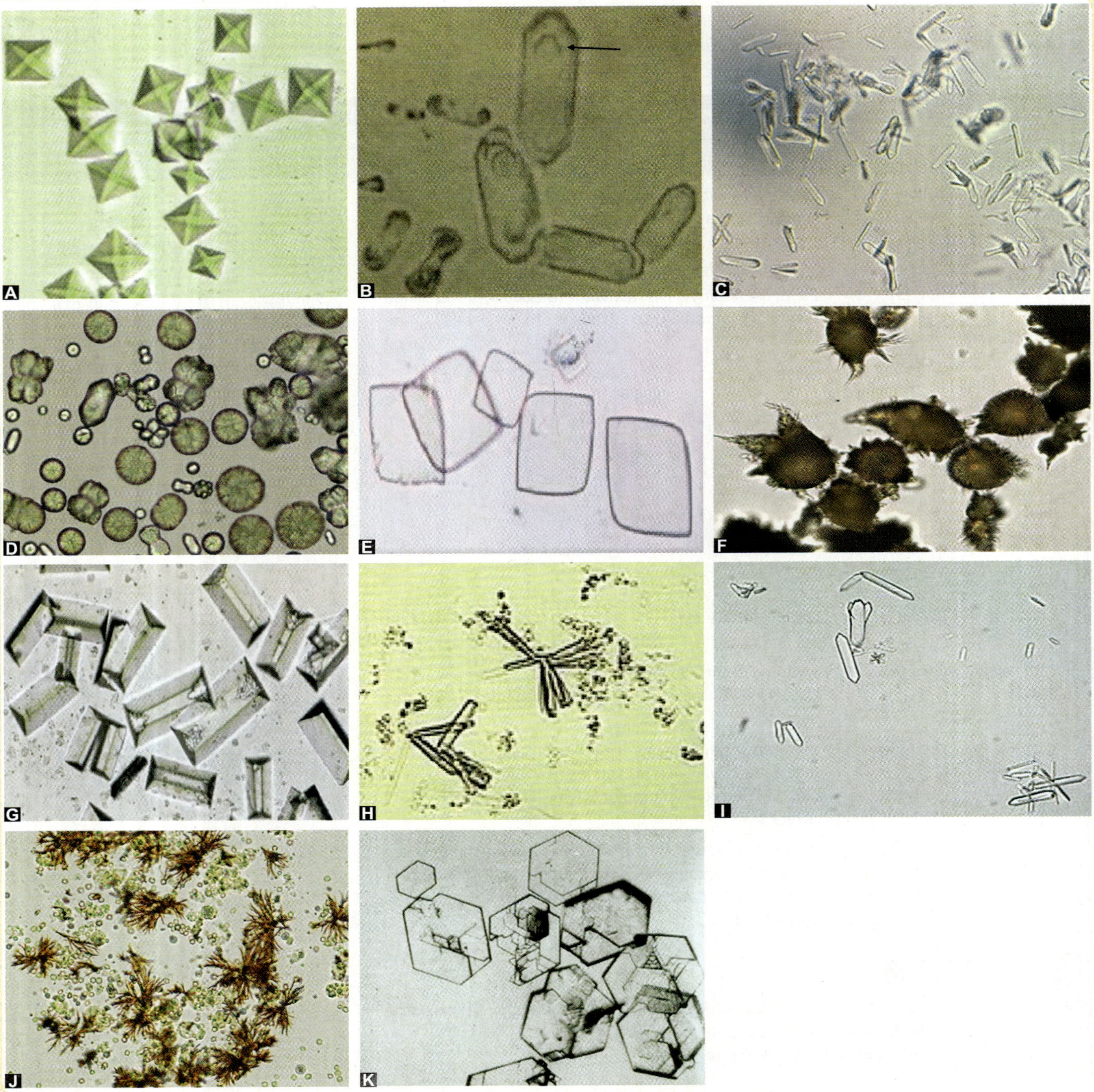

URINARY CRYSTALS

Urinary Crystals			
Crystal	**Shape**	**Favorable pH**	**Comments**
A= Calcium Oxalate dihydrate	Colorless Octahedron (**Envelope shaped**), diamond shape	Acidic or pH insensitive in the physiologic pH range of 5 to 8	Artifact of storage (can develop in stored urine). Associated with food high in oxalate (tomatoes, asparagus, ascorbic acid
B= Calcium oxalate monohydrate	Colorless, Spindle (arrow), oval (**Hemp seed**), or dumbbell shape,	Acidic or pH insensitive in the physiologic pH range of 5 to 8	Associated with food high in oxalate (tomatoes, asparagus, ascorbic acid
C= Calcium oxalate monohydrate (picket fence)	A particular form of calcium oxalate monohydrate are flat, elongated, six-sided crystals ("**picket fences**") which are the larger crystals	Acidic or pH insensitive in the physiologic pH range of 5 to 8	Seen in ethylene glycol toxicosis
D= Calcium Carbonate	Yellow to colorless **dumbbells or spheres with radial striations**	Alkaline urine	Usually large crystals and can be readily observed at low magnification.
E= Uric Acid	Amber in color, Rhombic, 4 sided plates, prism, oval with pointed ended	5-5.5 (Acidic Urine)	
F= Ammonium biurate	Brown or yellow-brown spherical bodies with irregular protrusions ("**thorn-apples**").	Alkaline pH	Can be observed under low magnification,
G= Struvite crystals (magnesium ammonium phosphate, triple phosphate)	Colorless, three-dimensional, prism-like crystals ("**coffin lids**")	Neutral and Alkaline pH is favorable.	UTI with urease positive bacteria promote struvite crystalluria
H= Calcium phosphate	Large flat-shaped plates or wedge-shaped prisms in rosettes. Single prisms are usually blunt on one end and pointed on the other end.	Alkaline urine	
I= Hippuric acid	Colorless prisms, plates, or needle-like often conglomerated into masses		
J= Bilirubin crystals	Yellow-brown **needles or granules**. Form from conjugated bilirubin.		They are frequently attached to the surface of cells. Bilirubin crystals are seen in several hepatic disorders
K= Cystine crystals	Flat colorless, thin, **hexagonal** plates with equal or unequal sides	Acidic urine	Cystine crystals are found in the inherited condition, **cystinuria**. Cystine crystals are the most frequent cause of kidney stones in children.

Footnote:
- All abnormal crystals precipitate in the urine at acidic pHs.
- Crystals by drugs are often caused by sulphadiazine (appearance of sheaves of wheat), acyclovir (birefringent, needle-sharp crystals) and Vitamin C.

PATHO PLATE 3

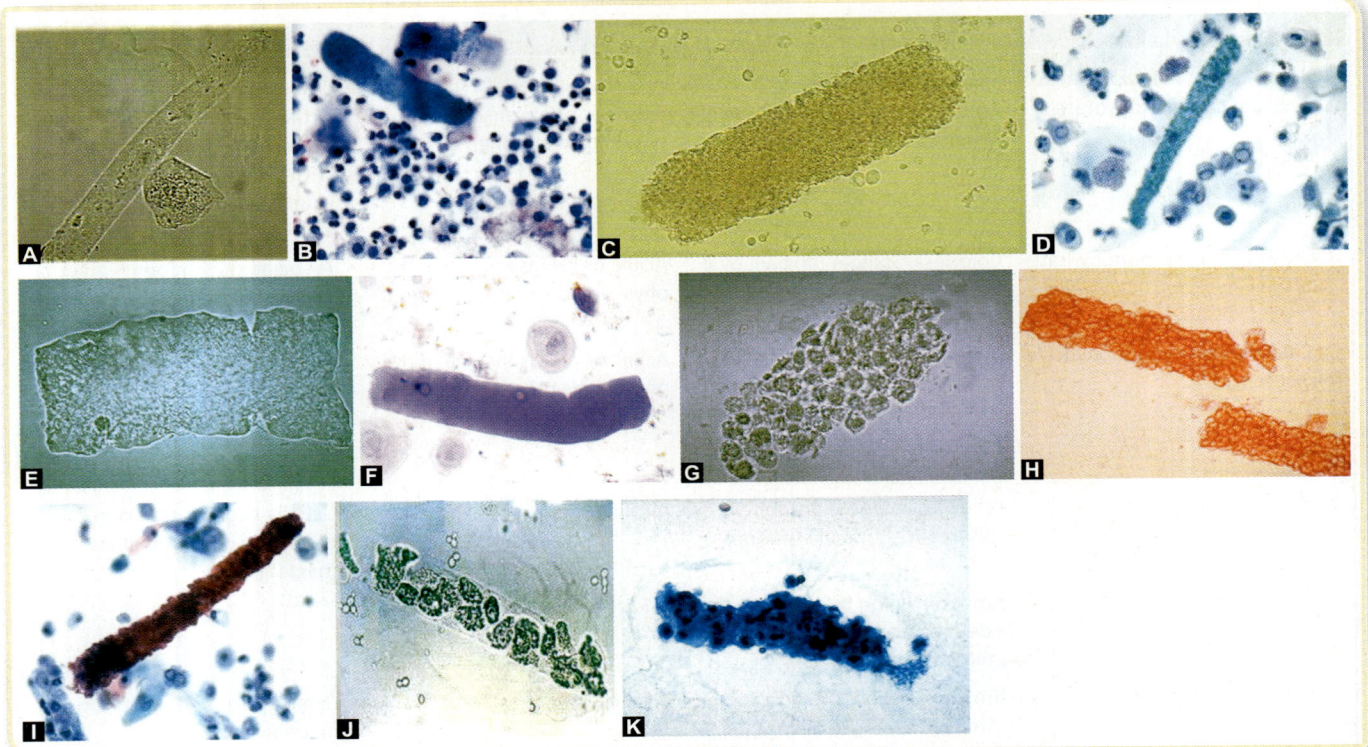

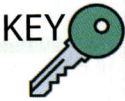

URINARY CASTS

A. **Hyaline cast urine microscopy (Unstained):** Colorless, homogeneous, transparent. Parallel sides with clear margins and blunted ends
B. **Hyaline cast urine microscopy Papanicolaou stain**
C. **Granular cast urine microscopy (Unstained):** Rectangular shape, often with rounded extremities. True casts can be differentiated from these artefacts by their parallel sides. Granular casts that contain fine granules may appear grey or pale yellow in color. Granular casts that contain larger coarse granules are darker. Granular and waxy casts are be believed to derive from renal tubular cell casts.
D. **Granular cast urine microscopy Papanicolaou stain**
E. **Waxy cast urine microscopy (Unstained):** Appear yellow, grey, or colorless. Note that ends that the edges are sharp or broken and there are serrations/ cracks" in this cast. Waxy casts result from the degeneration of granular casts. Granular and waxy casts are be believed to derive from renal tubular cell casts.
F. **Waxy cast urine microscopy Papanicolaou stain**
G. **Fatty cast urine microscopy (Unstained):** A typical fatty cast contains both large and small fat droplets. The small fat droplets are yellowish-brown in color.
H. **RBC cast urine microscopy (Unstained):** Red blood cells may stick together and form red blood cell casts
I. **RBC cast urine microscopy Papanicolaou stain**
J. **WBC cast urine microscopy (Unstained)**
K. **WBC cast urine microscopy Papanicolaou stain**

Urinary casts are formed only in the distal convoluted tubule (DCT) or the collecting duct (distal nephron). The proximal convoluted tubule (PCT) and loop of Henle are not locations for cast formation. Hyaline casts are composed primarily of a mucoprotein (Tamm-Horsfall protein) secreted by tubule cells. The Tamm-Horsfall protein secretion (green dots) is illustrated in the diagram below, forming a hyaline cast in the collecting duct:

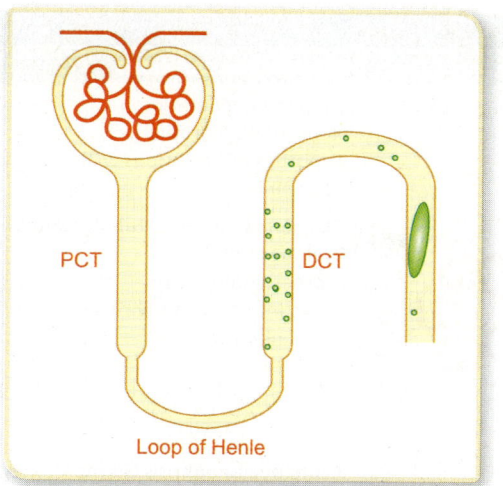

Horsfall mucoprotein, although albumin and some globulins are also incorporated. An example of glomerular inflammation with leakage of RBC's to produce a red blood cell cast is shown in the diagram as follows:

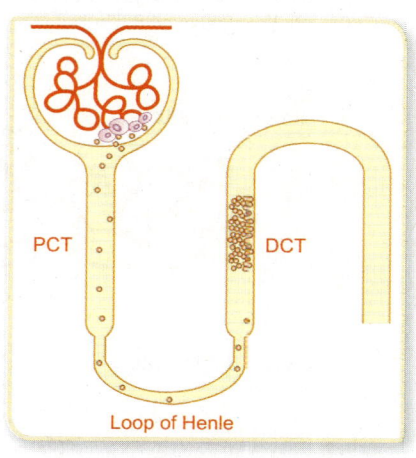

Even with glomerular injury causing increased glomerular permeability to plasma proteins with resulting proteinuria, most matrix or "glue" that cements urinary casts together is Tamm-

Urinary Cast		
Casts	**Comments**	**Associated conditions**
Hyaline casts	Most common type of casts which are composed of solidified Tamm-Horsfall mucoprotein. The factors which favor protein cast formation are low flow rate, high salt concentration, and low pH, all of which favor protein denaturation and precipitation, particularly that of the Tamm-Horsfall protein.	Normal individuals Dehydration Heavy exercise
Granular casts	Various cell types (Degeneration of cellular casts, Aggregates of plasma proteins or immunoglobulin light chains) When cellular casts remain in the nephron for some time before they are flushed into the bladder urine, the cells may degenerate to become a coarsely granular cast, later a finely granular cast, and ultimately, a waxy cast.	After strenuous exercise Chronic renal diseases Acute tubular necrosis
Waxy casts *(renal failure casts)*	Various cell types (Final stage of degeneration of cellular cast)	They are associated with severe, often ESRD. Renal amyloidosis

Contd...

Urinary Cast		
Casts	Comments	Associated conditions
Fatty casts	Lipid droplets within the protein matrix of the cast. Due to fatty degeneration of the tubular epithelium	Tubular degeneration Nephrotic syndrome Hypothyroidism, Lupus & Toxic renal poisoning
RBC Casts	Red Blood Cells Red blood cell cast	Glomerular, or renal tubular injury, Pyelonephritis Glomerulonephritis Acute interstitial nephritis Lupus nephritis
WBC Casts	White Blood Cells White blood cell cast	Acute pyelonephritis Glomerulonephritis
Epithelial Cell Casts	Renal Tubular Epithelial Cells	▫ Renal tubular necrosis ▫ Viral Diseases ▫ Kidney transplant rejection
Bacterial Cell Casts	Bacterial Cells	▫ Acute pyelonephritis ▫ Intrinsic renal infection

Types of Epithelial Cells in Urine

Renal tubular epithelial cells, usually larger than granulocytes, contain a large round or oval nucleus and normally slough into the urine in small numbers. However, with nephrotic syndrome and in conditions leading to tubular degeneration, the number sloughed is increased. This renal tubular cell cast suggests injury to the tubular epithelium.

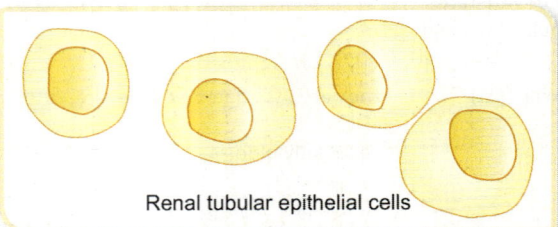
Renal tubular epithelial cells

Transitional epithelial cells from the renal pelvis, ureter, or bladder have more regular cell borders, larger nuclei, and smaller overall size than squamous epithelium. Renal tubular epithelial cells are smaller and rounder than transitional epithelium, and their nuclei occupy more of the total cell volume.

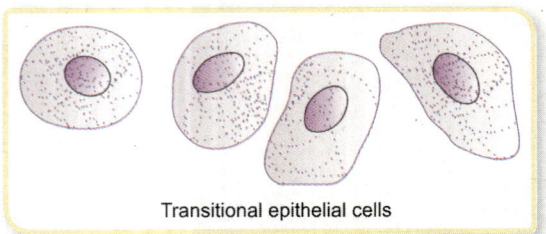
Transitional epithelial cells

Squamous epithelial cells from the skin surface or from the outer urethra can appear in urine. Their significance is that they represent possible contamination of the specimen with skin flora.

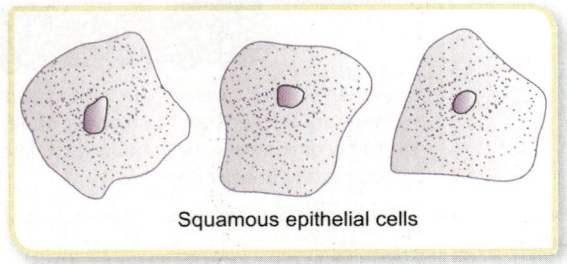
Squamous epithelial cells

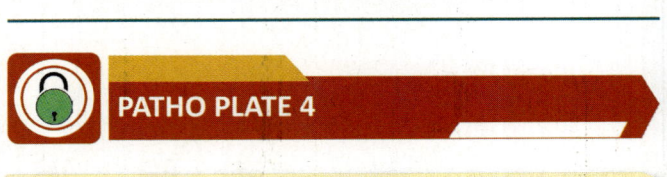
PATHO PLATE 4

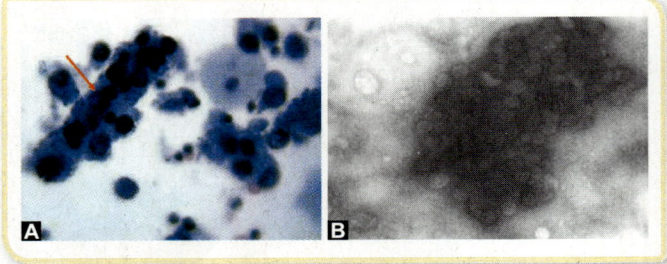

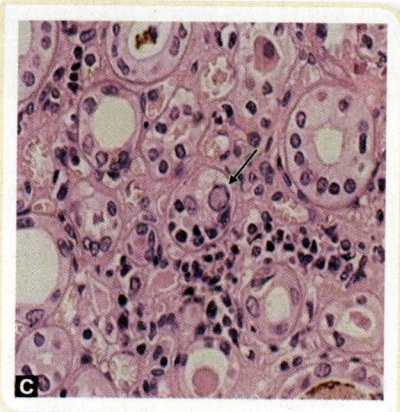

German= heap, hive, pile) in the urine accurately predicts BK polyomavirus nephropathy. Haufen detection was correlated with pathology in concomitant renal biopsies and BK viruria (decoy cell shedding and viral load assessments by PCR) and BK viremia (viral load assessments by PCR). Haufen originated from renal tubules containing virally lysed cells, and the detection of Haufen in the urine correlated tightly with biopsy confirmed BK polyomavirus nephropathy (concordance rate 99%).

C. **BK Virus Nephropathy:** Amphophilic large intranuclear inclusions with a dense peripheral chromatin ring in the nuclei of tubular epithelial cells. Variable degree of interstitial inflammation, fibrosis and atrophy. Similar appearance to cellular rejection.

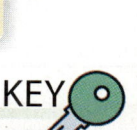 KEY

PATHO PLATE 5

PLATE LEGENDS

A. **Decoy cell in Urine Papanicolaou stain:** Disperse decoy cells and cellular cylinders containing compacted decoy cells. When they appear, these cylinders are pathognomic of kidney damage. Decoy cells are renal tubular or uroepithelial cells with intranuclear BK Virus inclusion bodies.

Note that the Decoy cell aggregates in the form of cylinders looks like Hyaline cast. Decoy cells are seen by three methods
- Electron microscopy
- Phase contrast microscopy and
- Papanicolaou stain

B. **Urine Electron Microscopy with Haufen:** There are no accurate, noninvasive tests to diagnose BK polyomavirus nephropathy, But recently Electron microscopic qualitative detection of cast-like, three-dimensional polyomavirus aggregates (**"Haufen"**

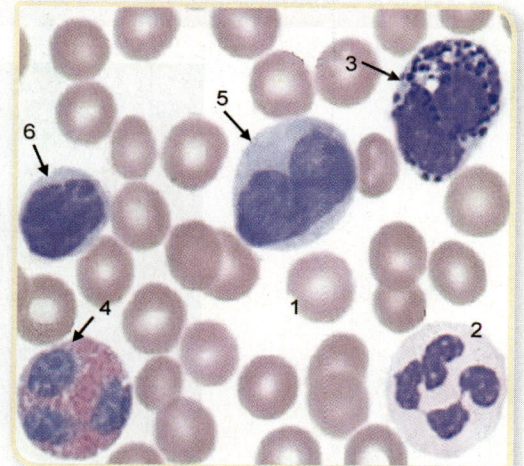

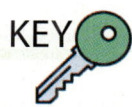 KEY

CELLS OF PERIPHERAL SMEAR

1. RBC
2. Basophil
3. Monocytes
4. Neutrophil
5. Eosinophil
6. Lymphocytes

Cells of Peripheral Smear					
Cells	Description	Cells/ mm³ of blood	Duration of development & life span	Function
Erythrocytes (RBC) (Marked as 1)	Biconcave, anucleate disc, salmon Colored, diameter 7-8μm	4-6 millions	D-15 days LS- 100-120 days	Transport oxygen and CO_2
Leukocytes (WBC)	Spherical Nucleated Cell	4000-11000		
Granulocytes				
☐ Neutrophil (Marked as 2)	Multilobed nucleus, inconspicuous cytoplasmic granules, diameter 10-12 μm	3000-7000	D- 14 days LS- 14 hrs to few days	Phagocytize bacteria
☐ Eosinophil (cell 4)	Bilobed nucleus, red cytoplasmic granules, diameter 10-14 μm	100-400	D- about 14 days LS- about 5 days	Kills parasitic worms, complex role in allergy and asthma
• Basophil (Marked as 3)	Bilobed nucleus, large purplish-black cytoplasmic granules, diameter 10-14 μm	20-50	D- about 1-7 days LS- a few hours to few days	Release histamine and other mediators of inflammation; contain heparin and anticoagulant

Contd...

Cells of Peripheral Smear				
Cells	Description	Cells/ mm³ of blood	Duration of development & life span	Function
Agranulocytes				
☐ Lymphocyte (Marked as 6)	Spherical or indented nucleus, pale blue cytoplasm, diameter 5-17 µm	1500- 3000	D- days to weeks LS- hours to years	Mount immune response by direct cell attack or via antibodies
☐ Monocyte (Marked as 5)	U or kidney shaped nucleus, grey-blue cytoplasm, diameter 14-24 µm	100-700	D- about 2-3 days LS- months	Phagocytosis; develop into macrophages in the tissue
Platelets	Discoid cytoplasmic fragments containing granules, stain deep purple, diameter 2-4 µm	150,000-400,000	D- 4-5 days LS- 5-10 days	Seal small tears in blood vessels, instrumental in blood clotting

PATHO PLATE 6

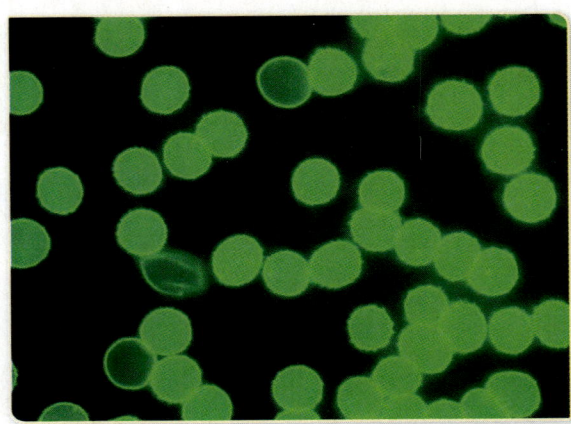

HUMAN RBC WITH FLUORESCENT MICROSCOPY
Human red blood cells (RBC, erythrocytes) stained with Fluorescent microscopy

PATHO PLATE 7

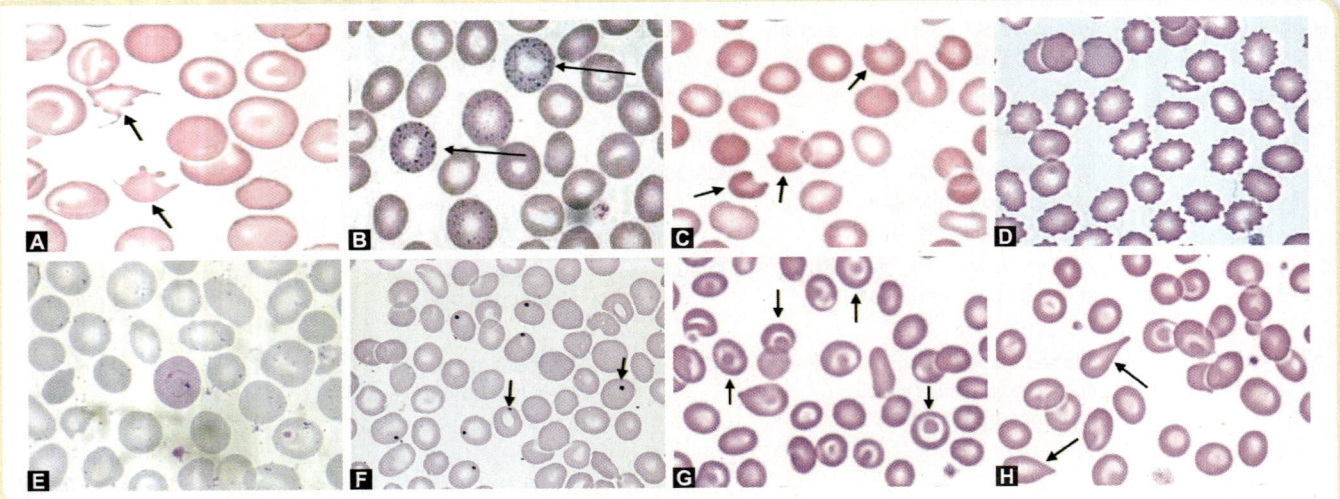

PATHOLOGIC RED CELLS IN BLOOD SMEAR

A. Acanthocytes
B. Basophilic stippling
C. Bite cells
D. Burr cells
E. Cabot Rings
F. Howell-Jolly bodies
G. Target cells
H. Teardrop cells

Pathologic Red Cells in Blood Smears

Red cell type	Description	Underlying change	Disease state associations
Acanthocyte (spur cell)	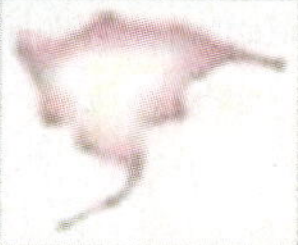 Irregularly spiculated red cells with projections of varying length and dense center	Altered cell membrane lipids	Abetalipoproteinemia, parenchymal liver disease, postsplenectomy
Basophilic stippling	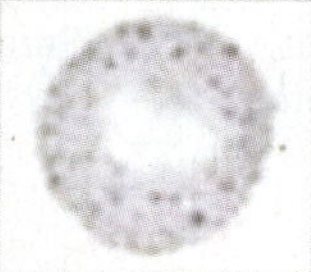 Punctuate basophilic inclusions	Precipitated ribosomes (RNA)	Coarse stippling: Lead intoxication, thalassemia Fine stippling: A variety of anemias
Bite cell (degmacyte)	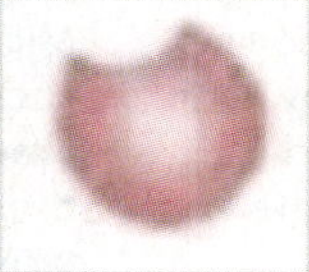 Smooth semicircle taken from one edge	Heinz body pitting by spleen	Glucose-6-phosphate dehydrogenase deficiency, drug-induced oxidant hemolysis
Burr cell (echinocyte) or crenated red cell	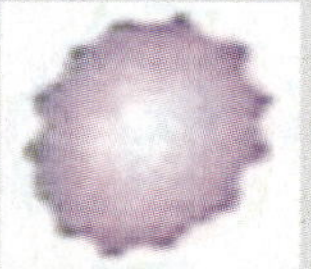 Red cells with short, evenly spaced spicules and preserved central pallor	May be associated with altered membrane lipids	Usually artifactual; seen in uremia, bleeding ulcers, gastric carcinoma
Cabot rings	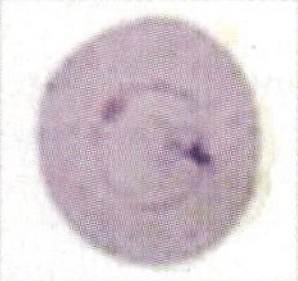 Circular, blue, threadlike inclusion with dots	Nuclear remnant	Postsplenectomy, hemolytic anemia, megaloblastic anemia
Ovalocyte (elliptocyte)	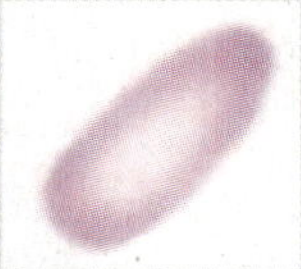 Elliptically shaped cell	Abnormal cytoskeletal proteins	Hereditary elliptocytosis
Howell-Jolly bodies	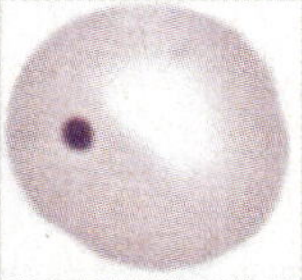 Small, discrete, basophilic, dense inclusions; usually single	Nuclear remnant (DNA)	Postsplenectomy, hemolytic anemia, megaloblastic anemia
Hypochromic red cell	Prominent central pallor	Diminished hemoglobin synthesis	Iron deficiency anemia, thalassemia, sideroblastic anemia
Macrocyte	Red cells larger than normal (>8.5 μm), well filled with hemoglobin	Young red cells, abnormal red cell maturation	Increased erythropoiesis; oval macrocytes in megaloblastic anemia; round macrocytes in liver disease

Contd...

Pathologic Red Cells in Blood Smears

Red cell type	Description	Underlying change	Disease state associations
Microcyte	Red cells smaller than normal (<7.0 µm)	—	Hypochromic red cell
Pappenheimer bodies	Small, dense, basophilic granules	Iron-containing siderosome or mitochondrial remnant	Sideroblastic anemia, postsplenectomy
Poly chromatophilia	Grayish or blue hue often seen in macrocytic RBC lacking central pallor.	Ribosomal material	Reticulocytosis, premature marrow release of red cells
Rouleaux	Red cell aggregates resembling stack of coins	Red cell clumping by circulating paraprotein	Paraproteinemia
Schistocyte (helmet cell)	Distorted, fragmented cell; two or three pointed ends	Mechanical distortion in microvasculature by fibrin strands, disruption by prosthetic heart valve	Microangiopathic hemolytic anemia (disseminated intravascular coagulation, thrombotic thrombocytopenic purpura, prosthetic heart valves, severe burns)
Sickle cell (drepanocyte)	Bipolar, spiculated forms, sickle shaped, pointed at both ends	Molecular aggregation of HbS	Sickle cell disorders, not including S trait
Spherocyte	Spherical cell with dense appearance and absent central pallor, usually decreased diameter	Decreased membrane surface area	Hereditary spherocytosis, immunohemolytic anemia
Stomatocyte	Mouth or cuplike deformity	Membrane defect with abnormal cation permeability	Hereditary stomatocytosis, Alcoholism, immunohemolytic anemia
Target cell (AKA- Mexican hat cells/ codocyte)	Target like appearance, often hypochromic	Increased redundancy of cell membrane	Liver disease, postsplenectomy, thalassemia, hemoglobin C disease

Contd...

Pathologic Red Cells in Blood Smears

Red cell type	Description	Underlying change	Disease state associations
Teardrop cell (dacryocyte)	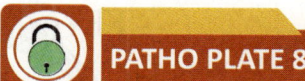 Distorted, drop-shaped cell	—	Myelofibrosis, myelophthisic anemia, Thalassemia

PATHO PLATE 8

 KEY

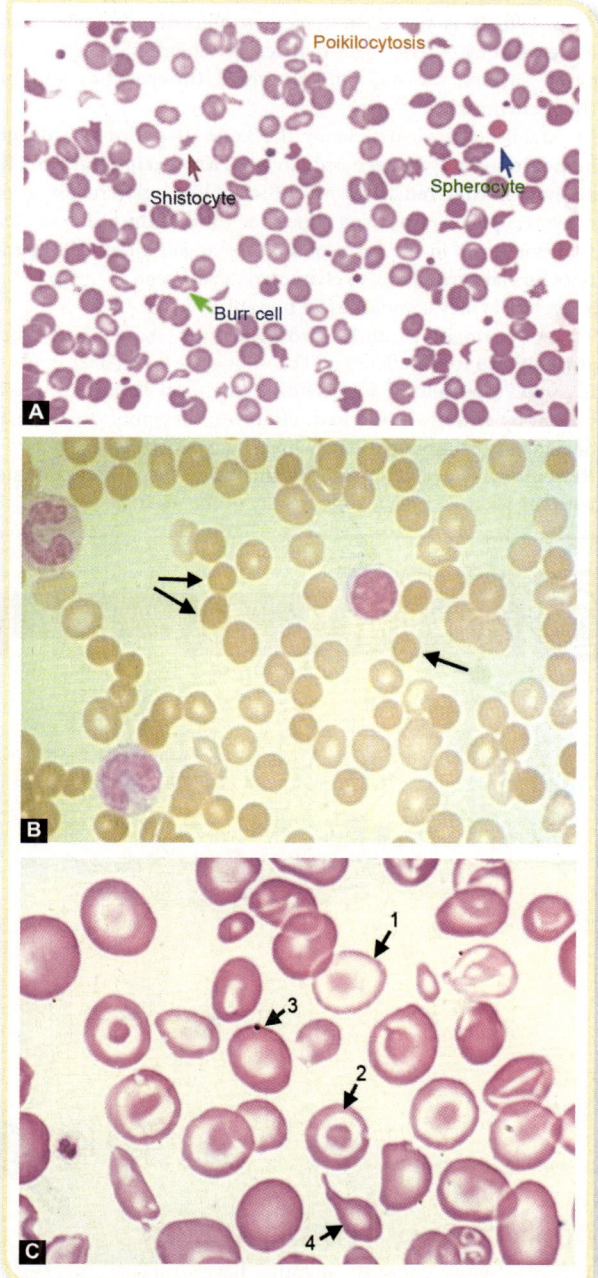

PLATE LEGENDS

A. Blood picture of hemolytic anemia:
- Certain changes are seen in hemolytic anemias regardless of cause or type.
- Compensatory increases in erythropoiesis result in a **prominent reticulocytosis** in the peripheral blood. The phagocytosis of red cells leads to hemosiderosis, which is most pronounced in the spleen, liver, and bone marrow. If the anemia is severe, extramedullary hematopoiesis can appear in the liver, spleen, and lymph nodes. With chronic hemolysis, elevated biliary excretion of bilirubin promotes the formation of pigment gallstones (cholelithiasis).
- When reticulocytes are increased, polychromatophilia and **fine basophilic stippling** are apparent on routinely stained smears of blood.
- **Macrocytosis** is found in association with most hemolytic disorders because of erythropoietin-mediated stimulation of Hb synthesis and because prematurely released (shift) reticulocytes are larger than normal erythrocytes. Exceptions occur in hereditary spherocytosis and sickle cell anemia, diseases in which the intrinsic defect of the cell tends to decrease its size.

B. Blood picture of hereditary spherocytosis:
- Erythrocyte morphology in HS is variable. **The most specific morphologic finding is spherocytosis** (arrow) apparent on smears as abnormally small, dark-staining (**hyperchromic**) *red cells lacking the central zone of pallor.* Their **mean cell diameter is decreased,** and they appear **more intensely hemoglobinized**
- Spherocytosis is distinctive but **not pathognomonic,** since other forms of membrane loss, such as in autoimmune hemolytic anemias, also cause the formation of spherocytes
- Other features are common to all hemolytic anemias includes **reticulocytosis**
- Less commonly, patients present with only a few spherocytes on the film or, at the other end of the spectrum, with numerous small, dense spherocytes and bizarre erythrocyte morphology with anisocytosis and poikilocytosis.
- Rarely, **spherostomatocytes** are seen.
- Specific morphologic findings have been identified in patients with certain membrane protein defects, such as **pincered erythrocytes (band 3) or spherocytic acanthocytes (β-spectrin).**

C. Blood picture of homozygous b thalassemia:
- Microcytic and hypochromic RBCs (1)
- Nucleated red cells, anisopoikilocytosis, target cells (2), Howell Jolly Bodies (3), Tear drop cells (4)

Note

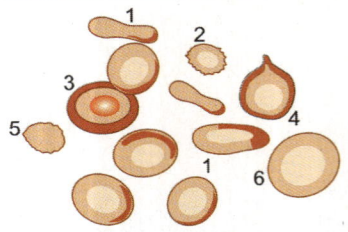

- Poikilocytic red cells (elliptocytes (1), schistocytes (2), target cells (3), tear drop (4), spherocytes (5) and hypochromic (6) usually present in Thalassemia Major.

PATHO PLATE 9

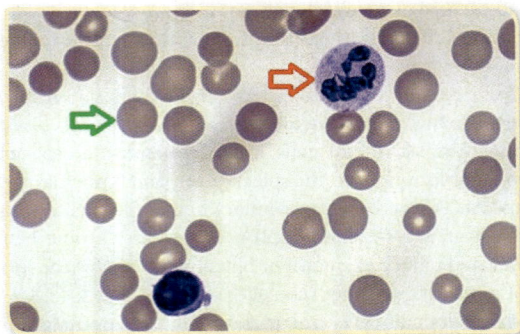

KEY

BLOOD PICTURE MEGALOBLASTIC ANEMIA

- Certain peripheral blood findings are shared by all megaloblastic anemias. **The presence of red cells that are macrocytic and oval (macro-ovalocytes) is highly characteristic** (Green arrow).
- Because they are larger than normal and contain ample hemoglobin, most macrocytes lack the central pallor of normal red cells and even appear **"hyperchromic,"** but the MCHC is not elevated.
- Examination of the blood smear often reveals the **two most valuable findings for differentiating megaloblastic from nonmegaloblastic anemia: Neutrophil hypersegmentation and oval macrocytes**
- There is marked variation in the size (**anisocytosis**) and shape (**poikilocytosis**) of red cells.
- The **reticulocyte count is low**.
- Nucleated red cell progenitors occasionally appear in the circulating blood when anemia is severe. Neutrophils are also larger than normal (**macropolymorphonuclear**) and **hypersegmented,** having five or more nuclear lobules instead of the normal three to four (Red arrow). Typically, more than 5 percent of the neutrophils have five lobes
- **Neutrophile hypersegmentation is one of the most sensitive and specific signs of megaloblastic anemia**
- Megaloblastic granulocyte precursors are larger than normal. They show **nuclear-cytoplasmic asynchrony**, with cytoplasm that looks less mature than the cytoplasm of their normal counterparts. A characteristic cell is the **giant metamyelocyte**, which has a large horseshoe-shaped nucleus, sometimes irregularly shaped, containing ragged open chromatin.

PATHO PLATE 10

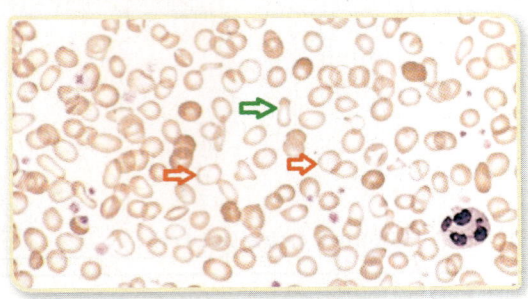

KEY

BLOOD PICTURE OF IRON DEFICIENCY ANEMIA

- **Anisocytosis** is the earliest recognizable morphologic change of erythrocytes in iron-deficiency anemia In peripheral blood smears, the red cells are small (**microcytic**) **and pale (hypochromic).**
- In established iron deficiency the **zone of pallor is enlarged; hemoglobin may be seen only in a narrow peripheral rim (Red arrow)** (Normal red cells with sufficient hemoglobin have a zone of central pallor measuring about one third of the cell diameter).
- **Poikilocytosis** in the form of small, elongated red cells (**pencil cells- green arrow**) is also characteristically seen
- **Target cells** may sometimes be present.
- Thrombocytopenia and thrombocytosis have both been attributed to iron deficiency. Thrombocytosis has been reported in 50 to 75 percent of adults with classic iron-deficiency anemia caused by chronic blood loss. However, thrombocytosis usually occurs only in those patients who are actively bleeding.
- **Reticulocytes are often mildly increased**, a finding consistent with the increased erythroid activity of the marrow.

PATHO PLATE 11

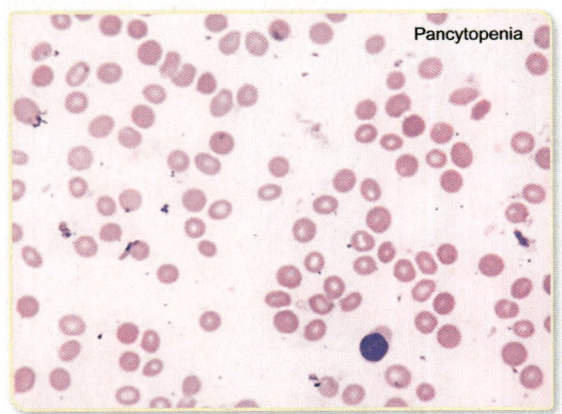

KEY

BLOOD PICTURE OF APLASTIC ANEMIA

- Patients with aplastic anemia have varying degrees of **pancytopenia**.
- Anemia is associated with a **low reticulocyte index**.

- The *relative reticulocyte count is usually less than 1 percent* and may be zero despite the high levels of erythropoietin.
- Absolute reticulocyte counts are usually fewer than 40,000/μL (40 x 10⁹/L).
- **Macrocytes** may be present.
- The absolute neutrophil and monocyte count are low. An absolute neutrophil count fewer than 500/μL (0.5 x 10⁹/L) along with a platelet count fewer than 30,000/μL (30 x 10⁹/L) is indicative of severe disease and a neutrophil count below 200/μL (0.2 x 10⁹/L) denotes very severe disease
- A **hypocellular bone marrow** is required for the diagnosis of aplastic anemia.

PATHO PLATE 12

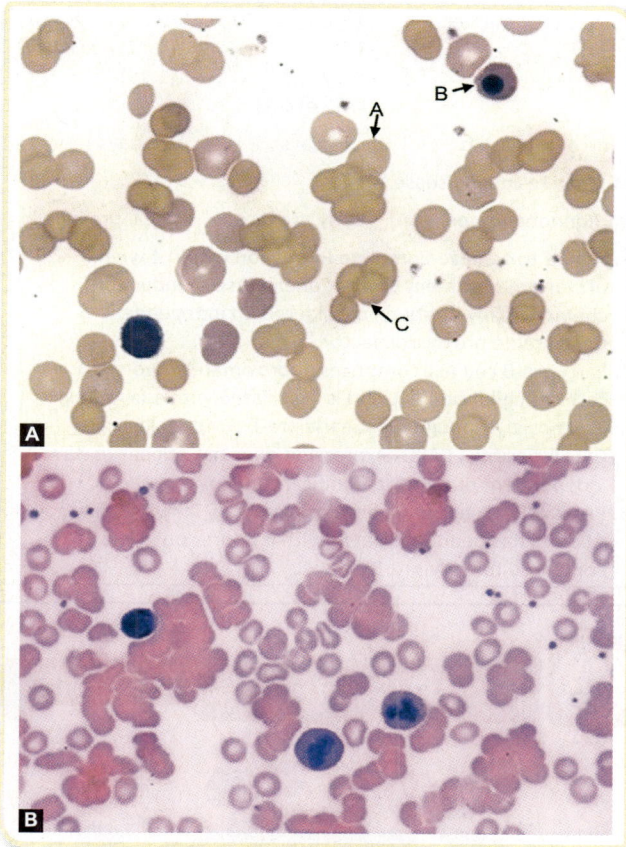

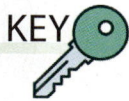

PLATE LEGENDS

A. **Warm AIHA:** Peripheral blood smear showing microspherocytosis (A), nucleated red cell (B) and red cell clumps (C) in a patient with immune-mediated hemolysis. The spherocytes lack a central halo of normal red cells and they are smaller than the nucleus of a normal lymphocyte.

B. **Cold AIHA:** Peripheral blood smear showing marked RBC agglutination into irregular clamps. The background of the smear is bluish because of high protein content, which contains IgM hemagglutinin.

PATHO PLATE 13

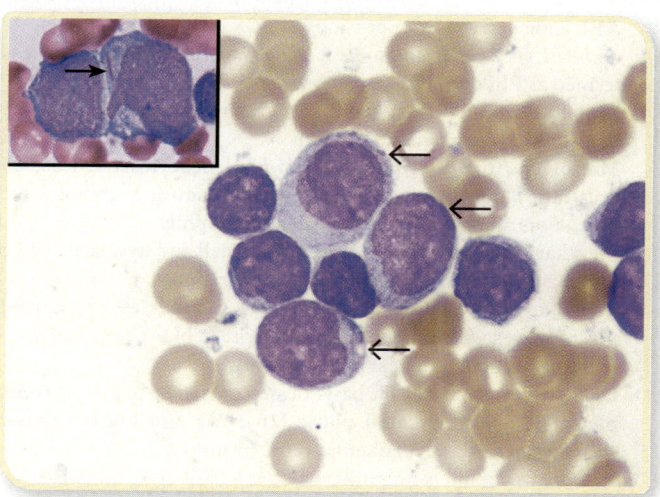

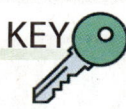

ACUTE MYELOID LEUKEMIA (AML)

- It is a tumor of hematopoietic progenitors caused by acquired oncogenic mutations that impede differentiation leading to accumulation of immature myeloid blasts in the marrow.
- It leads to marrow failure and complications related to anemia, thrombocytopenia and neutropenia.
- Diagnosis is based on presence of **20% or more myeloid blasts in marrow**.
- **Blasts** (long arrows) have delicate chromatin, 2-4 nucleoli and more cytoplasm than lymphoblasts. They also show fine peroxidase positive azurophilic granules in the cytoplasm.
- **Auer rods** (needle like azurophilic granules) are a distinctive feature of myeloid blasts (insat). These are more abundant in APML (acute promyelocytic leukemia).
- Occasionally, blasts are totally absent from blood (aleukemic leukemia) hence marrow examination is essential to rule out acute leukemia in pancytopenic patients.
- Immunophenotyping plays important role in differentiating myeloblasts from lymphoblasts.
- Cytogenetics and molecular pathology are important in classification of AML as treatment differs according to type.

PATHO PLATE 14

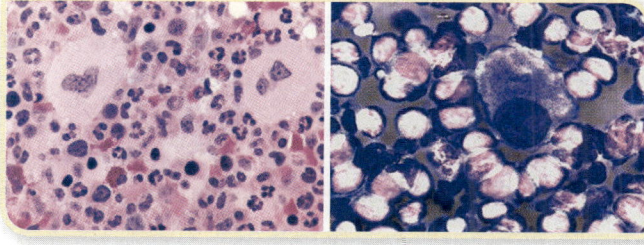

CHRONIC MYELOID LEUKEMIA (CML)

- It is a myeloproliferative disorder characterized by chimeric **BCR-ABL gene** derived from portions of *BCR gene on chromosome 22 and ABL gene on chromosome 9*. Presence of this chimeric gene is termed as **Philadelphia chromosome.**
- It directs production of a mutant tyrosine kinase, which is the basis of its systemic manifestations.
- Marrow picture is hypercellular with leucocytosis (>1,00,000 cells/mm³) due to massive increase in maturing granulocytic precursors along with eosinophils and basophils.
- Megakaryocytes are also increased but small and dysplastic while erythroid cells may be normal to slightly reduced.
- Characteristic finding- **'sea green histiocytes'** (scattered macrophages with abundant wrinkled green blue cytoplasm).
- Increased reticulin deposition in marrow.
- Divided into 3 phases on basis of percentage of blasts- **chronic phase (10%), accelerated phase (10-19%) and blastic phase/ conversion to acute leukaemia (20% or more).**
- Specific treatment is imatinib, which is a BCR-ABL inhibitor.

PATHO PLATE 15

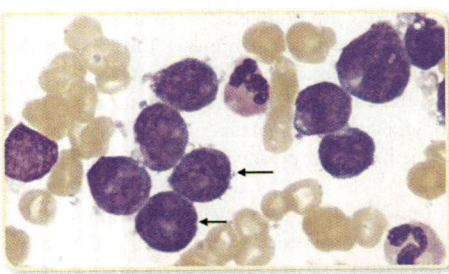

ACUTE LYMPHOID LEUKEMIA (ALL)

- These are neoplasms of immature B cells or T cells which are referred to as lymphoblasts (long arrows)
- 85% of all cases are B-ALLs which manifest typically as childhood acute leukemias while rest are T-ALLs which manifest as thymic 'lymphomas' in adolescents specially males.
- Marrow is hypercellular, packed with lymphoblasts, which replace the normal marrow elements.
- Blasts are larger, with scanty cytoplasm as compared to small lymphocytes.
- As compared to myeloid blasts, lymphoblasts have more condensed chromatin, less conspicuous or absent nucleoli and lesser cytoplasm without granules.
- However morphological differentiation is not absolute and definitive diagnosis is based on immunohistochemistry.
- Histochemical stains are also helpful as lymphoblasts are **MPO negative** and show **PAS positive** cytoplasmic granules.
- ALL is the commonest cancer in children but it has about 95% remission rate with aggressive chemotherapy and 75-85% complete cure rates.
- Yet it is the leading cause of cancer deaths in children.

Prognostic Factors of All		
Determinants	Favorable	Unfavorable
WBC count / µL	Low (<50000)	High (>100000)
Age	2-10 yrs	<1 & > 10yrs
Sex	Female	Male
Race	White	Black
Hepatosplenomegaly and lymphadenopathy	Absent	present
Testicular involvement	Absent	Present
CNS	Absent	Overt
FAB classification	L1	L2
PLOIDY	Hyperdiploidy (>50 chromosomes)	Hypodiploidy (<45 chromosomes)
Cytogenetic markers	Trisomy 4, 10, 17 t(12:21) (TEL:AML1)	t(9:22) (BCR:ABL) t(4:11) (MLL AF4) t(1:19)
Time of remission	<14 days	>28 days
Minimal residual disease	<10^{-4}	>10^{-3}
Immunophenotype	Early pre B cell	T cell, pre B cell

1. Failure to achieve Complete Remission within 4 weeks of starting treatment or after one course of induction chemotherapy has been considered an independent unfavorable prognostic factor
2. Early pre-B cell ALL comprises approximately two-thirds of cases of childhood ALL and is associated with a favorable prognosis. Although most early pre-B lymphoblasts are CALLA positive, CALLA expression does not appear to have independent prognostic significance.
3. Pre-B cell ALL accounts for approximately 20% of childhood ALL and has been associated with a poorer outcome compared to early pre-B cell ALL.

PATHO PLATE 16

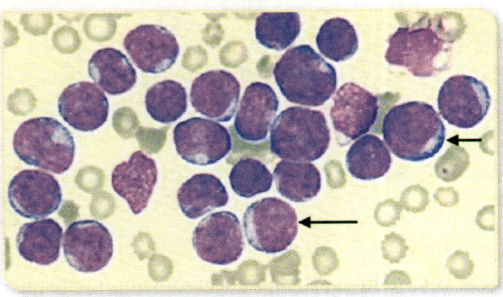

CHRONIC LYMPHOID LEUKEMIA (CLL)

- Although the diagnosis of CLL previously required a lymphocytosis of >5×10^9/L, it has more recently been suggested that the diagnosis can be made with the presence of a chronic absolute increase in blood lymphocytes having the typical morphologic and immunophenotypic features

- Commonest adult leukemia in the Western world.
- Median age of diagnosis is 60 years and 2:1 male preponderance.
- Lymph nodes are diffusely effaced with **atypical small lymphocytes admixed with larger active lymphocytes** (long arrows) **in loose aggregates (proliferation centers)** which are pathognomonic for CLL.
- In peripheral smears, the small lymphocytes may be disrupted in the smearing process producing smudge cells.
- **Smudge cells** (basket cells or shadow cells of Gumprecht) are commonly seen in the blood smear and appear to be caused by a decrease in vimentin (223,224). A recent study suggests that patients with ≥30% smudge cells are more likely to have mutated IgVH and have a better prognosis than those with <30% smudge cells
- A number of other conditions can produce peripheral lymphocytosis, but a careful examination of the blood smear and immunophenotyping can differentiate these disorders
- Distinct immunophenotype-express pan–B-cell surface antigens, such as **CD19 and CD20 well as CD23 and CD5. CLL B cells also express CD27**
- Chromosomal translocations rare in CLL.
- Generally, manifestations are non specific like anorexia and weight loss or sometimes it may be completely asymptomatic.
- Conversion to aggressive forms may occur. Commonly it is converted to prolymphocytic form. Less commonly into diffuse large B cell lymphoma, called as **Richter syndrome.**
- Most symptomatic patients have **enlarged lymph nodes as well as splenomegaly**. Enlargement of the cervical and supraclavicular nodes occurs more frequently than axillary or inguinal lymphadenopathy. The lymph nodes are usually discrete, freely movable, and nontender. Painful enlarged nodes usually indicate superimposed infection, which may be bacterial or viral. There is usually only mild to moderate enlargement of the spleen, and splenic infarction is uncommon. Less common manifestations are enlargement of the tonsils, abdominal masses due to mesenteric or retroperitoneal lymphadenopathy, and skin infiltration

an inflammatory condition that affects the genitourinary tract. Michaelis–Gutmann bodies are thought to represent remnants of phagosomes mineralized by iron and calcium deposits. In many macrophages there is central core and a targetoid appearance (Green arrow), in others appearance is homogenous (Blue arrow). In some cells, there are several inclusions (red arrow) and occasionally this bodies can be seen extracellular.

PATHO PLATE 18

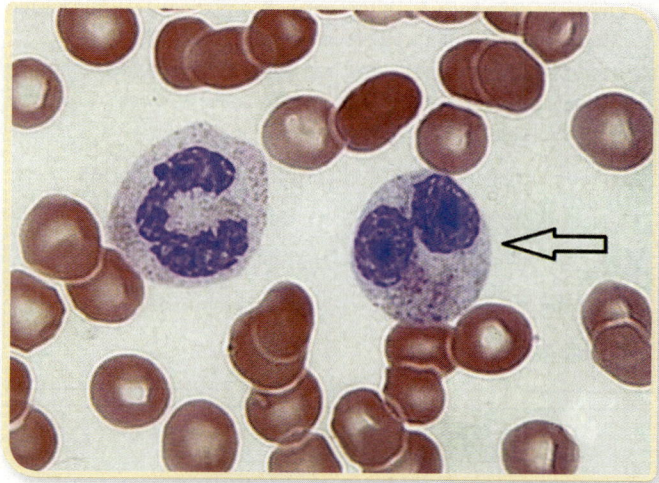

KEY

PELGER-HUËT ANOMALY

It is characterized by distinctive shapes of the nuclei of leukocytes, **hyposegmented neutrophils**, and coarseness of the chromatin of the nuclei of neutrophils, lymphocytes, and monocytes. The nuclei appear rod-like, dumbbell shaped, peanut shaped, and **spectacle like ("pince-nez")** with smooth, round, or oval individual lobes, contrasted with the irregular lobes seen in normal neutrophils.

PATHO PLATE 17

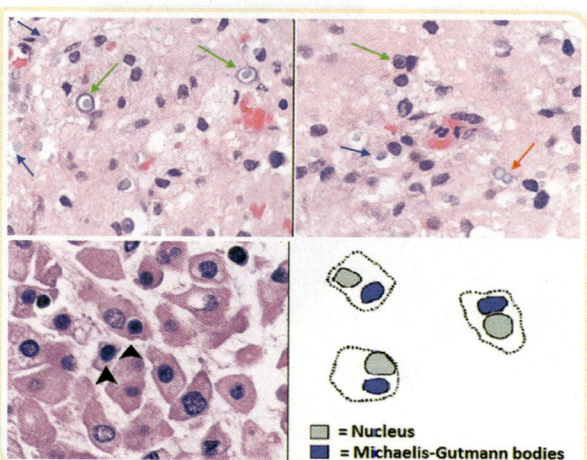

KEY

MICHAELIS–GUTMANN BODIES

Michaelis–Gutmann bodies are concentrically layered basophilic inclusions bodies that are pathognomonic feature of *malakoplakia*,

PATHO PLATE 19

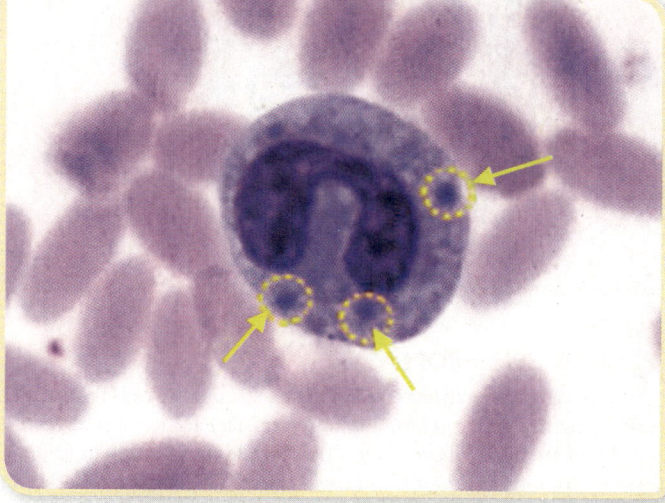

115

PATHO PLATE 20

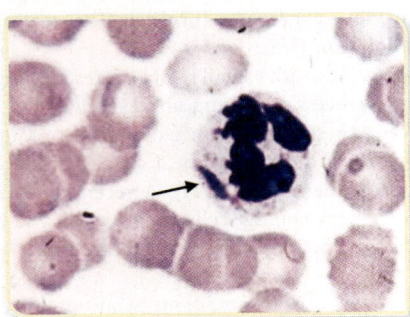

DOHLE BODIES

Dohle bodies are single or multiple round, oval, or filamentous sky-blue inclusions (Yellow arrow) with Romanowksy stains found at the periphery of the cytoplasm of neutrophils.

- Dohle bodies represents **lamellar aggregates of rough endoplasmic reticulum** on electron microscopic studies
- They are associated with toxicity and may be seen together with toxic granulations in scarlet fever, severe infections, burns, administration of cytotoxic agents like cyclophosphamide
- Dohle bodies must be differentiated with May Hegglin bodies which are morphologically identical.

Dohle Bodies	May Hegglin Anomaly
Mostly multiple	Always single
Rounded inclusion	Crescent shaped inclusion
Myeloid series shift to left	No shift to left
Elevated TLC	Normal TLC
Toxic granulation	No toxic granulation
Vacuolization in cytoplasm	Giant platelet

MAY-HEGGLIN INCLUSION

Neutrophil containing a typical **May-Hegglin inclusion** (arrow). The May-Hegglin anomaly is a rare, dominantly inherited disorder characterized by large (2 to 5 μm), well-defined, basophilic and pyroninophilic inclusions in granulocytes (neutrophils, eosinophils, basophils, monocytes) and accompanied by variable thrombocytopenia and giant platelets containing few granules. See previous plate to see difference from Dohle bodies.

PATHO PLATE 21

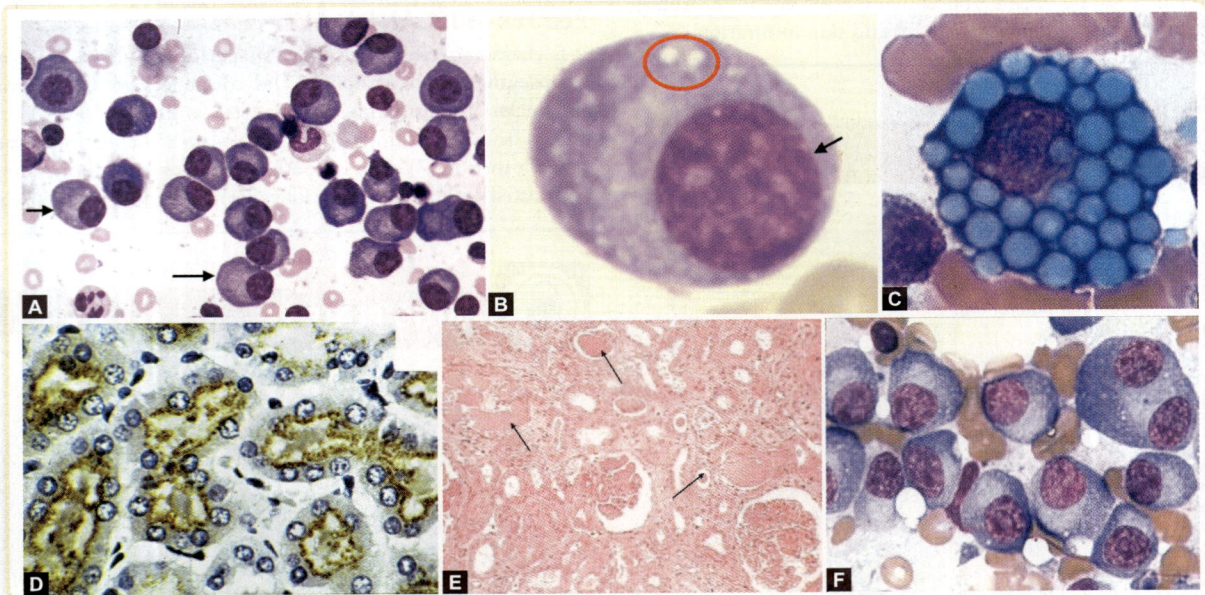

PLASMA CELL NEOPLASMS

These B-cell proliferations contain neoplastic plasma cells that virtually always secrete a monoclonal Ig or Ig fragment. Collectively, the plasma cell neoplasms (often referred to as dyscrasias) account for about 15% of the deaths caused by lymphoid neoplasms. The most common and deadly of these neoplasms is multiple myeloma. Multiple myeloma (plasma cell myeloma), the most important monoclonal gammopathy, usually presents as tumorous masses scattered throughout the skeletal system. Solitary myeloma (plasmacytoma) is an infrequent variant that presents as a single mass in bone or soft tissue.

A. Plasma cell have **basophilic cytoplasm** containing pale zones of extensive **Golgi apparatus** and an **eccentric nucleus** with heterochromatin in a characteristic **cartwheel or clock face arrangement.** The plasma cells are well differentiated morphologically. The more mature cells have clumped nuclear chromatin, abundant cytoplasm, low nuclear-cytoplasmic ratio
B. **Plasma cell high definition (classical):** Basophilic (blue) cytoplasm, Cartwheel eccentric nucleus (arrow), and pale Golgi apparatus in cytoplasm (red circle).

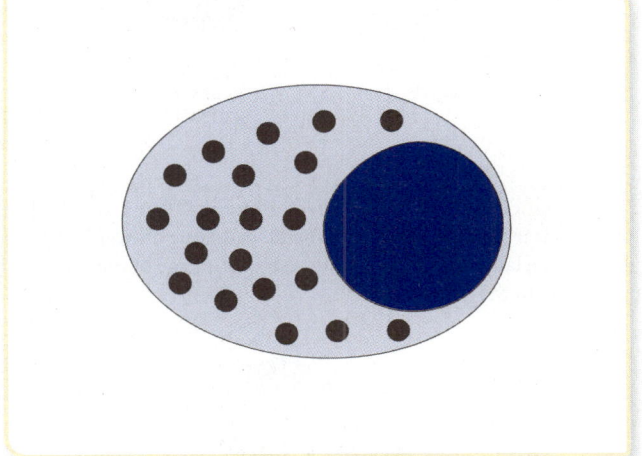

C. Plasma cell myeloma, morphologic variants based on cytoplasmic features. So-called **Mott cell with abundant "grape-like"** cytoplasmic inclusions of immunoglobulin.
D. **Plasma cell myeloma:** Section of kidney showing renal tubular lambda deposition with casts reflecting renal tubular Bence Jones protein reabsorption (**Immunoperoxidase, anti-lambda light chain**). Immunohistochemical stains on marrow biopsy sections are often valuable to essential in the diagnosis of plasma cell neoplasms. They may be used to:
   - Assess the quantity of plasma cells in marrow biopsies
   - Identify monoclonal plasma cell proliferations
   - Distinguish myeloma from other neoplasms
E. **Bence Jones cast nephropathy** in multiple myeloma is associated with glassy, fracturing casts occluding the tubular lumina (arrows). Multinucleated giant cells surround some casts.
F. **Bone marrow biopsy in multiple myeloma:** plasma cells with basophilic cytoplasm, eccentric nuclei, and "clock face" chromatin.

PATHO PLATE 22

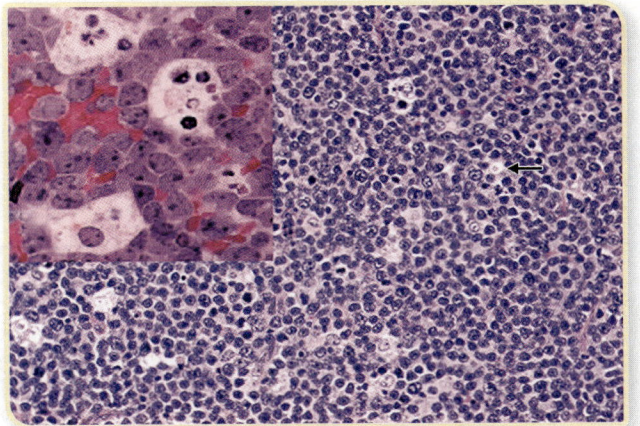

BURKITT'S LYMPHOMA

- Classified into- Endemic (African) type, Non endemic (sporadic) type, HIV associated aggressive type
- BL tumor cells are intermediate in size (Medium size) and typically have round or oval nuclei and two to five distinct nucleoli. There is a moderate amount of basophilic or amphophilic cytoplasm that often contains small, lipid-filled vacuoles (a feature appreciated only on smears).
- Medium-sized lymphoma cells (**Burkitt cells**) have a very high proliferative rate and frequent mitotic figures. The rate of proliferation, as determined with **Ki-67 staining**, is at or above 95 percent
- These cells are characterized by a high rate of spontaneous apoptosis with interspersed macrophages engorged with cellular debris as a result of the high cell turnover rate (high rate of apoptosis and cell proliferation) leading to the characteristic **"starry sky" pattern** in marrow and lymph nodes
- Nuclear contours are round to oval without cleaves or folds, a key feature in the distinction from diffuse large cell lymphoma
- Nuclear remnants are phagocytosed by benign macrophages (**tangible body macrophages**)
- BL cells are mature B cells, **positive for CD19, CD20, CD22, and CD79a, and have monotypic surface IgM; they lack CD5 and CD23.**
- BL cells also show immunologic similarity to germinal center cells of B-cell follicles rather than activated B cells, being positive for BCL6, CD10, Tcl1, and CD38, and negative for Mum-1, CD44, CD138, and Bcl-2.
- All forms are associated with **c-MYC gene translocations on chromosome 8.** Most translocations fuse MYC with the IgH gene on chromosome 14, but variant translocations involving the κ and λ light chain loci on chromosomes 2 and 22, respectively, are also observed. The net result of each is the same—the dysregulation and overexpression of **MYC protein.**
- Essentially all endemic type and about 20% of sporadic cases tumors are latently infected by **EBV**. It was the first tumor to be etiologically associated with a virus
- Most tumors occur at extra nodal sites- commonest presentation for endemic type is a mass involving mandible and for sporadic type, mass involving the ileocaecum and peritoneum.
- Very aggressive tumor but responds well to intensive chemotherapy.
- Most children and young adults have very high rates of complete cure but prognosis is guarded in adults.

PATHO PLATE 23

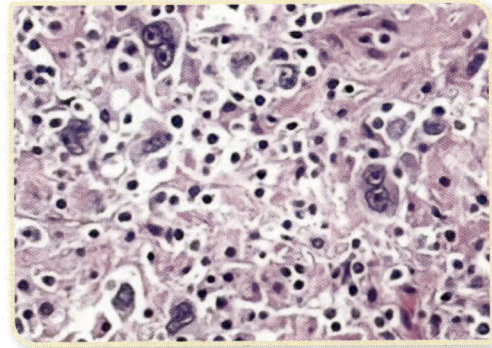

HODGKINS LYMPHOMA

- **Essential for the diagnosis of Hodgkin lymphoma is the Reed-Sternberg (RS) cell**, a very large cell (15 to 45 μm in diameter) with an enormous multilobate nucleus, exceptionally prominent nucleoli and abundant, usually slightly eosinophilic cytoplasm. Particularly characteristic are cells with two mirror-image nuclei or nuclear lobes, each containing a large (inclusion-like) acidophilic nucleolus surrounded by a clear zone, features that impart an **owl-eye appearance**. The nuclear membrane is distinct.
- Typical RS cells and variants have a characteristic immunophenotype, as they **express CD15 and CD30 and fail to express CD45** (common leukocyte antigen), B cell antigens, and T cell antigens. As we shall see, "classic" RS cells are common in the mixed-cellularity subtype, uncommon in the nodular sclerosis subtype, and rare in the lymphocyte predominance subtype; in these latter two subtypes, other characteristic RS cell variants predominate.
- The events that transform Reed Sternberg cells and alter their appearance and gene expression programs are still unclear. One clue stems from the involvement of EBV. **EBV is present in the RS cells in as many as 70% of cases of the mixed-cellularity subtype and a smaller fraction of other "classical" forms of Hodgkin lymphoma.** More important, the integration of the EBV genome is identical in all RS cells in a given case, indicating that infection precedes (and therefore may be related to) transformation and clonal expansion.
- Thus, as in Burkitt lymphoma and B cell lymphomas in immunodeficient patients, EBV infection probably is one of several steps contributing to tumor development, particularly of the mixed-cellularity subtype.

KEY

Reed-sternberg cells (and variants) are large cells with very striking "Inclusion-like" eosinophilic nucleoli. Try and identify them using the following diagram:

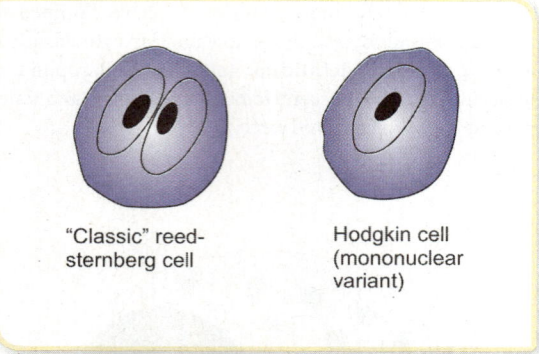

"Classic" reed-sternberg cell | Hodgkin cell (mononuclear variant)

The lacunar cell variant has a folded or multilobulated nucleus lying within a clear space with fine pink bands radiating outwards from the nucleus; the latter are artifacts caused by shrinkage of the cell during processing in the laboratory.

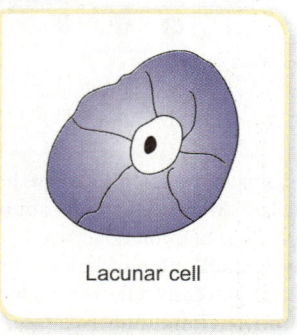

Lacunar cell

Subtypes of Hodgkin's Lymphoma

Subtype	Morphology and immunophenotype	Typical clinical features
Nodular sclerosis	Frequent **lacunar cells** and occasional diagnostic **RS cells**; background infiltrate composed of T lymphocytes, eosinophils, macrophages, and plasma cells; fibrous bands dividing cellular areas into nodules. RS cells CD15+, CD30+; usually EBV-	**Most common subtype**; usually stage I or II disease; frequent mediastinal involvement; equal occurrence in males and females (F = M), most patients young adults
Mixed cellularity	Frequent mononuclear and diagnostic RS cells; background infiltrate rich in T lymphocytes, eosinophils, macrophages, plasma cells; RS cells CD15+, CD30+; 70% EBV+	More than 50% present as stage III or IV disease; M greater than F; biphasic incidence, peaking in young adults and again in adults older than 55
Lymphocyte predominance	Frequent mononuclear and diagnostic RS cells; background infiltrate rich in T lymphocytes; RS cells CD15+, CD30+; 40% EBV+	Uncommon; M greater than F; tends to be seen in older adults
Lymphocyte depletion	Reticular variant: Frequent diagnostic RS cells and variants and a paucity of background reactive cells; RS cells CD15+, CD30+; most EBV+	Uncommon; more common in older males, HIV-infected individuals, and in developing countries; often presents with advanced disease
Lymphocyte predominance	Frequent L&H (popcorn cell) variants in a background of follicular dendritic cells and reactive B cells; RS cells CD20+, CD15-, C30-; EBV-	Uncommon; young males with cervical or axillary lymphadenopathy; mediastinal

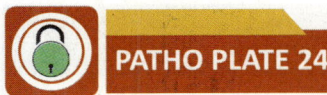

PATHO PLATE 24

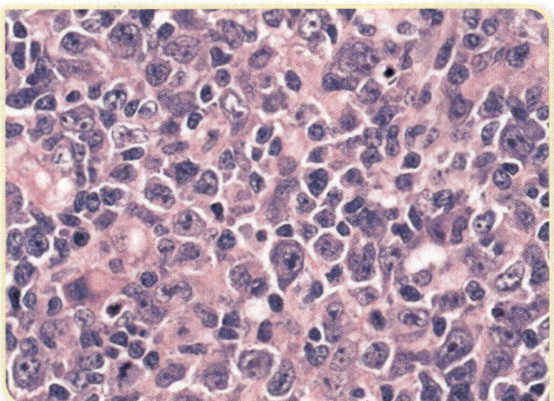

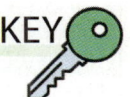

In **Gaucher disease,** the degradation stops at the level of **glucocerebrosides,** which accumulate in the phagocytes. These phagocytes—the Gaucher cells— become enlarged, with some reaching a diameter as great as 100 μm, because of the accumulation of distended lysosomes, and acquire a pathognomonic cytoplasmic appearance characterized as **"wrinkled tissue paper".** No distinct vacuolation is present.

PATHO PLATE 26

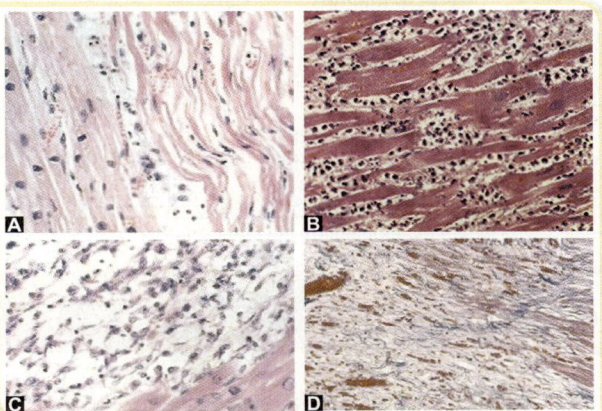

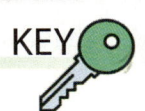

INFECTIOUS MONONUCLEOSIS

Characteristic morphological features of **infectious mononucleosis** cases. Ulceration of tonsillar mucosa and geographic ulcer. Focal distortion of normal tissue architecture. Polymorphous infiltrates consisting of scattered immunoblasts in a background of numerous small mature lymphocytes and plasma cells.

PATHO PLATE 25

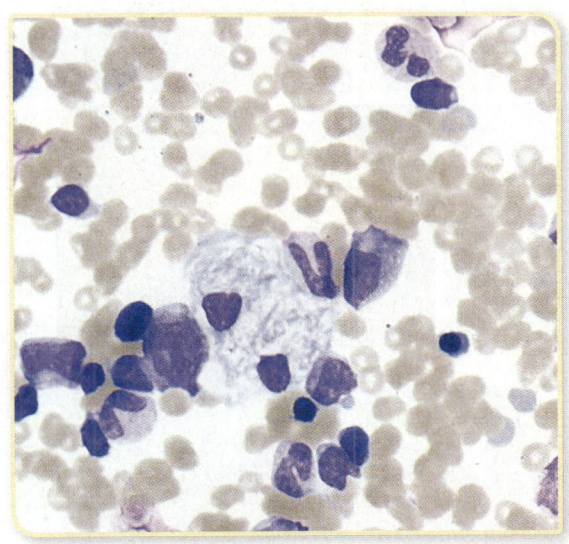

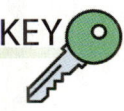

MICROSCOPIC FEATURES OF MYOCARDIAL INFARCTION

Microscopic features of **myocardial infarction** and its repair.

A. **< 24 hour old infarct:** Showing **coagulative necrosis along with wavy fibers** (elongated and narrow) as compared with adjacent normal fibers (at left). Widened spaces between the dead fibers contain edema fluid and scattered neutrophils.

B. **1-3 days old infarct:** Reperfusion contraction band/ coagulative necrosis with Dense polymorphonuclear leukocytic infiltrate in area of acute myocardial infarction

C. **3 to 7 days old infarct:** Dead myocytes begin to disintegrate and are removed by macrophages and enzyme proteolysis. There is proliferation of fibroblasts with formation of granulation tissue, which progressively replaces necrotic tissue. Nearly complete removal of necrotic myocytes by phagocytosis (approximately 7 to 10 days).

D. **> 2 Weeks old infarct:** Granulation tissue characterized by loose collagen and abundant capillaries.

Evolution of Morphologic Changes in Myocardial Infarction			
Time	Gross features	Light microscope	Electron microscope
Reversible injury			
0–½ hr	None	None	Relaxation of myofibrils; glycogen loss; mitochondrial swelling
Irreversible injury			
½–4 hr	None	Usually none; variable **waviness of fibers** at border may be present	Sarcolemmal disruption; mitochondrial amorphous densities

Contd...

Evolution of Morphologic Changes in Myocardial Infarction

Time	Gross features	Light microscope	Electron microscope
4–12 hr	Dark mottling (occasional)	**Early coagulation necrosis (loss of nuclei) with wavy fibers**; edema; hemorrhage	
12–24 hr	Dark mottling	Ongoing **coagulation necrosis with wavy fibers**; pyknosis of nuclei; myocyte hypereosinophilia; marginal **contraction band necrosis**; early neutrophilic infiltrate	
1–3 days	Mottling with yellow-tan infarct center	Coagulation necrosis, with loss of nuclei and striations; **brisk interstitial infiltrate of neutrophils**	
3–7 days	Hyperemic border; central yellow-tan softening	Beginning disintegration of dead myofibers, with dying neutrophils; early phagocytosis of dead cells by macrophages at infarct border	
7–10 days	Maximally yellow-tan and soft, with depressed red-tan margins	Well-developed phagocytosis of dead cells; early formation of fibrovascular granulation tissue at margins	
10–14 days	Red-gray depressed infarct borders	Well-established granulation tissue with new blood vessels and collagen deposition	
2–8 wk	Gray-white scar, progressive from border toward core of infarct	Increased collagen deposition, with decreased cellularity	
>2 mo	Scarring complete	Dense collagenous scar	

PATHO PLATE 27

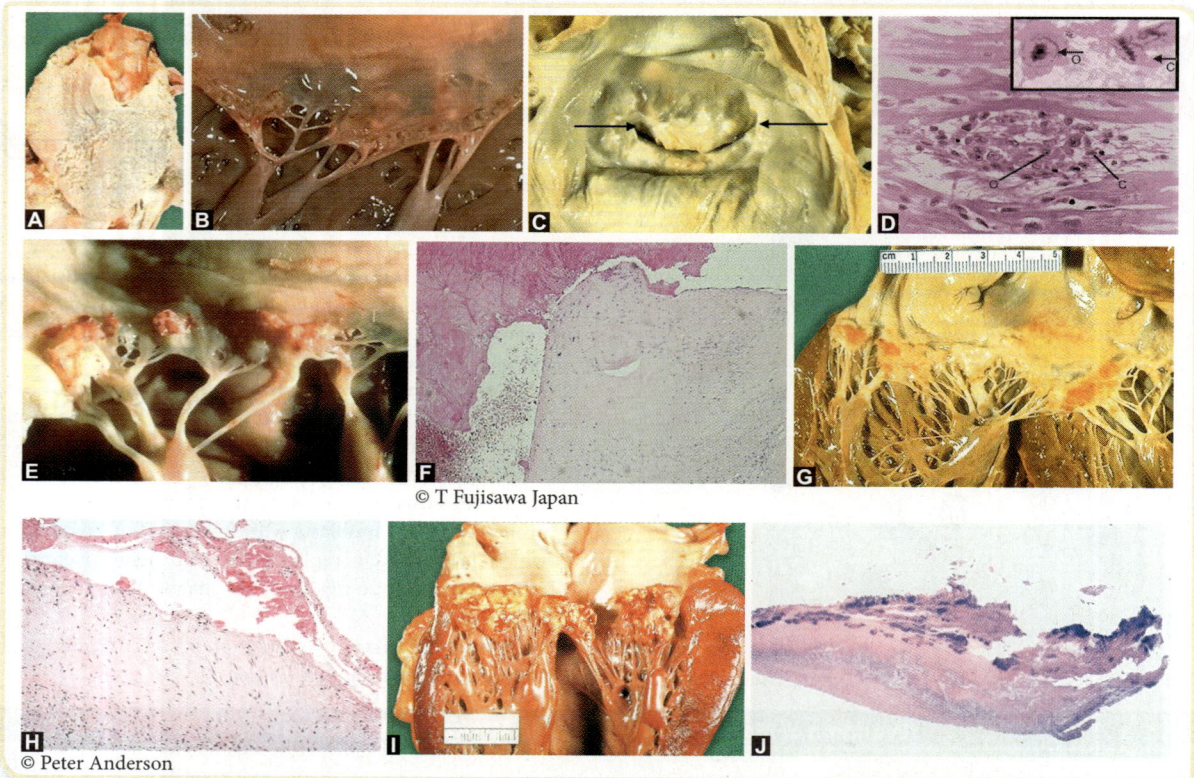

PLATE LEGENDS

A. **Rheumatic Heart disease Gross:** Bread and Butter pericarditis
B. **Rheumatic Heart disease Gross:** Valvular vegetation- **Irregular, warty, firm**, along the line of closure of valves
C. **Rheumatic Heart disease Gross:** Fibrous bridging across the valves and calcification causes **"Fishmouth" or "Buttonhole" stenosis**

D. **Rheumatic Heart disease HPE: Aschoff bodies or Rheumatic granuloma** demarcated by
   - **Anitschkow cells** (Specialized Histiocytes which appears caterpillar like in cross section- marked as C and owl's eye in longitudinal section- marked as O) associated with fibrinoid necrosis
   - Scattered Plasma cells and T lymphocytes
   - Aschoff cells (Inflammatory Giant cells)

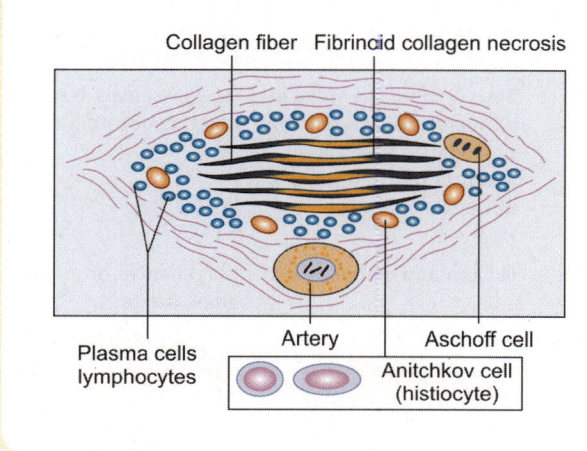

E. **Non bacterial thrombotic endocarditis Gross:** Bland thrombi that are loosely attached to the underlying valve along the line of closure of the leaflets or cusps.
F. **Non bacterial thrombotic endocarditis HPE:** Bland thrombus, with virtually no inflammation thrombus is only loosely attached to the cusp. Vegetation made up of a web like mesh of fibrin and platelets with numerous RBC trapped within it
G. **Libman sack's endocarditis Gross:** Irregular, granular, small (1–4 mm in diameter), sterile, pink vegetations that often have a warty (verrucous) appearance
H. **Libman sack's endocarditis histology:** Atrial surface of mitral valve with small fibrin thrombus representing Libman Sacks endocarditis. Vegetations consist of a finely granular, fibrinous eosinophilic material that may contain hematoxylin bodies, homogeneous remnants of nuclei.
I. **Infective endocarditis Gross:** Irregular, Friable, bulky, potentially destructive vegetations that extends to chordae. Vegetations sometimes erode into the underlying myocardium and produce an abscess (**ring abscess**).
J. **Infective endocarditis HPE:** Valve in infective endocarditis demonstrates friable vegetations of fibrin and platelets (pink) mixed with inflammatory cells and bacterial colonies (blue). Vegetations often have granulation tissue indicative of healing at their bases. With time, fibrosis, calcification, and a chronic inflammatory infiltrate can develop.

	Types of Endocarditis			
	Rheumatic fever	**Non bacterial thrombotic endocarditis**	**Libman sack's endocarditis**	**Infective endocarditis**
Seen in	Rheumatic fever	AKA- **Marantic endocarditis** Hypercoagulable state, AML-M3, Cancer	SLE	Infective endocarditis
Size	Small	Small	Medium	Large
Gross	☐ Bread and Butter pericarditis ☐ Myocarditis (With Aschoff bodies/ Rheumatic granuloma) ☐ Endocarditis (With Fibrinoid necrosis) ☐ Valvular vegetation- **Irregular, warty, firm**, along the line of closure of valves ☐ Fibrous bridging across the valves and calcification causes **"Fishmouth" or "Buttonhole" stenosis**	Composed of bland thrombi that are loosely attached to the underlying valve. Single or Multiple vegetation 1-5 mm in size, along the line of closure of the leaflets or cusps. Not invasive and do not elicit any inflammatory reaction	Irregular, granular, small (1–4 mm in diameter), sterile, pink vegetations that often have a warty (verrucous) appearance	Irregular, Friable, bulky, Potentially destructive vegetations that extends to chordae. Vegetations sometimes erode into the underlying myocardium and produce an abscess (**ring abscess**).
Histopathology	**Aschoff bodies or Rheumatic granuloma** demarcated by ☐ **Anitschkow cells** (Specialized Histiocytes which appears caterpillar like in cross section and owl's eye in longitudinal section) associated with fibrinoid necrosis ☐ Scattered Plasma cells and T lymphocytes ☐ Aschoff cells (Inflammatory Giant cells)	Bland thrombus, with virtually no inflammation thrombus is only loosely attached to the cusp. Vegetation made up of a web like mesh of fibrin and platelets with numerous RBC trapped within it	Vegetations consist of a finely granular, fibrinous eosinophilic material that may contain hematoxylin bodies, homogeneous remnants of nuclei damaged by anti-nuclear antigen bodies	Valve demonstrates friable vegetations of fibrin and platelets (pink) mixed with inflammatory cells and bacterial colonies (blue). Vegetations often have granulation tissue indicative of healing at their bases. With time, fibrosis, calcification, & a chronic inflammatory infiltrate can develop.
Friability	Friable (but less than NBTE)	Friable	Not friable	Friable
Sterility	Sterile	Sterile	Sterile	Non sterile

Contd...

Types of Endocarditis

	Rheumatic fever	Non bacterial thrombotic endocarditis	Libman sack's endocarditis	Infective endocarditis
Composition	Fibrin only	Bland thrombus, no inflammation	Fibrinous eosinophilic material, hematoxylin bodies	Fibrin, bacteria, platelets, inflammatory cells
Valve Location	Left sided valve (Mitral valve > Mitral + Aortic > Aortic alone > Mitral + Aortic + Tricuspid)	Right sided valve (Tricuspid, Pulmonary)	Mitral valve is more frequently involved than the aortic valve	Left sided- aortic and mitral valves are the most common sites (right sided in IV drug users)
Location on the valve	Located along the lines of closure	Along lines of closure of valves	Seen on both the surfaces, although more commonly on undersurface, mural endocardium and valve pockets may also be involved	On valve cusps, less on mural endocardium
Emboli	Embolization not common	Uncommon embolization	Uncommon embolization	Max chances of embolization
	RHD	NBTE	LSE	IE

PATHO PLATE 28

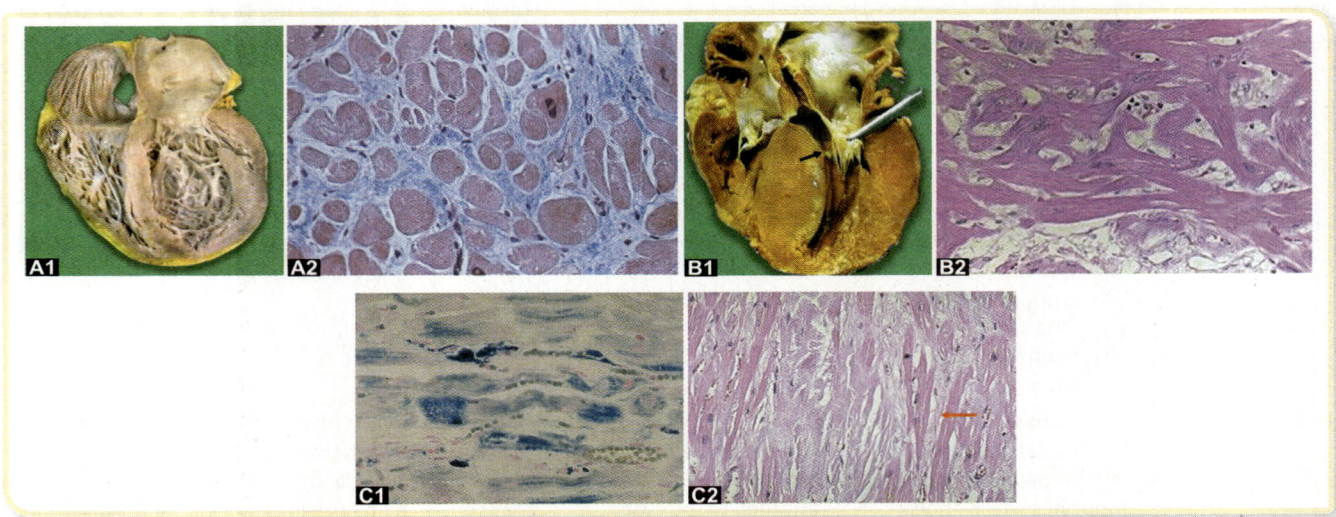

KEY

Types of Cardiomyopathy

	Dilated	Restrictive	Hypertrophic
Ejection fraction (normal >55%)	Usually <30% when symptoms severe	25-50%	>60%
Left ventricular diastolic dimension (normal <55 mm)	>60 mm	>60 mm (may be decreased)	Often decreased

Contd...

Types of Cardiomyopathy

	Dilated	Restrictive	Hypertrophic
Left ventricular wall thickness	Decreased	Normal or increased	Markedly increased
Atrial size	Increased	Increased; may be massive	Increased; related to abnormal
Valvular regurgitation	Related to annular dilation; mitral appears earlier, during decompensation; tricuspid regurgitation in late stages	Related to endocardial involvement; frequent mitral and tricuspid regurgitation, rarely severe	Related to valve-septum interaction; mitral regurgitation
Common first symptoms	Exertional intolerance	Exertional intolerance, fluid retention early	Exertional intolerance; may have chest pain
Congestive symptoms*	Left before right, except right prominent in young adults	Right often dominates	Left-sided congestion may develop late
Physical examination	Moderate to severe cardiomegaly; S3, S4, Atrioventricular valve regurgitation, especially mitral	Mild to moderate cardiomegaly; S3 or S4, Atrioventricular valve regurgitation; inspiratory increase in venous pressure (**Kussmaul sign**)	Mild cardiomegaly Apical systolic thrill and heave; brisk carotid upstroke, S4 common, Systolic murmur that increases with Valsalva maneuver
Chest radiograph	Moderate to marked cardiac enlargement, especially left ventricular Pulmonary venous hypertension	Mild cardiac enlargement Pulmonary venous hypertension	Mild to moderate cardiac enlargement Left atrial enlargement
Electrocardiograph (ECG)	Sinus tachycardia Atrial and ventricular arrhythmias ST-segment and T wave abnormalities Intraventricular conduction defects	Low voltage Intraventricular conduction defects Atrioventricular conduction defects	Left ventricular hypertrophy ST-segment and T wave abnormalities Abnormal Q waves Atrial and ventricular arrhythmias
Arrhythmia	Ventricular tachyarrhythmia; conduction block in Chagas' disease, and some families. Atrial fibrillation.	Ventricular uncommon except in sarcoidosis conduction block in sarcoidosis and amyloidosis. Atrial fibrillation.	Ventricular tachyarrhythmias; atrial fibrillation
Echocardiography	Left ventricular dilation and dysfunction Abnormal diastolic mitral valve motion secondary to abnormal compliance and filling pressures	Increased left ventricular wall thickness and mass Small or normal-size left ventricular cavity Normal systolic function Pericardial effusion	Asymmetric septal hypertrophy Narrow left ventricular outflow tract Systolic anterior motion of the mitral valve Small or normal-sized left ventricle
Radionucleotide studies	Left ventricular dilation and dysfunction (RVG)	Infiltration of myocardium (^{201}Tl) Small or normal-sized left ventricle (RVG) Normal systolic function (RVG)	Small or normal-sized left ventricle (RVG) Vigorous systolic function (RVG) Asymmetric septal hypertrophy (RVG or ^{201}Tl)
Cardiac catheterization	Left ventricular enlargement and dysfunction Mitral and/or tricuspid regurgitation Elevated left- and often right-sided filling pressures Diminished cardiac output	Diminished left ventricular compliance "Square root" sign in ventricular pressure recordings Preserved systolic function Elevated left- and right-sided filling pressures	Diminished left ventricular compliance Mitral regurgitation Vigorous systolic function Dynamic left ventricular outflow gradient
Valvular regurgitation	Related to annular dilation; mitral appears earlier, during decompensation; tricuspid regurgitation in late stages	Related to endocardial involvement; frequent mitral and tricuspid regurgitation, rarely severe	Related to valve-septum interaction; mitral regurgitation
Mechanism of heart failure	Impairment of contractility (**Systolic Dysfunction**)	Impairment of compliance (**diastolic Dysfunction**)	Impairment of compliance (**diastolic Dysfunction**)

Contd...

Types of Cardiomyopathy

	Dilated	Restrictive	Hypertrophic
Gross changes	**A-1:** All 4 chambers are dilated, most severe in the left ventricle which appears globular. Heart is usually enlarged and flabby (weighing approx 2-3 times from normal heart). The wall thickness may be normal as the hypertrophy is masked by the dilatation.	Ventricles are of approximately normal size or slightly enlarged, cavities are not dilated, myocardium is firm and non compliant.	**B-1:** Marked left ventricular hypertrophy, with asymmetric bulging of a very large interventricular septum into the left ventricular chamber (aka asymmetric septal hypertrophy)
Microscopic changes	**A-2:** Most muscle cells are hypertrophic with enlarged nuclei but some are attenuated, stretched and irregular. Interstitial and endocardial fibrosis of variable degree- blue on Trichome stain	There may be only patchy or diffuse interstitial fibrosis. Etiology specific findings can be seen.	**B-2:** Most important histologic features of myocardium in HCM are: ☐ Extensive **myocyte hypertrophy** to a degree unusual in other conditions. ☐ **Haphazard disarray** of bundles of myocyte, individual monocyte and sarcomere within cells (termed myofiber disarry) ☐ **Interstitial fibrosis.**
Etiology	**Most common:** Alcoholic or Idiopathic **Infective:** Viral (Coxsackie, adenovirus, HIV, hepatitis C) Parasitic (T. Cruzi- Chagas' disease, toxoplasmosis) Bacterial (diphtheria), Spirochetal (Borrelia burgdorferi- Lyme disease) Rickettsial- (Q fever), Fungal (with systemic infection) **Noninfective:** Granulomatous inflammatory disease (Sarcoidosis, Giant cell myocarditis) Hypersensitivity myocarditis, Polymyositis, dermatomyositis, Collagen vascular disease Peripartum cardiomyopathy, Transplant rejection **Toxic:** Alcohol, Catecholamines: amphetamines, cocaine, Chemotherapeutic agents: (anthracyclines, trastuzumab), Interferon Other therapeutic agents (hydroxychloroquine, chloroquine), Drugs of misuse (emetine, anabolic steroids), Heavy metals: lead, mercury, Occupational exposure: hydrocarbons, arsenicals **Metabolic:** Nutritional deficiencies (thiamine, selenium, carnitine), Electrolyte deficiencies (calcium, phosphate, magnesium) Endocrinopathy (Thyroid disease Pheochromocytoma, Diabetes), Obesity, Hemochromatosis **Inherited Metabolic Pathway Defects:** (few) **Familial:** Skeletal and cardiac myopathy Dystrophin-related dystrophy (Duchenne's, Becker's), Mitochondrial myopathies (e.g., Kearns-Sayre syndrome), Arrhythmogenic ventricular dysplasia, Hemochromatosis	**Most common:** Amyloidosis **Infiltrative (Between Myocytes):** Amyloidosis (Primary- light chain amyloid, Familial- abnormal transthyretin, Senile- normal transthyretin or atrial peptides), Inherited metabolic defects **Storage (Within Myocytes):** Hemochromatosis (iron), *Inherited metabolic defects* (Pompe's, Forbes, Carnitine transport defect, Fabry's disease, Gaucher disease, Danon's disease (lysosome associated membrane protein, LAMP2), Hemochromatosis, Familial amyloidosis, Barth syndrome, Friedreich's ataxia) **Fibrotic:** Radiation, Scleroderma Endomyocardial: Tropical endomyocardial fibrosis Hypereosinophilic syndrome (Löffler's endocarditis), Carcinoid syndrome, Radiation, Drugs: e.g., serotonin, ergotamine **Overlap with Other Cardiomyopathies:** Hypertrophic cardiomyopathy/"pseudohypertrophic, Minimally dilated" cardiomyopathy (Early stage dilated cardiomyopathy, Partial recovery from dilated cardiomyopathy), Sarcoidosis **Idiopathic**	**Most common:** Idiopathis Hypertrophic subaortic stinosis (IHSS) **Genetic:** This is the best characterized genetic cardiomyopathy, for which more than 400 individual mutations have been identified in 11 sarcomeric genes. More than 80% of the mutations are in the beta-myosin heavy chain, the cardiac myosin-binding protein C, or cardiac troponin T **Pseudohypertrophic:** inherited metabolic diseases **Secondary hypertrophy:** cardiovascular causes

Contd...

Types of Cardiomyopathy		
Dilated	Restrictive	Hypertrophic
Overlap with Restrictive Cardiomyopathy: Minimally dilated cardiomyopathy", Hemochromatosis, Amyloidosis, Hypertrophic cardiomyopathy ("burned-out") **Idiopathic:** **Miscellaneous:** Arrhythmogenic right ventricular dysplasia (may also affect left ventricle), Left ventricular noncompactiona, Peripartum cardiomyopathy **Tako-Tsubo Cardiomyopathy**		

Note: Restrictive cardiomyopathy is not a pathological entity but rather a description of hemodynamic condition due to stiffness of ventricles. Hearth size and walls are essentially normal on gross.

RVG = Radionuclide ventriculogram; 201Tl = thallium-201.

- Left-sided symptoms of pulmonary congestion; dyspnea on exertion, orthopnea, paroxysmal nocturnal dyspnea. Right-sided symptoms of systemic versus congestion: discomfort on bending, hepatic and abdominal distention, peripheral edema.

Footnote:
- **Stress cardiomyopathy "tako-tsubo" or "broken heart syndrome":** An acute dilated cardiomyopathy can be provoked by a stressful or emotional situation
- Well-recognized in hypertrophic cardiomyopathy, heritability is present in at least 30% of dilated cardiomyopathy without other clear etiology.
- Inherited Defects in Metabolic Pathways Associated With Cardiomyopathy are usually Restrictive or Pseudohypertrophic Phenotype
- Restrictive cardiomyopathy is not a pathological entity but rather a description of hemodynamic condition due to stiffness of ventricles. Hearth size and walls are essentially normal on gross.

HEMOCHROMATOSIS AND AMYLOIDOSIS

- **C-1: Hemochromatosis,** with excessive iron deposition, can occur in the heart as shown here microscopically with Prussian blue iron stain. The excessive deposition of iron leads to heart enlargement and failure similar to a cardiomyopathy, making hemochromatosis a form of **"restrictive" cardiomyopathy.**
- **C-2:** This section of myocardium shows amorphous deposits of pale pink material between myocardial fibers. This is characteristic for amyloid. **Amyloidosis** is a cause for an "infiltrative" or **"restrictive" form of cardiomyopathy.** It is a nightmare for anesthesiologists when intractable arrhythmias occur during surgery on such patients.

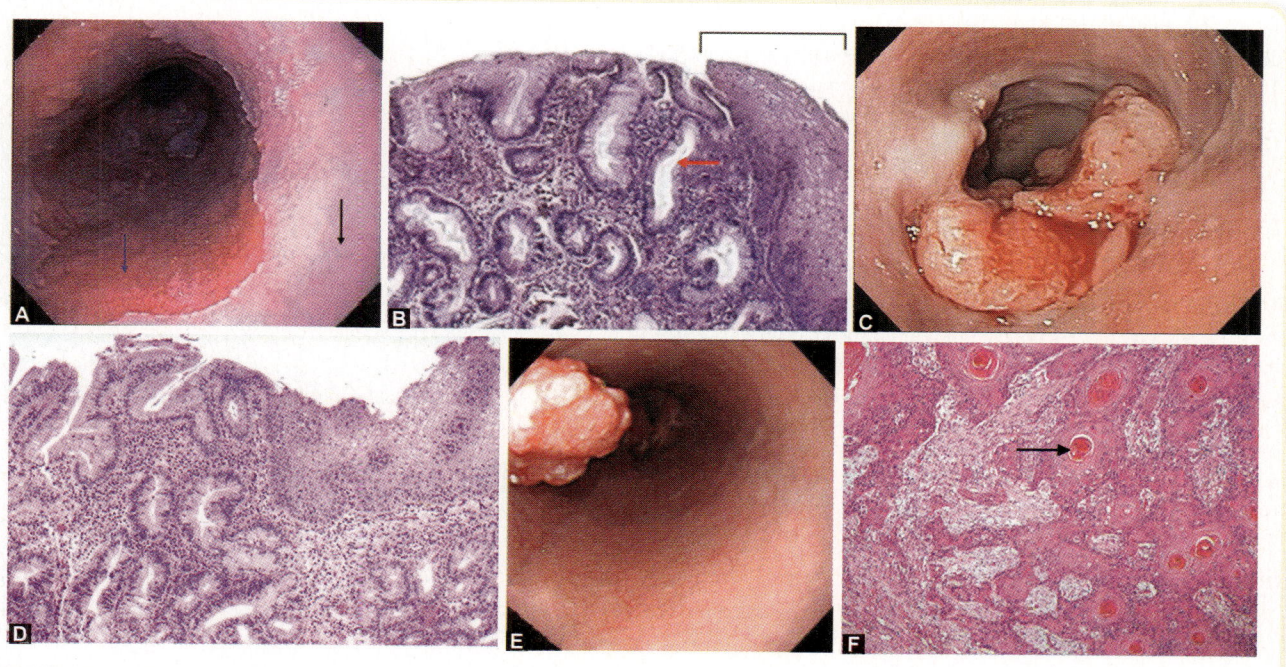

PATHO PLATE 29

PLATE LEGENDS

A. **Barrett esophagus endoscopy:** Esophageal squamous epithelium (Black arrow) is replaced by metaplastic columnar epithelium (Blue arrow- **Salmon Colored mucosa in Endoscopy**)

B. **Barrett esophagus histopathology:** Esophageal squamous epithelium is replaced by metaplastic columnar epithelium containing intestinal goblet cells (Red arrow). Note the squamous epithelium on the right side and collumnar epithelium on the left side.

C. **Adenocarcinoma Esophageal endoscopy:** Upper-gastrointestinal endoscopy showing lower-esophageal ulceroproliferative tumor measuring 2.5 cm × 2.5 cm. Lower third esophageal cancers are mostly adenocarcinoma.

D. **Adenocarcinoma of Esophagus Histopathology:** Microscopically, Barrett esophagus is frequently present adjacent to the tumor. Right half of this slide is Barrett esophagus and left half is Adenocarcinoma. Tumors most commonly produce mucin and form glands, often with intestinal-type morphology; less frequently tumors are composed of diffusely infiltrative signet-ring cells (similar to those seen in diffuse gastric cancer)

E. **Squamous cell carcinoma esophagus endoscopy:** In contrast to adenocarcinoma, half of squamous cell carcinomas occur in the middle third of the esophagus. Early lesions appear as small, gray-white, plaque-like thickenings. It is polypoid or exophytic and protrude into and obstruct the lumen. Alternatively, it can either ulcerated or diffusely infiltrate. These may invade surrounding structures including the respiratory tree, causing pneumonia; the aorta, causing catastrophic exsanguination; or the mediastinum and pericardium.

F. **Squamous cell carcinoma esophagus Histopathology:** Typical keratinizing conventional, well differentiated squamous cell carcinoma with keratin pearls (arrow). Most squamous cell carcinomas are moderately well-differentiated. Squamous cell carcinoma begins as an in situ lesion termed **squamous dysplasia**.

Barrett Esophagus

- Barrett esophagus is a complication of long standing gastroesophageal reflux, occurring over time in up to 10% of patients with symptomatic GERD.
- It is single most important risk factor of esophageal adenocarcinoma
- In Barrett esophagus distal squamous mucosa is replaced by metaplastic columnar epithelium as a response to prolonged injury (**columnar metaplasia; AKA Intestinal Metaplasia**)
- Two criteria are required for the diagnosis of Barrett esophagus:
  1. Endoscopic evidence of columnar epithelium lining above the gastroesophageal junction
  2. Histological evidence of intestinal metaplasia in biopsy specimen from columnar epithelium

Locations of Goblet cells

Goblet cells are glandular simple columnar epithelial cells whose sole function is to secrete mucin, which dissolves in water to form mucus. They use both apocrine and merocrine methods for secretion. They are found scattered among the epithelial lining of organs, such as the intestinal and respiratory tracts. They are found inside the trachea, bronchus, and larger bronchioles in respiratory tract, small intestines, the colon, and conjunctiva in the upper eyelid. They may be an indication of metaplasia, such as in Barrett's esophagus.

Staining of Goblet cell- Alcian Blue

- Common "routine" stain (not an immunohistochemical stain) to detect mucins
- At pH 2.5, detects acidic mucins, At pH 1.0, detects highly acidic mucins
- Stained parts are blue to bluish-green
- PAS-Alcian blue may be best pan mucin combination; PAS also stains glycogen, but predigestion with diastase will remove the glycogen
- Alcian blue-high iron diamine detects sulfomucins (brown) and sialomucins (blue)

PATHO PLATE 30

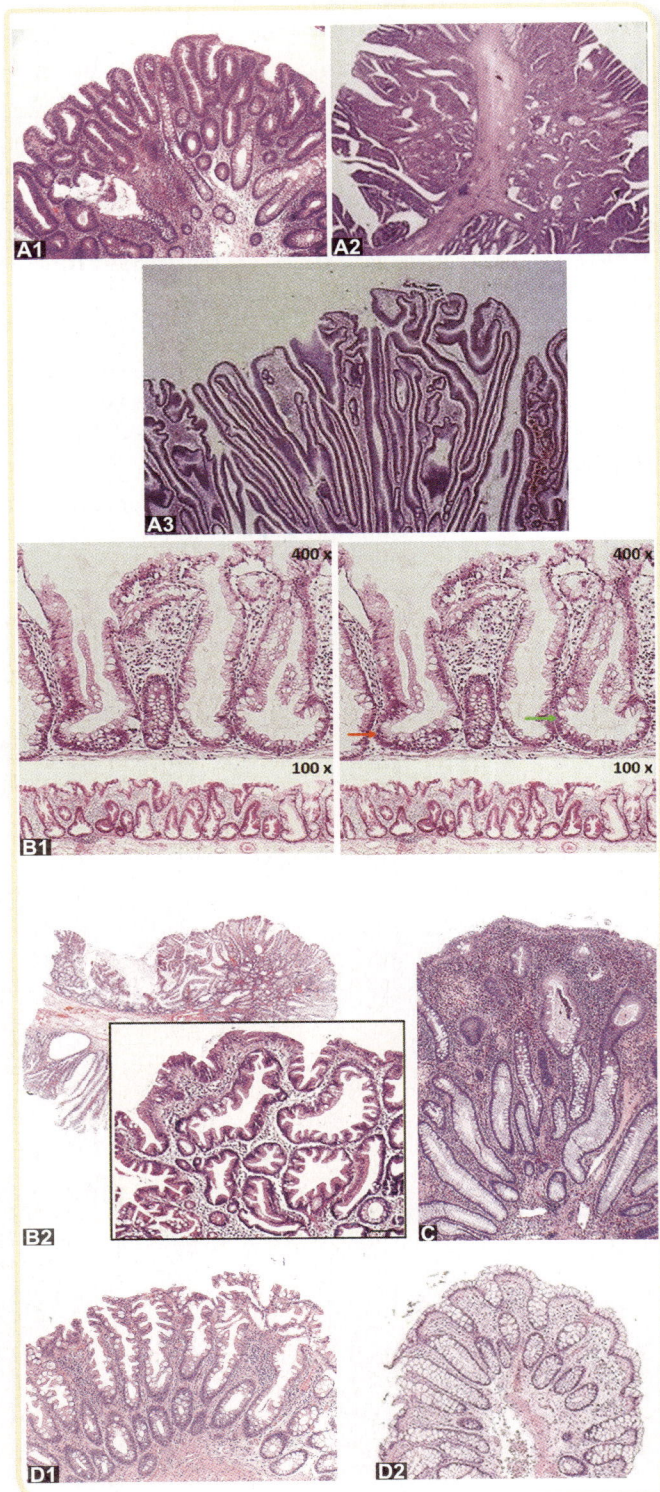

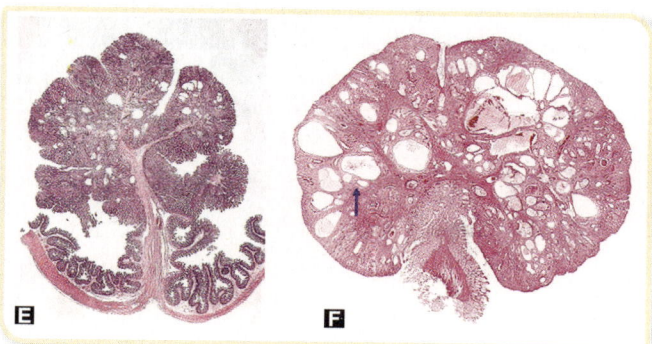

elongated stalk, it is said to be pedunculated. If no stalk is present, it is said to be sessile. Polyps are most common in the colon but may occur in the esophagus, stomach, or small intestine.

Classification: In general, intestinal polyps can be classified as non-neoplastic or neoplastic in nature. The most common neoplastic polyp is the adenoma, which has the potential to progress to cancer. The non-neoplastic polyps can be further classified as inflammatory, hamartomatous, or hyperplastic.

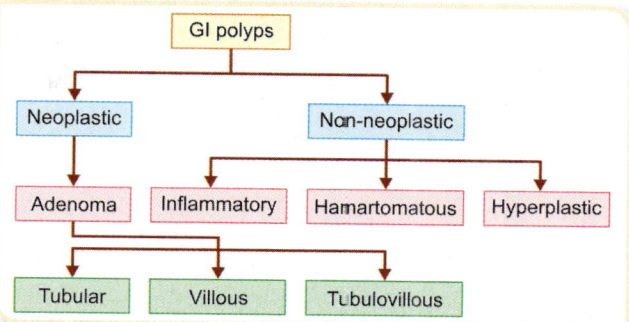

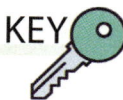

INTESTINAL POLYPS

Definition: A polyp is an abnormal growth of tissue projecting from a mucous membrane. If it is attached to the surface by a narrow-

Intestinal Polyps

Polyp	Histologic appearance	Risk of malignancy	Comments
Adenoma	0.3 to 10 cm in diameter often pedunculated or large sessile, with the surface of both types having a texture resembling velvet or a raspberry, due to the abnormal epithelial growth pattern	Characterized by the presence of epithelial dysplasia, precursors to colorectal cancer	Sub classified as **A-1: tubular** (small, pedunculated, small rounded, or tubular, glands), < 20% villous element **A-2: tubulovillous** (mixture of tubular and villous elements) **A-3: villous** (larger sessile covered by slender villi) based on their architecture. > 80% villous element
Serrated adenoma (Serrated = Saw tooth)	**Serrated architecture** throughout the full length of the glands, **including the crypt base**, Overlap histologically with hyperplastic polyps (see Footnote), but are more commonly found in the right/proximal colon. Horizontalization of the crypts, **L shaped** (red arrow) **or inverted T shaped** (green arrow) base branching of the crypt	Malignant potential but lack typical cytologic features of dysplasia that are present in other adenomas	Subtypes are: **(B-1) Sessile serrated adenoma/polyp,** showing asymmetrical serrated crypts and dilated crypts. **(B-2) Traditional serrated adenoma,** with prominent complex serration and hypereosinophilic cells. Mostly found at rectosigmoid junction.
Inflammatory (C)	Dilated glands, epithelial hyperplasia, superficial erosions, inflammatory infiltrate and lamina propria fibromuscular hyperplasia	No malignant potential	Forms as part of the solitary rectal ulcer syndrome
Hamartomatous polyp	Can present in different forms depending on the syndrome they are seen in (i.e. Juvenile polyp/ Peutz Jeghers). Sporadic hamartomatous polyp has overlapping histology with Peutz Jeghers type Hamartomatous polyp	No malignant potential	Peutz-Jeghers syndrome, Cowden syndrome, Bannayan Ruvalcaba Riley syndrome, Cronkhite-Canada syndrome are syndromic Hamartomatous polyps
Hyperplastic polyp	Subtytes are: **(D-1) Microvesicular hyperplastic polyp:** Serrations are limited to 1/2 to 2/3 of crypts (base is spared), mostly found in left/ distal colon and rectum. Cells have microvesicular mucin droplets **(D-2) Goblet cell rich Hyperplastic polyp:** Typically less than 5 mm... Delayed shedding and crowding of goblet cells. Mucosal thickening	No malignant potential	Hyperplastic polyposis syndrome. They must be distinguished from sessile serrated adenomas, a histologically similar lesions that have malignant potential (see footnote)

Contd...

Intestinal Polyps

Polyp	Histologic appearance	Risk of malignancy	Comments
Peutz-Jeghers type Hamartomatous Polyp (E)	Multiple GI **hamartomatous polyps**. Large and pedunculated with a lobulated contour. Characteristic **arborizing network** of connective tissue, smooth muscle, lamina propria, and glands lined by normal-appearing intestinal epithelium. The arborization **(Christmas tree appearance)** and presence of smooth muscle intermixed with lamina propria are helpful in distinguishing polyps of Peutz-Jeghers syndrome from juvenile polyps.	Increased risk	Peutz-Jeghers syndrome
Juvenile Polyp (Juvenile type Hamartomatous polyp) (F)	Sporadic are solitary, < 3 cm in diameter, typically pedunculated, smooth surfaced, reddish lesions. A typical juvenile polyp demonstrate multiple mucus retention cysts/ gland dilatation (blue arrow), inflammatory cell infiltrate and **unlike PJS absence of smooth-muscle proliferation**.	Dysplasia may develop. Juvenile polyposis syndrome is associated with increased risk of colonic adenocarcinoma	Autosomal dominant **Juvenile polyposis syndrome (JPS);** > 3 hamartomatous polyps in colorectum or polyps throughout GIT or any number of polyp with family history of JPS

Footnote:
Serrated Adenoma has 2 of the 6 criteria in at least 2 well serrated crypts: (difference from hyperplastic polyp)
- Serrations at the base of the crypt
- Horizontalization of the crypts (L shaped or inverted T shaped crypt Base branching of the crypt)
- Dilatation of the crypts
- Increased epithelial stromal ratio > 50%
- Mitosis on the surface of the crypts
- Cellular atypia.

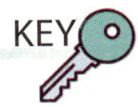
KEY

NUTMEG LIVER; LIVER WITH CHRONIC PASSIVE CONGESTION AND HEMORRHAGIC NECROSIS

Morphology

The cut surfaces of congested tissues are often discolored due to the presence of high levels of poorly oxygenated blood. Microscopically, **acute pulmonary congestion** exhibits engorged alveolar capillaries often with alveolar septal edema and focal intra-alveolar hemorrhage. In **chronic pulmonary congestion** the septa are thickened and fibrotic, and the alveoli often contain numerous hemosiderin-laden macrophages called **heart failure cells**. In **acute hepatic congestion**, the central vein and sinusoids are distended; centrilobular hepatocytes can be frankly ischemic while the periportal hepatocytes—better oxygenated because of proximity to hepatic arterioles—may only develop fatty change. In **chronic passive hepatic congestion,** the centrilobular regions are grossly red-brown and slightly depressed (because of cell death) and are accentuated against the surrounding zones of uncongested tan liver (**nutmeg liver**- so-called because it resembles the cut surface of a nutmeg). Microscopically, there is centrilobular hemorrhage, hemosiderin-laden macrophages, and degeneration of hepatocytes. Because the centrilobular area is at the distal end of the blood supply to the liver, it is prone to undergo necrosis whenever the blood supply is compromised.

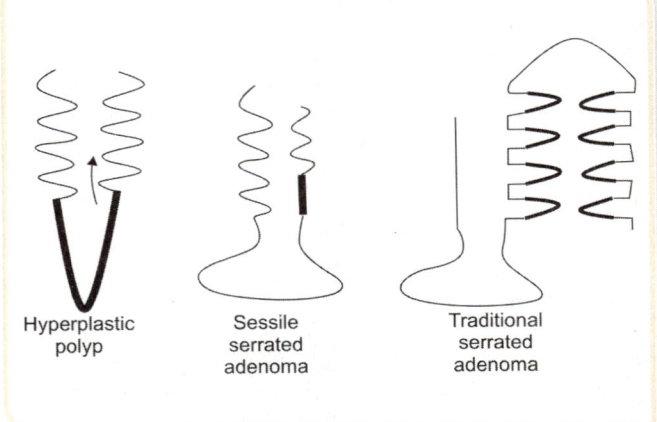

Hyperplastic polyp · Sessile serrated adenoma · Traditional serrated adenoma

Note

- Conditions associated with hepatic venous congestion causing nutmeg liver include:
  - Hepatic veno-occlusive disease
  - Budd-Chiari syndrome
  - Congestive hepatopathy - Right-sided cardiac decompensation (**Right heart failure**) constrictive pericarditis
- Nutmeg is the seed of the tree in genus **Myristica**, roughly egg-shaped

PATHO PLATE 31

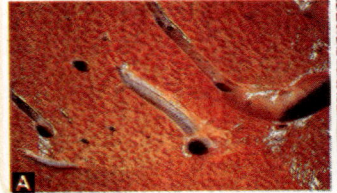
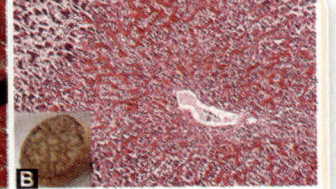

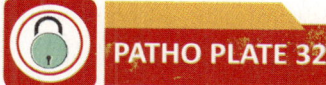

PATHO PLATE 32

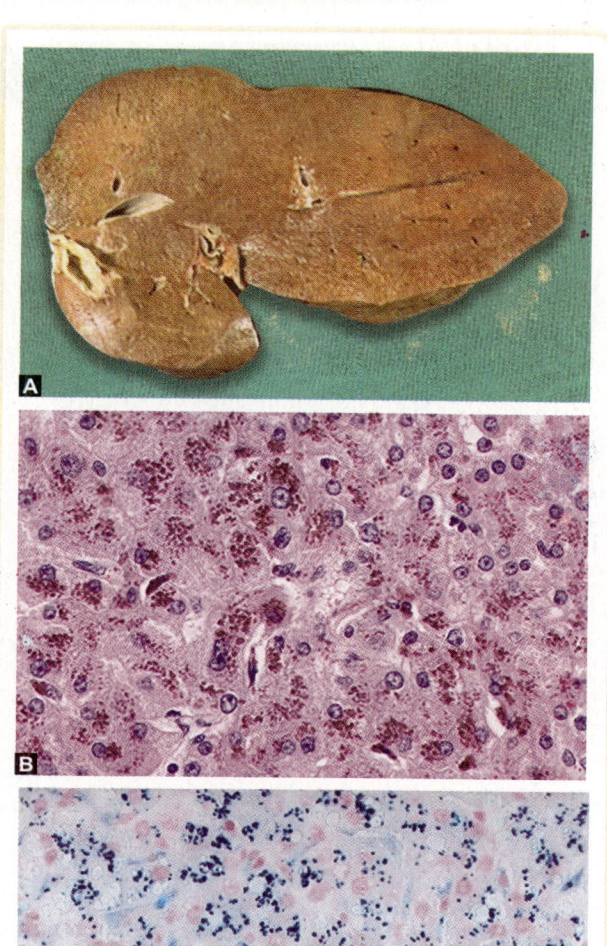

A. **Hemochromatosis Liver Gross:** The dark brown color of the liver on sectioning is due to extensive iron deposition in hereditary hemochromatosis (HHC). HHC results from a mutation involving the hemochromatosis gene (HFE) that leads to increased iron absorption from the gut.

B. **Hemochromatosis Liver Histopathology H & E staining:** The hepatocytes and Kupffer cells here are full of *granular brown deposits* of hemosiderin from accumulation of excess iron in the liver. The iron accumulation may lead to a micronodular cirrhosis (so called "pigment" cirrhosis).

C. **Hemochromatosis Liver Histopathology Prussian Blue staining:** A Prussian blue iron stain demonstrates the blue granules of hemosiderin in hepatocytes and Kupffer cells. In the liver, iron becomes evident first as *golden-yellow hemosiderin* granules in the cytoplasm of periportal hepatocytes, which stain *blue* with the **Prussian blue stain.**

PATHO PLATE 33

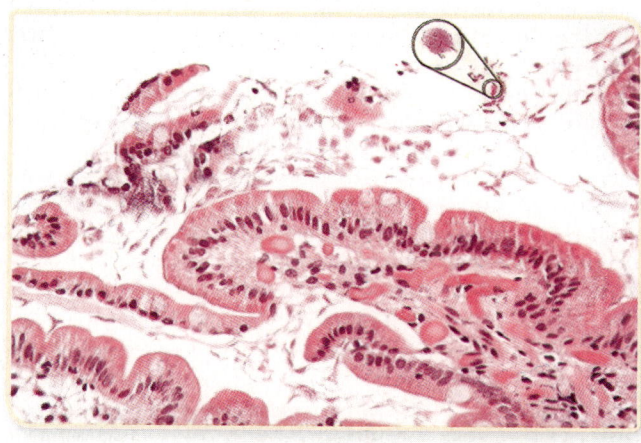

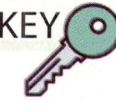

GIARDIA HISTOPATHOLOGY

The small **pear-shaped trophozoites** live in the duodenum and become infective cysts that are excreted. They produce a watery diarrhea. A useful test for diagnosis of infectious diarrheas is stool examination for ova and parasites. Although pathologists usually encounter Giardia in duodenal biopsy specimens, the organism has been found in the gastric antrum, ileal specimens, and even colonic biopsy specimens. The small-bowel mucosal histology in biopsy specimens is usually normal; however, a patchy villous abnormality of variable severity can be observed. The histologic diagnosis rests on the demonstration of trophozoites either along the surface of epithelial cells in biopsy specimens or in touch preparations. The organism is approximately the same size as the enterocyte nucleus. In profile, the trophozoite of G. lamblia is **sickle-shaped; seen en face**, it has a characteristic **pear shape** with a tapered posterior region. It has prominent paired nuclei, paired median rods, a curved median body, and four pairs of flagellae. These morphologic features are most easily recognized on Giemsa-stained or trichrome-stained touch preparations.

HEMOCHROMATOSIS

The morphologic changes in hereditary hemochromatosis are all responses to the **deposition of hemosiderin** in the following organs (in decreasing order of severity): liver, pancreas, myocardium, pituitary, adrenal, thyroid and parathyroid glands, joints, and skin.

The term **"hemosiderosis"** is used to denote a relatively benign accumulation of iron. The term **"hemochromatosis"** is used when organ dysfunction occurs. Hemochromatosis can be primary (the cause is probably an autosomal recessive genetic disease) or secondary (excess iron intake or absorption, liver disease, or numerous transfusions). Hemochromatosis leads to bronze pigmentation of skin, diabetes mellitus (from pancreatic involvement), and cardiac arrhythmias (from myocardial involvement).

PATHO PLATE 34

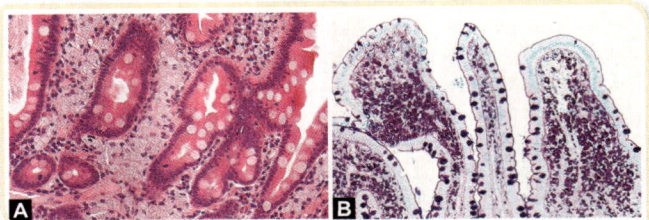

WHIPPLE'S DISEASE

A. **Whipple's disease high magnification H&E stain, Duodenal biopsy:** The images show the characteristic foamy macrophages are present in the lamina propria.

B. **Whipple's disease PAS stain, Duodenal biopsy:** Duodenum villi of Whipples disease with Foamy infiltrate in lamina propria on a PAS stain

Whipple disease, a chronic systemic illness with numerous gastrointestinal features such as diarrhea and malabsorption, is caused by Tropheryma whippleii, a rod-shaped microorganism. The diagnosis of Whipple disease is usually based on the identification of **PAS-positive**, diastase-resistant inclusions in small-intestinal biopsy specimens. Positive gut mucosal biopsy specimens demonstrate infiltration of the lamina propria; muscularis mucosae; and, in some cases, submucosa by macrophages with a *foamy gray-blue cytoplasm*. The number of intraepithelial lymphocytes is not increased.

PATHO PLATE 35

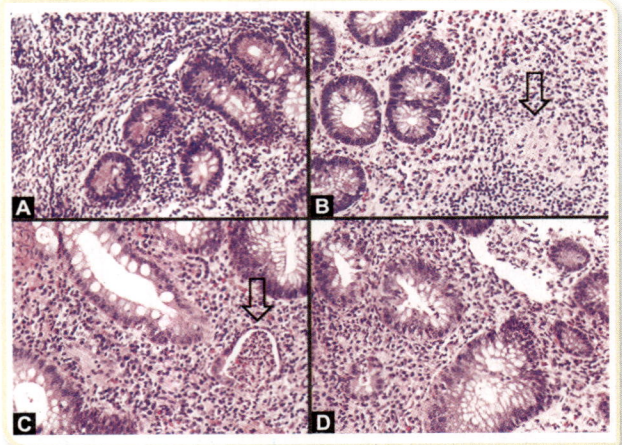

CROHN'S DISEASE

Histopathology of lower GI biopsies demonstrating Crohn's disease.
A. Terminal ileum showing mild active ileitis, with lymphocytic and neutrophilic infiltration into glands
B. Chronic active colitis with **granuloma formation** (arrow) in the ascending colon.

C, D. Descending colon with chronic active colitis with **crypt abscess** (arrow) formation (C) and cryptitis (D).

PATHO PLATE 36

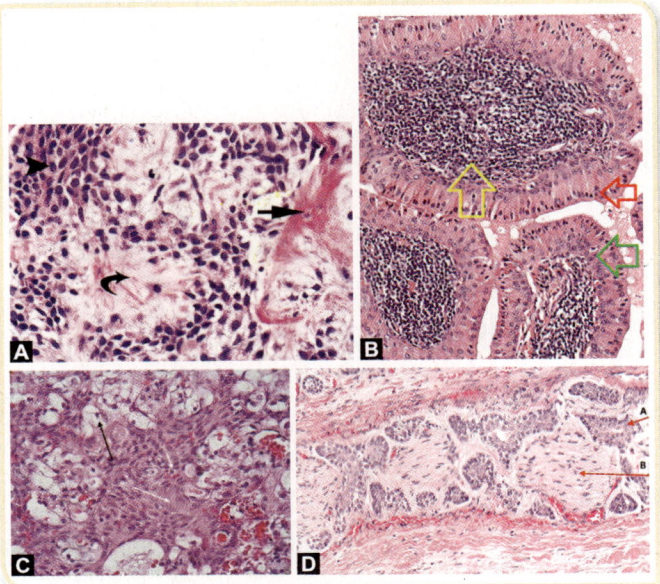

SALIVARY GLAND TUMORS

A. **Pleomorphic Adenoma**
   Morphology. Most pleomorphic adenomas present as rounded, well-demarcated masses rarely exceeding 6 cm in the greatest dimension. Although they are **encapsulated**, in some locations (particularly the palate) the capsule is not fully developed, and expansile growth produces protrusions into the surrounding gland, rendering enucleation of the tumor hazardous. The cut surface is gray-white with myxoid and blue translucent areas of chondroid.

   The dominant histologic feature is the great **heterogeneity** mentioned. In the typical morphology epithelial/myoepithelial areas (right arrowhead) are punctuated by myxochondroid areas (arrows). The **epithelial elements** resembling ductal cells or myoepithelial cells are arranged in duct formations, acini, irregular tubules, strands, or sheets of cells. These elements are typically dispersed within a mesenchyme-like background of loose myxoid tissue containing islands of **chondroid** and, rarely, foci of bone. Sometimes the epithelial cells form well-developed ducts lined by cuboidal to columnar cells with an underlying layer of deeply chromatic, small **myoepithelial cells**. In other instances, there may be strands or sheets of myoepithelial cells. Islands of well-differentiated squamous epithelium may also be present. In most cases, there is no epithelial dysplasia or evident mitotic activity.

B. **Warthin's Tumor**
   Most Warthin tumors are round to oval, encapsulated masses, 2 to 5 cm in diameter, usually arising in the superficial parotid gland, where they are readily palpable. Transection reveals a pale gray surface punctuated by narrow cystic or cleftlike spaces filled with a mucinous or serous secretion.

   On microscopic examination there is **Papillary projections** lined by a double layer of neoplastic epithelial cells resting on a dense lymphoid stroma sometimes bearing germinal centers. **Outer oncocytic layer** of columnar cells having an abundant, finely granular, eosinophilic cytoplasm (red arrow). Secretory cells are dispersed in the columnar cell layer, accounting for the secretions within the cystically dilated lumens. **Inner oncocytic layer** of cuboidal to polygonal cells (green arrow) resting on lymphoid stroma (yellow arrow)

C. **Mucoepidermoid Carcinoma**

Mucoepidermoid carcinomas can grow as large as 8 cm in diameter and although they are apparently circumscribed, they lack well-defined capsules and are often infiltrative at the margins. Pale and gray-white on transection, they frequently contain small, mucin-containing cysts. The basic histologic pattern is that of cords, sheets, or cystic configurations three distinct cell lines of **squamous/ epidermoid cells** (long white arrow), **mucous cells** (black arrow), or **intermediate cells** (short white arrow). The hybrid cell types often have squamous features, with small to large **mucus-filled vacuoles**, best seen when highlighted with mucin stains. The tumor cells may be regular and benign appearing or, alternatively, highly anaplastic and unmistakably malignant. Accordingly, mucoepidermoid carcinomas are subclassified into low, intermediate, or high grade.

D. **Adenoid Cystic Carcinoma**

In gross appearance, they are generally small, poorly encapsulated, infiltrative, gray-pink lesions. On histologic evaluation, they are composed of multiple basaloid epithelial cells having dark, compact nuclei and scant cytoplasm arranged in cribriform architecture (arrow A) with perineural invasion (arrow B). The spaces between the tumor cells are often filled with a **hyaline material** thought to represent excess basement membrane.

PATHO PLATE 37

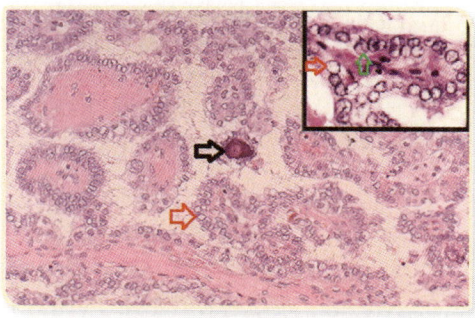

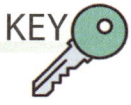
KEY

PAPILLARY CARCINOMAS OF THYROID

Papillary carcinomas of thyroid are solitary or multifocal lesions. Some tumors may be well circumscribed and even encapsulated; others may infiltrate the adjacent parenchyma with ill-defined margins. The lesions may contain areas of fibrosis and calcification and are often cystic. The cut surface sometimes reveals papillary foci that may point to the diagnosis. The microscopic hallmarks of papillary neoplasms include the following:

1. Papillary carcinomas can contain **branching papillae** having a fibrovascular stalk covered by a single to multiple layers of cuboidal epithelial cells.
2. The nuclei of papillary carcinoma cells contain finely dispersed chromatin, which imparts an optically clear or empty appearance, giving rise to the designation **ground-glass or Orphan Annie eye nuclei** (red arrow)
3. In addition, invaginations of the cytoplasm may in cross-sections give the appearance of intranuclear inclusions (**"pseudo-inclusions"**) or **intranuclear grooves** (inset green arrow). The diagnosis of papillary carcinoma is made based on these nuclear features, even in the absence of papillary architecture.
4. Concentrically calcified structures termed **psammoma bodies** (black arrow) are often present within the lesion, usually within the cores of papillae. These structures are almost never found in follicular and medullary carcinomas, and so, when present in fine-needle aspiration material, they are a strong indication that the lesion is a papillary carcinoma.

Below is the hand drawn illustration of Orphan Annie-eye nuclei reveals large nuclei cleared out in the center with powdery chromatin marginated to the periphery along with few open- and close-faced nuclei.

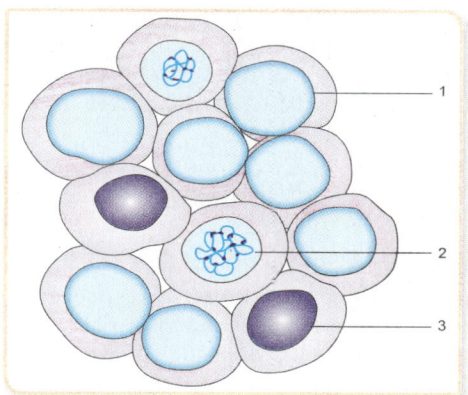

1 = Orphan Annie-eye nuclei, 2=open-faced nuclei, 3=closed faced nuclei

Note

- The term Orphan Annie eye was coined by Dr. Nancy E. Warner (Professor of Pathology at University of Southern California, USA) upon noticing tumor cells with empty nuclei or those showing just a thin rim of peripheral chromatin in sections of papillary thyroid carcinoma. The appearance of these abnormal nuclei to Dr. Nancy Warner, resembled the "Eyes Of Orphan Annie". Little Orphan Annie was a daily comic strip created by American cartoonist Harold Gray which was quite popular in the period of 1894-1968.
- Another histopathological sign of papillary carcinoma of the thyroid are Psammoma bodies. Psammoma bodies are whorled collection of calcium that builds up within certain neoplasms. The presence of Psammoma bodies is one of the points of distinction between follicular and papillary carcinoma of the thyroid gland. Now the word Psammoma is derived from the Greek word psammos which means SAND, which is almost similar to the name of Annie's accompanying dog. Coincidence? probably not!

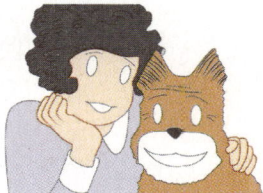

- Orphan Annie-eye nuclei are characteristically seen in:
  - Papillary thyroid carcinoma
  - Polymorphous low grade adenocarcinoma
  - Cribriform adenocarcinoma of tongue
  - Autoimmune thyroiditis: Hashimoto's disease, Grave's disease, and nodular goiter.

PATHO PLATE 38

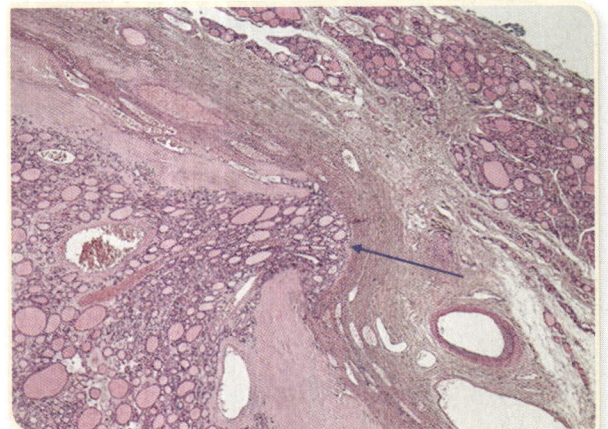

MEDULLARY CARCINOMA OF THYROID

Sporadic medullary thyroid carcinomas present as a solitary nodule while bilaterality and multicentricity are common in familial cases. The tumor tissue is firm, pale gray to tan, and infiltrative. There may be foci of hemorrhage and necrosis in the larger lesions.

Microscopically, these tumors typically show a solid pattern of growth and do not have connective tissue capsules. Histology demonstrates abundant **deposition of acellular amyloid** (arrow), visible here as homogeneous extracellular material, derived from calcitonin molecules secreted by the neoplastic cells. Medullary carcinomas are composed of polygonal to spindle-shaped cells, which may form nests, trabeculae, and even follicles.

Calcitonin is readily demonstrable within the cytoplasm of the tumor cells as well as in the stromal amyloid by immunohistochemical methods. One of the peculiar features of familial medullary cancers is the presence of multicentric C-cell hyperplasia in the surrounding thyroid parenchyma, a feature that is usually absent in sporadic lesions.

FOLLICULAR CARCINOMAS OF THYROID

Follicular carcinomas of Thyroid are single nodules that may be well circumscribed or widely infiltrative. Sharply demarcated lesions may be exceedingly difficult to distinguish from follicular adenomas by gross examination. Larger lesions may penetrate the capsule and infiltrate well beyond the thyroid capsule into the adjacent neck. They are gray to tan to pink on cut section and, on occasion, are somewhat translucent due to the presence of large, colloid-filled follicles. Degenerative changes, such as central fibrosis and foci of calcification, are sometimes present

Microscopically, most follicular carcinomas are composed of fairly uniform cells forming small follicles containing colloid, quite reminiscent of normal thyroid. The follicles of the adenoma contain colloid, but there is greater **variability in size than normal.** In other cases, follicular differentiation may be less apparent, and there may be nests or sheets of cells without colloid.

Diagnosis is made by observing **capsular invasion (arrow),** requiring the pathologist to carefully inspect the whole capsule. For this reason, diagnosis is usually made on paraffin section, as determining capsular invasion is very difficult at frozen section. There can also be difficulty following fine-needle aspiration to distinguish traumatic capsular rupture from true foci of capsular invasion.

PATHO PLATE 39

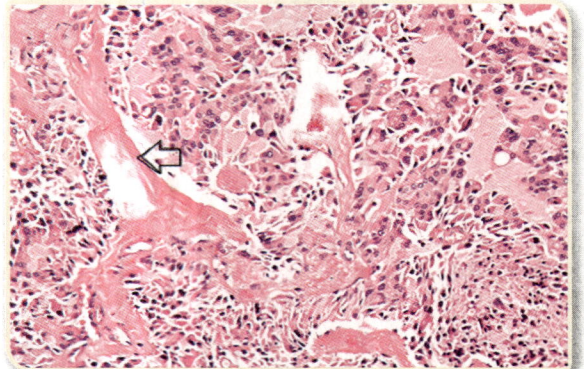

PATHO PLATE 40

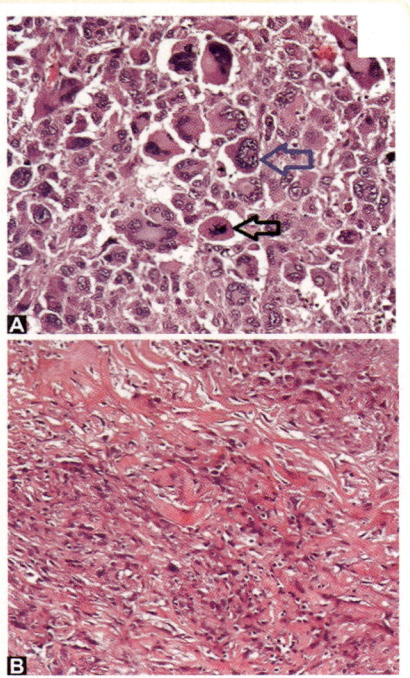

ANAPLASTIC THYROID CARCINOMA

Anaplastic thyroid carcinoma showing marked cellular pleomorphism. Microscopically, these neoplasms are composed of highly anaplastic cells, with variable morphology, including:
A. Large, pleomorphic **Bizzare giant cells (black arrow),** including occasional osteoclast-like multinucleate giant cells (blue arrow)
B. Anaplastic thyroid carcinoma with a prominent **spindle cell component** with a sarcomatous appearance.
C. Mixed spindle and giant cells. (no slide is given here)

	Thyroid Carcinoma					
	Papillary carcinoma	**Follicular carcinoma**	**Hurthle cell ca**	**Anaplastic carcinoma**	**Medullary carcinoma**	**Lymphoma**
Prevalence	80% (MC)	10% (2nd MC)	3%	1%	5%	<1%
Mean Age group	30-40 yrs	> 50 yrs	60-75 yrs	Elderly (7th to 8th decade)	Familial c- young age, Sporadic- 50-60 yrs	Older pts (Late 60's)
Sex prevalence	F:M ratio 2:1	F:M 3:1	F>M	F>M	F:M ratio 1.5:1	F:M ratio 2:1
Mutation	(N-Ras, gsp, c-myc, p53)- worse prognosis. TRK1, (RET/PTC rearrangements) MET PTEN (rare)	MET, RAS PTEN (asso. With Cowden's disease)	P53 RAS	P53 P21/WAF LOH	RET protooncogene (sporadic & familial) APC	
Risk Factors	**External radiation** especially <5 yrs of age (usually 5 years after exposure)	Geographical distribution with **Iodine deficiency** causing long standing goitre	Radiation to neck, Iodide deficiency	Dedifferentiation in setting of previous thyroid pathology (**preexisting goiter**, FTC, PTC)	**Familial MEN 2A or 2B**, C cell hyperplasia may be premalignant	Hashimoto's disease
Cell type	Follicular	Follicular	Follicular, oxyphilic cells	wide variety of cell types	Parathyroid C cells	Non Hodgkin's B cell type
Pathology	Very seldom encapsulated, well-defined follicles with only minimal papillary architecture, **Orphan Annie eye nuclei, Psammoma bodies**	Majority are encapsulated Follicles containing colloid are present	Variant of Follicular, Abundant, granular, eosinophilic cytoplasm due to abundant mitochondria (**Hurthle / Askanazy cells**), vascular or capsular invasion	Regions of spontaneous necrosis and hemorrhage. **Angioinvasion**, Spindle cell, giant cell (osteoclast like) with intranuclear cytoplasmic invaginations	Neuroendocrine neoplasms, Presence of **amyloid stroma**, MCT is associated with the secretion of **calcitonin** (but not associated with hypocalcemia)	
Origin	Solitary or multifocal	Solitary mostly	Often multifocal & bilateral (about 30%)		Familial cases are multicentric	
Clinical features	Slow growing painless thyroid mass, cervical lymphadenopathy is a common initial presentation	Painless thyroid mass, 1% cases maybe associated with hyperthyroidism, cervical lymphadenopathy is an uncommon initial presentation (about 5%),	Painful palpable thyroid mass (MC clinical sign). Symptoms more suggestive of malignancy (dysphagia, dyspnea, coughing, choking spells, hoarseness)	Dysphonia, Dysphagia, Dyspnea, cervical tenderness, and a painful, rapidly enlarging neck mass. Early fixity to adjacent structures is characteristic. SVC syndrome can also be part of the findings	The presence of both neck mass and an elevated calcitonin level is virtually diagnostic of MCT, Unilateral (80%) in sporadic disease, bilateral in 90% of familial patients. Palpable cervical lymphadenopathy (15 to 20%). Diarrhea may be seen in some cases (due to secretion of 5HT)	Rapidly growing painless mass (Goitre) in a short period Respiratory distress, hoarseness, fever, dysphagia
Metastasis	Lymph node (**Lateral aberrant thyroid**) Blood borne (less common, occur esp. If extra thyroidal, i.e infiltrated capsule) to lungs	Lymph node involvement is unusual & occurs in <10% of cases. Blood borne distant spread is more common (**Osteolytic bone mets**, lung, liver)	Unlike PTC & FTC, spread to lymph nodes is a poor prognosis (70% mortality), More invasive than FTC, metastasize more frequently to bones	Direct spread	Early spread to lymphatics, Later **Osteoblastic** to bones	Lymphatic

Contd...

	Thyroid Carcinoma					
	Papillary carcinoma	**Follicular carcinoma**	**Hurthle cell ca**	**Anaplastic carcinoma**	**Medullary carcinoma**	**Lymphoma**
Investigations	FNAC of mass or lymph node, Tumor marker: **Thyroglobulin** (no prognostic value pre surgical)	In 1% cases, warm nodule may be seen on scintiscan FNAC doesn't differentiate bn follicular ca & adenoma (Hence frozen section may be required) **Thyroglobulin** positive	a. Do not take up RAI b. Vascular or capsular invasion and can, therefore, not be diagnosed by FNAB **thyroglobulin** positive	FNAC Positive for epithelial markers like cytokeratin but negative for thyroglobulin	a. FNAC b. Tumour markers: Calcitonin b. Do not take up RAI c. Serum calcium: hyperparathyroidism d. Urinary catecholamines-pheochromocytoma e. CEA & calcitonin gene related peptide	a. FNAC, Large needle (Trucut) biopsy, b. USG-classic pseudocystic pattern
Recurrence	Less thyroglobulin levels used for monitoring recurrence	More common. Serum thyroglobulin levels used for monitoring recurrence	Presently Recurrent tumours are incurable	Lethal hence pts do not survive in the first place		
Prognosis	Excellent (93 % 10 yr survival rate for most favourable stages) Thyroglobulin is used as prognostic indicator for recurrence post surgically	Poorer than papillary better than Hurthle cell, although this disparity is more prominent after 10-15 years, (Poorly differen-tiated FTC and well-differentiat-ed FTC have 60% & 85% 10-year survival rates)	Poor	Very poor	MEN 2A usually has a more favorable long-term outcome than MEN 2B or sporadic MCT	Good
Comments	Least malignant, Asso. With dystrophic calcification	Pulsatile secondaries are seen	Highest incidence of metastasis amongst differentiated thyroid cancers	Most malignant, Radiotherapy required along with surgery	Rule out pheochromocytoma & hyperparathyroidism	May be assoociated With generalized NonHodgkin's lymphoma

PATHO PLATE 41

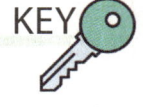 KEY

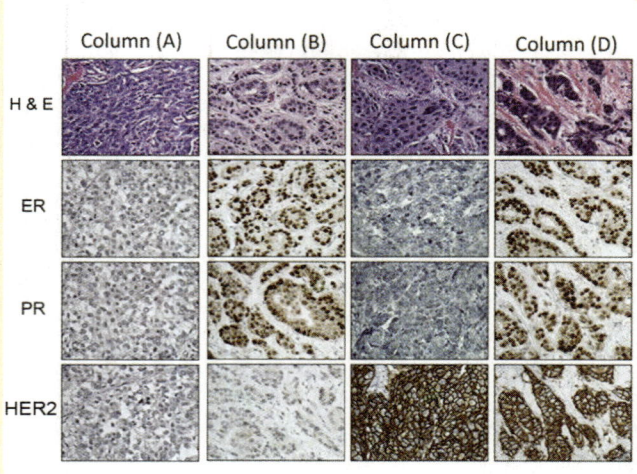

BREAST TISSUE BIOPSY

ER and PR (on any tissue of the body) are stained brown in the "nucleus" on the other hand HER2 is stained brown in the membrane (peripheries)

Column (A): ER (-), PR (-), HER2 (-) [TRIPLE NEGATIVE]
Column (B): ER (+), PR (+), HER2 (-)
Column (C): ER (-), PR (-), HER2 (+)
Column (D): ER (+), PR (+), HER2 (+)

Reporting Guidelines

ASCO and the CAP have issued recommendations for reporting the results of immunohistochemical assays for ER and PR. Studies using both IHC and the ligand binding assay suggest that patients with higher hormone receptor levels have a higher probability of response to hormonal therapy, but expression as low as 1% positive staining has been associated with clinical response. As a result, the guidelines recommend classifying all cases with at least 1% positive cells as receptor positive. For patients with low ER expression (1% to 10% weakly positive cells), the decision on endocrine therapy should be based on an analysis of its risks and potential benefits.

Quantification of ER and PR

There is a wide range of receptor levels in cancers as shown by the biochemical ligand binding assay and as observed with IHC. Patients whose carcinomas have higher levels have improved survival when treated with hormonal therapy. Quantification systems may use only the proportion of positive cells or may include the intensity of immunoreactivity:

1. **Number of positive cells:** The number of positive cells can be reported as a percentage or within discrete categories.

2. **Intensity:** Refers to degree of nuclear positivity (i.e., pale to dark). The intensity can be affected by the amount of protein present, as well as the antibody used and the antigen retrieval system. In most cancers, there is heterogeneous immunoreactivity with pale to darkly positive cells present.

PATHO PLATE 42

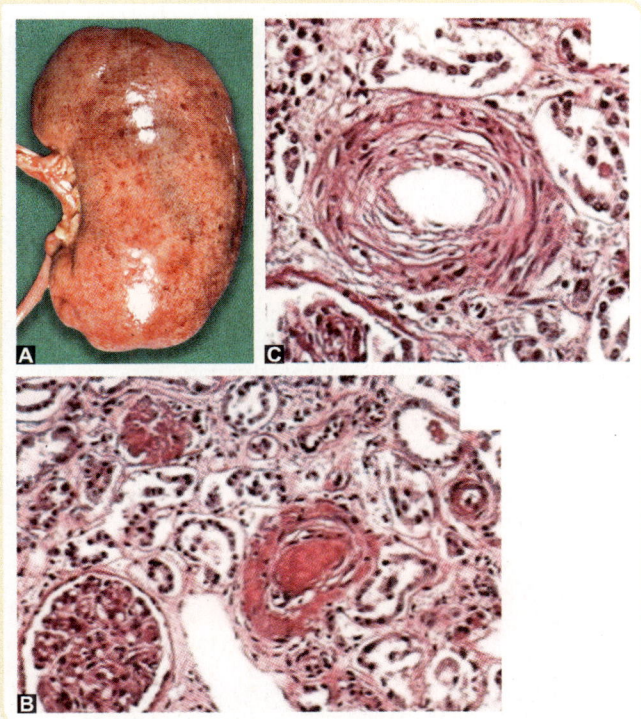

 KEY

MALIGNANT HYPERTENSION AND ACCELERATED NEPHROSCLEROSIS

Malignant nephrosclerosis is the form of renal disease associated with the malignant or accelerated phase of hypertension

A. On gross inspection, the kidney size depends on the duration and severity of the hypertensive disease. Small, pinpoint petechial hemorrhages may appear on the cortical surface from rupture of arterioles or glomerular capillaries, giving the kidney a peculiar **"flea-bitten" appearance.**

Two histologic alterations characterize blood vessels in malignant hypertension

B. **Fibrinoid necrosis of arterioles.** This appears as an eosinophilic granular change in the blood vessel wall, which stains positively for fibrin by histochemical or immunofluorescence techniques. This change represents an acute event; it may be accompanied by limited inflammatory infiltrate within the wall, but prominent inflammation is not seen. Sometimes the glomeruli become necrotic and infiltrated with neutrophils, and the glomerular capillaries may thrombose.

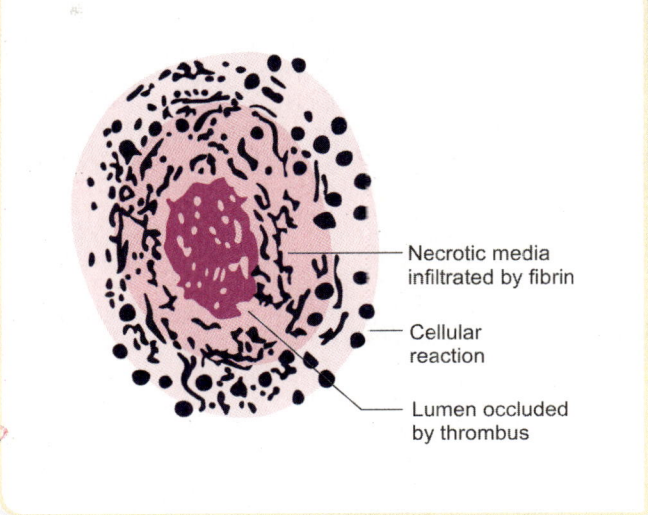

C. **Hyperplastic arteriolitis (onion-skin lesion):** In the interlobular arteries and arterioles, there is intimal thickening caused by a proliferation of elongated, **concentrically arranged smooth muscle cells,** together with fine concentric layering of collagen and accumulation of pale-staining material that probably represents accumulations of proteoglycans and plasma proteins. This alteration has been referred to as onion-skinning because of its concentric appearance. The lesion, also called hyperplastic arteriolitis, correlates well with renal failure in malignant hypertension. There may be superimposed intraluminal thrombosis. The arteriolar and arterial lesions result in considerable narrowing of all vascular lumens, ischemic atrophy and, at times, infarction distal to the abnormal vessels.

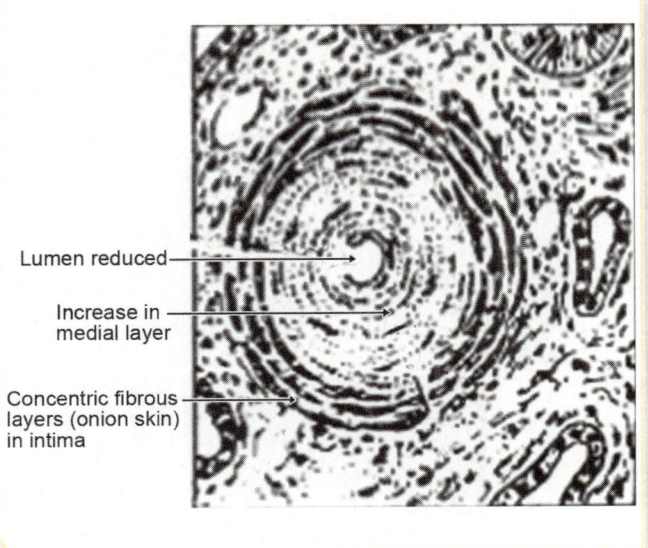

Vascular Pathology of Hypertension

	Hyaline arteriosclerosis	Hyperplastic arteriosclerosis
Renal condition	In kidney it is called is **Benign Nephrosclerosis**	In Kidney it is called as **Malignant Nephrosclerosis**
Etiology	Characteristic of **benign Hypertension**. May also occur in Diabetes and Ageing	Characteristic of **malignant hypertension**
Pathogenesis	Two processes participate in the arterial lesions: 1. Medial and intimal thickening, as a response to hemodynamic changes, aging, genetic defects, or some combination of these 2. Hyaline deposition in arterioles, caused partly by extravasation of plasma proteins through injured endothelium and partly by increased deposition of basement membrane matrix in response to chronic hemodynamic stress. In diabetic microangiography the underlying etiology is hyperglycemia-induced endothelial cell dysfunction	Result from long standing benign hypertension, with eventual injury to arteriolar walls, or the initiating injury may spring de novo from arteritis, a coagulopathy, or some injury causing acute exacerbation of the hypertension. In any case, the result is increased permeability of the small vessels to fibrinogen and other plasma proteins, endothelial injury, focal death of cells of the vascular wall, and platelet deposition. This leads to the appearance of **fibrinoid necrosis** of arterioles and small arteries, swelling of the vascular intima, and intravascular thrombosis. Mitogenic factors from platelets (e.g., PDGF), plasma, and other cells cause hyperplasia of intimal smooth muscle of vessels, resulting in the **hyperplastic arteriolosclerosis** that is typical of malignant hypertension and further narrowing of the lumens.
Gross	Either normal or moderately reduced in size. Fine, leathery granularity of the surface	Kidney size depends on the duration & severity of hypertensive disease. Small, pinpoint petechial hemorrhages may appear on the cortical surface from rupture of arterioles or glomerular capillaries, giving the kidney a peculiar **"flea-bitten" appearance.**
Microscopy	Homogenous pink, Hyaline thickening of arteriolar wall with luminal narrowing. Medial hypertrophy, reduplication of the elastic lamina, and increased myofibroblastic tissue in the intima, which combine to narrow the lumen. This change, called fibroelastic hyperplasia, often accompanies hyaline arteriolosclerosis	Two histologic alterations characterize blood vessels in malignant hypertension: a. **Fibrinoid necrosis of arterioles.** This appears as an eosinophilic granular change in the blood vessel wall, which stains positively for fibrin by histochemical or immunofluorescence techniques. b. **Concentric, laminated, onion skinned** thickening of arteriolar wall with luminal narrowing. The laminations consist of smooth muscle cells with thickened, reduplicated basement membranes The lesion, also called hyperplastic arteriolitis, correlates well with renal failure in malignant hypertension. There may be superimposed intraluminal thrombosis. The arteriolar and arterial lesions result in considerable narrowing of all vascular lumens, ischemic atrophy and, at times, infarction distal to the abnormal vessels.

PATHO PLATE 43

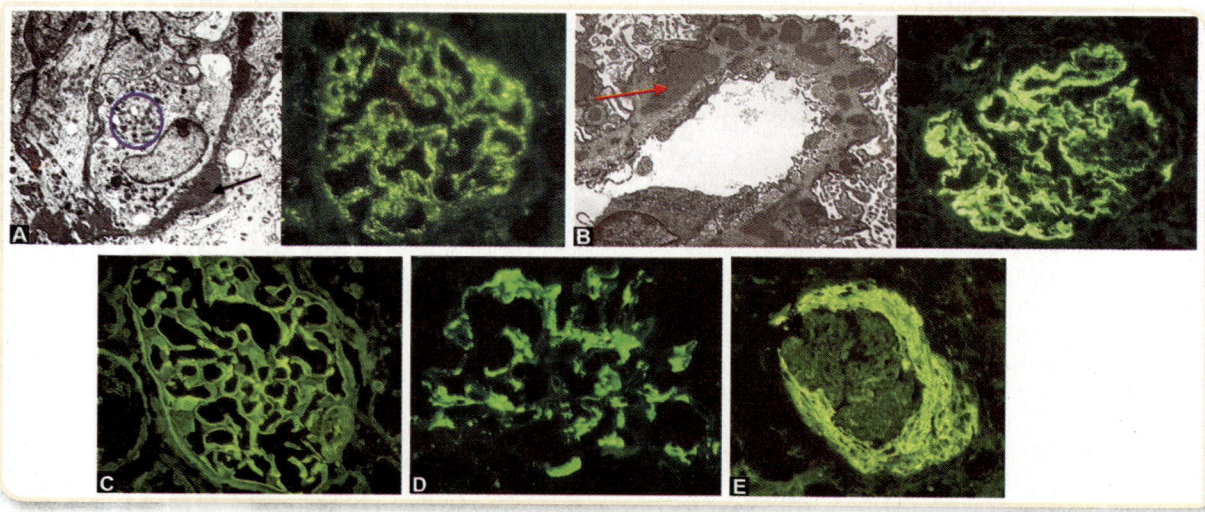

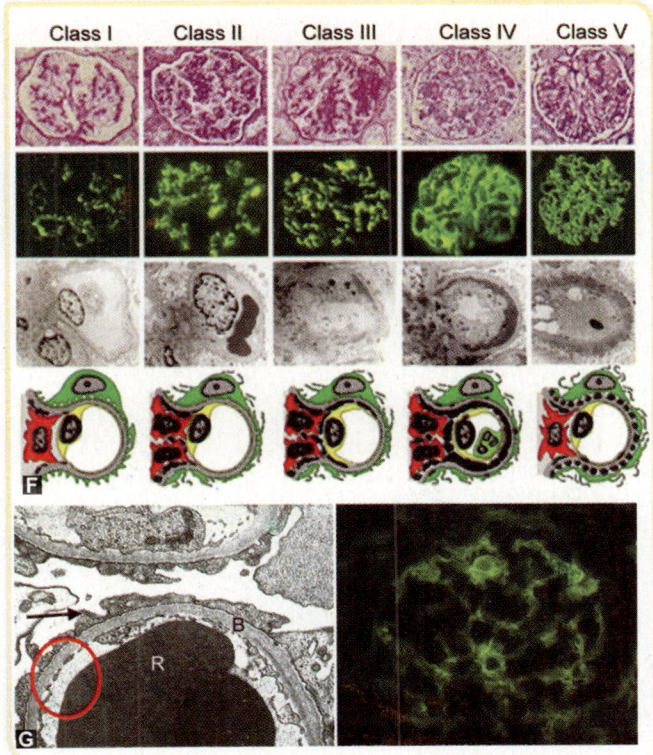

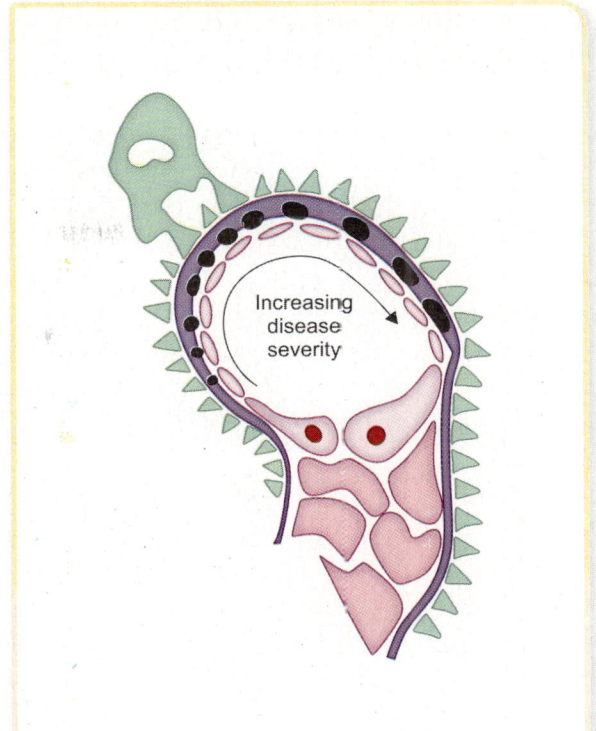

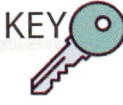

PLATE LEGENDS

Two patterns of deposition of immune complexes as seen by immunofluorescence microscopy:
1. Granular, characteristic of circulating and in situ immune complex nephritis
2. Linear, characteristic of classic anti-GBM disease

A. **Post-infectious glomerulonephritis** is immunologically mediated, and the immune deposits are widely distributed within the capillary loops. The deposits are seen here with bright green fluorescence in a **granular, bumpy pattern** because of the focal nature of the immune complex deposition process. In type III hypersensitivity, antigen-antibody complexes tend to filter out and become trapped along basement membranes, such as those in glomerular capillaries.

   Electron microscopy: The immune deposits of post-infectious glomerulonephritis are predominantly subepithelial, as seen above with electron dense subepithelial "humps" above the basement membrane (arrow) and below the epithelial cell. The capillary lumen is filled with a leukocyte demonstrating cytoplasmic granules (circle)

B. **Membranous nephropathy** is an immunologically mediated disease in which deposits of mainly IgG and complement collect in the basement membrane and appear in a **diffuse granular** by immunofluorescence, as seen here.

   Electron Microscopy: Immune complexes (black dots on picture below) are deposited in a thickened basement membrane creating a **"spike and dome"** appearance on electron microscopy. Darker electron dense immune deposits are seen scattered within the thickened basement membrane. The "spikes" seen with the silver stain represent the intervening matrix of basement membrane between the deposits.

C. **Goodpasture syndrome:** This immunofluorescence pattern shows positivity with antibody to IgG and has a **smooth, diffuse, linear pattern** that is characteristic for deposition of glomerular basement membrane antibody with Goodpasture syndrome. Serologic testing for anti-GBM in patient serum is often positive.

D. **IgA nephropathy,** and the immunofluorescence pattern demonstrates positivity with antibody to IgA. Note that the pattern is that of mesangial deposition in the glomerulus. Some viruses and bacteria express N-acetylgalactosamine on their cell surfaces so that infection may promote anti-glycan antibody formation. IgA nephropathy may initially appear in association with an upper respiratory or gastrointestinal infection. Some of these patients progress slowly to chronic renal failure. Early in the course, there may be gross hematuria, often within 3 days following a respiratory tract infection.

E. **RPGN:** This immunofluorescence micrograph of a glomerulus demonstrates positivity with antibody to fibrinogen. With a **rapidly progressive GN**, the glomerular damage is so severe that fibrinogen leaks into Bowman's space, leading to proliferation of the epithelial cells and formation of the bright crescent shown here.

F. **Lupus glomerulonephritis classes:** on microscopy, Immunofluorescence, Electron microscopy and Demonstrative. Note the increasing granularity on immunofluorescence. It's a type of MGN.

G. **Minimal change disease:** No deposit of complement or immunoglobulins are recognized (nil deposit disease)

   Electron microscopy: Minimal change disease (MCD) is characterized by effacement of the epithelial cell (podocyte) foot processes and loss of the normal charge barrier such that albumin selectively leaks out and proteinuria ensues. The capillary loop in the lower half contains two electron dense RBC's (marked as R). Fenestrated endothelium is present (marked by circle), and the basement membrane is normal (marked as B).

PATHO PLATE 44

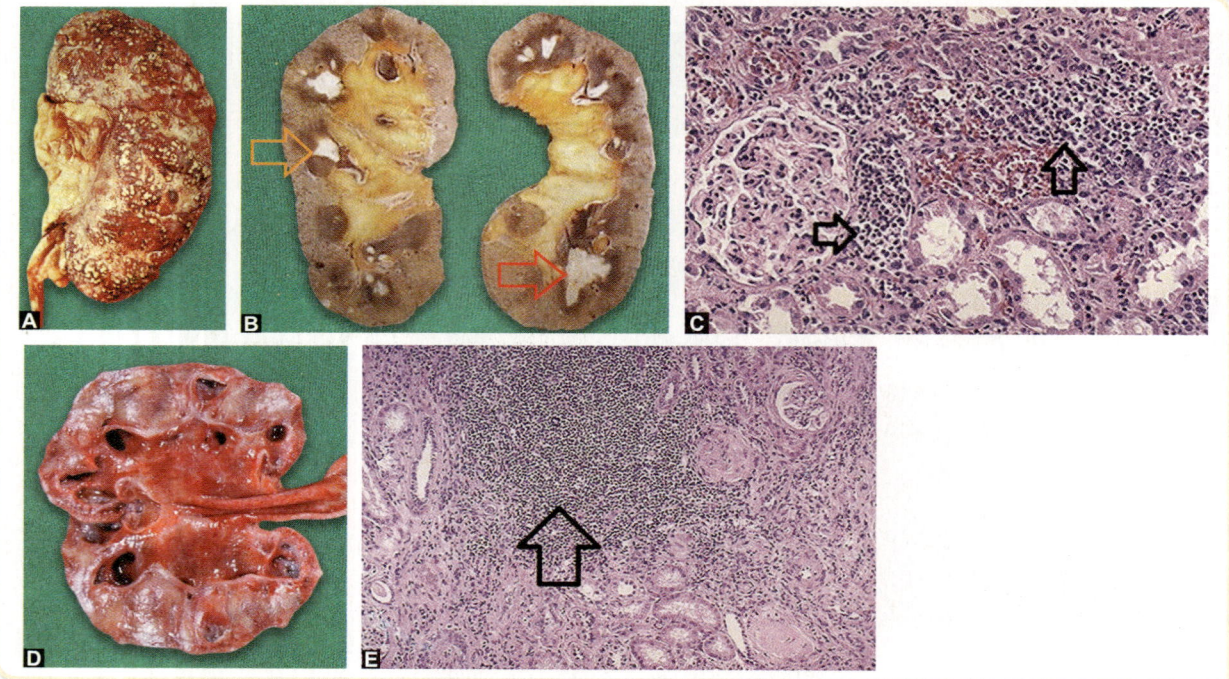

 KEY

PYELONEPHRITIS

Pyelonephritis is a renal disorder affecting the tubules, interstitium, and renal pelvis and is one of the most common diseases of the kidney. It occurs in two forms. Acute pyelonephritis is caused by bacterial infection and is the renal lesion associated with urinary tract infection. Chronic pyelonephritis is a more complex disorder; bacterial infection plays a dominant role, but other factors (vesicoureteral reflux, obstruction) are involved in its pathogenesis.

Acute pyelonephritis is an acute suppurative inflammation of the kidney caused by bacterial and sometimes viral (e.g., polyomavirus) infection, whether hematogenous and induced by septicemic spread or ascending and associated with vesicoureteral reflux. Acute pyelonephritis is generally caused by ascending bacterial infection, rarely fungal infection, and is usually preceded by infection and inflammation of the urinary tract, including the renal pelvis. In hematogenously disseminated infection, highly virulent pathogenic bacteria and fungi are the causative agents, but the renal pelvis is usually not involved. Thus, the term acute pyelonephritis is nosologically incorrect; diffuse suppurative nephritis is more appropriate terminology in such cases, especially if there is abscess formation. The term acute infectious tubulointerstitial nephritis has been introduced in those cases

Chronic pyelonephritis can be divided into two forms: chronic reflux-associated and chronic obstructive. Reflux Nephropathy is by far the more common form of chronic pyelonephritic scarring.

A. **Acute Pyelonephritis (Gross):** In ascending infection, the kidney has yellow striping in the medulla and medullary rays, with scattered abscess (suppuration) formation throughout the renal parenchyma. In hematogenous spread, there are scattered and usually small abscesses (often glomerulocentric) throughout the cortex, with sparing of the medulla. The suppuration may occur as discrete focal abscesses involving one or both kidneys, which can extend to large wedge-shaped areas of suppuration. The distribution of these lesions is unpredictable and haphazard, but in pyelonephritis associated with reflux, damage occurs most commonly in the lower and upper poles.

B. **Acute pyelonephritis (Gross) with papillary necrosis:** The pale white areas involving some or all of many renal papillae are areas of papillary necrosis (arrow). This is an uncommon but severe complication of acute pyelonephritis, particularly in persons with diabetes mellitus. Papillary necrosis may also accompany analgesic nephropathy.

C. **Acute pyelonephritis microscopic:** This is an ascending bacterial infection leading to acute pyelonephritis. Numerous PMN's are seen filling renal tubules across the center and right of this picture (arrow). These leukocytes may form into a cast within the tubule. Casts appearing in the urine originate in the distal renal tubules and collecting ducts.

D. **Chronic pyelonephritis (Gross):** The kidneys usually are irregularly scarred; if bilateral, the involvement is asymmetric. This contrasts with chronic glomerulonephritis, in which both kidneys are diffusely and symmetrically scarred. The hallmarks of chronic pyelonephritis are coarse, discrete, corticomedullary scars overlying dilated, blunted, or deformed calyces, and flattening of the papillae. In obstructive chronic pyelonephritis, there is dilation (hydronephrosis) and deformation of the renal pelvis and calyces, with atrophy and scarring of the overlying renal parenchyma. In advanced nonobstructive chronic pyelonephritis, the kidneys are similar; however, initially, they may not show generalized caliceal dilatation. In early stages, there is dilatation and deformation of a limited number of calyces (usually upper or lower pole), with retraction and destruction of the renal papillae (usually affecting the complex concave rather than normal convex papillae). There are characteristic secondary, deep, broad-based, U-shaped scars of the overlying cortex (as a result of destruction of the medullary ducts of Bellini). For this reason, it is important to bisect the kidney in such a manner as to see the entire pyelocalyceal system (papillae).

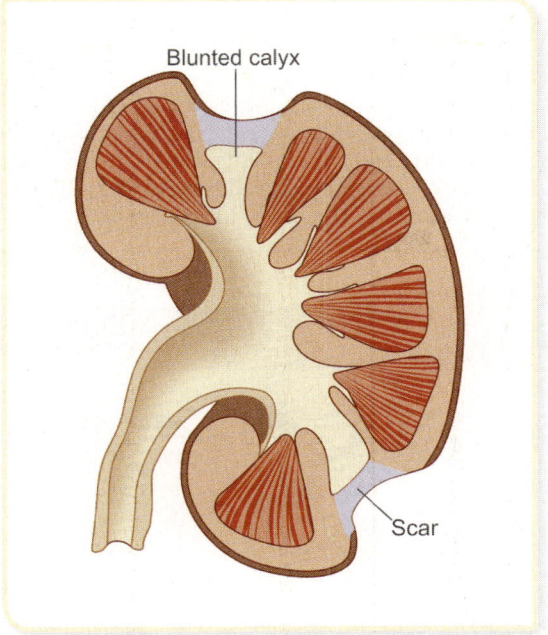

wall, narrowing them (Large arrow). Congo red is a special staining, elective for amyloid. Renal involvement gives rise to proteinuria that may be severe enough to cause the nephrotic syndrome. Progressive obliteration of glomeruli in advanced cases ultimately leads to renal failure and uremia. Renal failure is a common cause of death

B. **Polarized light microscopy** of renal amyloidosis showing **Apple green birefringence** (arrow)

Tissue/substance		Stain	Comment
Amyloid	Gross staining	Lugol's iodine	
	Light microscopy	H & E , Congo red	(Pink Color)
	Polarized light	Congo red	(Apple green birefringence)
	Metachromatic stain	Methyl violet, crystal violet	(Pink Color)
	Fluorescent stain	Thioflavin T	
	Non specific stain	PAS, Toluidine blue, Alcian blue	

E. **Chronic pyelonephritis microscopy:** The microscopic changes involve predominantly tubules and interstitium. The tubules show atrophy in some areas and hypertrophy or dilation in others. Dilated tubules with flattened epithelium may be filled with colloid casts (thyroidization). There are varying degrees of chronic interstitial inflammation and fibrosis in the cortex and medulla. In the presence of active infection, there may be neutrophils in the interstitium and pus casts in the tubules. It is important to emphasize that chronic pyelonephritis is not a diagnosis that can be made on LM evidence, particularly if only a needle renal biopsy specimen is available for examination.

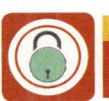

PATHO PLATE 45

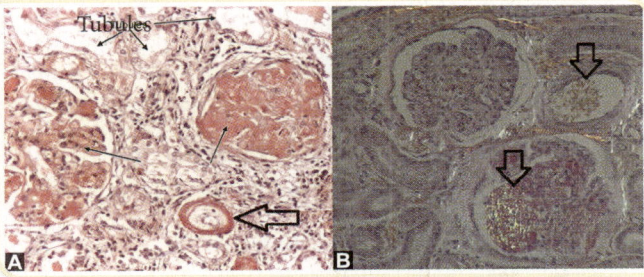

RENAL AMYLOIDOSIS

A. **Congo red staining of renal amyloidosis:** Amyloid (an abnormal protein) accumulates as extra-cellular deposits, nodular or diffuse, as pink, amorphous material. Initially, the deposits appear in the glomeruli: within the mesangial matrix and along the basement membranes of the capillary loops. The glomerular architecture is almost totally obliterated by the massive accumulation of amyloid (arrow heads). Continuous accumulation of the amyloid will compress and obliterate the capillary tuft. With progression, amyloid deposits appear also peritubular and within the arteriolar

PATHO PLATE 46

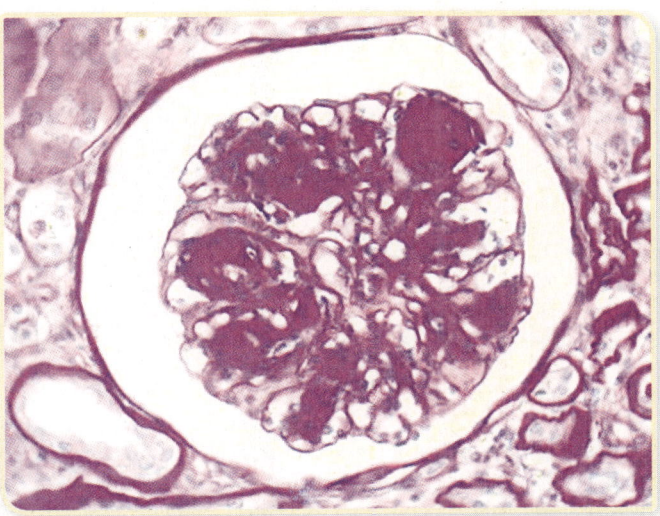

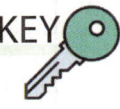

KIMMELSTIEL WILSON LESION IN DIABETIC NEPHROPATHY

- Nodular glomerulosclerosis describes a glomerular lesion made distinctive by ball-like deposits of a laminated matrix situated in the periphery of the glomerulus.
- These nodules are PAS-positive and usually contain trapped mesangial cells. This distinctive change has been called the **Kimmelstiel-Wilson lesion**, after the two pathologists who first described it.
- Nodular glomerulosclerosis is encountered in approximately **15% to 30% of persons with long-term diabetes** and is a major contributor to morbidity and mortality.
- Diffuse mesangial sclerosis also may be seen in association with old age and hypertension; by contrast, the nodular form of glomerulosclerosis, once certain unusual forms of nephropathies have been excluded, is essentially pathognomonic of diabetes.

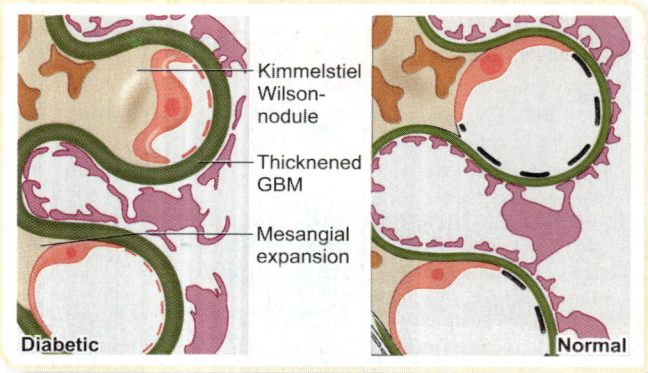

- The silver is in a form readily able to precipitate as metallic silver (diamine silver solution) The Optimal pH for maximum uptake of silver ions is pH 9.0.
- A reducing agent, formalin, causes deposition of silver in the form of metal. Any excess silver in the unprecipitated state is removed by treating with hypo.
- Gold chloride treatment renders the preparation permanent and produces a neutral black Color of high intensity.

PATHO PLATE 48

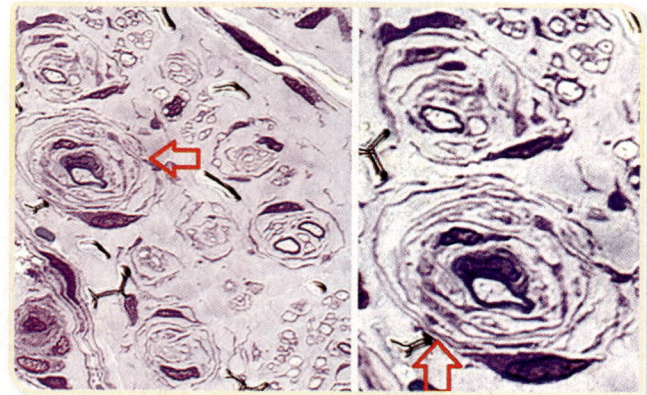

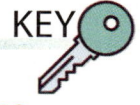

PATHO PLATE 47

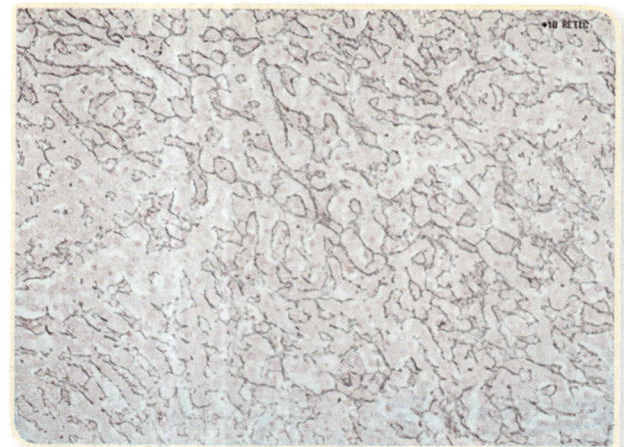

RETICULIN STAIN

In pathology, the reticulin stain, is a popular staining method in histology. It is used to visualize reticular fiber and used extensively in liver histopathology. Gordon & Sweet's Staining Protocol for Reticulin is commonly used.

- A silver impregnation technique that demonstrates reticular fibers. Reticulum is a support function of the body and is abundant in liver, spleen, and kidney. In a normal liver the fibers are will defined strands, but necrotic and cirrhotic liver show discontinuous patterns. Reticulum also forms characteristic patterns in relationship to certain tumor cells.
- **Principle:** The tissue is oxidized and then sensitized with the iron alum, which is replaced with silver. The silver is reduced with formalin to its visible metallic state.
- Reticulin fibers have little natural affinity for silver solutions so, they must be treated with potassium permanganate to produce sensitized sites on the fibers where silver deposition can be initiated.

CHRONIC INFLAMMATORY DEMYELINATING POLYRADICULONEUROPATHY (CIDP)

Chronic inflammatory demyelinating polyneuropathy (CIDP), first recognized by Austin in 1958, is clinically a heterogeneous disorder. The classical form is a symmetric, predominantly proximal, demyelinating motor polyneuropathy, but several variants like predominantly distal, axonal, or sensory forms, and asymmetric or focal presentations are described. It follows a subacute or chronic course, usually with relapses and remissions over a period of several years, rather than the acute course of Guillain-Barré syndrome. In these cases, there is often a symmetric, mixed sensorimotor polyneuropathy, although some patients have predominantly sensory or motor impairment. Clinical remissions may occur with steroid treatment and plasmapheresis. Biopsies of sural nerves show evidence of

1. Recurrent demyelination and remyelination
2. Well-developed **onion bulb structures** (defined as more than one concentric supernumery Schwann cell lamella surrounding the entire circumference of a myelinated axon) (Red arrow).
3. Subperineural edema

PATHO PLATE 49

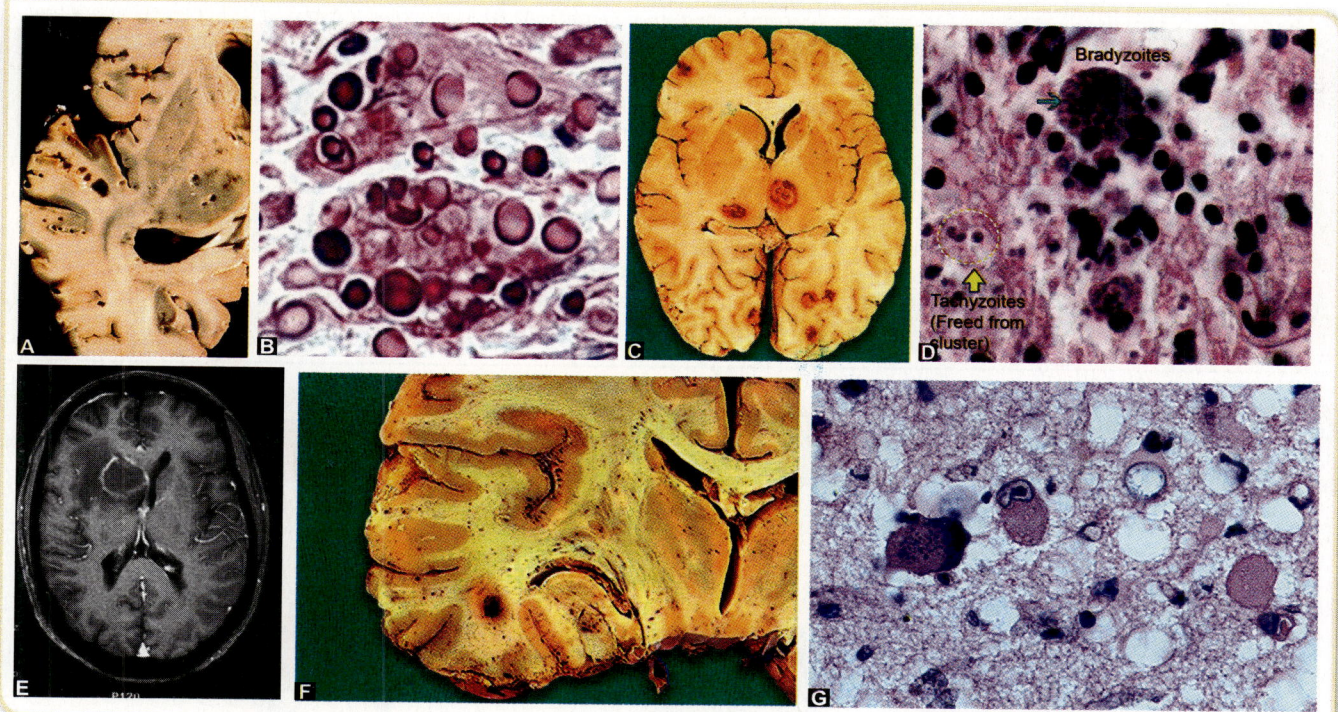

INFECTION OF BRAIN (HISTOPATHOLOGY)

A. **Cryptococcus infection of Brain (Gross):** Multiple small cystic lesion of brain giving a Swiss cheese appearance.
B. **Cryptococcus infection of Brain Histopathology:** Cryptococcus (an encapsulated yeast) appears as a spherical, encapsulated structure, which is surrounded by large empty spaces. Confirmed on India ink preparation
C. **Toxoplasmosis infection of Brain (Gross):** Showing multiple hemorrhagic necrosis
D. **Toxoplasmosis infection of Brain Histopathology:** showing Bradyzoites and Tachyzoites. T. gondii is considered to have three stages of infection; the tachyzoite stage of rapid division, the bradyzoite stage of slow division within tissue cysts, and the oocyst environmental stage. Host's immune system causes T. gondii tachyzoites to convert into bradyzoites, the semidormant, slowly dividing cellular stage of the parasite. Inside host cells, clusters of these bradyzoites are known as tissue cysts
E. **Toxoplasmosis infection of Brain CT scan:** Hypodense focal area with ring enhancement on contrast and local edema.
F. **Herpes simplex encephalitis (Gross):** The hemorrhages seen here in the temporal lobe are due to Herpes simplex virus infection. Viral infections produce mononuclear cell infiltrates microscopically.
G. **Herpes simplex encephalitis Histopathology:** Intranuclear inclusions are seen mainly in neurons. Vacuolated neuropil and mild gliosis are associated.

	Herpes	**Toxoplasma Gondi**	**Cryptococcus Neoformans**
Gross (Brain)	Advanced HSV encephalitis shows diffuse softening and edema, accentuated by **hemorrhagic necrosis of the inferior frontal and temporal lobes.**	Multiple foci of **Hemorrhagic necrosis** with 3-5 nm tachyzoites (cysts). Focal, variable in size but generally large, of irregular borders and can affect any part of the brain, with strong predilection to basal ganglia and brainstem.	Gelatinous grayish material within the subarachnoid space & multiple small cysts within the parenchyma giving a **Swiss cheese appearance**, especially prominent at basal ganglia. As the infection spreads the perivascular space (**Virchow Robin**) may become distended & filled with same mucoid, gelatinous material originated from the cryptococcal capsule

Contd...

	Herpes	Toxoplasma Gondi	Cryptococcus Neoformans
Histopathology	**Cowdry A amphophilic intranuclear inclusions of 90-nm to 100-nm "target" capsids.** Without treatment, extensive necrosis, macrophage reaction & neovascularization develop. The degree of Necrosis (especially in the frontal & temporal lobes, frequently bilateral) & inflammatory & reactive changes are more severe than any other viral encephalitis and can be detected by imaging.	Histologically, acute lesions differ from chronic abscesses. ☐ **Acute lesions**: poorly circumscribed, contain necrotic & hemorrhagic areas with scanted inflammatory cells & abundant intracellular tachyzoites & parenchymal oocysts. ☐ **Chronic lesions** developed after treatment, well demarcated cysts with microglial nodules and macrophages in the adjacent brain parenchyma, where parasites are difficult to find	Cystic lesions in the basal ganglia consist of aggregates of organisms confined to the **Virchow-Robin spaces**, which are enlarged. In tissue sections, the Cryptococcus appears as a **spherical, encapsulated structure**, which is surrounded by large empty spaces result of the abundant mucoid material secreted by the yeasts. The **capsule of Cryptococcus** can be visualized more clearly with special staining methods and silver impregnations, such as Gomori methenamine and Grocott, PAS and mucicarmine.

PATHO PLATE 50

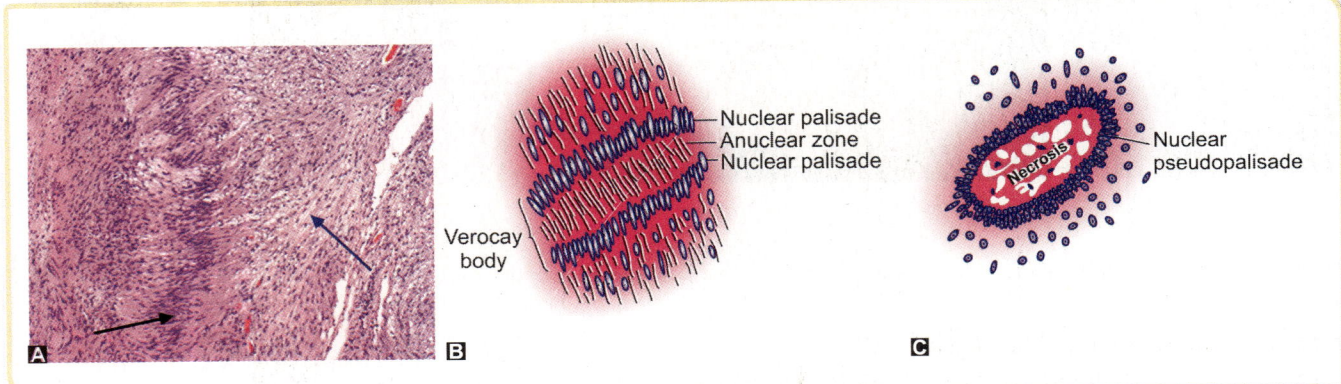

The black arrow represents nuclear Palisading called verocay Bodies in Antomi A patter of Schwannoma

SCHWANNOMA

Schwannomas are well-circumscribed, encapsulated masses that are attached to the nerve but can be separated from it. Tumors form firm, gray masses that may have areas of cystic and xanthomatous change. The defining histomorphologic features of schwannomas are eponymously named after the individuals who described them during the process of classification: in 1910, the Uruguyan neuropathologist Jose Verocay described the phenomenon of opposing rows of palisaded nuclei separated by eosinophilc, anuclear fibrillary processes now known as "**Verocay bodies**," and a decade later in 1920, the Swedish neurologist Nils Antoni described the characteristic mixed architectural pattern of schwannomas:

☐ In the **Antoni A pattern** of growth, elongated cells with cytoplasmic processes are arranged in fascicles in areas of moderate to high cellularity and scant stromal matrix; the "**nuclear-free zones**" of processes that lie between the regions of nuclear palisading are termed Verocay bodies. (Black arrow PATH PLATE 2 A)

☐ In the **Antoni B pattern** of growth, the tumor is hypocellular and consists of a loose meshwork of cells, microcysts and myxoid stroma. (Blue arrow PATH PLATE 2 A)

In both areas, the individual cells have an elongated shape and regular oval nuclei. Electron microscopy shows basement membrane deposits encasing single cells and collagen fibers. Because the lesion displaces the nerve of origin as it grows, silver stains or immunostains for neurofilament proteins demonstrate that axons are largely excluded from the tumor, although they may become entrapped in the capsule. The Schwann cell origin of these tumors is borne out by their **S-100 immunoreactivity.** A variety of degenerative changes may be found in schwannomas, including nuclear pleomorphism, xanthomatous change, and vascular hyalinization. Malignant change is extremely rare, but local recurrence can follow incomplete resection.

What are Palisades and Pseudopalisades?

A palisade is a strong fence or protective perimeter made of a row of wooden poles or stakes driven into the ground. Pathologists examining the microscopic appearance of certain tumors noted arrangements of elongated nuclei stacked in neat rows and attached the descriptive term "**palisades**" on the basis of their resemblance to the forts. Nuclear palisades may be considered "**primary**" (**plate 2B**) when they reflect a natural tendency of the nuclei to develop this distinctive pattern of growth or "**secondary**" (**plate 2C**) when the alignment forms as a response to external influences such as necrosis. The latter have been termed "**pseudopalisades**" to distinguish them from primary palisades. Although not pathognomonic, palisades are most often seen in schwannomas, whereas pseudopalisades are typical of glioblastomas.

PATHO PLATE 51

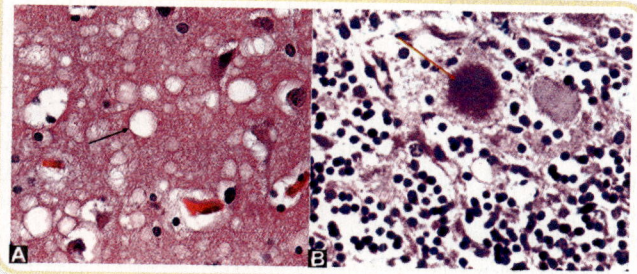

TRANSMISSIBLE SPONGIFORM ENCEPHALOPATHIES (PRION DISEASES)
Morphology

The progression of the dementia in CJD is usually so rapid that there is little if any grossly evident brain atrophy. On microscopic examination, the pathognomonic finding is a **spongiform transformation** of the cerebral cortex (A) and, often, deep gray-matter structures (caudate, putamen); this multifocal process results in the uneven formation of small, apparently empty, *microscopic vacuoles* (Black arrow in A) of varying sizes within the neuropil and sometimes in the perikaryon of neurons. In advanced cases there is severe *neuronal loss*, reactive gliosis, and sometimes expansion of the vacuolated areas into cystlike spaces ("*status spongiosus*"). No inflammatory infiltrate is present. Electron microscopy shows the vacuoles to be membrane-bound and located within the cytoplasm of neuronal processes.

Kuru plaques (Red arrow in B) are extracellular deposits of aggregated abnormal protein; they are *Congo red- and PAS positive* and usually occur in the cerebellum although they are present in abundance in the cerebral cortex in cases of vCJD, surrounded by the spongiform changes. In all forms of prion disease immunohistochemical staining demonstrates the presence of proteinase K–resistant PrP^{sc} in tissue. In a minority of cases of prion disease in the central nervous system, the misfolded *prion proteins* aggregate in the extracellular space and acquire the structural and staining characteristics of amyloid protein. Therefore, prion diseases are sometimes considered examples of **local amyloidosis.**

PATHO PLATE 52

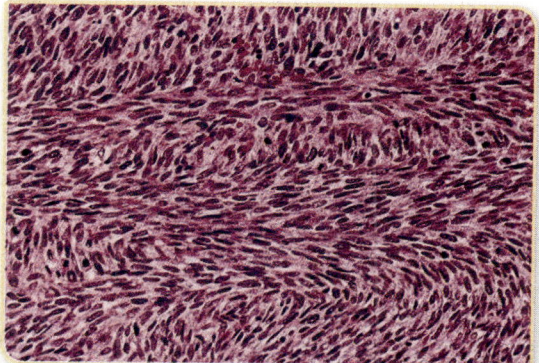

FIBROSARCOMAS

Fibrosarcomas occur anywhere in the body, but are most common in the deep soft tissues of the extremities. Fibrosarcomas are aggressive tumors, recurring in more than 50% of cases and metastasizing in more than 25%. Typically these neoplasms are unencapsulated, infiltrative, soft, fish-flesh masses often having areas of hemorrhage and necrosis. Better differentiated lesions may appear deceptively encapsulated. Histologic examination discloses all degrees of differentiation, from slowly growing tumors that closely resemble cellular fibromatosis and sometimes having spindled cells growing in a herringbone fashion, to highly cellular neoplasms dominated by **architectural disarray, pleomorphism**, frequent mitoses, and areas of necrosis. The **herringbone pattern** V-shaped twill weaved pattern, so named for a fancied resemblance to the skeleton of a fish such as a herring.

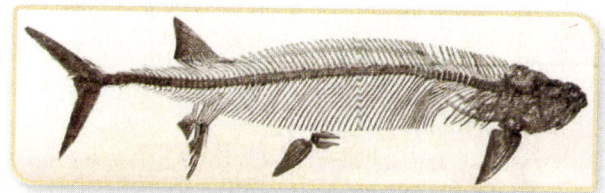

PATHO PLATE 53

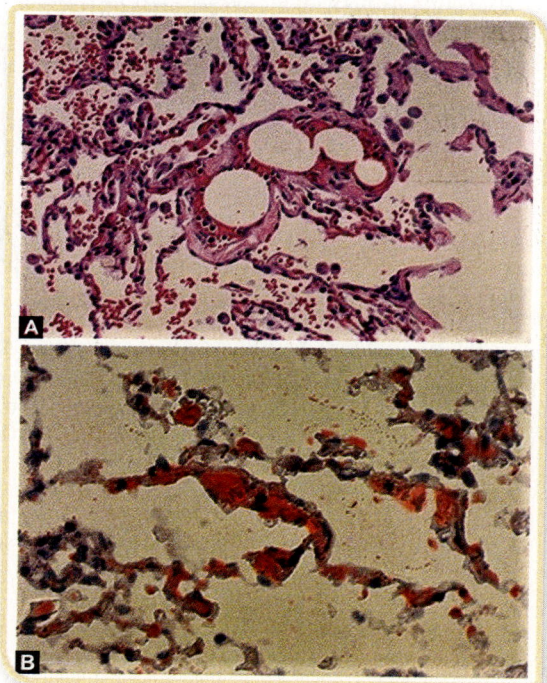

FAT EMBOLISM

A. Fat embolism Histopathology: The clear rounded holes in the small pulmonary arterial branch in this section of lung are characteristic for fat embolism. Fat embolism syndrome is most often a consequence of trauma with long bone fractures.

B. **An oil red O stain demonstrates the fat globules within the pulmonary arterioles.** The globules stain reddish-orange. The cumulative effect of many of these gobules throughout the lungs is similar to a large pulmonary embolus, but the onset of dyspnea is usually 2 to 3 days following the initiating event, such as blunt trauma with bone fractures.

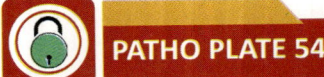

PATHO PLATE 54

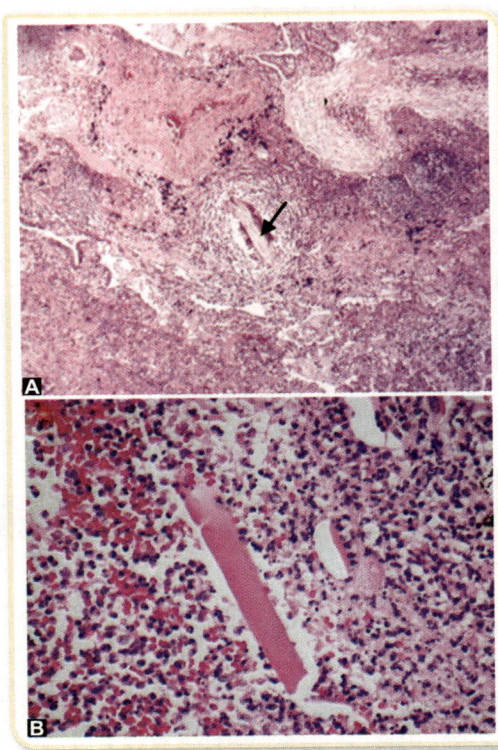

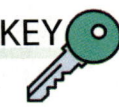

ASPIRATION PNEUMONIA

A. **Aspiration Pneumonia due to Vegetative matter:** Dense granulocytic infiltrate with Giant cells surround vegetable matter (arrow) in purulent exudates, organizing pneumonia (Top right corner) and Hyperemic capillaries.

B. **Aspiration pneumonia showing skeletal muscle**

Most commonly food aspiration are due to vegetable matter (seeds), skeletal muscle, fat tissue, or fragments of bone. The most common vegetable matter seen in chronic aspiration is the starch grain or granule, found in legumes, including peas, beans, and lentils. The starch granule is about 100 μ in length, is eosinophilic and well demarcated and oval, and eventually degenerates as macrophages engulf the material. If foreign material is not present, a histologic diagnosis of aspiration pneumonia cannot be made. Acute exudative response in <24 h. Chronic changes include foreign body giant cell reaction and organizing pneumonia. Fibrosis and calcification can occur at later stages. Recurrent aspiration can lead to diffuse bronchiolitis in a miliary form.

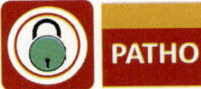

PATHO PLATE 55

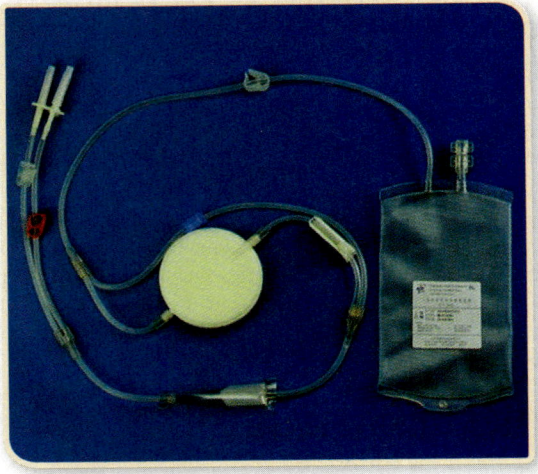

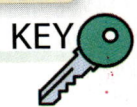

BLOOD BAG WITH LEUKOREDUCTION FILTER[AIIMSPG]

Leukoreduction or Leucodepletion is a technical term for the removal of leucocytes (white blood cells) from blood components using special filters. 3rd generation filters may eliminate up to 99.9% WBC in one unit of blood. Leukoreduced blood reduces the incidence of CMV transmission, febrile reactions and alloimmunization to HLA antigen.

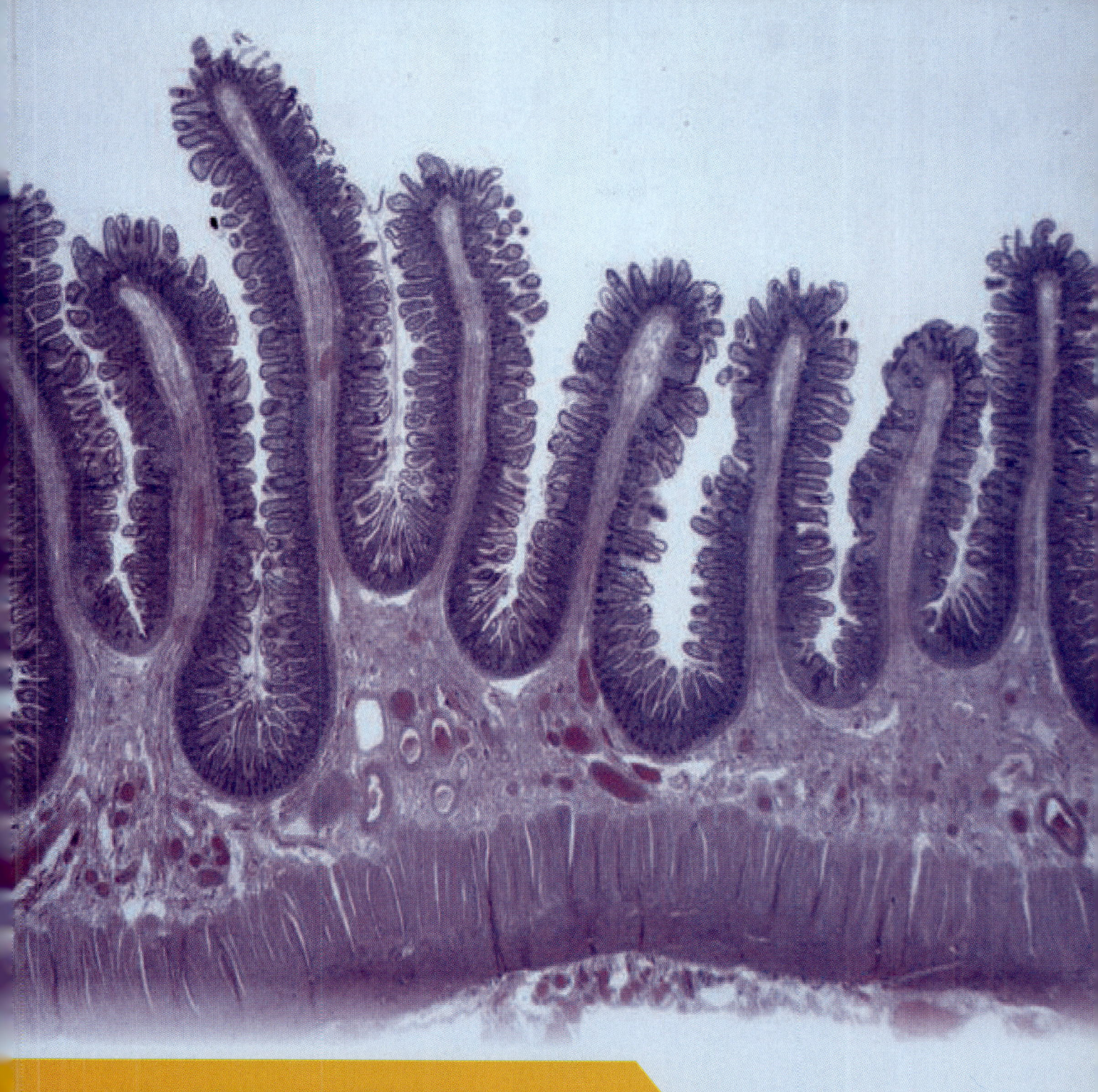

HISTOLOGY

HISTOLOGY PLATE 1

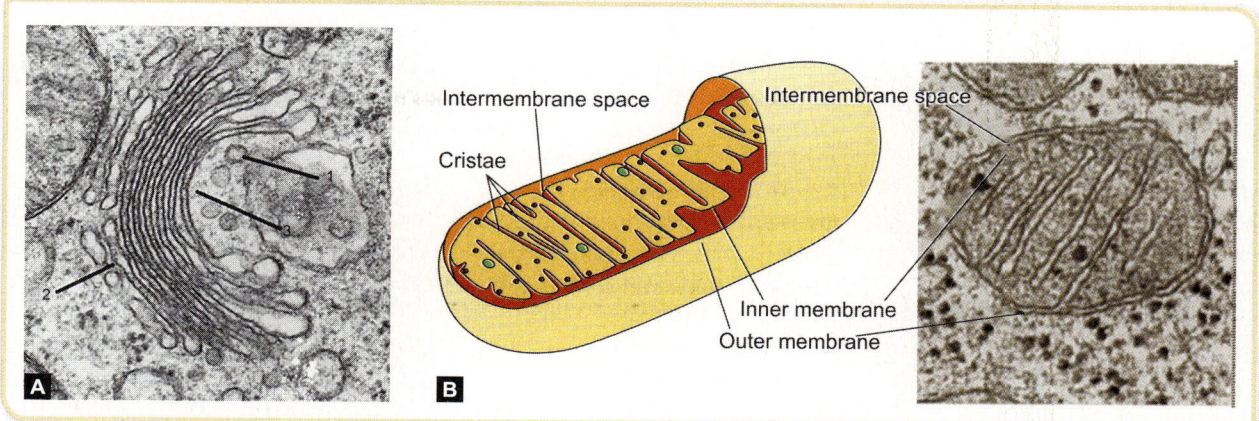

A. ELECTRON MICROSCOPIC PICTURE OF GOLGI APPARATUS

The Golgi apparatus was named after Camillo Golgi (Nobel Prize 1906), who discovered this cell structure in nerve cells (1898) and assigned it the role of a cell organelle.

- The Golgi apparatus (GA) is a **lamellar membranous structure** near the nucleus of almost all cells.
- The basic unit of the Golgi apparatus is the **dictyosome** or Golgi field; curved parallel series of flattened saccules that are often expanded at their ends
- It consists of a stack of 3–8 smooth (i.e., ribosome-free) slightly arcuate stacked membranes in close proximity to each other.
- Golgi cisternae are always accompanied by Golgi vesicles (Marked 1), which deliver and export material (transport vesicles). The Golgi apparatus has therefore two faces, **a convex (cis-), or forming face** (Marked 2) and a concave **trans-(secretory) face** pointing away from the nucleus (marked 3)
- The GA serves for regeneration of the cell membrane and modification of proteins (e.g. joining of proteins and glucuronic acids). Vesicles of the RER fuse on the **cis-part** of the GA while so called Golgi-vesicles are released on its **trans-part**.

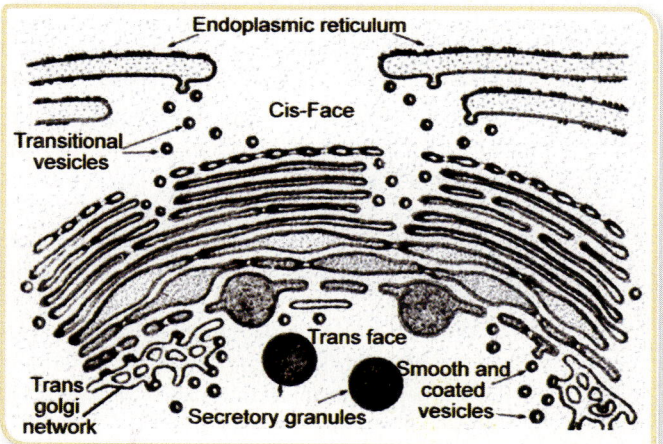

B. ELECTRON MICROSCOPIC PICTURE OF MITOCHONDRIA

Altmann discovered and described mitochondria, the power plant organelle of cells, as granular, rod-like stringy cell components. In 1898, C. Benda introduced the term mitochondria for these "threaded bodies". The mitochondria stand out as long, black-brown rods, which line up in the basal cytoplasm to almost parallel rows. The cell nuclei are not visible; their positions appear as gaps.

The basic structure follows the same principle layout in all mitochondria.

- An outer membrane (outer mitochondrial membrane) separates the mitochondrion from the cytoplasm.
- Inside this outer membrane (border) lies the inner membrane. It forms septum-like folds (cristae mitochondriales), which extend to various lengths across the organelle (crista-type mitochondria).
- The inner and outer membranes separate two cell compartments. Between the outer and inner membrane, separated by about 8nm, lies the outer compartment (outer metabolic compartment, intermembrane space), which extends into the crevices of the cristae.
- The inner membrane and its cristae forms the border around the inner compartment (inner metabolic space). It contains a homogeneous or granular matrix of variable density.
- The inner mitochondrial matrix often contains granules, the granula mitochondrialia or matrix granules, which have a size of 30–50nm and are rich in Ca^{2+} and other ions.

Cell Organelle

Name	Prokaryotic/ plant/ animal	Description	Function
Cell membrane	Pro, A, P	Flexible boundary that surrounds the cell, Bi-layer of proteins and lipids	Separates the cell from outside environment, Selectively permeable
Cell wall	Pro, P	Rigid Structure outside plasma membrane, Made of cellulose	Additional support, protection, Gives cell its shape
Nucleus	A, P	Contains DNA, Surrounded by double membrane, visible on light microscopy	Controls the cell activities
Nuclear membrane/ envelope	A, P	Double membrane layer that surrounds nucleus	Allows material to move into and out of Nucleus (RNA pass through pores)
Nuclear pores	A, P	1000s of pores in nuclear envelope	Allow material to move into and out of Nucleus
Chromatin	A, P	Granular material within nucleus, DNA bound to protein	Condenses to form chromosome at the time of cell division
Chromosome	A, P	☐ Distinct thread like ☐ Contains genetic info	Blueprint - controls cell activity Pass on genetic info to next generation
Nucleolus	A, P	Small dense dark stained region inside in nucleus	Site of transcription of RNA, Assembly of ribosomes take place here
Cytoplasm	Pro, A, P	Clear Gelatinous (jelly) fluid inside the cell	Chemical reactions take place here
Cytoskeleton	A, P	☐ Network of protein filaments	Helps the cell to maintain its shape and 3 D structure, Cell movement
Cilia/ flagella	A	Short/long projections of microtubules	Cell Movement
Microtubule	A, P	Hollow tubes of protein	Maintain cell shape, Form cilia/flagella, Separate chromosomes in cell division
Microfilament	A, P	Long thin fibers	Maintain cell shape Cell movement and support
Ribosome	Pro, A, P	Tiny round structures found on the surface of the RER or free in the cytoplasm, Made of RNA and Protein	Translation of RNA and protein synthesis
Endoplasmic Reticulum	A, P	Highly folded membrane in cytoplasm. Internal membrane surrounding a lumen Rough E.R. (ribosome) Smooth E.R. (no ribosomes)	RER – protein synthesis SER – lipid biosynthesis
Golgi Apparatus	A, P	Pancake like stacks of membrane bound sacs called cisternae. Found near cell membrane. Has a cis and a trans face	Collects, sorts, packages, and secretes proteins. Proteins are taken in by the cis side and exit from the trans side
Lysosome	A	Tiny round vesicles containing digestive enzymes	Digests food, bacteria, worn out organelle
Vacuole	P, A (small or none)	Sac (membrane bound)	☐ Stores food, enzyme, and other material ☐ Support
Mitochondrion	A, P	Double membrane bound organelle. The inner membrane has folds called cristae	Power house of cell – produces energy for growth, development, and movement
Centrioles/ Basal bodies	A	Small structure outside nucleus formed from microtubules	☐ Helps in cell division (mitosis) ☐ Helps in forming flagella and cilia
Chloroplast	P	☐ Double membrane bound organelle ☐ Pigment chlorophyll is present in inner membrane	☐ Captures light and converts it into chemical energy ☐ Pigment chlorophyll (photosynthesis)

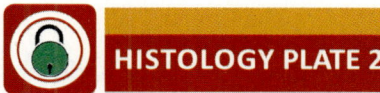

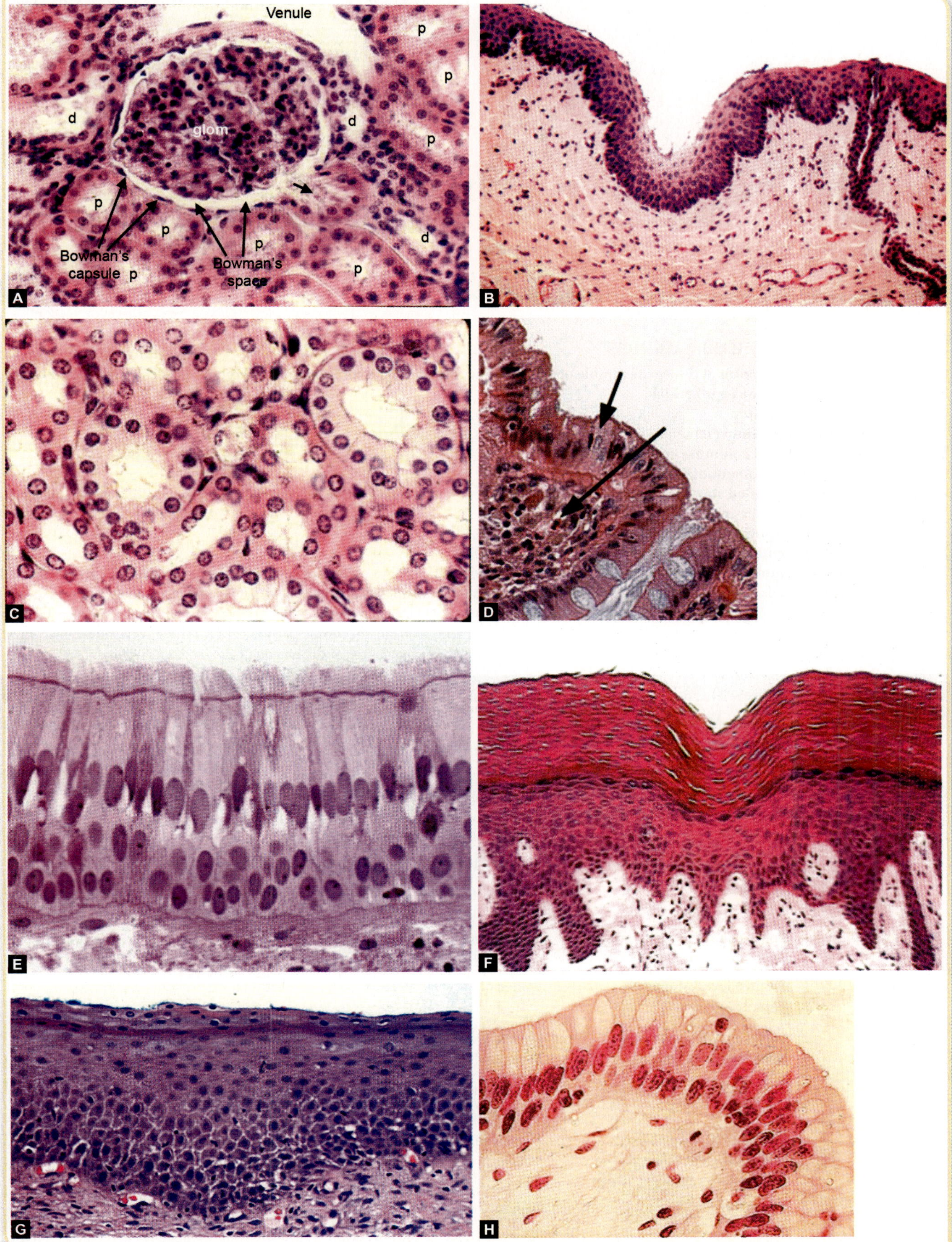

HISTOLOGY PLATE 2

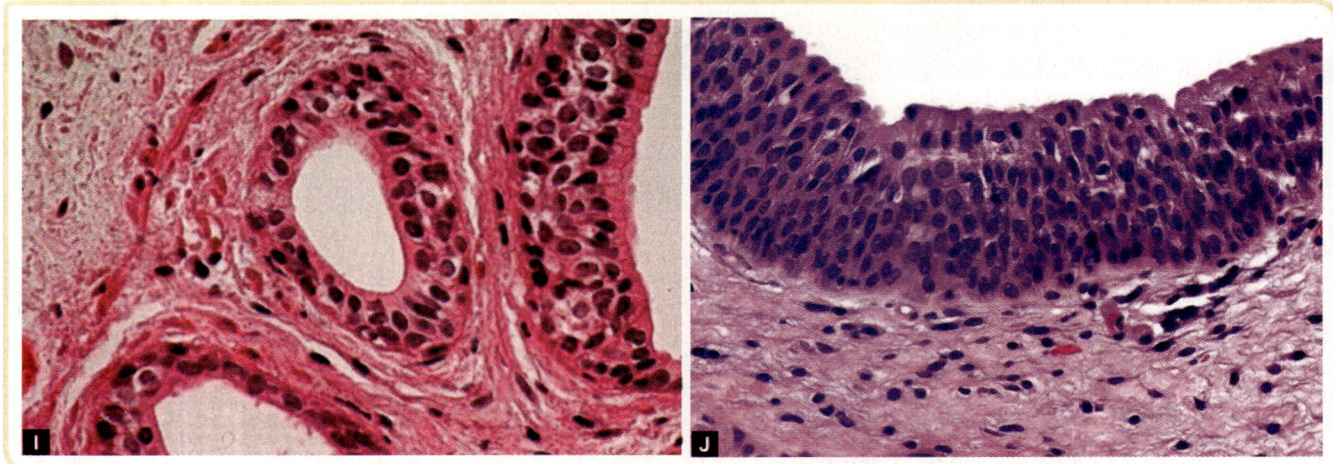

SOME IMPORTANT EPITHELIUM LININGS

A. **Simple squamous epithelium** of Bowman's capsule of Kidney (long arrow). P = proximal convoluted tubule, d= distal convoluted tubule
B. **Simple stratified squamous epithelium**
C. **Simple cuboidal epithelium**
D. **Simple columnar epithelium** (short arrow) over the connective tissue (long arrow)
E. **Pseudostratified ciliated columnar epithelium**
F. **Keratinizing stratified squamous epithelium**
G. **Non–Keratinizing stratified squamous epithelium:** Multiple layers of flattened cells, basal cells typically are cuboidal, while apical cells are squamous. Surface cells are alive and kept moist.
H. **Stratified columnar epithelium** - Multiple layers of columnar cells
I. **Stratified cuboidal epithelium** - Multiple layers of cube-shaped cells
J. **Transitional epithelium:** It is a multilayered epithelium, the lowermost cells are columnar or cuboidal, the middle cells are polyhedral and the uppermost cells are almost umbrella shaped. This is typical of transitional epithelium which is seen in urothelium. Transitional epithelium is found in the renal pelvis and calyces, the ureter, the urinary bladder, and part of the urethra. The wall of the urinary bladder consists of urothelium, lamina propria, muscularis propria, serosa, and, in some locations, perivesical fat. The normal urothelial lining varies in thickness from two layers to seven layers of cells, depending upon the degree of distension of the bladder.

Some Important Epithelium Linings (Classification Wise)			
Type	**Cell form**	**Examples of distribution**	**Main function**
Simple	Squamous	Lining of vessels (endothelium)	Facilitates the movement of the viscera (mesothelium), active transport by pinocytosis (mesothelium and endothelium), secretion of biologically active molecules (mesothelium)
		Serous lining of cavities; pericardium, pleura, peritoneum (mesothelium)	
	Cuboidal	Covering the ovary, thyroid	Covering, secretion
	Columnar	Lining of intestine, gallbladder.	Protection, lubrication, absorption, secretion
Pseudostratified	Some columnar and some cuboidal	Lining of trachea, bronchi, nasal cavity	Protection, secretion; cilia-mediated transport of particles trapped in mucus
Stratified	Surface layer squamous keratinized (dry)	Epidermis	Protection; prevents water loss
	Surface layer squamous nonkeratinized (moist)	Mouth, esophagus, larynx, vagina, anal canal	Protection, secretion; prevents water loss
	Cuboidal	Sweat glands, developing ovarian follicles	Protection, secretion
	Transitional: Domelike to flattened, depending on the functional state of the organ	Urinary Bladder, ureters, renal calyces	Protection, distensibility
	Columnar	Conjunctiva	Protection.

Contd...

HISTOLOGY COLOR PLATES

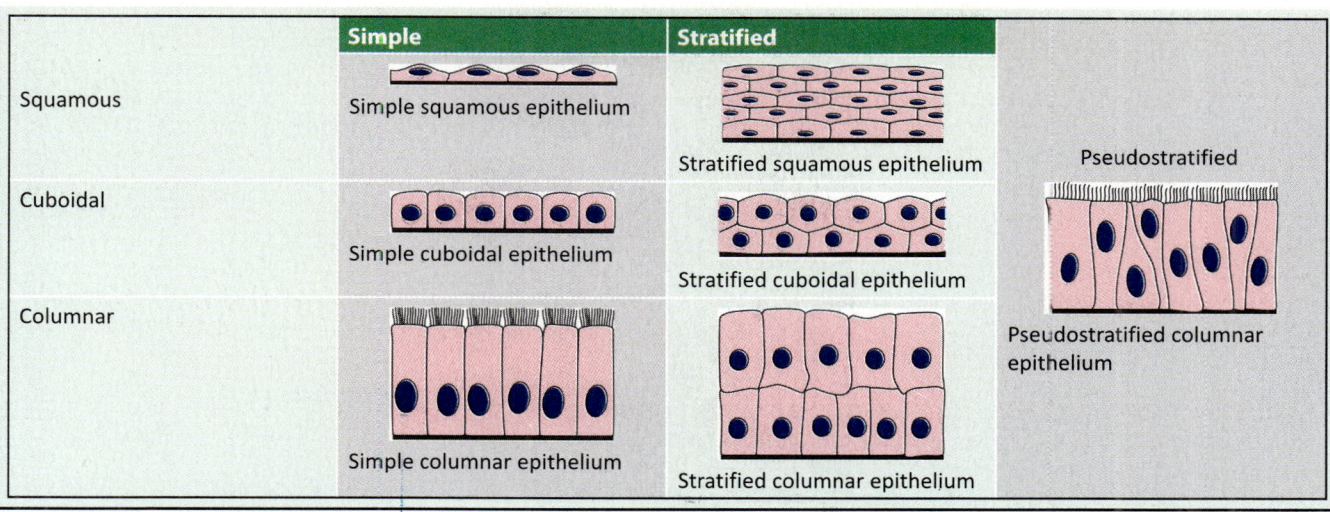

HISTOLOGY PLATE 3

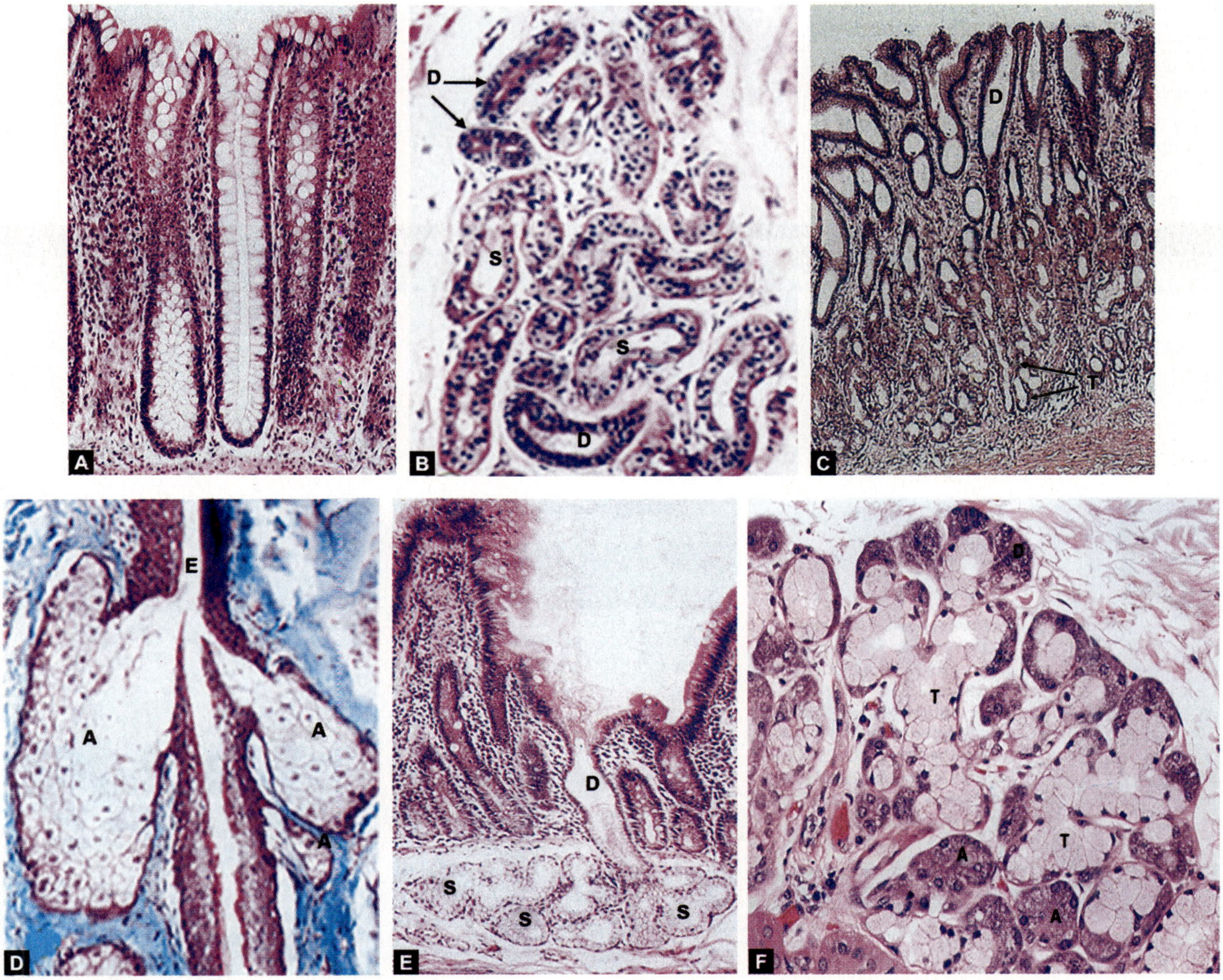

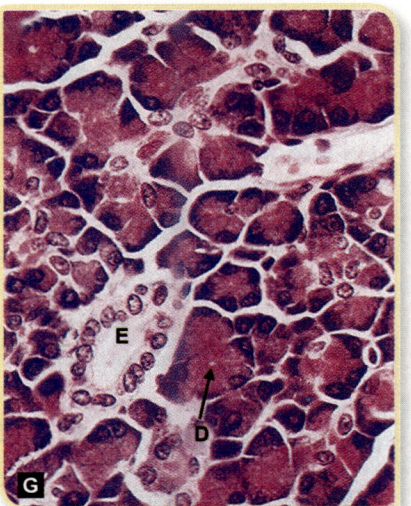

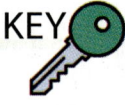

Abbreviations: d = duct, t = tube, A = acini, S = secretory cells

PLATE LEGENDS
A. Simple tubular gland
B. Simple coiled tubular
C. Simple branched tubular
D. Simple branched acinar
E. Compound branched tubular
F. Compound tubuloacinar
G. Compound acinar

Structural Classifications of Exocrine Glands			
Duct system	Secretory portion	Example	
Simple	Tubular	Intestinal crypts of Lieberkuhn	
Simple	Coiled tubular	Eccrine sweat glands of the skin	
Simple	Branched tubular	Fundic glands of the stomach	

Contd...

Structural Classifications of Exocrine Glands

Simple	Branched acinar	Sebaceous glands of the skin	
Compound	Tubular	Cardiac glands of the stomach	
Compound	Tubuloacinar	Submandibular salivary glands	
Compound	Acinar	Exocrine pancreas	

HISTOLOGY PLATE 4

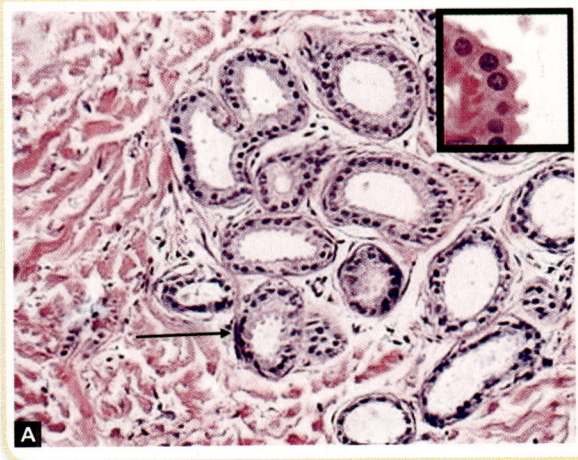
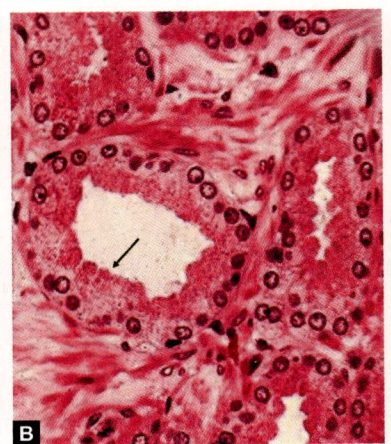
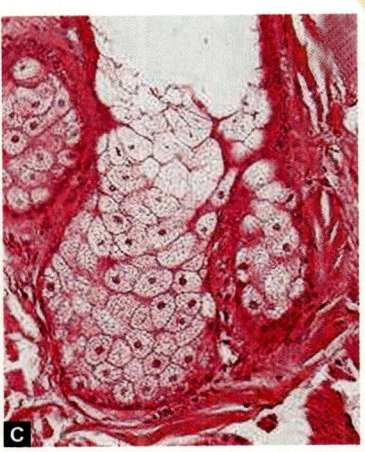

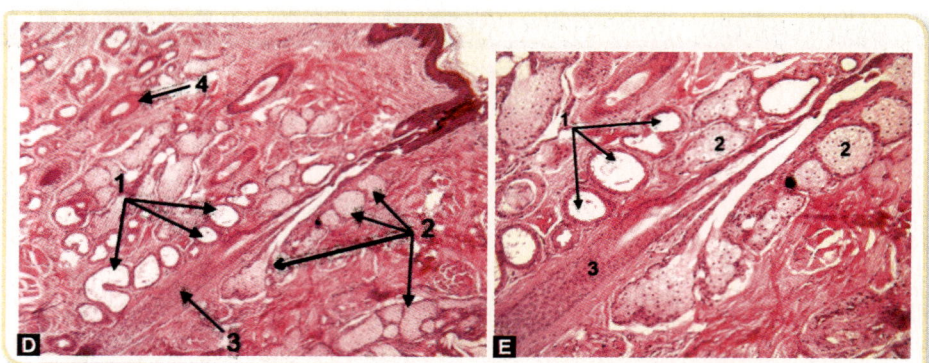

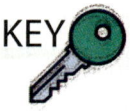

EXOCRINE GLANDS

A. **Apocrine gland:** Apocrine sweat glands are typically larger and more productive than Merocrine (eccrine) glands. They are characterized by a simple cuboidal epithelium and widely dilated lumen that stores the secretory product. Secretion from apocrine glands contains protein, lipid, carbohydrate, ammonium and other organic compounds. The ducts of the glands empty into an adjacent hair follicle. **The bleb** (insat) on the apical surface of the secretory cells suggested that the cell underwent apocrine secretion

B. **Merocrine (Eccrine) gland:** Merocrine sweat glands are simple tubular glands. However, the secretory units and the beginnings of the duct are coiled. The coiled mass is seen as numerous closely arranged tubular sections. Most merocrine glands have their main portions in the dermis, but some may reach even the hypodermis. In this picture note the dense connective tissue of the reticular dermis around the gland.

C. **Holocrine gland:** Sebaceous glands are holocrine glands. Their secretion, sebum, is an oily material. In this picture, note the outer cells comparable to the basal layer. As the cells grow they move inwards and accumulate their secretion. The fatty secretion is lost in processing leaving behind a spongy framework of other cytoplasmic elements. The cells are very similar to brown fat cells in appearance.
   In the deepest part of the gland you can see cells without nuclei disintegrating. The entire cell dies in releasing the sebum. Sebum travels to the surface along a hair shaft.

D. **40x Magnification; Sweat and Sebaceous gland**
   1. Apocrine Sweat glands
   2. Sebaceous glands (Holocrine)
   3. Hair follicle
   4. Duct of Sweat gland

E. **100x Magnification; Sweat and Sebaceous gland**
   1. Apocrine Sweat glands
   2. Sebaceous glands (Holocrine)
   3. Hair follicle

	Classification of Exocrine Glands on the Basis of Mechanism of Secretion		
	Merocrine	**Apocrine**	**Holocrine**
Greek	Gr. meros, part, + krinein	Gr. apo, away from, + krinein	Gr. holos, whole, + krinein
Mode of secretion	The secretory granules leave the cell by exocytosis with no loss of other cellular material most common mechanism of secretion	The secretory product is discharged together with parts of the apical cytoplasm	The product of secretion is shed with the whole cell, a process that involves destruction of the secretion filled cells
Example	Pancreas Eccrine Sweat gland	Lactating mammary glands, Apocrine glands of skin, Apocrine sweat glands, Ciliary (Moll's) glands of eyelids Ceruminous glands of external auditory meatus	Sebaceous glands Tarsal (Meibomian) glands of eyelids
Representative diagram	Merocrine gland — Secretory product in lumen of gland, Intact cell, A vesicle releasing its contents	Apocrine gland — Pinched off portions of cells releasing secretory product, Pinched off portions of cells apocrine gland	Holocrine gland — A disintegrating cell releasing its contents, Cell with secretory product, New cells forming

HISTOLOGY PLATE 5

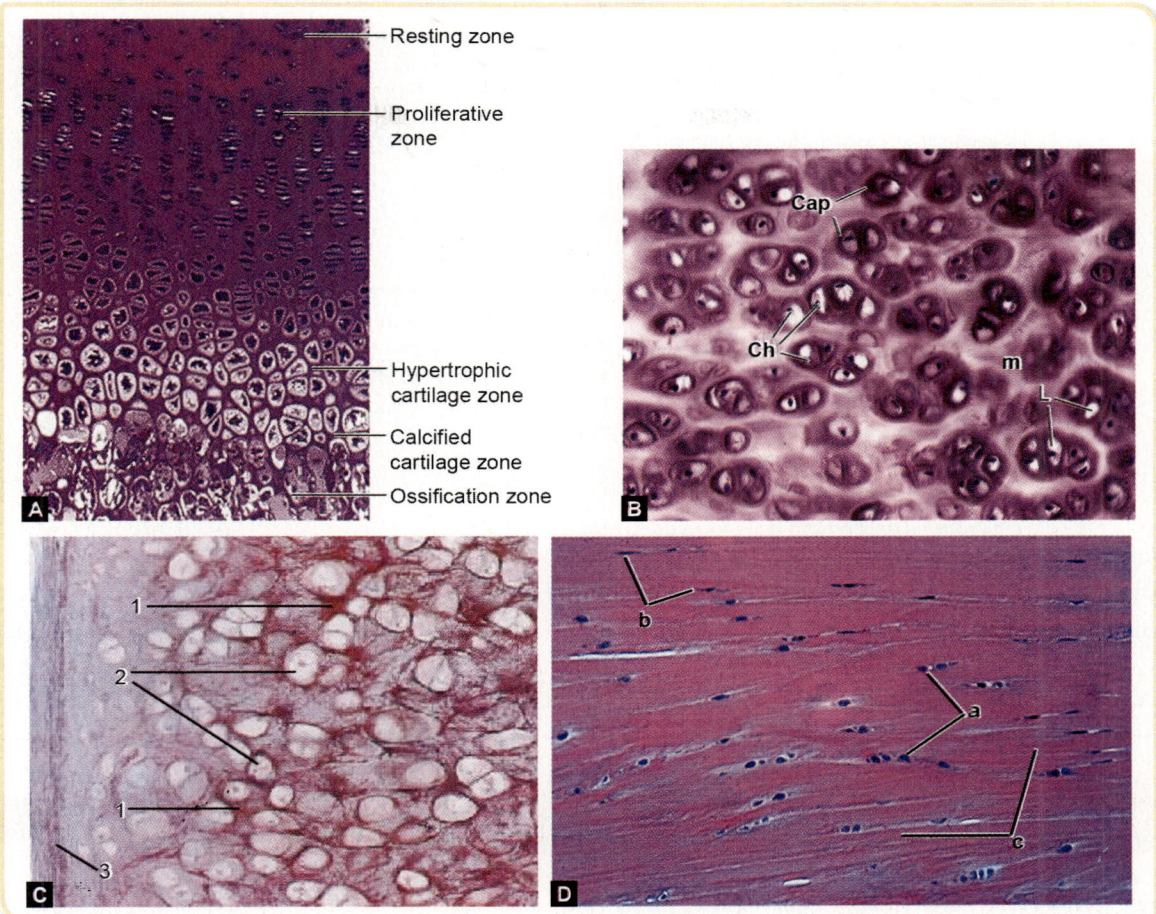

TYPES OF CARTILAGES

A. **Hyaline cartilage (Low power; Epiphysis): Meta-epiphyseal cartilage** is divided into five zones, starting from the epiphyseal side of cartilage:
  1. The resting zone consists of *hyaline cartilage* without morphologic changes in the cells.
  2. In the proliferative zone (columnar), chondrocytes divide rapidly and form columns of stacked cells parallel to the long axis of the bone.
  3. The hypertrophic cartilage zone contains large chondrocytes whose cytoplasm has accumulated glycogen. The resorted matrix is reduced to thin septa between the chondrocytes.
  4. Simultaneous with the death of chondrocytes in the calcified cartilage zone, the thin septa of cartilage matrix become calcified by the deposit of hydroxyapatite.
  5. In the ossification zone, endochondral bone tissue appears.
  Blood capillaries and osteoprogenitor cells formed by mitosis of cells originating from the periosteum invade the cavities left by the chondrocytes. The osteoprogenitor cells form osteoblasts, which are distributed in a discontinuous layer over the septa of calcified cartilage matrix. Ultimately, the osteoblasts deposit bone matrix over the three-dimensional calcified cartilage matrix.
B. **Hyaline cartilage (High power):** The word hyaline is derived from the Greek word "hyalos" which means glass. Enzymatic digestion of the ground substances in the cartilage matrix can unmask the collagen fibrils and render them visible.
  Cap = capsule, Ch = chondrocytes, L = lacuna, m = avascular matrix
C. **Elastic cartilage:** The matrix of elastic cartilage contains nonmasked elastic fiber networks (marked 1). In principle, the rest of the elastic cartilage structure is like that of hyaline cartilage. Like hyaline cartilage, it contains masked collagen fibers. The round or oval spaces (lacuna) contain the cartilage cells or Chondrocytes (marked 2), which are only slightly stained. At the left edge of the figure is the perichondrium (marked 3), with it's fine elastic fibers parallel to the surface.
D. **Fibrocartilage:** Fibrocartilage (connective tissue cartilage) expresses the structures and attributes of two types of tissue, dense regular connective tissue and hyaline cartilage. The extracellular matrix consists mostly of collagen fibers (type I and type II collagen), which are not masked and therefore visible after staining (collagen fiber cartilage). Bundles of collagen fibrils run in the direction, which is determined by the mechanical stress vector. Between the unmasked collagen fibers (marked c) are single cartilage cells or small groups of **chondrocytes** (marked a) and fibroblast nucleus (marked b). The ovoid to spherical chondrocytes occur singly or often one after the other in a row.

Types of Cartilages

	Hyaline cartilage	Elastic cartilage	Fibrocartilage
Composition	Type II collagen Chondroitin sulfate	Type II collagen Elastin fibers	Type I collagen
Perichondrium	Present (Except articular cartilage, covering the bony ends and Epiphyseal plate)	Present	Absent
Function	Resist compression, provide cushioning smooth and low friction surface for joints, Provides structural support in respiratory system, Forms foundation of fetal skeleton	Provides flexible support	Resist deformation under stress
Example	Fetal skeletal tissue Articular cartilage Larynx (Arytenoid, Thyroid and Cricoid cartilage) Tracheal rings and Bronchi Epiphyseal growth plate Nasal cartilage Costal cartilage of ribs	Auricle/ Pinna of external ear External auditory meatus External auditory canal Auditory/Eustachian tube Larynx (Epiglottis, Corniculate and Cuneiform cartilage)	Articular discs Intervertebral discs Menisci Pubic symphysis Glenoid labrum Acetabular labrum Insertion of tendons
Undergoes calcification	Yes (during enchondral bone formation and ageing process)	No	Yes (during bone repair)
Main cell type	Chondroblasts and chondrocytes	Chondroblasts and chondrocytes	Chondrocytes and Fibroblasts
Extracellular matrix	Type 2 collagen and Aggrecan (most important proteoglycan)	Type 2 collagen, Elastic fibers and Aggrecan	Type 1, Type 2 collagen fibers and Versican (a proteoglycan secreted by fibroblast)

HISTOLOGY PLATE 6

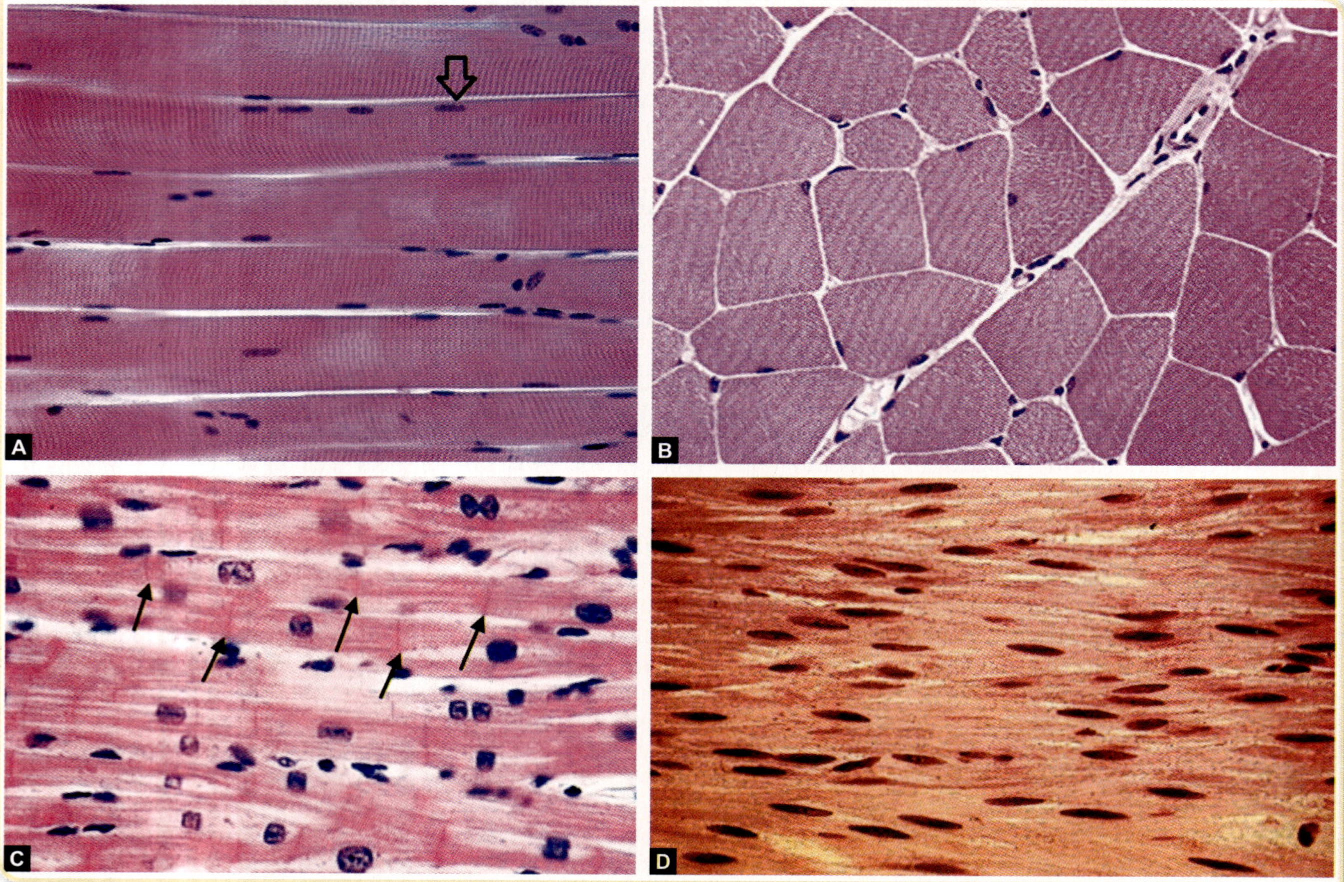

MUSCLE CELL'S TYPES

A. **Longitudinal section of skeletal muscle** (See striations perpendicular to the length of muscle fibers and the peripherally placed nucleus- arrow)
B. **Transverse/Cut section of skeletal muscle** (Striations are not visible on Transverse section but peripherally placed nuclei are seen)
C. **Cardiac muscle histology:** Striations are visible perpendicular to the length of muscle fibers. Branching of the fibers can be seen (yellow circle). Nuclei is centrally placed. Intercalated disc is visible (arrow).
D. **Smooth muscle histology:** Spindle shaped cells with centrally placed nucleus

	Muscle Cells Types		
	Skeletal	Cardiac	Smooth
Histology	**Striated, Nonbranching,** cylindrical, long (cant see ends in slide) and tubular shape of the cell. Multinucleate syncitium is seen in cells. Peripheral position of the elongate nuclei just inside of the sarcolemma (plasma membrane)	**Striated** muscle with tubular cells. **Branching** of fibers may be seen. Centrally placed nucleus. Mononucleated or bi nucleated cells. Contains **intercalated discs** which are seen as dark staining lines between myocytes. The discs always lie opposite the I-bands.	Non striated, Spindle shaped cells, Centrally located nucleus
Nuclei	Multinucleated, peripherally located	Single nuclei, Centrally located	Single nuclei, Centrally located
Banding	Actin and myosin form distinctive bands	Actin and myosin form distinctive bands	Actin and myosin; No distinctive bands
Z-disks	Present	Present	Absent, cytoplasmic dense bodies are present
T tubules	T tubules at A-I junction; triads present	T tubules at Z disk; diads present	No T tubules; no triads
Cellular junctions	No junctional complexes	Intercalated disks	Gap junctions
Neuromuscular junctions	Present	Not present; contraction is intrinsic	Not present; contraction is intrinsic, neural, or hormonal
Ca$^+$ binding	Troponin	Troponin	Calmodulin
Regeneration	Limited; satellite cells	None	High

HISTOLOGY PLATE 7

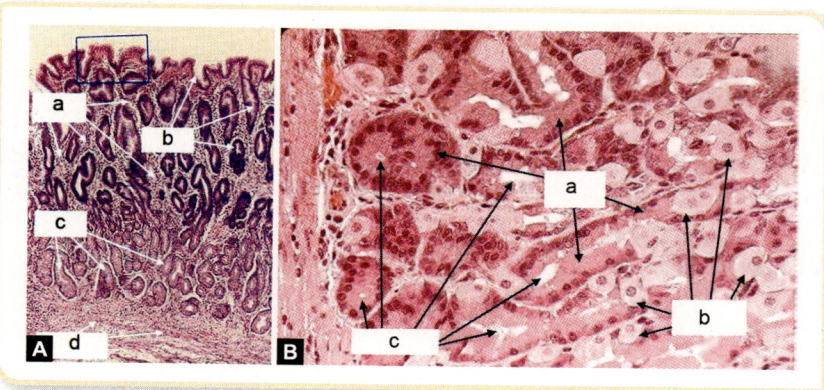

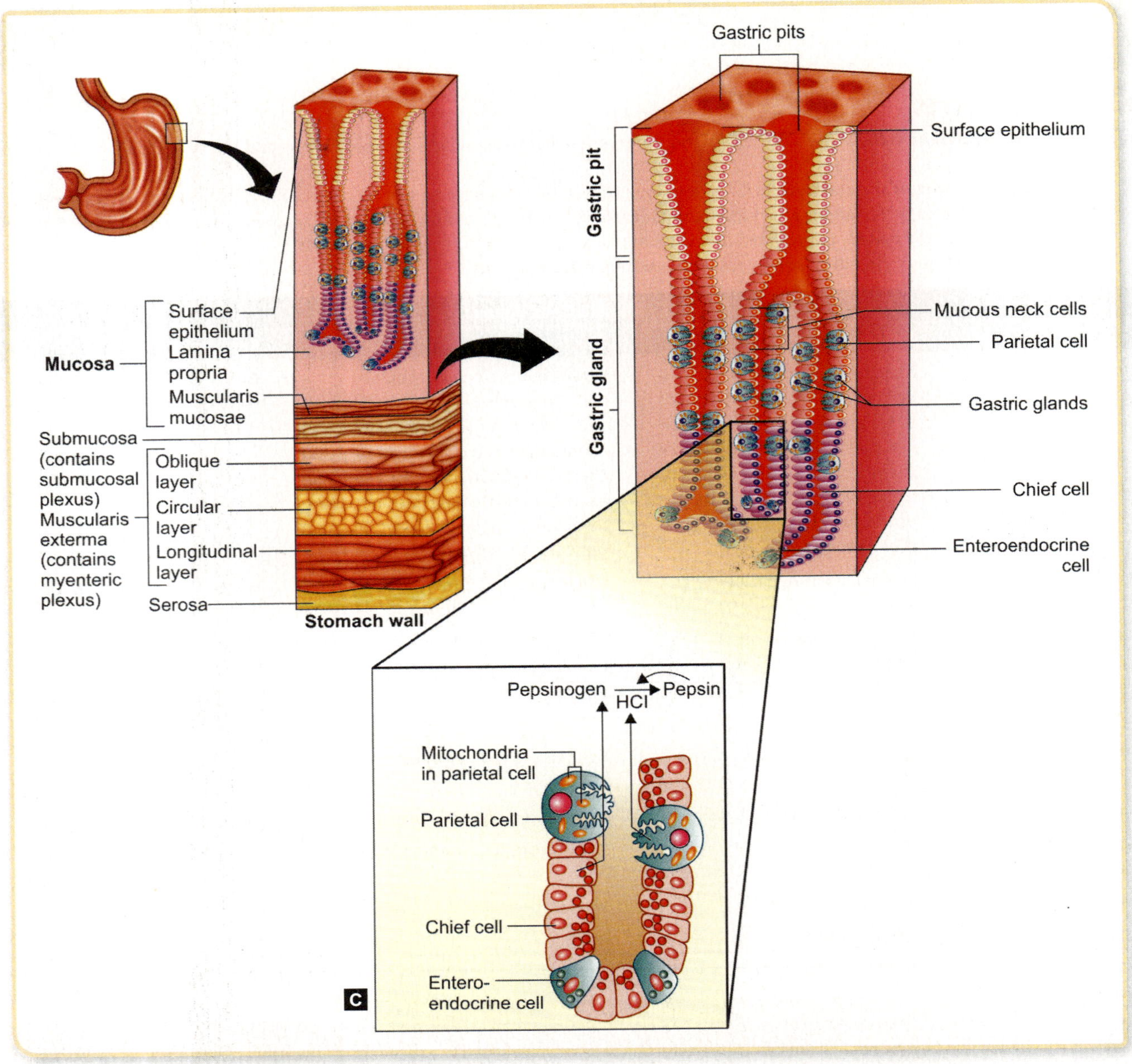

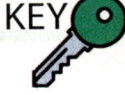

A. GASTRIC MUCOSA HISTOLOGY LOW POWER
a. Lamina Propria
b. Gastric Pits: gastric pits of the pyloric stomach are quite deep, extending more than halfway through the thickness of the mucosa
c. Pyloric Glands: the pyloric glands lie above the muscularis mucosae, in the mucosa
d. Muscularis mucosae

B. GASTRIC MUCOSA HIGH POWER
a. Chief cells
b. Parietal cells
c. Glandular lumen

Gastric Glands

They can be divided into three groups-the cardiac, principal (in the body and fundus) and pyloric glands

Principal glands: ☐ Located in body and fundus ☐ In the walls of the gland are at least five distinct cell types: chief, parietal, mucous neck, stem and neuroendocrine	Chief cells	Source of pepsinogen, rennin and lipase. Contain zymogens, contain abundant RNA and hence intensely basophilic
	Parietal (oxyntic) cells	Are the source of gastric acid and of intrinsic factor
	Neuroendocrine cells	These cells synthesize a number of biogenic amines and polypeptides important in the control of motility and glandular secretion. In the stomach they include cells designated as G cells secreting gastrin, D cells (somatostatin), and ECL (enterochromaffin-like) cells (histamine).
Pyloric glands		Pyloric glands are mostly populated with mucus-secreting cells, parietal cells are few and chief cells scarce. In contrast, neuroendocrine cells are numerous, especially G cells, which secrete gastrin when activated by appropriate mechanical stimulation (causing increased gastric motility and secretion of gastric juices)
Cardiac glands		Mucus-secreting cells predominate and parietal and chief cells, although present, are few **Note:** There are other cells that secrete mucus (as in the foveolar cells of the stomach), but they are not usually called "goblet cells" because they do not have this distinctive shape.

Gastric Mucosa Cells

Name		Location	Secretion	Appearance
Mucous neck cell		Common to all type of gastric glands specially neck of glands at Fundus and Body	Gastric mucous (Mucin)	Lightly eosinophilic or clear cytoplasm and bubbly PAS positive neutral mucin
Zymogenic, or chief		Gastric glands of body and fundus	Pepsinogen and gastric lipase	Basophilic cytoplasm due to abundant rough endoplasmic reticulum
Parietal (oxyntic) cells		Gastric glands of body and fundus	HCL and Intrinsic factor	Eosinophilic due to abundant mitochondria
Endocrine (APUD) cells	Gastrin cells or G cells (60%)	Antrum only	Gastrin, GABA	Small condensed nucleus with clear cytoplasm
	D cell (20%)	Antrum and Fundus	Somatostatin	
	Enterochromafin (EC) cells	Antrum and Fundus	Enterostatin, serotonin	
	Enterochromafin like (ECL) Cells	Fundus only	Histamine	

HISTOLOGY PLATE 8

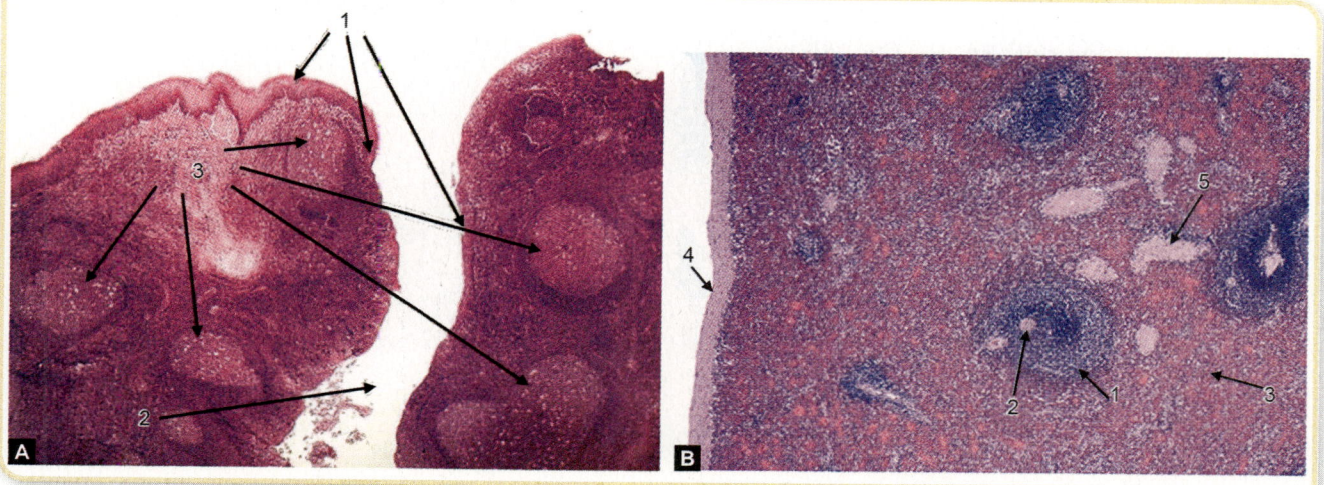

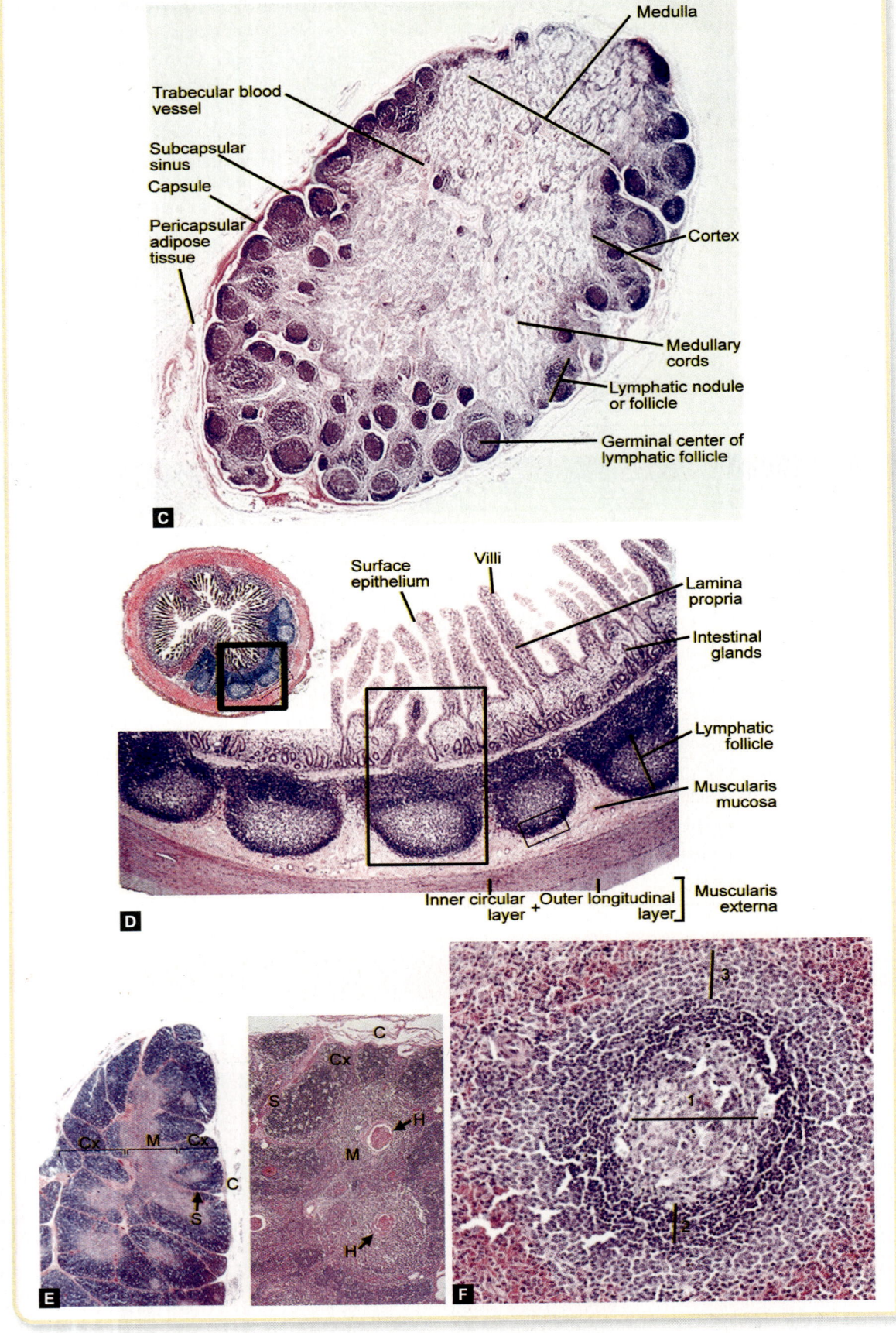

LYMPHATIC ORGANS

The characteristic feature of all lymphatic tissue is a lymphatic nodule which is nothing but a collection of lymphocytes. Each Lymphatic tissue has a unique feature which helps in its identification

A. **Tonsil histology:** stratified squamous epithelium lining (marked as 1), tonsillar crypt (marked as 2), Lymph nodules (marked as 3)
B. **Spleen histology:** This is the normal appearance of the spleen at low power with white pulp (lymphocytes) (marked as 1) surrounding a central arteriole (marked as 2). The red pulp (marked as 3) forms the bulk of the splenic parenchyma. The splenic capsule (marked as 4) is seen at the left, and connective tissue is also present within the spleen as trabeculae (marked as 5) that carry the arteries, veins, and nerves from the hilum. Eccentric arteriole in the lymphatic nodule
C. **Lymph node histology:** Note the characteristic Subcapsular sinus
D. **Peyer's patches histology:** lymphatic nodes in ilieum, so features of gastrointestinal tract are seen. Mucosa, submucosa, muscularis and adventitia.
E. **Thymus histology:** Characteristic Hassall's corpuscles are seen. Loose collagenous capsule, **C**, from which short interlobular septa, **S**, containing blood vessels radiate into the substance of the organ. The thymic tissue is divided into two distinct zones, a deeply basophilic outer cortex, **Cx**, and an inner eosinophilic medulla, **M**; distinction between the two zones is most marked in early childhood as is represented in this specimen. The cortex, **Cx**, is packed with lymphocytes, accounting for its basophilia, whereas the medulla, **M**, contains fewer lymphocytes. In the center of the medulla are eosinophilic, lamellated structures known as **Hassall's corpuscles**, **H**, representing degenerate epithelial reticular cells.
F. **Lymphatic follicle:** It is common to all Lymphatic organs. When these nodules become activated, the B-cells in the center of the nodule undergo maturation, many becoming plasma cells. Since plasma cells have a much larger cytoplasm-to-nucleus ratio, the center of the nodule becomes lighter-staining. This center area of lightness is referred to as the **germinal center (marked 1)**. Surrounding the germinal center is a ring of small, dark, tightly-packed B cells which comprise the **mantle zone (marked 2)**. Directly outsize of the mantle zone is the **marginal zone (marked 3)**, which is also comprised of B-cells. Lymphomas can arise from each of these areas, and are thus classified as follicular (germinal center), mantle zone, or marginal zone lymphomas.

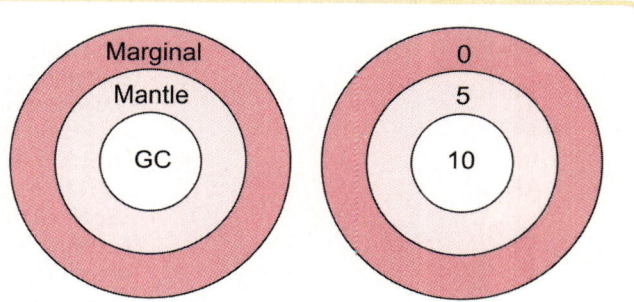

Germinal centre or Follicular CD 19+, CD 20+, CD 10+, CD 5-
Mantle cell: CD 19+, CD20+, CD 10-, CD 5+
Marginal zone: CD 19+, CD 20+, CD 10-, CD 5-

Lymphatic Organs: Distinctive Morphological Features				
Organ	Capsule and connective tissue septa	Parenchyma	Vessels	Other features
Lymph node	Well-developed capsule, clearly visible trabeculae	Lymphoreticular, compact cortex with lymph follicles, lighter medulla with medullary cords	Afferent vessel, marginal sinus, intermediary sinus, medullary sinus, efferent vessel; in the lumina of all sinuses: a bow-net (weir) system of reticular fibers and reticular cells, no blood cells	Surrounded by loosely organized connective tissue and adipose tissue; lymph vessels with valves often exist in the vicinity; no surface epithelium
Spleen	Very well-developed capsule, strong trabeculae	Lymph nodes and lymphoreticular Sheaths around the central artery = **white pulp**. The **red pulp** is not part of the lymphatic system	Characteristic blood vessels (laminar vessels, central artery, Penicillary arteriole, splenic sinus with gaps, muscle-free pulp and laminar veins); blood cells in the lumen of the splenic sinus	Single layered flat peritoneal epithelium forms a sheath around the capsule
Tonsils	Well-developed capsule, weak trabeculae (palatine tonsils), Not developed capsule, thin or no trabeculae (Pharyngeal and Lingual tonsil)	Lymphoreticular nodes (lymph follicles) surround 10–15 branched, Narrow epithelial invaginations (fossulae tonsillares with tonsillar crypts)	-	-

Contd...

Lymphatic Organs: Distinctive Morphological Features				
Organ	Capsule and connective tissue septa	Parenchyma	Vessels	Other features
Thymus	Well developed capsule, partitioning into lobes by connective tissue septa	Lymphoepithelial; no lymph follicles; denser cortex, more loosely organized medulla with interspersed lymphocytes; epithelial Hassall bodies in the medulla	-	Involution after puberty; adipose tissue Gradually replaces the parenchyma; in senescence: adipose tissue with Parenchyma islets
Peyer's patches	No capsule or connective tissue septa	The patches are regions of concentrated B lymphocyte follicles covered in a 'dome' of a specialized follicle associated epithelium (FAE) which consists of follicle associated enterocytes and M (microfold or multifold) cells. M-cells are a specialized epithelial cell that reside above Peyer's patches and take up antigen from the lumen of the intestine		Peyer's patches are lymphoid tissues found in the wall of the small intestine. They are part of the mucosal associated lymphoid tissues (MALT) and more specifically gut associated lymphoid tissue (GALT)

HISTOLOGY PLATE 9

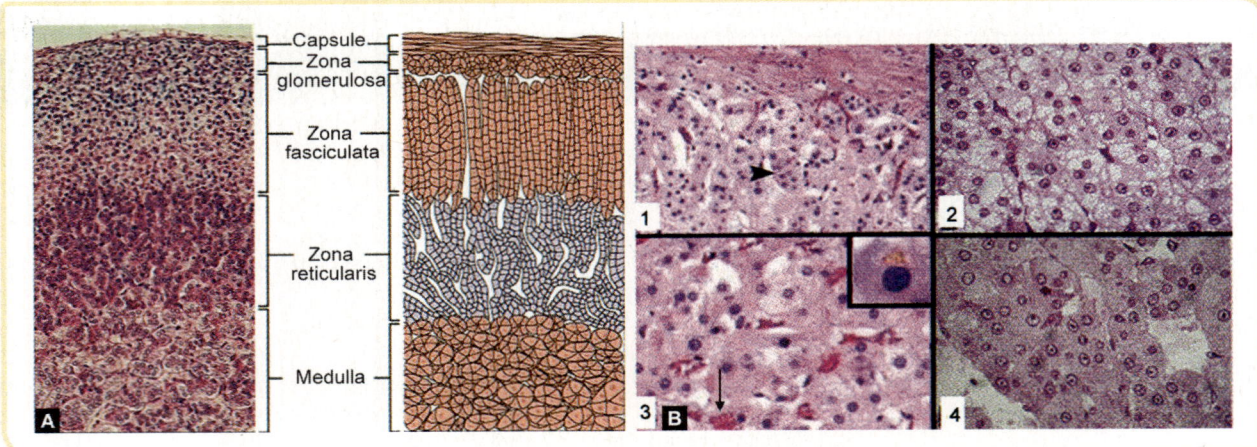

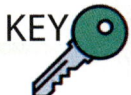

PLATE LEGENDS
A. **Histology of Adrenal gland (low power):** Labelled along with representative illustration.
B. **Histology of Adrenal zones (high power):**
1. **Zona glomerulosa:** Capsule is visible in right upper quadrant; cells are arranged in rounded clusters like glomeruli (arrow head). Minimal or no vaculation.
2. **Zona fasciculata:** Cells are arranged in long cords that runs perpendicular to capsule. Abundant lipid vacuoles (containing mainly glucocorticoids), round uniform nuclei
3. **Zona reticularis:** small cells with anastomosing network, some ageing cells contain the yellow-brown pigment lipofuscin (brown, see Insat), Blood capillaries run between cell plates (Arrow)
4. **Adrenal medulla**: The medulla consists of anastomosing cords and trabecuale of groups of cells (arrow) separated by venous sinusoids. Minimal or no vaculation. In addition to pheochromocytes, medulla contains single or groups of sympathetic ganglions (Visible in High HD)

Adrenal Gland

Part	Comments	Factors acting on gland	Hormone secreted
Cortex: Zona Glomerulosa	Outermost, Thinnest, 15% of adrenal, 20% of cortex, columnar or pyramidal cells are arranged in round to oval clusters that resemble renal glomeruli, and hence called "glomerulosa. Cells contains numerous mitochondria	Angiotensin and Corticotropin (ACTH)	Mineralocorticoids (Aldosterone)
Cortex: Zona Fasciculata	Middle and widest layer, 65% of adrenal, 80% of cortex, columnar or polyhedral cells in 1-2 cell thick long cords that run at right angles to the surface of the organ, Cytoplasm loaded with vacuoles and lipid droplets, hence cells are also called **spongyocytes**. Mitochondria are large and contain numerous vesicular cristae	Corticotropin (ACTH)	Glucocorticoids (Cortisol and Corticosterone), Some androgens
Cortex: Zona Reticularis	Innermost layer, 7% of adrenal, 10% of cortex, Irregularly shaped cells smaller than other layers forming irregular cords that form an anastomosing network, Blood capillaries run between cell plates, Mitochondria are large and have vesicular cristae, no vacuoles and fat droplets in cytoplasm. Some aged cells have **Lipofuscin pigment** granules **Pyknotic nuclei** suggesting cell death are often found in this layer	Corticotropin (ACTH)	Androgens (dehydroepiandrosterone-DHEA), Some glucocorticoids
Medulla	13% of adrenal, polygonal cells (pheochromocytes) nests are arranged in anastomosing cords separated by large venous sinusoids/ muscular veins. Due to their affinity to chromium salts, the cells are often called **chromaffin or pheochrome cells**.		Catecholamines (adrenaline or noradrenaline)

Footnote:
- Adrenals are made of two concentric layers: a yellow peripheral layer, the adrenal cortex; and a reddish-brown central layer, the adrenal medulla
- The *adrenal cortex and the adrenal medulla can be considered two organs with distinct origins, functions, and morphological characteristics* that became united during embryonic development. They arise from different germ layers. The cortex arises from the coelomic epithelium, whereas the cells of the medulla derive from the neural crest, from which sympathetic ganglion cells also originate.

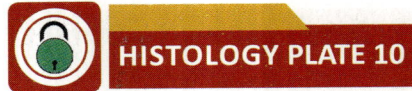

HISTOLOGY PLATE 10

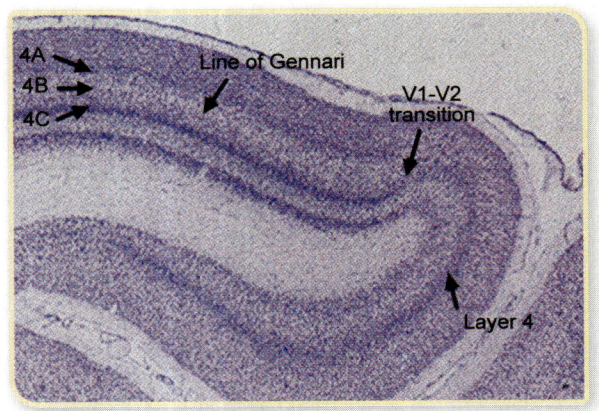

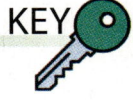

PRIMARY VISUAL CORTEX

Is also called visual area I or striate cortex because of the highly striated appearance. The primary visual (VI) cortex is mostly located on the medial aspect of the occipital lobe, and is coextensive with the **subcortical nerve fibre stria of Gennari** in layer IV, hence its alternative name, the **striate cortex**.

It occupies the upper and lower lips and depths of the posterior part of the calcarine sulcus and extends into the cuneus and lingual gyrus. Posteriorly it is limited by the lunate sulcus, and by polar sulci above and below this sulcus. It extends to the occipital pole.

The primary visual cortex receives afferent fibres from the lateral geniculate nucleus via the optic radiation. The latter curves posteriorly and spreads through the white matter of the occipital lobe. Its fibres terminate in strict point-to-point fashion in the striate area

The primary visual cortex is divided into six functionally distinct layers, labeled 1 through 6. Layer 4, which receives most visual input from the lateral geniculate nucleus (LGN), is further divided into 4 layers, labelled 4A, 4B, 4Cα, and 4Cβ. Sublamina 4Cα receives most magnocellular input from the LGN, while layer 4Cβ receives input from parvocellular pathways. The striate cortex is granular.

Layer IV, bearing the **stria of Gennari,** is commonly divided into three sublayers. Passing from superficial to deep, these are *IVA, IVB (which contains the stria), and IVC*. The densely cellular IVC is further subdivided into a superficial IVCα and a deep IVCβ. Layer IVB contains only sparse, mainly non-pyramidal, neurons. The input to area 17 from the lateral geniculate nucleus terminates predominantly in layers IVA and IVC.

HISTOLOGY PLATE 11

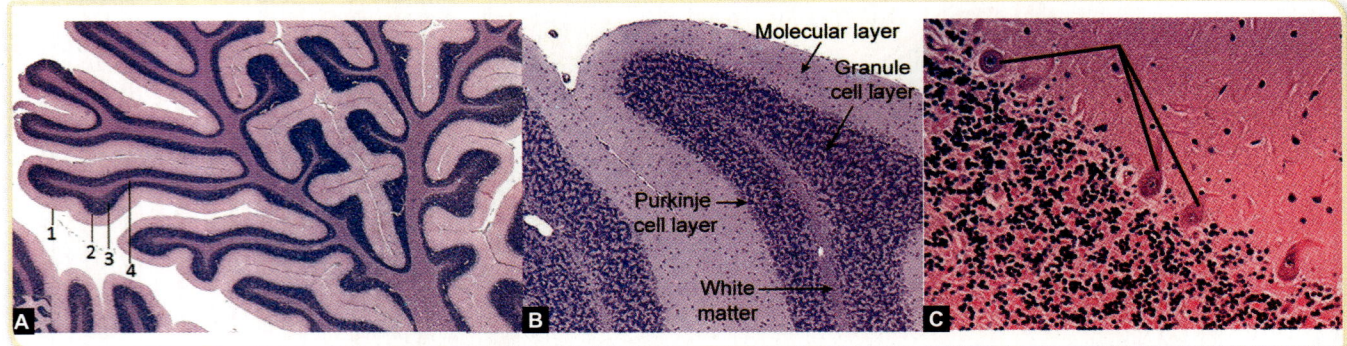

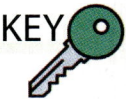

HISTOLOGY OF CEREBELLUM

A. Histology of cerebellum H & E staining 4X view
  1. Molecular layer
  2. Purkinje cell layer
  3. Granular cell layer
  4. White matter

B. Histology of cerebellum H & E staining 10 X view

C. Histology of cerebellum H & E staining 100 X view: Arrow marked structures are Purkinjee cells between dense Granular cell layer (left inferior) and Molecular cell layer (Right anterior)

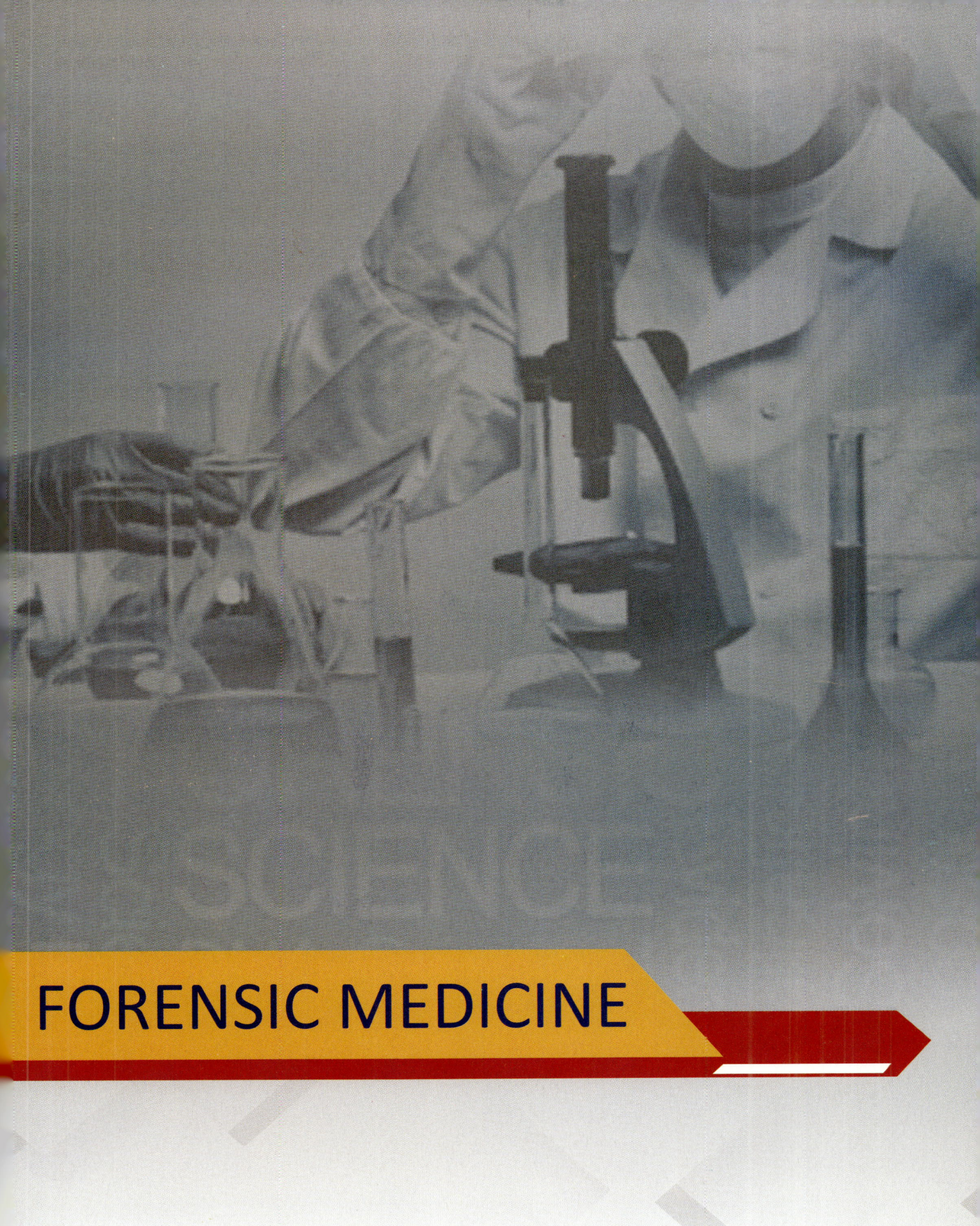

FORENSIC MEDICINE

FMT PLATE 1

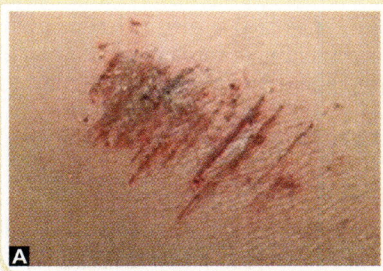
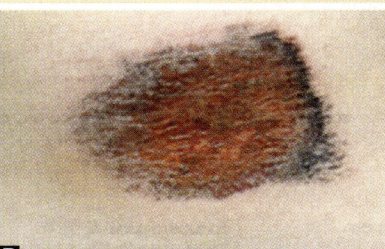
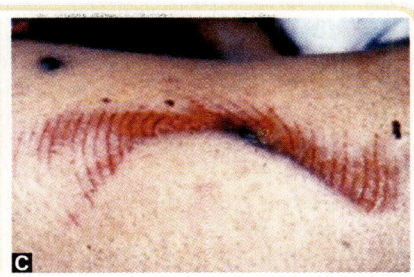

TYPES OF ABRASION
A. Scratch abrasion[AIIMS PG]
B. Graze abrasion
C. Imprint/ pattern abrasion

> **Note**
> Cleaning and dressing is the best way to manage abrasions[AIIMS PG]

	Types of Abrasions	
Scratch	Linear injury by sharp object like pin, thorn.	Direction of injury is indicated by sharp edge initially and heaping up epithelium at the end.
Graze	When broad surface of skin slides or scraps against a rough surface.	A.K.A **Brush burn, Friction burn** because it is caused by frictional force and resembles burn after drying
Imprint/ Pressure/ Contact abrasion	Direct impact or pressure or contact with object which stamps reproduction of its shape and surface marking.	A.K.A **Patterned abrasion,** e.g. – Ligature mark in hanging, Tyre mark in RTA.

FMT PLATE 2

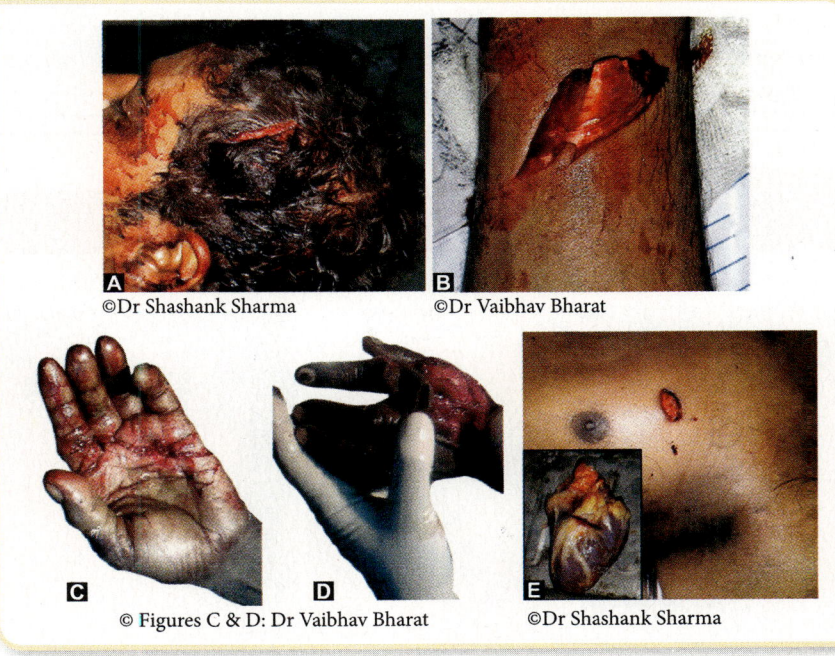

© Figures A: Dr Shashank Sharma
© Figure B: Dr Vaibhav Bharat
© Figures C & D: Dr Vaibhav Bharat
© Figure E: Dr Shashank Sharma

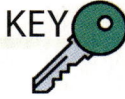

TYPES OF WOUND

A. **Typical Incised wound of the scalp:** With clean cut averted margins from a sharp object, linear shape and length more than depth
B. **Atypical Incised wound of the forearm,** a lacerated looking incised wound due to slightly irregular margins, which may be inverted (contrary to averted margins of typical incised wound). Cut tendon can be seen in the wound. Caused by hick sharp object like glass. In this case, the person slipped and accidently put his hand on the broken glass.
C. **Lacerated wound of Hand:** With irregular shape and margins (contrary to incised wound), Length greater than depth (contrary to chop wound).
D. **Flaying of the hand:** Type of laceration in which skin and subcutaneous tissues are separated from underlying tissues is called avulsion laceration. This type of laceration over a large area is known as **flaying** and is due to shearing force, which produces this type of laceration, e.g., tyre run over, long hairs caught in a rotating machine cause flaying over scalp. Flaying (Skinning) is also a method of torture or execution.
E. **Stab wound of the chest:** With regular margins and shape. Depth of the wound is greater than the length (contrary to both incised and lacerated wound). In the 'Insat' the post mortem finding of the heart of the same patient can be seen, the stab puncturing the heart.

Difference Between Incised, Lacerated and Stab Wounds

Trait	Incised wound	Lacerated wound	Stab wound
Manner of production	By sharp objects or weapons	By blunt objects or weapons	By pointed, sharp or pointed blunt weapon
Site	Anywhere	Usually over bony prominences	Anywhere, usually chest and abdomen
Margins	Smooth, even, clean-cut and averted	Irregular and often undermined, serrated, minute tears in margins	Clean- cut parallel edges, smooth → pointed sharp Lacerated → pointed blunt
Abrasions on edges	Absent	Usually present	negative Present with Handle bruise
Bruising	No adjacent bruising of soft tissues	Bruising of surrounding and underlying	Rare
Shape	Linear or spindle shaped; tail and head present	Varies: Usually irregular, shallow tail	Linear or irregular; fish tail may be present
Dimensions	Usually longer than deep; often after gaping	Usually longer than deep	Depth greater than length and breadth
Depth of wound	Structures deeply cut to the depth of the wound	Small strands of tissue at the bottom bridge across margins	Structures cleanly cut
Hemorrhage	Usually profuse and external Spurting of blood may be seen	Slight except scalp and external	Varies, usually internal
Hair bulbs	Cleanly cut	Crushed or torn	Usually clean cut
Bones	May be cut	May be fractured	May be punctured
Foreign bodies	Absent	Usually present	Usually absent
Clothes	May be cut	May be torn	May be cut

Note: A thick glass produces atypical incised wound which might look like a Lacerated wound

FMT PLATE 3

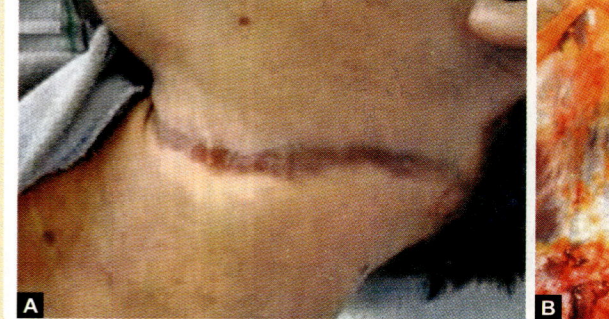
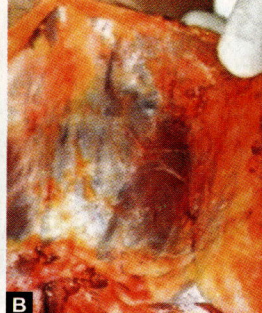
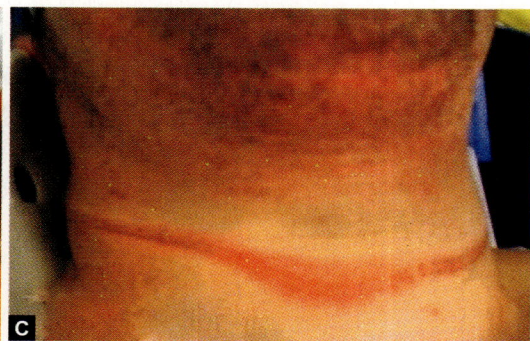

A B C

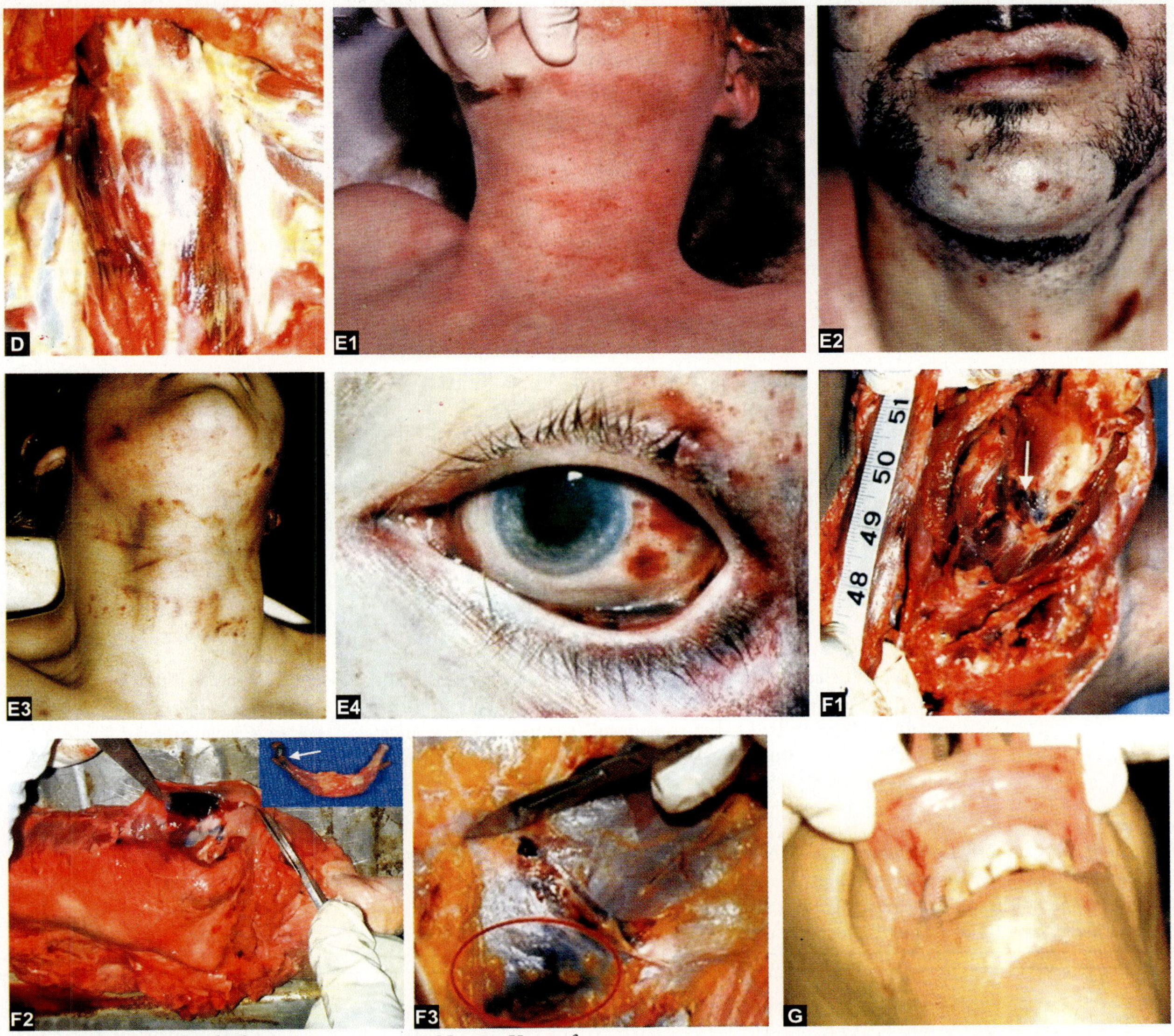

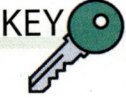
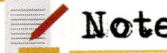
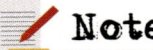

SIGNS OF ASPHYXIAL DEATH

A. **Hanging External:** Ligature mark is oblique, incomplete and high in neck.
B. **Hanging Internal:** Underlying tissue pale white glistening, no bruising, hemorrhage/ hematoma of underlying structures.
C. **Ligature strangulation external:** Ligature mark, which is transverse, circular, complete, in lower neck.
D. **Ligature strangulation internal:** Anterior neck "strap" muscle hemorrhage in a strangulation case.
E1. **Manual strangulation/Throttling external:** Injuries to the neck in homicidal manual strangulation deaths may be quite subtle. A mark semilunar mark of thumb or nail is often visible below the chin or high in the neck. Fingerprint abrasions are visible on the neck.
E2. **Manual strangulation/Throttling external:** This is a case of manual strangulation. One can notice semilunar fingernail abrasions on the chin and a contusion on the left and right angle of the lower lip together with multiple nail abrasions on the right side of the neck and a big abraded contusion over the left clavicle. Such lesions indicate attempted smothering while manually strangulating the victim.
E3. **Manual strangulation/Throttling external:** Multiple irregular unpatterned abrasions on the neck.
E4. **Manual Strangulation/Throttling external:** Conjunctival hemorrhages/petechiae in manual strangulation.

> **Note**
> **Tardieu spots** were first described by French police surgeon Ambroise Augustae Tardieu as minute hemorrhages on the surfaces of the lungs, heart, conjunctiva and other body parts. Its pathognomonic sign of asphyxial deaths.

F1. **Manual strangulation/Throttling internal:** Arrow pointing hematoma
F2. **Manual strangulation/Throttling internal:** Forceps pointing hematoma and Hyoid bone fracture in Insat
F3. **Manual strangulation/Throttling internal:** Hematoma visible without deep dissection
G. **Smothering external:** Bruising of inside of mouth.

> **Note**
> Note that the Bruising and/or laceration of oral mucosa in Smothering needs to be differentiated from the Petechial hemorrhage, which is seen in all cases of asphyxia death

Signs of Asphyxial Death

Condition	External finding/ligature mark	Autopsy/internal finding	Other significant findings
Hanging	Oblique, incomplete, high- between thyroid and hyoid cartilage or above hyoid **Note**: Running noose may cause horizontal ligature mark	Underlying tissue pale white glistening, no bruising, hemorrhage/hematoma of underlying structures	Swollen cyanosed face Dribbling of saliva, semen at meatus, suicide note, **Amussat sign** (tears in intima of carotids)
Ligature strangulation	Transverse/Horizontal, circular, complete, across the middle or lower part of neck, at or below the level of thyroid cartilage. May be oblique if person is strangled or dragged.	Bruising, hemorrhage of the subcutaneous tissue and muscles of neck, especially underneath the ligature and knot. There may be bruising or laceration of the sheath of carotid arteries. Fracture thyroid cartilage. (Picture will show distinctly visible red bleeding point)	Face is congested, swollen and cyanosed. **Tardieu's spots** more abundant, bitten tongue, blood stained froth
Manual strangulation, throttling	Abrasions and bruises on the front and sides of the neck.	Bruise: Oval or round and 1.5–2 cm in size. Bruises made by tips of thumbs are more prominent than with other fingers. Multiple abrasions are present due to struggle.	Extravasation of blood in subcutaneous tissues underneath the external marks of bruising and abrasions is the most significant internal sign. Inward compression **fracture of hyoid bone** is the most diagnostic finding of throttling
Smothering	Abrasions and bruises around the mouth, inner side of mouth, gums, tongue, lips, nostrils, chin, border of mandible. Fracture nasal none/cartilage	Injuries on the inside of the lips from pressure of teeth are seen. Bruising of gums or sometimes tears of delicate tissues are seen.	Most common mode is by plastic bag in suicidal and Pillow in homicidal. Minimal facial injury if pillow or soft material used.

Summary:
- Ligature mark + underlying hematoma with or without Thyroid fracture = **Ligature strangulation**
- Ligature mark without underlying hematoma with or without hyoid fracture = **Hanging**
- Nail marks/no marks, no ligature with underlying hematoma of neck muscles = **Throttling**
- Signs of asphyxia + facial injury/fracture nasal bone/cartilage along with injury inner side of lips = **Smothering**

FMT PLATE 4

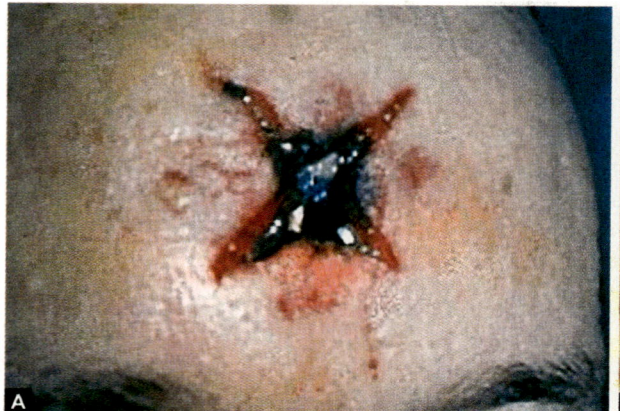
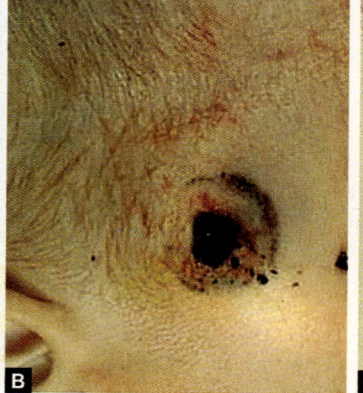
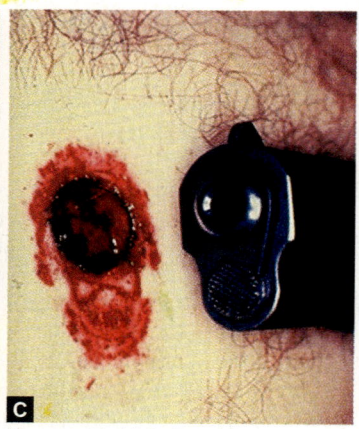

(*Source:* Todd C. Grey University of Utah)

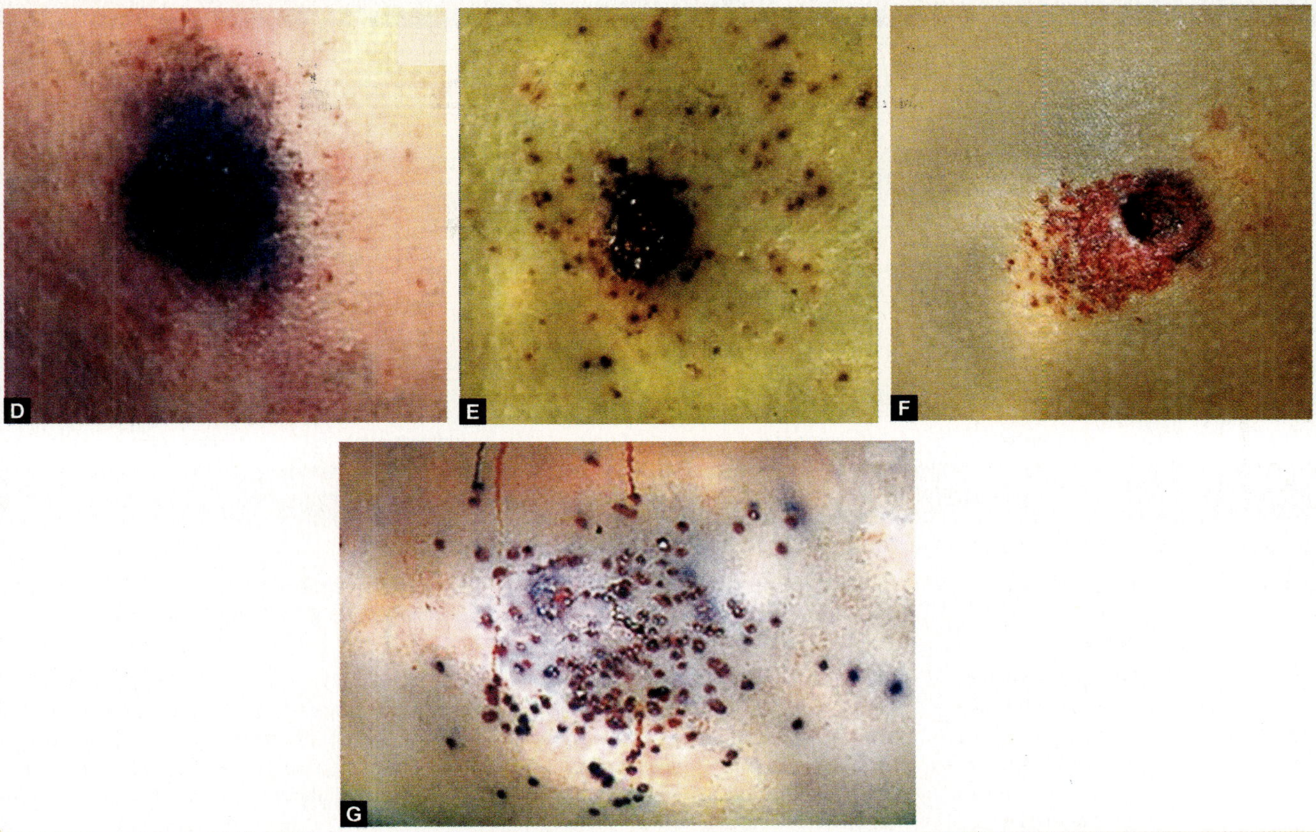

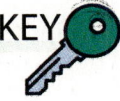

SHOTGUN FIREARM INJURIES

A. **Contact shotgun bullet entry wound:** Since the barrel contacts the skin, the gases released by the fired round go into the subcutaneous tissue and caused the star shaped laceration. Note the grey black soot and faint abrasion ring.
B. **Contact shotgun bullet entry wound:** An abrasion ring, formed when the force of the gases entering below the skin blow the skin surface back against the muzzle of the gun, is seen here in this contact range gunshot wound to the right temple.
C. **Contact shotgun bullet entry wound:** The abrasion ring, and a very clear muzzle imprint, are seen in this contact range gunshot wound.
D. **Close range shotgun bullet entry wound** with dark circular soot deposition and minor stippling after that, but no independent Tattooing.
E. **Intermediate range shotgun bullet wound** which is not angled, with powder tattooing but no soot/ blackening.
F. **Intermediate range shotgun bullet wound** which is angled, with powder tattooing but no soot/ blackening.
G. **Distant range shotgun bullet wound:** Widespread pattern of pellet wounds as all pellets show independent entry wound from 4 meters onwards. Both soot and tattooing is absent.

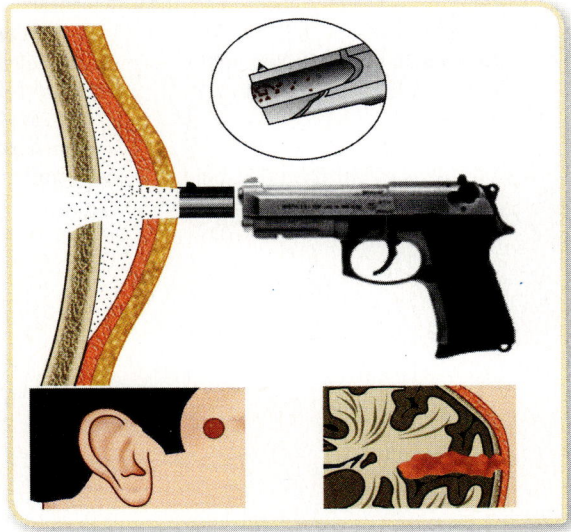

Fig: Contact range gun shot

Shotgun Firearm Injuries

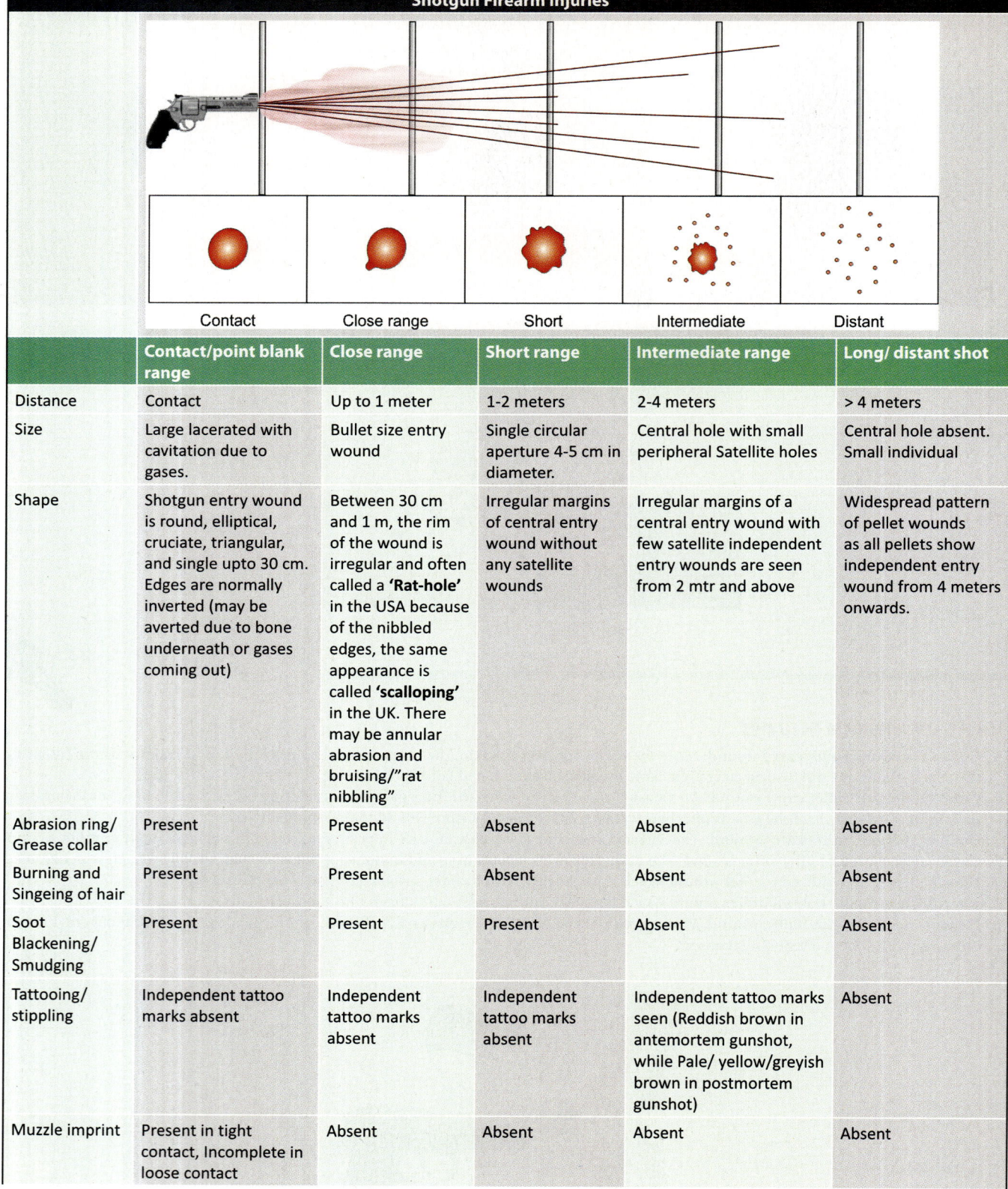

	Contact/point blank range	Close range	Short range	Intermediate range	Long/ distant shot
Distance	Contact	Up to 1 meter	1-2 meters	2-4 meters	> 4 meters
Size	Large lacerated with cavitation due to gases.	Bullet size entry wound	Single circular aperture 4-5 cm in diameter.	Central hole with small peripheral Satellite holes	Central hole absent. Small individual
Shape	Shotgun entry wound is round, elliptical, cruciate, triangular, and single upto 30 cm. Edges are normally inverted (may be averted due to bone underneath or gases coming out)	Between 30 cm and 1 m, the rim of the wound is irregular and often called a **'Rat-hole'** in the USA because of the nibbled edges, the same appearance is called **'scalloping'** in the UK. There may be annular abrasion and bruising/"rat nibbling"	Irregular margins of central entry wound without any satellite wounds	Irregular margins of a central entry wound with few satellite independent entry wounds are seen from 2 mtr and above	Widespread pattern of pellet wounds as all pellets show independent entry wound from 4 meters onwards.
Abrasion ring/ Grease collar	Present	Present	Absent	Absent	Absent
Burning and Singeing of hair	Present	Present	Absent	Absent	Absent
Soot Blackening/ Smudging	Present	Present	Present	Absent	Absent
Tattooing/ stippling	Independent tattoo marks absent	Independent tattoo marks absent	Independent tattoo marks absent	Independent tattoo marks seen (Reddish brown in antemortem gunshot, while Pale/ yellow/greyish brown in postmortem gunshot)	Absent
Muzzle imprint	Present in tight contact, Incomplete in loose contact	Absent	Absent	Absent	Absent

Contd...

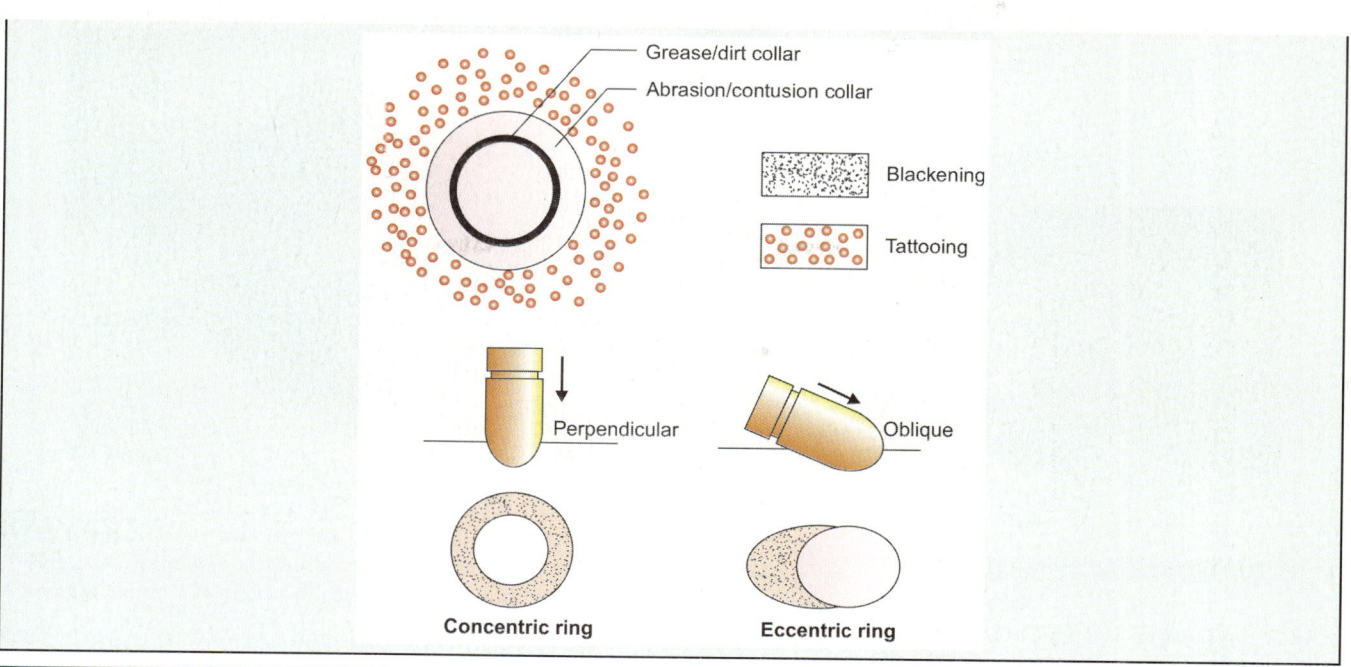

FMT PLATE 5

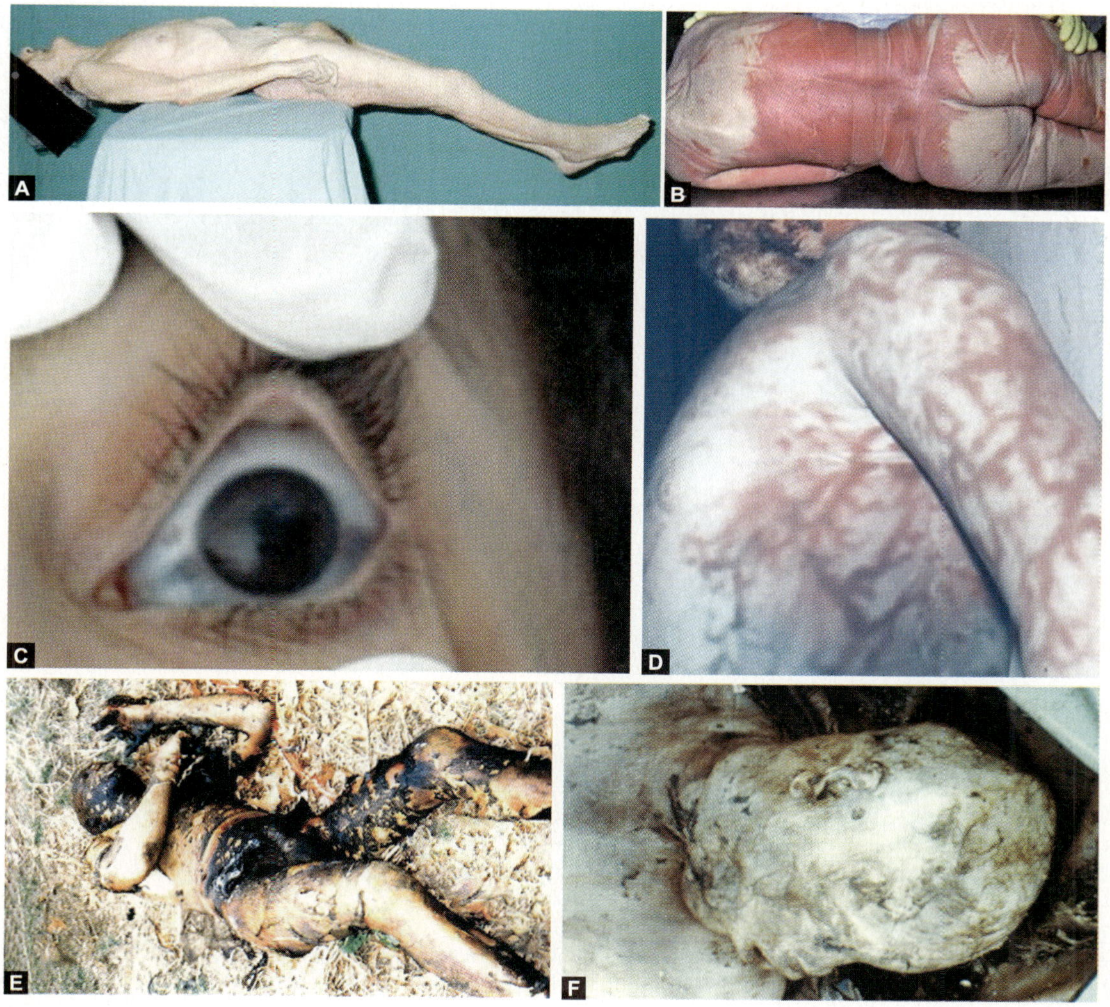

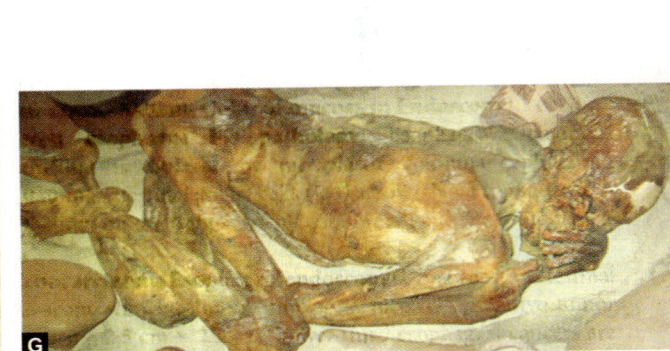
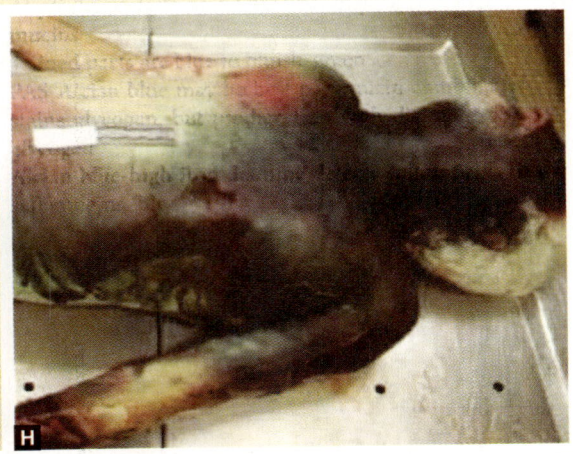

EARLY AND LATE SIGNS OF DEATH

A. Rigor Mortis[NEET PG]

Rigor Mortis

- After death muscles of the body pass through three stages
  - Primary relaxation or flaccidity (lasts for 1-2 hours)
  - Rigor mortis or cadaveric rigidity
  - Secondary relaxation or flaccidity
- **Nysten's law:** After French Pathologist Pierre Hubert Nysten who proposed the law in 1811. Is applicable to **voluntary muscles only.** It states that the muscles closest to the brain goes into Rigor mortis first and those which are farthest goes into Rigor mortis last. Hence it is also known as **Proximodistal progression of Rigor Mortis**. It appears in the order of (**Mnemonic**- in the multiples of 3)
  - Eyelids (orbicularis oculi) [2 hrs]
  - *Jaw first and then facial muscles* [3 hrs] (since temporalis and masseter are placed high on face but effect is seen on jaw so jaw shows RM first and then facial muscles)
  - Neck, thorax [4-5 hrs]
  - Upper limb (from shoulder to the hand) [6 hrs]
  - Abdomen, lower limb (from the hip to the foot) [9 hrs]
  - Small muscles of fingers and toes [12 hrs]

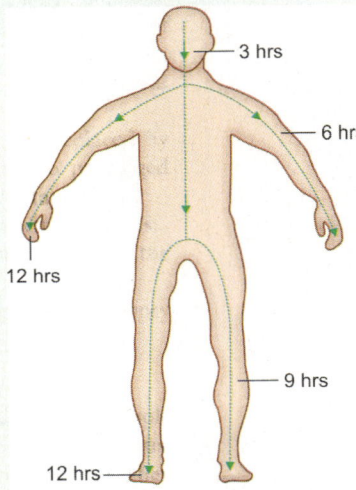

Nysten's rule: Proximo-distal progression of Rigor Mortis

- Rigor mortis does not develop in a fetus of < 7 months of intrauterine age. It is moderate in children, emaciated and mild in elderly people
- Conditions simulating rigor mortis:
  - **Heat stiffening:** When a body is exposed to temperatures above 65°C a rigidity is produced, which is much more marked than that found in rigor mortis. The stiffening remains until the muscles and ligaments soften from decomposition and the normal rigor mortis does not occur.

Contd...

Rigor Mortis

- Boxing attitude/Pugilistic attitude/Fencing posture is due to **heat stiffening**.
- The legs are fixed at hip and knees, arms are flexed at elbows, and fingers are hooked like claws.
- This attitude is present when a living or dead body is burnt and therefore **has no clinical significance. (Can be seen in both ante mortem or post mortem burns)**
- The condition is due to coagulation of proteins other than those affected by rigor mortis.
- It is **permanent** and does not pass off (unlike rigor mortis).
- **Cold stiffening:** When a body is exposed to freezing temperatures, the tissues become frozen and stiff due to freezing of the body fluids and solidification of subcutaneous fat simulating rigor. If the body is placed in warm atmosphere; the stiffness disappears and after a time, the normal rigor mortis occurs.
- **Cadaveric spasm** or instantaneous rigor Cadaveric spasm is a rare condition. The muscles that were contracted during life become stiff and rigid immediately after death without passing into the stage of primary relaxation. As such the change preserves the exact attitude of the person at the time of death for several hours. It originates by normal nervous stimulation of the muscles. This is usually limited to a single group of muscles and frequently involves the hands. Very great force is required to overcome stiffness. It passes without interruption into normal rigor mortis and disappears when rigor disappears.

B. **Postmortem Lividity/Livor Mortis/Suggillation**[AIIMS PG]: Livor mortis has been variously named as postmortem hypostasis, post-mortem lividity, post-mortem staining, suggillations, vibices, and so on

C. **Tache noir:** Triangular (base at limbus) discoloration of sclera seen after 3-4 hrs of death that develops when the eyes remain open after death. Exposure to the environment leads to clouding of the cornea and dryness of the sclera between the eyelids. It appears as a yellowish band of discoloration running horizontally across the eye, which become brownish black with time. It may be mistaken for a traumatic eye injury.

D. **Marbling of Skin**[NEETPG, AIIMSPG]: The blood vessels provide an important route through which the bacteria can spread with ease throughout the body. Their passage is marked by the decomposition of hemoglobin to sulphmethemoglobin in the blood vessels, which causes a greenish or reddish-brown staining of the inner walls of the superficial vessels. This is seen as linear branching patterns, which gives a 'marbled' ('road map') appearance of the skin.
   Areas where visible: It appears first in the shoulder, roots of the limbs, thighs, sides of abdomen, chest and neck.
   Onset: In summers, 'marbling' is seen in 36–48 h after death.

E. **Pugilistic attitude / Boxers / Defense/ Fencing attitude**[NEETPG]: Given photograph shows a charred/burnt body with degloving (peeling off) of skin at hands and various parts, i.e., this is a case of thermal death by dry heat/flame burn. Most common post mortem muscle change in such cases is Pugilistic attitude/Boxers/Defense/Fencing attitude. It is due to heat stiffening which causes coagulation of muscle proteins and dehydration. Legs are flexed at hips and knees, arms are flexed at elbows and held out in front of the body and fingers are hooked as claws. Flexor muscles being bulkier contract more and causes an attitude of generalized flexion. Can occur in both antemortem and postmortem burns. Dead bodies while being cremated attain a posture of "sit up and beg" due to this phenomenon. Rigor mortis spreads uniformly and sequentially in non-thermal deaths. Cadaveric spasm takes place in a single group of muscles. Post mortem caloricity cannot be shown in the picture.

F. **Adipocere**[AIIMSPG]: Conversion of fatty tissues into fatty acids. Rancid smell. Gains moisture and undergo hydrolysis. Ideal conditions are warm temperature, moisture (hot and humid) less air, bacteria, and fat splitting enzymes. Time required = 1 week (5-15 days)

G. **Mummification:** Dehydration or desiccation. Odorless. Ideal conditions are High temperature, dry condition, and free circulation of air 3–12 months.

Adipocere vs Mummification		
Feature	Adipocere	Mummification
Definition	Conversion of fatty tissues into fatty acids	Dehydration or desiccation
Smell	Rancid smell	Odorless

Contd...

Adipocere vs Mummification		
Feature	Adipocere	Mummification
Moisture	Gains moisture and undergo hydrolysis	Loses moisture
Ideal conditions	Warm temperature, moisture, (hot and humid) less air, bacteria, and fat splitting enzymes	High temperature, dry condition, and free circulation of air
Time required	1 week (5-15 days)	3-12 months

Note:
- Adipocere: Liver is well preserved
- Adipocere and mummification: Facial features (identification) and injuries well preserved
- Adipocere mummification and rigor mortis: Not seen in fetus less than 7 months

H. **Putrefaction:**
- Rate of putrefaction in different medium is determined by **(Casper's Dictum)** AIR > WATER > EARTH (8:2:1)
- First internal sign of putrefaction is "Greenish discoloration of under surface of liver"
- First external sign of putrefaction is "Greenish discoloration of flank over caecum" because it is here that the contents of the bowel are more fluid and full of bacteria. The discoloration varies from green to black and is due to formation of **sulphamethhemoglobin**
- Larynx and trachea are first organs to putrefy
- Bone is the last tissue to putrefy
- Prostate and non-gravid uterus are relatively resistant to putrefaction (last to putrefy if bone is not available in options)

Putrefaction is delayed in poisoning of:
1. Arsenic
2. Antimony
3. Cerebra thevatia (Yellow oleander)
4. Carbolic acid
5. Strychnine (Nux vomica)
6. Zinc oxide
7. Nicotine/tobacco
8. Hyocyamus niger/Scopolamine/Henbane

Signs of Death		
Immediate signs of death	Early signs of death	Late signs of death
▫ Loss of sensation of pain, temperature, touches, etc. ▫ Loss of muscle power ▫ Cessation of respiration and circulation ▫ Loss of EEG and ECG	▫ Algor mortis (cooling) ▫ Rigor mortis ▫ Eye and Skin changes ▫ Postmortem lividity	▫ Putrefaction ▫ Adipocere formation ▫ Mummification

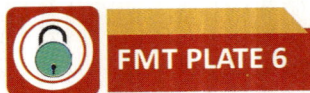

FMT PLATE 6

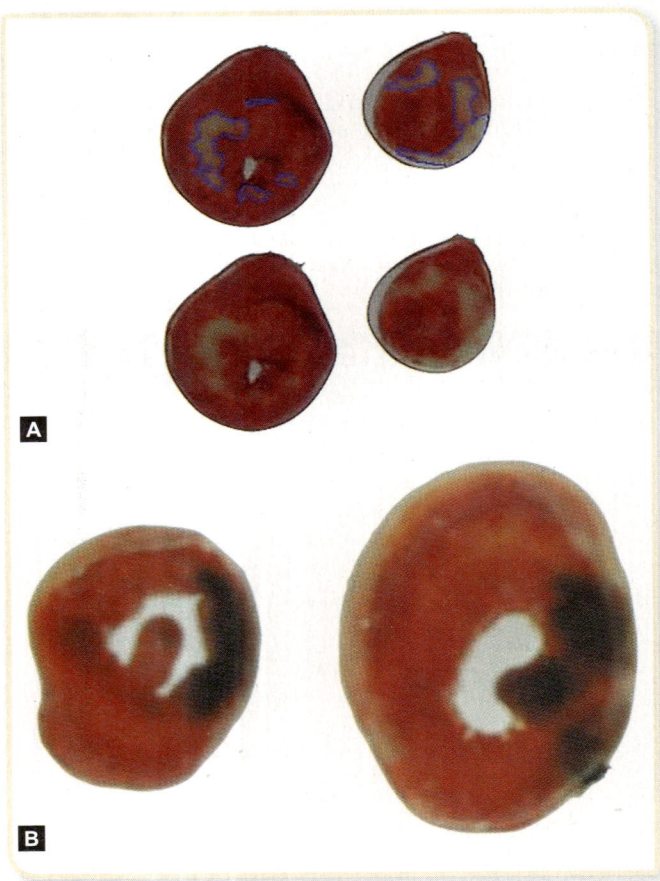

Autopsy Staining of Myocardium		
	NBT (Nitro Blue Tetrazolium chloride)	**TTC (Triphenyl Tetrazolium Chloride)**
Cost of chemical	100 dollars/gm	4 dollars/ gm
Characteristic	Cannot cross cell membrane	can cross cell membrane
Clinical use	Not cross membranes and therefore can only be used with sliced tissue. The slicing disrupts enough cells that the nitroblue will react with the exposed cytosol	Can cross cell membrane, hence it can be used to both stain slices as well as perfusate. TTC is quite toxic and will cause the heart to stop beating instantly. Therefore the heart must be in a Langendorff apparatus where coronary perfusion will persist even if the heart stops beating. It cannot be used in the in situ heart
Normal myocardium	Blue	Brick red
Necrosed/ Infarcted myocardium	Pale yellow (unstained)	Pale yellow (unstained)
Perfused Infarct	Dark brown on adding formalin	Dark Brown on adding formalin

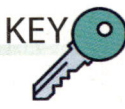

AUTOPSY STAINING OF MYOCARDIUM

A. **Staining of Sliced myocardium by TTC (Triphenyl Tetrazolium Chloride) stain on autopsy.**[AIIMSPG] The infarct is unstained/pale below and is being measured by perimetric software above (blue perimetry). Normal myocardium is red stained.

B. **Blood perfused myocardium slice** soaked with 10% formalin after tetrazolium staining which turns the blood a dark brown color.

There are two forms of tetrazolium:
1. Nitro blue tetrazolium (NBT)
2. Triphenyl tetrazolium chloride (TTC)

Myocardial infarction can be demonstrated by **Triphenyltetrazolium chloride** or by **Nitrobluetetrazolium dye test** in an unfixed and fresh heart by immersing the slices of heart from suspected area or different areas of heart in these chemical dyes. The color of infracted area remains pale yellow (unstained) and the normal heart with intact dehydronases stains red with TTC and Blue with NBT dye.

Immersion of tissue slices in a solution of **triphenyl tetrazolium chloride (TTC)** gives red color (Brick red in Robbins) to the healthy area (where Lactate dehydrogenase activity is preserved), but infarcted area appears pale if seen in about 4 hours the results are, however, inconsistent.

In blood-perfused hearts the infarct is often hemorrhagic. The extravasated blood is often in dark red color and difficult to differentiate from tetrazolium stain. For that reason, heart slices are soaked in 10% formalin after tetrazolium staining, which turns the blood a dark brown color.

FMT PLATE 7

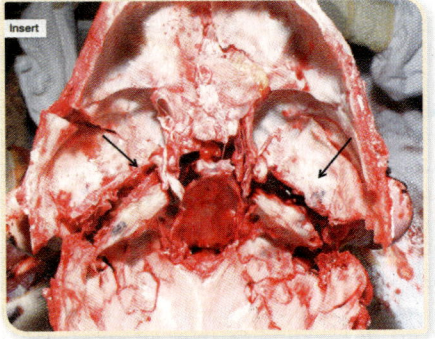

TRANSVERSE HINGE FRACTURE AKA- MOTORCYCLIST'S FRACTURE[AIIMSPG]

It is name given to a fracture of base of skull in which the skull base is broken down into two separate anterior and posterior halves and they move independently of each other. It is a type of hinge fracture. The fracture line runs on the base of middle cranial fossa following the petrous temporal bone.

Important fractures in forensic	
Ring fracture	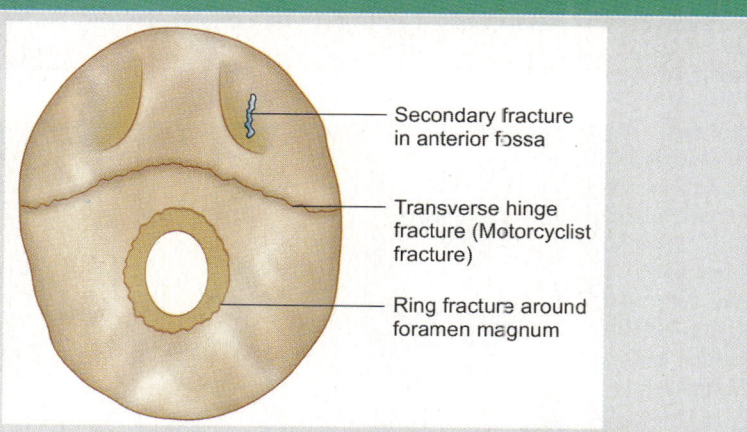 This is a type of fissure fracture that encircles the base of skull around the **foramen magnum,** running from the sella turcica, partly through petrous ridges and then going posteriorly and medially, joining in the posterior fossa. In the front, the fracture may pass through the middle ear and roof of the nose. As a result, the skull gets separated from the spine. In **feet-first impact,** forces transferred upward can result in significant pelvic trauma, as well as a 'ring fracture' of the skull, as forces drive the spinal column upward into the cranial cavity
Motorcyclist's fracture	It is name given to a fracture of base of skull in which the skull base is broken down into two separate anterior and posterior halves and they move independently of each other. It is a type of **hinge fracture**. The fracture line runs on the base of middle cranial fossa following the petrous temporal bone.
Depressed fracture/ Fracture *a la signature*	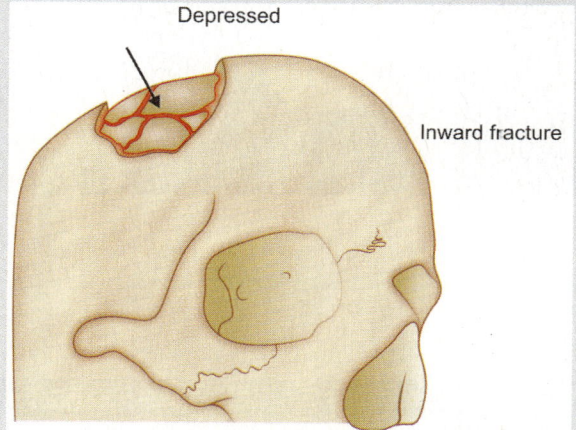 When a portion of fractured bone is driven inwards it is known as depressed fracture. It is also called *'fracture a la signature'* (**signature fracture**), as the shape often points towards the shape of the offending weapon. They are caused by blows with a heavy weapon having small striking surface, such as hammer, axe, brick or chopper.
Pond/Indented/ Ping pong ball fracture	This is a smooth concave depression without a fracture line resulting from in buckling of skull, occurring only in the elastic skull of **infants and children** (prior to 4 years of age). A dent is produced instead of cracking. May occur due to obstetric forceps
Comminuted/ spider-web/ mosaic fracture	Two or more intersecting lines of fracture divide the bone into three or more fragments. It is caused by blows with weapons having large striking surface, such as heavy iron bar, or from a bullet.
Blow out fracture	This is due to blunt trauma to the eye wherein the forces are transmitted via the globe to the bony orbit, causing disruption of the orbital walls. ***Teardrop sign***: The fracture is most commonly involves the thin medial wall and/or orbital floor that results in Radiographically, a soft tissue 'teardrop' or polypoid mass in the roof of the maxillary antrum.
Gutter fracture	Part of the thickness of the bone is removed to form a gutter, e.g. oblique bullet wounds. It is usually accompanied by comminuted depressed fracture of the inner table of skull
Countercoup injury	Occurs on the opposite side of impact
Fissured fracture	Caused by heavy weapon striking broad surface
Diastatic fracture	Separation of skull sutures
Undertaker's fracture	Rough handling of dead bodies by undertaker leads to fracture dislocation of C6-C7. This fracture dislocation is called **undertaker's fracture** and may resemble antemortem injury.

FMT PLATE 8

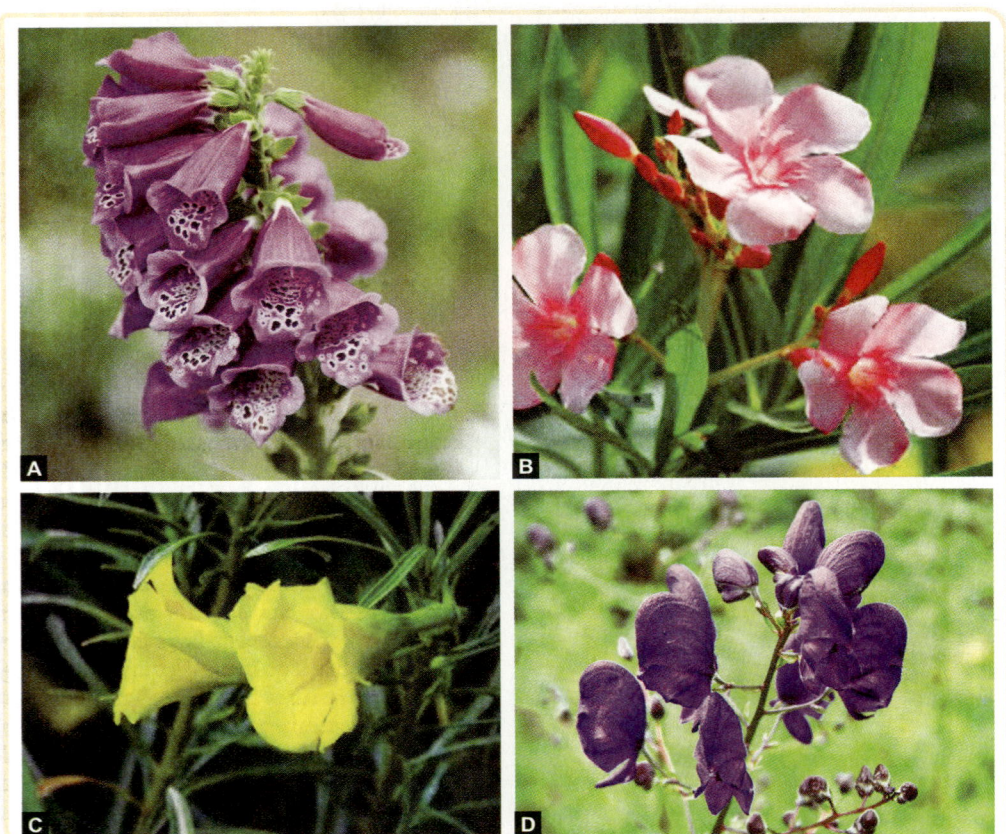

CARDIAC POISONS

	Cardiac poisons			
A. Digitalis purpurea/ Foxglove/Digitoxin/ Digitalin	Nausea, vomiting, abdominal pain, diarrhea, depression, headache, dizziness, Bradycardia, Heart block, Extrasystoles, coma, death	15-30 mg of digitalin 4 mg of digitoxin Half an hour to 24 hrs	Gastric lavage with tannic acid. K⁺ to ↓extrasystoles, Atropine for bradycardia, Propranolol/ Novocaine for arrhythmias, EDTA to ↓Ca, **Digibind**	▫ Mainly accidental, sometimes homicidal ▫ No suspicion of poisoning may arise in homicidal cases
B. Nerium odorum (True/white/pink oleander) C. Cerebra thevatia (Yellow oleander)	Vomiting, pain in abdomen, frothy salivation, **lock jaw**, muscular twitching followed by tetanic spasms, drowsiness, exhaustion, coma, death from cardiac failure	15 g of root can kill an adult in 24 hrs	Stomach wash, administration of anesthetic, morphine	▫ Active principle; **Nerium odorum-Nerin** (Neriodorin, Neriodorein, Karabin), **Cerbera thevetia-Thevetin, Thevotoxin, Cerberin** ▫ **Petechial hemorrhage of heart (characteristic)** ▫ Nerium can be detected even from a burnt body, Cerebra resists putrefaction ▫ Suicide, **Love philtre**, Cattle poison, Abortifacient

Contd...

	Cardiac poisons			
D. Aconite/Mitha bish/ Mitha zahar, Monk's hood, wolf's bane, women's bane, devil's helmet or blue rocket	Tingling and numbness in the oral cavity, salivation, nausea, vomiting, diarrhea, giddiness, impaired speech and vision, convulsions, low pulse, pupils alternately dilate and contract, become dilated later. Death from cardiac arrest or resp. paralysis	1 gm root, 250 mg extract, 25 drops tincture, 4 mg alkaloid. Average fatal period 6 hrs	No antidote. Supportive management. Gastric lavage with tannic acid/ $KMnO_4$, Atropine/ Novocaine Artificial resp. with O_2	▫ All parts are poisonous. Root is most poisonous. **Sweet taste (Mitha zahar)** ▫ Destroyed in the body hence difficult to detect after death ▫ Accidental/Homicidal poisoning ▫ Arrow poison, Cattle poison, Abortifacient

FMT PLATE 9

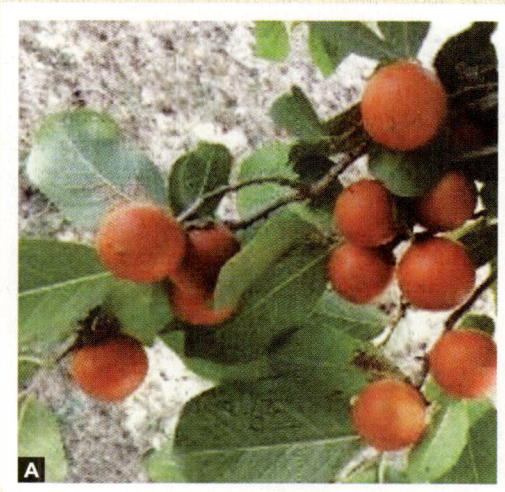
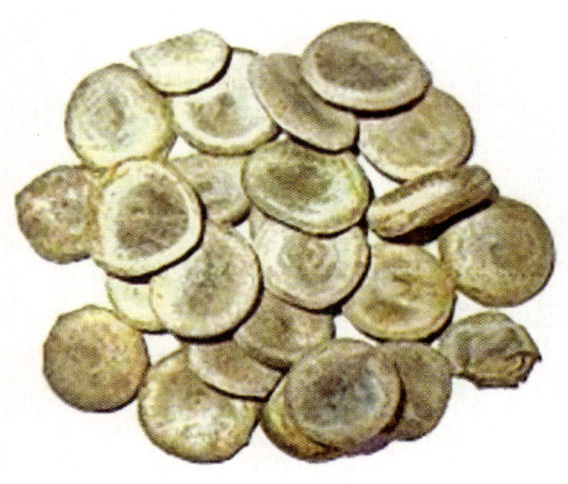

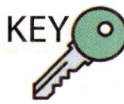
KEY

SPINAL POISONS (STRYCHINE/NUX VOMICA/KUCHILA)

	Spinal Poisons			
Strychnine/Nux vomica/ Kuchila A. Fruit B. Seed	Stiffness followed by 1st clonic and then tonic seizures. **Ophisthotonous** (arched forwards), or **pleurosthotonous** (arched sideways). **Risus sardonicus** (fixed grin). Death due respiratory paralysis and asphyxia	15–30 mg (1 seed) is fatal Usual fatal period is 1-2 hrs	Pt kept in a dark quiet room. Gastric lavage with $KMnO_4$. Barbiturate IV, Mephenesin (muscle relaxant) slow IV, Artificial respiration	▫ Active principle: **Brucine, Strychnine, Loganin.** ▫ Stimulates all parts of CNS especially anterior horn cells of the spinal cord causing ↑ reflex excitability ▫ Can be detected from exhumed putrefied bodies ▫ Cattle poison, arrow poison, Aphrodisiac

FMT PLATE 10

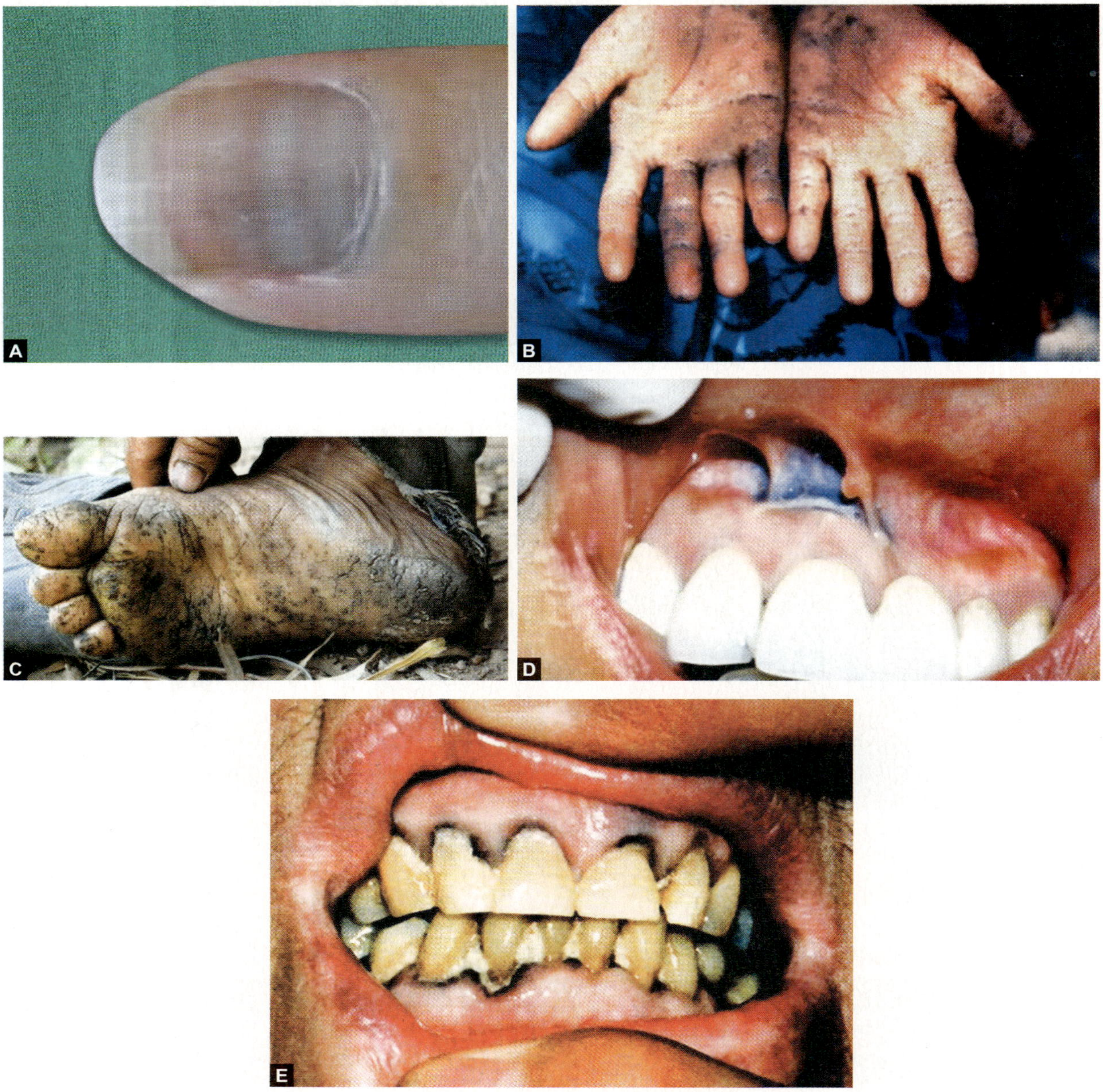

INORGANIC IRRITANT METAL POISONING SYMPTOMS

A. **Mee's lines** (white bands) in arsenic poisoning
B. **Raindrop pigmentation**[AIIMSPG] (Arsenic keratosis, so called "raindrops on a dusty road") in arsenic poisoning. Keratoses usually appears as small corn-like elevations, 0.4 to 1 centimeter (cm) in diameter. Arsenical hyperkeratosis occurs most frequently on the palms and soles. In severe cases, the pigmentation extends broadly over the chest, back, and abdomen. Pigment changes have been observed in population chronically consuming drinking water containing 400 ppb or more arsenic.
C. **Blackfoot disease** in Arsenic poisoning
D. **Bluish Black gum line** in Mercury poisoning, also called ad Amalgam Tattoo
E. **Bluish black gum line** in Lead poisoning along the margin of the gums

	Inorganic Irritants- Metals			
Arsenic	Burning pain, severe vomiting, tenesmus, bloody diarrhea with mucus shreds, cramps. **Red velvet gastric mucosa. Rain drop pigmentation. Mee's lines. Blackfoot Disease**	120-200mg 24hrs	Demulcents and Lavage, **Chelation-BAL (Antidote),** Freshly precipitated ferric hydroxide is no longer recommended.	Rigor mortis lasts longer. **Mimics cholera**. Arsenic neuritis resembles chronic alcoholism
Mercury	Grey-white discoloration of mucosa, bloody stools. **Chronic:** blue-black gum line (AKA **Amalgam tattoo**), penetrating ulcers, uremia, erethism, mercuria lentis, hatter's shakes	Corrosive sublimate 1-2 gms	Lavage, Egg white, Activated charcoal. **Chelation- EDTA> Penicillamine**, Alkaline fluids, Dialysis	▫ Selective action on large intestine, caecum ▫ **Metallic mercury not poisonous**
Lead (Plumbism/ Saturnism)	Intense thirst, paroxysmal colicky, constipation, cramps, convulsions. **Chronic:** facial pallor (1st, MC symptom), punctuate basophilia, **lead line** (stippled bluish black gum lines), wrist and foot drop, cardiorenal encephalopathy.	Fatal dose: Absorbed lead 0.5 gm, Acetate 20 gm, Carbonate 4 gm, Tetraethyl lead- few drops. Fatal period: Uncertain period	Lavage-1% Mg or Na sulfate. Morphine/ Atropine for colicy, Ca and vit D. **Chelator - (EDTA +BAL) > EDTA. DMSA for children**	Lead acetate is also known as **salt of saturn.** The term "**saturnine personality**" was introduced in 15th century to describe people born under the planet Saturn. These people were said to be gloomy (sad) with frequent headache, fatigue, irritability and depression. For the same reason lead poisoning is known as Saturnism. **Transverse opaque bands at ends of long bones in X-ray.**

FORENSIC MEDICINE COLOR PLATES

FMT PLATE 11

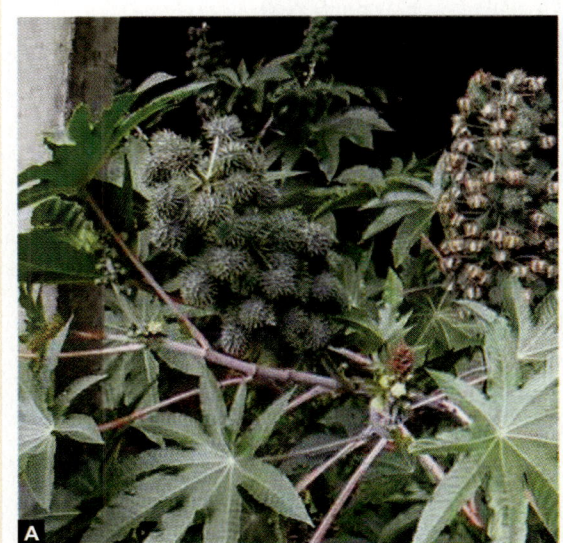

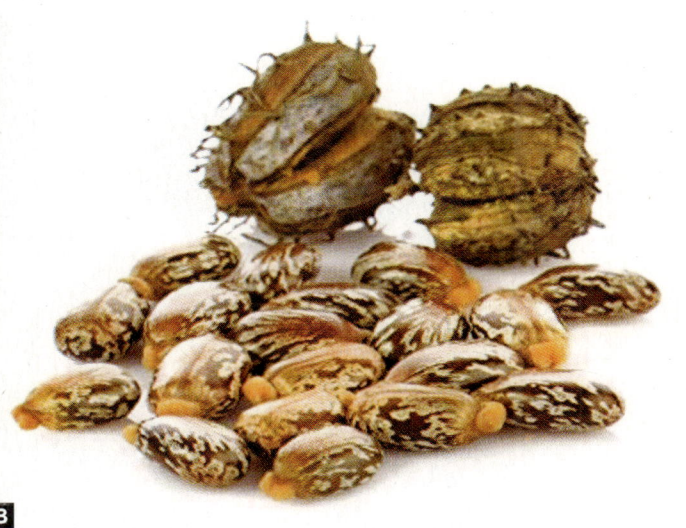

181

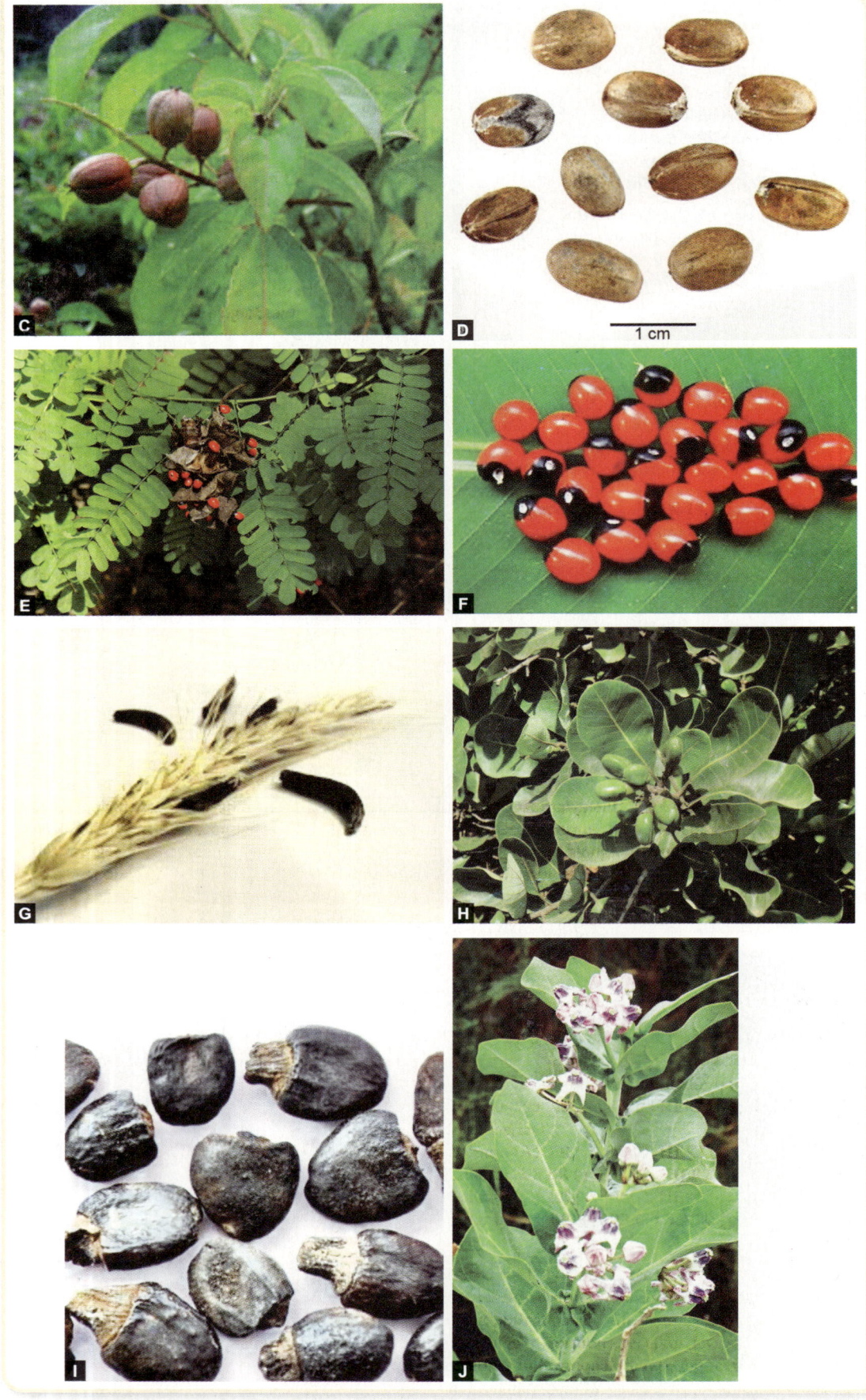

ORGANIC IRRITANTS – VEGETABLE ORIGIN

A. *Ricinus communis* (castor) plant
B. *Ricinus communis* (castor) seeds
C. *Croton tiglium* plant
D. *Croton tiglium* seed
E. *Abrus precatorius* plant
F. *Abrus precatorius* seed
G. Ergot (*Claviceps purpurea*) on rye: Poisoning due to consumption of ergot infected rye by humans as well as other mammals is referred to as ergotism. Although other grasses may also become infected with *C. purpurea*, it most commonly occurs on rye.
H. *Semicarpus anacardium* (Marking nut) plant
I. *Semicarpus anacardium* (Marking nut) seeds
J. Calotropis plant

KEY

FORENSIC MEDICINE COLOR PLATES

	Organic Irritants- Vegetable Origin			
Ricinus communis (Castor/ Arandi)	GI symptoms, cramps, collapse, coma, convulsions	6 gm ricin = 10 seeds, Several days	No specific antidote, General treatment	▫ Active principle: **Ricin (Toxalbumin)** ▫ Used in **George Markov's political assassination.**
Croton tiglium (Jamalgota, Nepala)	GI symptoms, cramps, collapse, coma, convulsions	4 seeds = 20 drops of oil, 4-6 hrs	Same as above	▫ Active principle: **Crotin (Toxalbumin)** ▫ **Seed resemble castor** ▫ Arrow poison
Abrus precatorius (Guncha, Rati, Indian Liquorice)	**Mimics: Viper bite**, If Injected-swelling, ecchymosis, necrosis, vertigo, arrhythmias, convulsions, If ingested- GI symptoms	1-2 seeds, 90-120 mg abrin inj, 3-5 days	Removal of sui. **Antiabrin**, General measures	▫ Active principle: **Abrin (Toxalbumin)** ▫ Made into **sui (needle).** ▫ Sui mark may be mistaken for snake bite
Ergot (*Claviceps pupurea*) (Ergotism AKA: St.Anthony's Fire, St.Vitus's Dance)	Acute: GI symptoms, colicky pain, tingling, cramps, hypoglycemia and anuria. Chronic Ergotism has two forms: gangrenous (St. Anthony's Fire) or convulsive (St. Vitus' Dance).	Uncertain dose and period	Lavage-tannic acid. Amyl nitrate inhalation. Vasodilators	▫ Active principle: **Ergotoxin, Ergotamine, Ergometrine** ▫ **Gangrenous ergotism resembles Raynaud's**
Semicarpus anacardium (Marking nut)	Painful Skin-blisters with acrid serum, **Artificial bruise**. If ingested-GI symptoms, dyspnea, cyanosis, tachycardia, coma	5-10 gm 12-24 hrs	Wash skin, apply bland liniment. Lavage-warm water.	▫ Active principle: **Bhilawanol, Semecarpol** ▫ **Abortifacient, Malingerer's conjunctivitis, Juice can be used for Vitriolage**
Calotropis (Madar, Akdo)	Skin-vesication, fulminant conjunctivitis, impaired vision. If ingestion- GI symptoms, Mydriasis, convulsions	Uncertain dose, 12 hrs	On general principles	Active principle: **Gigantin (most toxic), Uscharin, Calotoxin, Calotropin, Calacin** Juice is used by Tanners for hair removal from hides and decolorise them. **Juice can be used for Vitriolage**

183

FMT PLATE 12

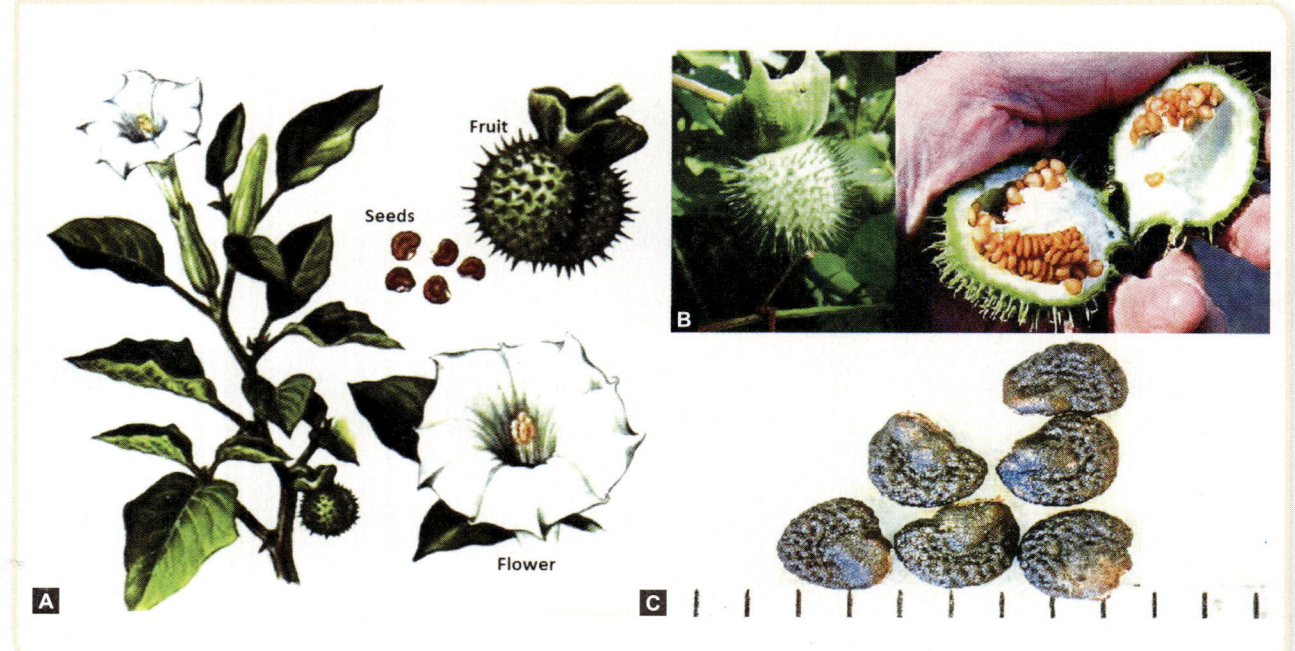

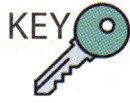

DELIRIANT POISONS

A. **Dhatura Plant:** All parts are toxic specially seeds.
B. **Dhatura Fruit:** Spherical with soft spines, contains 50-100 yellowish brown reniform (Kidney shaped) seeds.
C. **Dhatura seed:** Yellowish brown, kidney shaped, contains highest concentration of alkaloid, resembles chilly seeds

Deliriant Poisons				
Dhatura/Thorn apple/Devil's weed	**Anticholinergic Symptoms: Mnemonic = 9D** Dry skin, Dilatation of cutaneous vessels, Dilatation of pupils, Dry mouth, Delirium, Dysphagia, Drunken gait, Drowsiness, Difficulty in talking	100–125 seeds 60 mg alkaloid for adults, 4 mg for children 24 hrs	Gastric lavage with $KMnO_4$ or 5% tannic acid, Neostigmine 1-4 mg 1-2 hrly or Physostigmine 2.5 mg 3 hrly. Diazepam 10 mg i.v to allay excitement.	☐ Stupefying agent (robbery, kidnapping, rape) Hence AKA: **Road poison** ☐ Resemble chili seeds ☐ Resists putrefaction

Dhatura vs Capsicum Seeds		
Feature	**Dhatura seeds**	**Capsicum seeds**
Size	Large and thick	Small and thin
Shape	Kidney shaped	Rounded
Color	Dark brown (when dried)	Pale yellow
Convex border	Double edge	Single edge
Smell	Odorless	Pungent
Surface	Small depressions	Smooth
Taste	Bitter	Pungent
On cut section	Embryo curved outward	Embryo curved inward like "6"

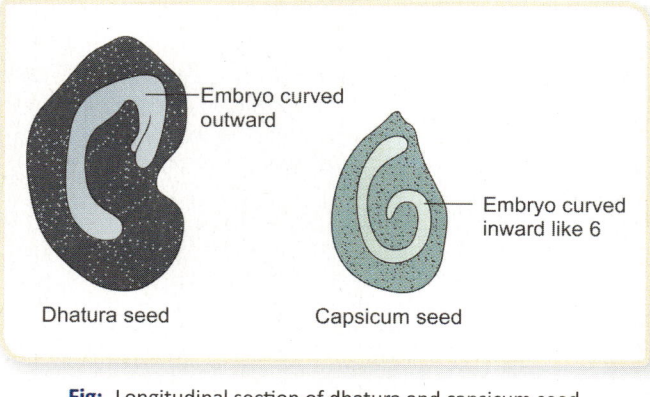

Fig: Longitudinal section of dhatura and capsicum seed

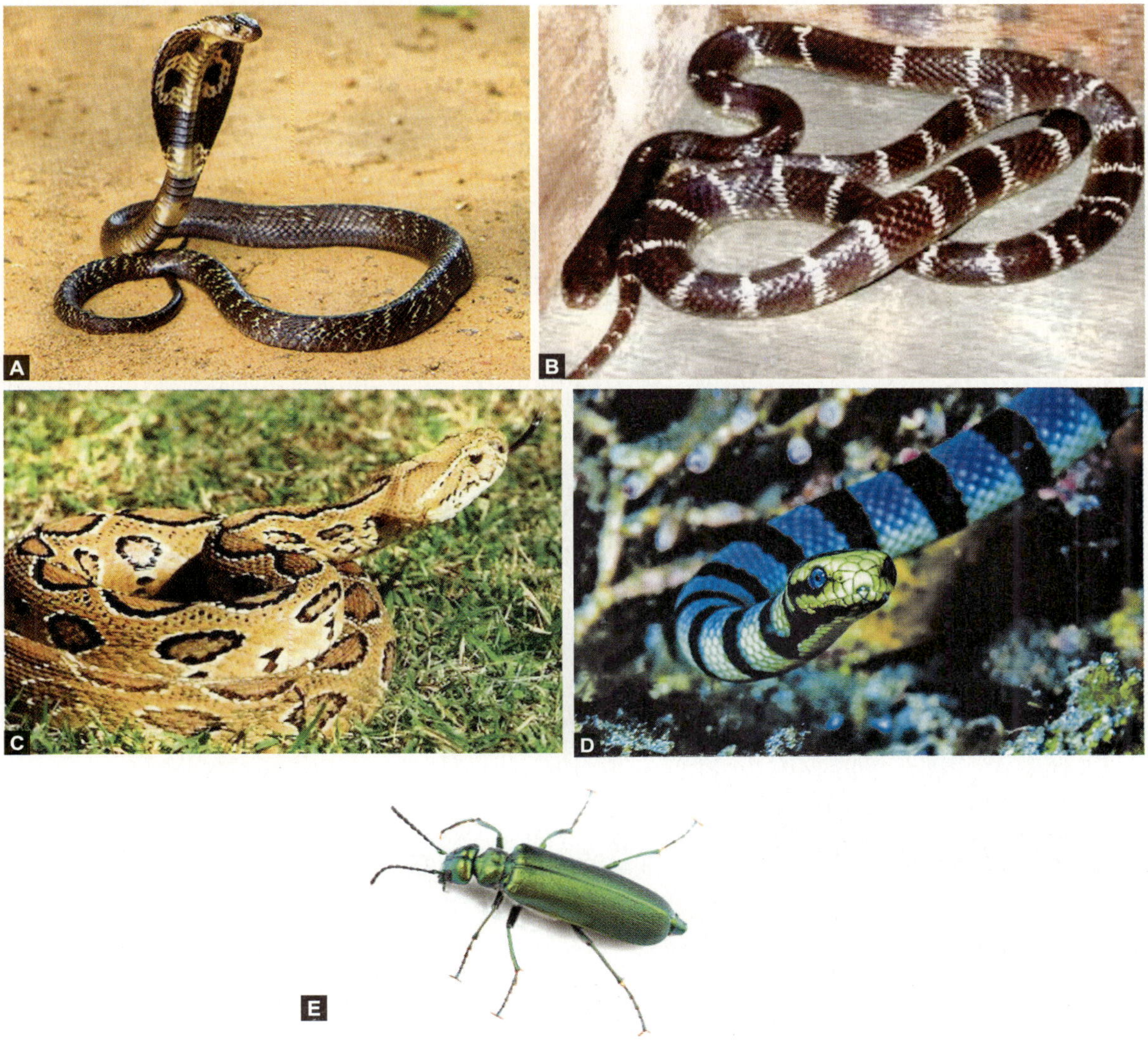

FMT PLATE 13

ANIMAL POISONS[NEETPG]

A. Cobra snake
B. Common krait
C. Russell viper
D. Sea snake
E. Spanish fly (*Cantharis vesicatoria*, blister beetle)

Animal Poisons				
Elapids (Cobra, Krait) -neurotoxic	Local burning, bite marks, muscle weakness, cramps, ptosis, paralysis, dysphagia, convulsions	Cobra-15mg Krait-6mg Few hrs	Clean and tourniquet, Specific/polyvalent antivenin (20 ml around bite, 20 ml IM, 20ml IV) Elapids specific - Atropine 0.6 mg + Neostigmine 0.5 mg (for Cobra only)	Fangs long, canalized so can give lethal dose through the clothes. Neurotoxins and cholinesterases are predominant in Elapid venom

Contd...

Animal Poisons					
Vipers (Russell's, Saw scaled)-**vasculotoxic**	Vomiting, hemolysis, hemorrhages, pupils dilated, renal tubular necrosis, collapse	Viper-40 mg Few days	General treatment same. Viper specific: heparin and fibrinogen	Fangs short, fixed, grooved so cannot bite effectively through clothes. Hemolysin and thromboplastin are predominant in viper venom
Sea Snakes-myotoxic	Generalized muscle pain, myoglobinuria, hyperkalemia	Uncertain. Not fatal.	General treatment same	
Spanish fly (*Cantharis vesicatoria*, blister beetle)	Locally irritant causing burning pain and vesicles. Pain abdomen, Nephrotoxic agent, Blood stained vomiting and micturition. Priapism, Abortion	Fatal dose: 15–30 mg of cantharidin or 1.5 g of powder. Fatal period: 24 h.	Gastric lavage, demulcents (but not fat) and symptomatic treatment	Active principle: **Cantharidin**

FMT PLATE 14

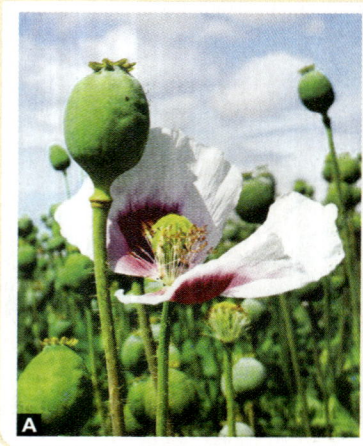
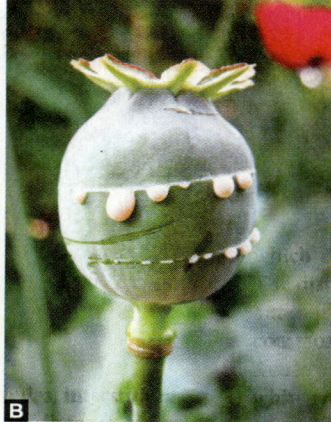
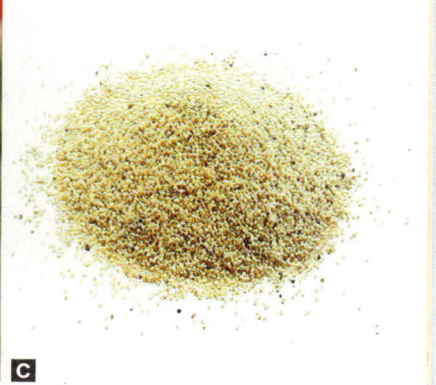

SOMNIFEROUS POISONS (OPIOIDS)

A. ***Papaver somniferum* plant:** Toxic part is unripe fruit capsule latex juice.
B. ***Papaver somniferum* fruit with latex:** Latex is obtained by scarring the immature seed pods; the latex leaks out and dries to form brown residue.
C. ***Papaver somniferum* seeds** are non-poisonous and are called 'khaskhas', which constitutes a condiment in cooking.

Somniferous Poisons (opioids)				
Opium (*Papaver somniferum*) and **Morphine**	Stage of Excitement, Stupor and Narcosis, similar to ethyl alcohol. ↓Temp, BP and RR. **Cheyne-Stokes breathing**, Respiratory depression, Cyanosis, ↓GI transit time (constipation), Pruritus, flushed skin, and urticaria may arise because of histamine release, **Pin point pupils**-dilate before death, Euphoria, Dysphoria, Seizure, coma	200 mg morphine, 2 mg opium 9-12 hrs	Gastric Lavage, Naloxone 0.4-0.8 mg IV/IM every 10-15 min till pupil dilates. Artificial respiration, O_2	▫ Raw flesh like smell ▫ Poison of choice for suicide ▫ High physical dependence
Heroin/ Smack/ Brown sugar (derived from *Papaver somniferum*, semisynthetic opioid)	Rapid development of tolerance. Withdrawal causes sweating, malaise, depression, anxiety, confusion, hallucinations, personality changes. **Heroin nephropathy** (FSGS- Focal segmental glomerulosclerosis)	Uncertain (high mortality)	Same as above	▫ Synthetic derivative of opium ▫ High addiction potential (more than morphine) ▫ Rapidly metabolized so not detected >30-60 min

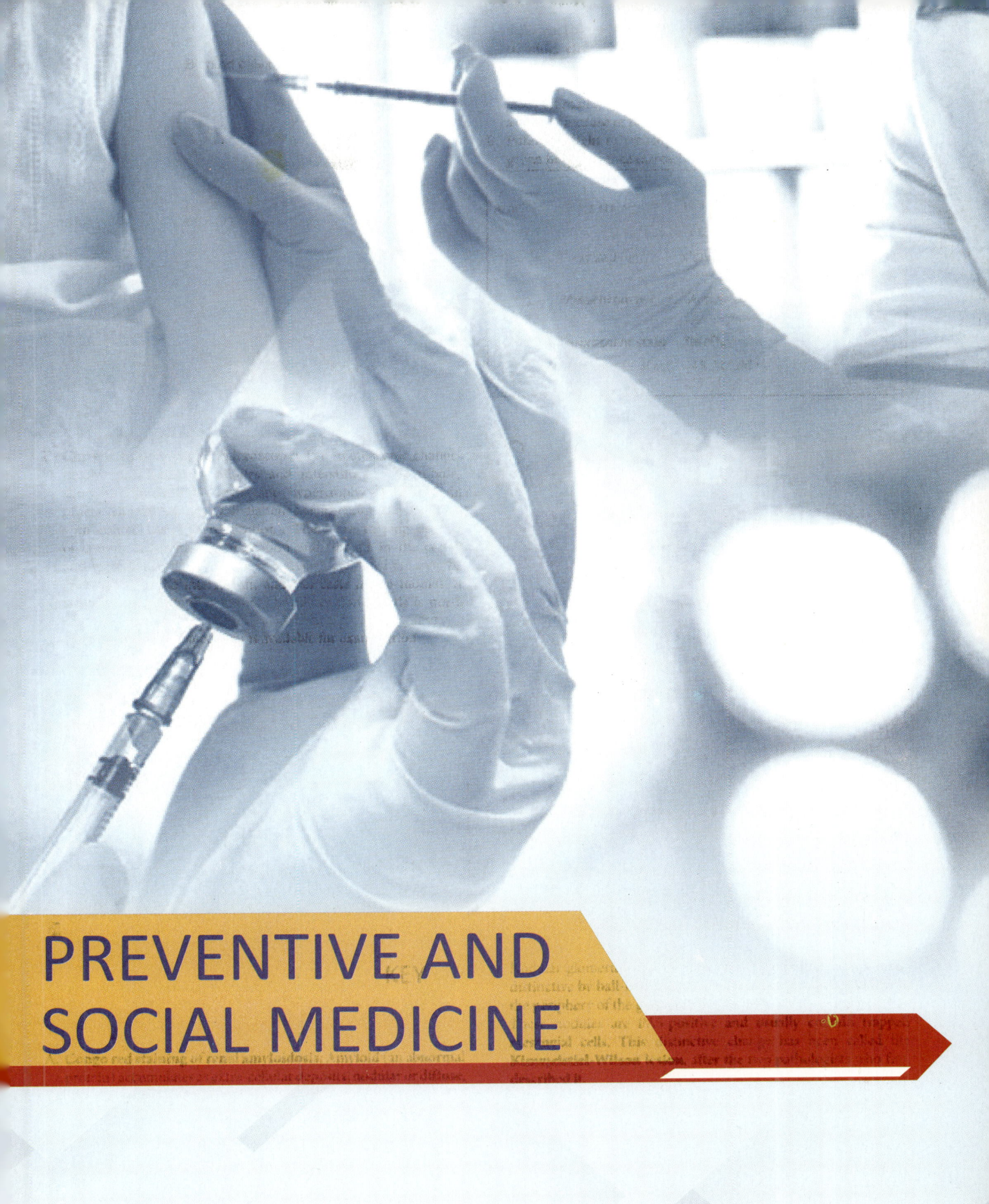

PREVENTIVE AND SOCIAL MEDICINE

PSM PLATE 1

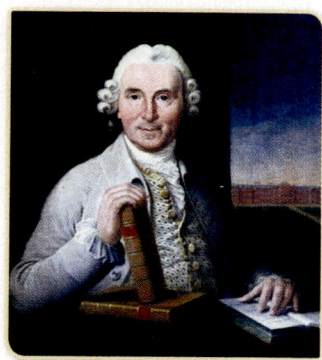

JAMES LIND

James Lind was a Scottish physician. He was a pioneer of naval hygiene in the Royal Navy. By conducting the **first ever clinical trial**, **he developed the theory that citrus fruits cured scurvy**. He argued for the health benefits of better ventilation aboard naval ships, the improved cleanliness of sailors' bodies, clothing and bedding, and below-deck fumigation with sulfur and arsenic. He also proposed that fresh water could be obtained by distilling sea water. His work advanced the practice of preventive medicine and improved nutrition.

In his book **"Treatise of the Scurvy"** (1753) James Lind did not decisively settle the questions of the causes and the treatment of scurvy, despite its presentation of experimental evidence that seemed to prove the efficacy of oranges and lemons in the cure of sea men suffering from scurvy.

PSM PLATE 2

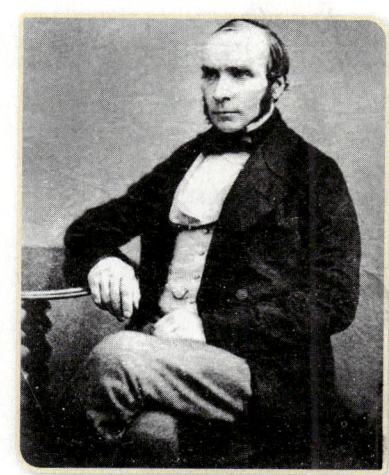

JOHN SNOW

John Snow (15 March 1813 – 16 June 1858) was an English physician and a leader in the adoption of anesthesia and medical hygiene. He is considered one of the **fathers of modern epidemiology**, in part because of his work in tracing <u>the source of a cholera outbreak in Soho, London, in 1854</u>.

Snow is best known for his **discovery that cholera is a water-borne infection**. His work on the *"Mode of Communication of Cholera"* was first published in 1849. The second edition (1855) contained statistical information on the case of Broad Street (an outbreak of cholera that caused 500 deaths in 10 days).

PSM PLATE 3

EMBLEMS AND LOGOS

	Emblems and Logos
A.	**Biological hazards**, also known as **biohazards**, refer to biological substances that pose a threat to the health of living organisms, primarily that of humans. This can include medical waste or samples of a microorganism, virus or toxin (from a biological source. It can also include substances harmful to animals. The term and its associated symbol is generally used as a warning, so that those potentially exposed to the substances will know to take precautions. The biohazard symbol was developed in 1966 by **Charles Baldwin.**
B.	**Ionizing radiation hazard:** The international radiation symbol (also known as trefoil) first appeared in 1946, at the University of California. At the time, it was rendered as magenta, and was set on a blue background. It is drawn with a central circle of radius R, an internal radius of 1.5R and an external radius of 5R for the blades, which are separated from each other by 60°. The trefoil is black in the international version. In general it is used for ionizing radiations like X rays, Gamma rays etc.

Contd...

Emblems and Logos

C.

Non ionizing radiation hazard
Non-ionizing (or non-ionising) radiation refers to any type of electromagnetic radiation that does not carry enough energy per quantum to ionize atoms or molecules. *Near ultraviolet, visible light, infrared, microwave, radio waves, and low-frequency radio frequency (longwave) are all examples of non-ionizing radiation*

D.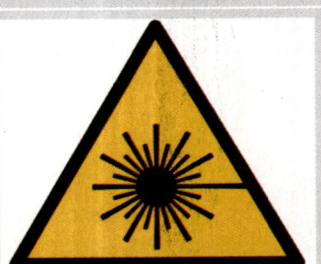

Laser hazard: Warning label for class 2 and higher

Class 1	Safe under all conditions of normal use. This means the maximum permissible exposure (MPE) cannot be exceeded when viewing a laser with the naked eye or with the aid of typical magnifying optics
Class 1M	Safe for all conditions of use except when passed through magnifying optics such as microscopes and telescopes.
Class 2	Safe because the blink reflex will limit the exposure to no more than 0.25 seconds. Intentional suppression of the blink reflex could lead to eye injury. Many laser pointers and measuring instruments are class 2.
Class 2M	Safe because of the blink reflex if not viewed through optical instruments
Class 3R	Safe if handled carefully, with restricted beam viewing
Class 3B	Hazardous if the eye is exposed directly, but diffuse reflections such as those from paper or other matter surfaces are not harmful. Used inside CD and DVD writers
Class 4	Highest and most dangerous class of laser, including all lasers that exceed the Class 3B. Most industrial, scientific, military & medical lasers are in this category

E.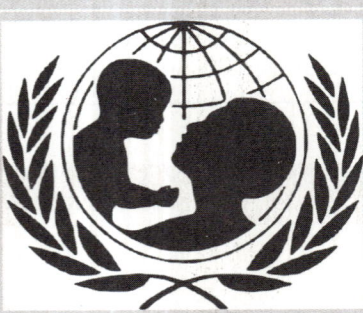

UNICEF Emblem: UNICEF *logo consists of four distinct elements*. These include the image of a mother and child, a globe, olive branches and the organization's name "UNICEF" in a very simple yet powerful lowercase typeface.
- **The olives** branches are a symbol for peace, which surround the globe.
- **The globe** represents the areas of interest in which the U.N. develops plans for peace and security, for all the people in the world, which is its main goal.
- **The mother and child** represent the nurturing of the children, caring and watching for their future and prosperity.

The use of **blue color** in the UNICEF logo stands for approachability, prosperity and grace of the organization, whereas the white color depicts nobility, peace and purity

The United Nations Children's Fund is a United Nations Programme **headquartered in New York City** that provides long-term humanitarian and developmental assistance to children and mothers in developing countries. It is one of the members of the United Nations Development Group and its Executive Committee. UNICEF was created by the United Nations General Assembly on **December 11, 1946**, to provide emergency food and healthcare to children in countries that had been devastated by World War II. In 1953, UNICEF became a permanent part of the United Nations System. UNICEF was awarded the **Nobel Peace Prize in 1965**

F.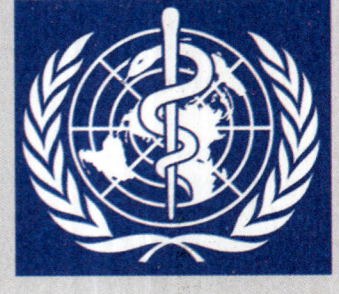

World Health Organization Emblem: WHO's emblem was chosen by the **first World Health Assembly in 1948.** The emblem consists of the United Nations symbol surmounted by a staff with a snake coiling round it. The *staff with the snake has long been a symbol of medicine and the medical profession*. It originates from the story of Asclepius who was revered by the ancient Greeks as a god of healing and whose cult involved the use of snakes. The World Health Organization (WHO) is a specialized agency of the United Nations (UN) that is concerned with international public health. It was **established on 7 April 1948**, with its **headquarters in Geneva, Switzerland.**
The **constitution of the World Health Organization** had been signed by all 61 countries of the United Nations by 22 July 1946, with the first meeting of the World Health Assembly finishing on **24 July 1948.**

Contd...

Emblems and Logos

G
The **NLEP Emblem** symbolizes beauty and purity in **lotus**: Leprosy can be cured and a leprosy patient can be a useful member of the society in the form of a **partially affected thumb**; a **normal fore-finger** and the **shape of house**; the symbol of hope and optimism in a **rising sun**. The Emblem captures the spirit of hope positive action in the eradication of Leprosy
The National Leprosy Eradication Programme is a centrally sponsored Health Scheme of the Ministry of Health and Family Welfare, Govt. of India.

H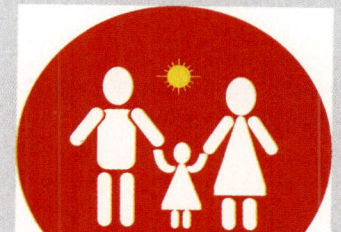
Emblem of NRHM with father, mother and child with rising sun above
The **National Rural Health Mission (NRHM) was launched in April 2005.** The NRHM focused especially on **18 states**, with poor infrastructure and low public health indicators, namely the eight Empowered Action Group (EAG) states - (Bihar, Jharkhand, Madhya Pradesh, Chhattisgarh, Uttar Pradesh, Uttaranchal, Odisha and Rajasthan), the eight North Eastern States (Assam, Arunachal Pradesh, Manipur, Mizoram, Meghalaya, Nagaland, Sikkim, Tripura) and two other states, namely, Himachal Pradesh and Jammu & Kashmir
The programme aimed at strengthening state Health systems with a special focus on **Reproductive and Child Health (RCH) services and Disease Control Programmes**. Though largely restricted to rural areas, components such as RCH services and entitlements such as the **Janani Suraksha Yojana (JSY)** and the **Janani Shishu Suraksha Karyakram (JSSK)** were extended to urban areas.

I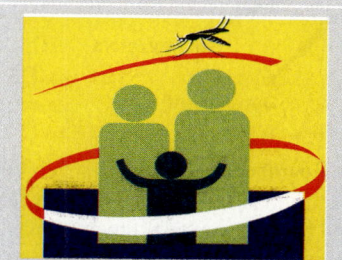
Emblem of NVBDCP with father, mother and child with protective shield around protecting from mosquito above. Directorate of **National Vector Borne Disease Control Programme (NVBDCP)** is the central nodal agency for the prevention and control of **vector borne diseases** i.e. Malaria, Dengue, Lymphatic Filariasis, Kala-azar, Japanese Encephalitis and Chikungunya in India. It is one of the Technical Departments of Directorate General of Health Services, Government of India.

J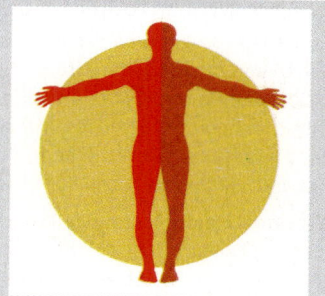
RNTCP or the Revised National Tuberculosis Control Program is the state-run tuberculosis control initiative of the Government of India. It incorporates the principles of directly observed treatment short course (DOTS), the global TB control strategy of the World Health Organization.
'DOTS: Pura course, pakka ilaaj': The element of 'Hinglish' is to bring some freshness into a communication that has been around for a long time. The DOTS strategy is cost-effective and is today the international standard for TB control programmes. To date, more than **180 countries** are implementing the DOTS strategy. India has adapted and tested the DOTS strategy in various parts of the country since **1993**, with excellent results, and by March 2006 nationwide DOTS coverage has been achieved.

K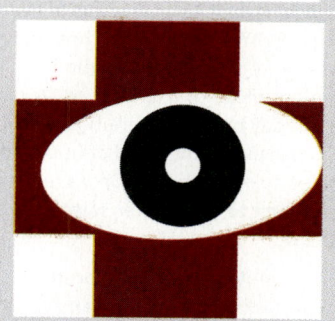
National Programme for Control of Blindness was launched in the year **1976 as a 100% Centrally Sponsored scheme** with the goal to reduce the prevalence of blindness from 1.4% to 0.3%
Main causes of blindness are as follows: - Cataract (62.6%) Refractive Error (19.70%) Corneal Blindness (0.90%), Glaucoma (5.80%), Surgical Complication (1.20%) Posterior Capsular Opacification (0.90%) Posterior Segment Disorder (4.70%), Others (4.19%)
Estimated National Prevalence of Childhood Blindness /Low Vision is 0.80 per thousand
The objectives of the programme are:
- To reduce the backlog of blindness through identification and treatment of blind.
- To develop Eye Care facilities in every district.
- To develop human resources for providing Eye Care Services.
- To improve quality of service delivery.
- To secure participation of Voluntary Organizations in eye care.

L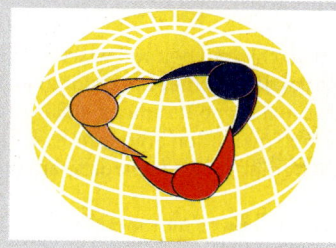
Integrated Disease Surveillance Project (IDSP) was launched with World Bank assistance in November 2004 to detect and respond to disease outbreaks quickly. The project was extended for 2 years in March 2010. From April 2010 to March 2012, World Bank funds were available for Central Surveillance Unit (CSU) at NCDC & 9 identified states (Uttarakhand, Rajasthan, Punjab, Maharashtra, Gujarat, Tamil Nadu, Karnataka, Andhra Pradesh and West Bengal) and the rest 26 states/UTs were funded from domestic budget. The Programme continues during 12th Plan under NRHM with outlay of Rs. 640 Crore from domestic budget only.

Contd...

Emblems and Logos

M

In August 1992, the National Goitre control programme (NGCP) was renamed as National Iodine Deficiency Disorders Control Programme (NIDDCP) with a view to emphasize wide spectrum disorders caused due to iodine deficiency. There is an increasing evidence of wide-spread distribution of environmental iodine deficiency not only in the Himalayan region but also in Sub Himalayan terai areas, riverine area and even the coastal regions.

Objectives: Realizing the magnitude of the problem the Government of India launched a 100 percent centrally assisted National Goitre Control Programme (NGCP) in 1962 with the following objectives:
- Initial surveys to assess the magnitude of the iodine deficiency disorders.
- Supply of iodized salt in place of common salt.
- Resurveys to assess the impact of iodized salt after every 5 years.

IDD being a National Public Health Problem it needs multisectoral approach with coming together of all stakeholders is important (as shown in the picture below)

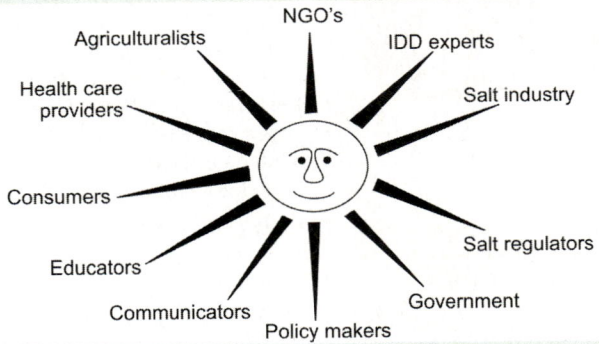

N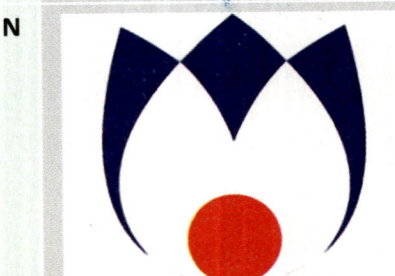

The **National Institute of Health and Family Welfare (NIHFW),** was established on 9th March, 1977 by the merger of two national level institutions, viz. the National Institute of Health Administration and Education (NIHAE) and the National Institute of Family Planning (NIFP). The NIHFW, an autonomous organization, under the Ministry of Health and Family Welfare, Government of India, acts as an 'apex technical institute' as well as a 'think tank' for the promotion of health and family welfare programmes in the country. The Institute addresses a wide range of issues on health and family welfare from a variety of perspectives through the departments of Communication, Community Health Administration, Education and Training, Epidemiology, Management Sciences, Medical Care and Hospital Administration, Population Genetics and Human Development, Planning and Evaluation, Reproductive Bio-Medicine, Statistics and Demography and Social Sciences

O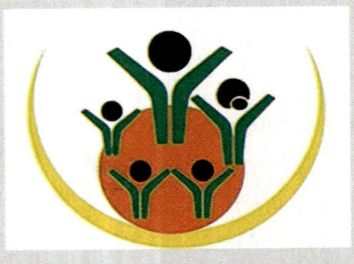

Rashtriya Swasthya Bima Yojana (RSBY), literally "National Health Insurance Programme" has been launched by Ministry of Labor and Employment, Government of India to provide health insurance coverage for Below Poverty Line (BPL) families. The objective of RSBY is to provide protection to BPL households from financial liabilities arising out of health shocks that involve hospitalization. Beneficiaries under RSBY are entitled to hospitalization coverage up to Rs. 30,000/- for most of the diseases that require hospitalization. Government has even fixed the package rates for the hospitals for a large number of interventions. Pre-existing conditions are covered from day one and there is no age limit. Coverage extends to five members of the family, which includes the head of household, spouse and up to three dependents. Beneficiaries need to pay only Rs. 30/- as registration fee while Central and State Government pays the premium to the insurer selected by the State Government on the basis of a competitive bidding.

P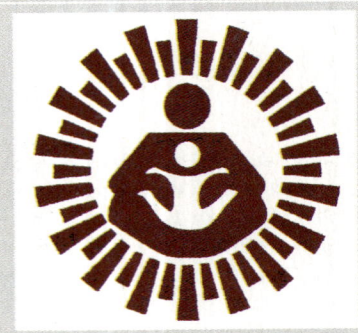

Integrated Child Development Services (ICDS), Government of India sponsored programme, is India's primary social welfare scheme to tackle malnutrition and health problems in children below 6 years of age and their mothers. The main beneficiaries of the programme were aimed to be the girl child up to her adolescence, all children below 6 years of age, pregnant and lactating mothers.

Objectives: The predefined objectives of ICDS are:
- To raise the health and nutritional level of poor Indian children below 6 years of age
- To create a base for proper mental, physical and social development of children in India
- To reduce instances of mortality, malnutrition and school dropouts among Indian Children
- To coordinate activities of policy formulation and implementation among all departments of various ministries involved in the different government programmes and schemes aimed at child development across India.
- To provide health and nutritional information and education to mothers of young children to enhance child rearing capabilities of mothers in country of India

Contd...

Emblems and Logos

Q	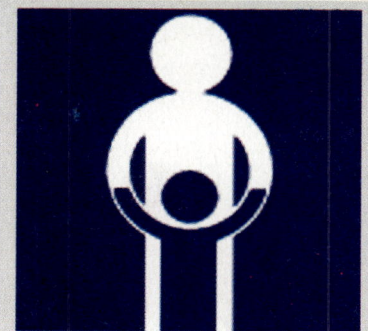	**Universal Immunization Programme** is a vaccination program launched by the Government of India in 1985. It became a part of Child Survival and Safe Motherhood Programme in 1992 and is currently one of the key areas under National Rural Health Mission (NRHM) since 2005. ▫ The program consists of vaccination for seven diseases- tuberculosis, diphtheria, pertussis (whooping cough), tetanus, poliomyelitis, measles and Hepatitis B. ▫ It is a Centrally sponsored scheme, so the total funding is managed by the Central Government.
R	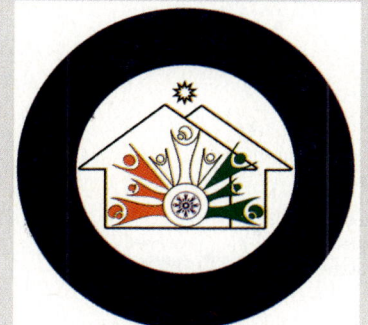	**Census of India 2011** is the largest exercise in human history to count and identify a billion people. Census of India has made all the preparations to count and identify the current Population of India. To present a unique identity to Census of India 2011, the government of India has come out with a logo for Census 2011.
S	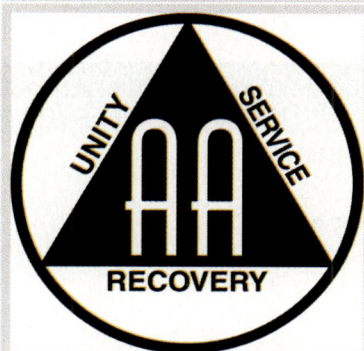	**Alcoholics Anonymous** is a fellowship of men and women who help each other with their common problem with alcoholism. It is the largest and oldest alcohol support group in the world.

PSM PLATE 4

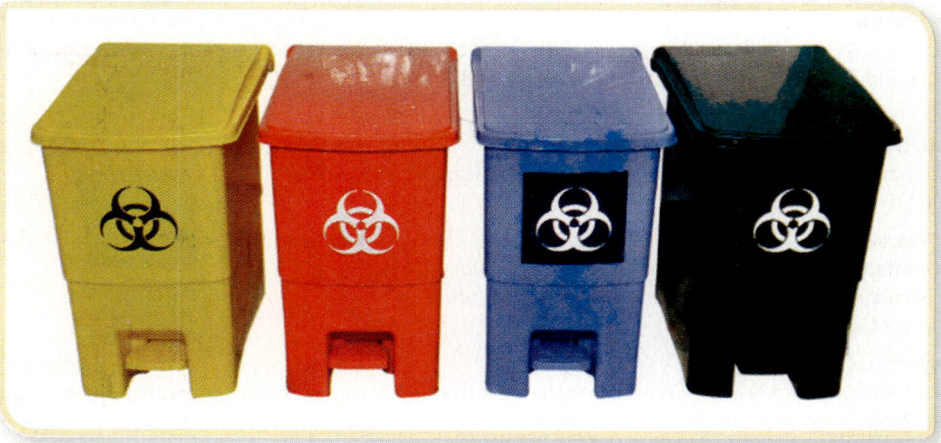

BIOMEDICAL WASTE CATEGORIES

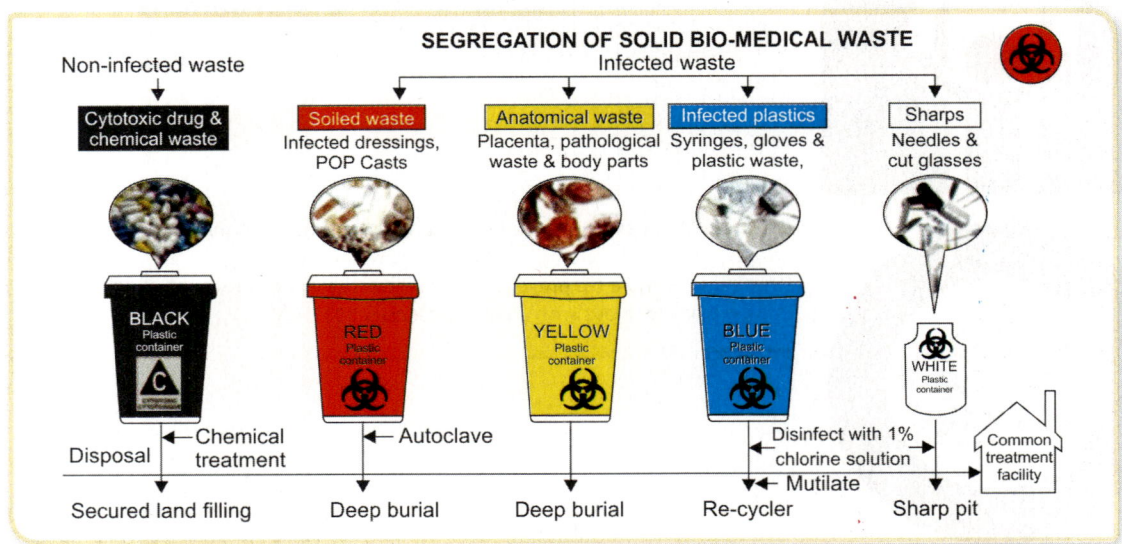

Note: Use any colored bin other than Black, Red, Yellow, blue & white for disposal of general waste.

Biomedical Waste Categories		
Category	**Waste category**	**Treatment and disposal**
Category 1	**Human Anatomical Waste** (human tissues, organs, body parts)	Incineration@/deep burial*
Category 2	**Animal Waste** (Animal tissues, organs, body parts carcasses, bleeding parts, fluid, blood and experimental animals used in research, waste generated by veterinary hospitals, colleges, discharge from hospitals, animal houses)	Incineration@/deep burial*
Category 3	**Microbiology & Biotechnology Waste** (Wastes from laboratory cultures, stocks or micro-organisms live or vaccines, human and animal cell culture used in research and infectious agents from research and industrial laboratories, wastes from production of biologicals, toxins, dishes and devices used for transfer of cultures)	Local autoclaving/microwaving/incineration@
Category 4	**Waste Sharps** (needles, syringes, scalpels, blade, glass, etc. that may cause puncture and cuts. This includes both used and unused sharps)	Disinfection (chemical treatment/ autoclaving/ microwaving and mutilation/shredding##
Category 5	**Discarded Medicines and Cytotoxic drugs** (Waste comprising of outdated, contaminated and discarded medicines)	Incineration@/destruction and drugs disposal in secured landfills
Category 6	**Soiled Waste** (items contaminated with blood, and body fluids including cotton, dressings, soiled plaster casts, lines, bedding, other material contaminated with blood)	Incineration@/ autoclaving/ microwaving
Category 7	**Solid Waste** (Waste generated from disposal items other than the sharps such a tubings, catheters, intravenous sets etc.)	Disinfection by chemical treatment@@ autoclaving/ microwaving and mutilation/shredding##
Category 8	**Liquid Waste** (Waste generated from laboratory and washing, cleaning, housekeeping and disinfecting activities)	Disinfection by chemical treatment@@ and discharge into drains
Category 9	**Incineration Ash** Ash from incineration of any bio-medical waste	Disposal in municipal landfill

Contd...

Biomedical Waste Categories

Category	Waste category	Treatment and disposal
Category 10	**Chemical Waste** (Chemicals used in production of biologicals, chemicals used in production of biologicals, chemicals used in disinfection, as insecticides, etc.)	Chemical treatment@@ and discharge into drains for liquids and secured landfill for solids

Note :

@ There will be no chemical pre-treatment before incineration. Chlorinated plastics shall not be incinerated.

* Deep burial shall be an option available only in towns with population less than five lakhs and in rural areas.

@@ Chemicals treatment using at least 1% hypochlorite solution or any other equivalent chemical reagent. It must be ensured that chemical treatment ensures disinfection.

Mutilation/shredding must be such so as to prevent unauthorised reuse.

Biomedical Waste Disposal

Colour code	Type of container	Waste category	Waste disposed	Treatment options
Black bag	Plastic bag	5, 9, 10	Noninfectious waste (papers, plastic covers), Discarded medicines & cytotoxic drugs	Disposal in secure land fills
Red bag	Plastic bag/ Disinfected container	3, 6, 7	Infected solid disposable wastes other than sharps (gloves, tunings, catheters, iv sets), Infected solid wastes contaminated with blood and body fluids (dressing, plaster, linen), Microbiology/ Biotech waste (vaccines, cultures)	Autoclave, Microwave, chemical treatment
Yellow bag	Plastic bag	1, 2, 3, 6	Human anatomical waste Animal waste, Microbiology/ Biotech waste (vaccines, cultures), Infected solid wastes contaminated with blood and body fluids (dressing, plaster, linen)	Incineration
Blue bag	Plastic bag/ Puncture proof container	4, 7	Solid sharps (needles, syringes, scalpels, blades), Infected solid disposable wastes other than sharps (gloves, tunings, catheters, iv sets)	Autoclave, Microwave, chemical treatment, destruction and shredding

PSM PLATE 5

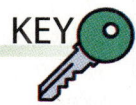 KEY

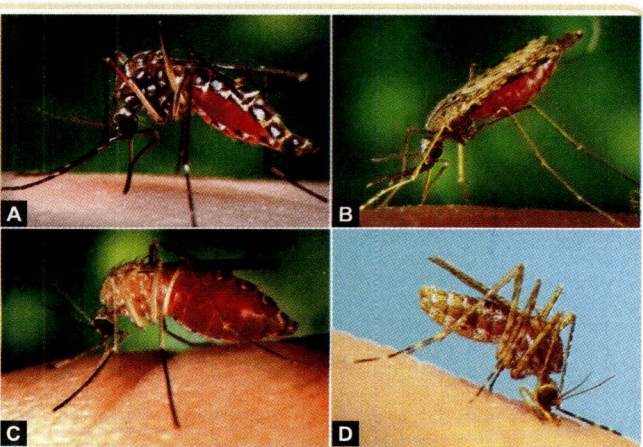

MOSQUITO VECTORS

A. **Aedes mosquito**
- AKA "Tiger mosquito" as the body is striped
- Pointed abdomen, short palpus (in females), and pale bands at the base of each segment on the abdomen
- Body parallel to surface at rest
- Wings not spotted.

B. **Anopheles mosquito**
- Body is not striped
- Body inclined with surface at rest
- Wings spotted
- Long palpi—they are about as long as the proboscis
- Long palpi in both sexes

C. **Culex mosquito**
- Cross veins on narrow wings, blunt abdomen, short palpus, and no prespiracular or postspiracular setae
- Body parallel to surface at rest
- Wings not spotted
- Short palpi in females

D. **Mansonia mosquito**
- Body parallel to surface at rest
- Wings not spotted
- Short palpi in females

	Mosquito Vectors			
	Anopheles	**Culex**	**Aedes**	**Mansonia**
Also known as		Nuisance mosquito	Tiger mosquito	
Egg laying	Singly on water	In small clusters of 200-300 on water	Singly on damp soil	In star shaped clusters/Rafts on under surface of aquatic plants
Egg shape	Boat shaped 2 Lateral floats + Trabeculated surface +	Raft shaped No lateral floats	Cigar shaped No lateral floats	Star shaped No lateral floats
Desiccation	Cannot survive	Cannot survive	Can survive	Cannot survive
Larva (Wrigglers) 5-7 days	Horizontal floating Surface feeders. No siphon tube	Head down at an angle of 45° parallel to the surface of water. Bottom feeders. Siphon tube @ 8th segment of abdomen	Head down at an angle of 45° parallel to the surface of water. Bottom feeders. Siphon tube @ 8th segment of abdomen	Head down at an angle of 45° parallel to the surface of water. Bottom feeders. Siphon tube @ 8th segment of abdomen
Pupa/Tumblers 1-2 days	Trumpet/siphon tube broad & short	Trumpet/siphon tube long & narrow	Trumpet/siphon tube long & narrow	Trumpet/siphon tube long & narrow
Adult (2 weeks)	Body inclined with surface at rest. Wings spotted Long palpi in both sexes.	Body parallel to surface at rest. Wings not spotted. Short palpi in females.	Body parallel to surface at rest. Wings not spotted. Short palpi in females.	Body parallel to surface at rest. Wings not spotted. Short palpi in females.
Feeding habit	Night biters	Night biters Biting peak at Midnight	Day time biters	Night biters
Breeding habit	Clean water	Dirty and polluted water	Artificial collection of water	Aquatic vegetation
Vector of	Malaria Filaria (not in India)	Bancroftian filariasis, Japanese encephalitis, west Nile fever	Yellow fever (not in India), Dengue, Chikungunya, Rift valley fever, Filaria (not in India)	Malayan (Brugian filariasis), Chikungunya
Larval Source reduction by Habitat modification	Appropriate engineering measures such as **filling and drainage**.	Abolition of domestic and peridomestic sources of breeding such as **cesspools & open ditches**;	Cleaned up/get rid of artificial water holding containers such as **discarded tins, empty pots, broken bottles, coconut shells**	**Aquatic plants** to which the larvae attach themselves should be removed or destroyed by herbicides.

Footnote:
- Eggs hatch in 48 hours
- Pupa is resting stage, moves actively but do not feed
- Eggs to adult = 7-10 days
- During growth, the larva molts (sheds its skin) four times. The stages between molts are called instars
- Life span of mosquito varies from 8-34 days (2 weeks average), males are short lived.
- Males never bite (feed on nectar). Females need blood meals every 2-3 days for development of eggs
- Life span of adult mosquito: 2 weeks
- Males have shorter life span
  Gonotrophic cycle: time between a blood meal and laying of eggs: 48 hours

Stages in Life History of Mosquito	
Stages	**Time span**
Egg	1 – 2 days
Larva	5 – 7 days
Pupa	1 – 2 days
Adult	2 weeks

PSM PLATE 6

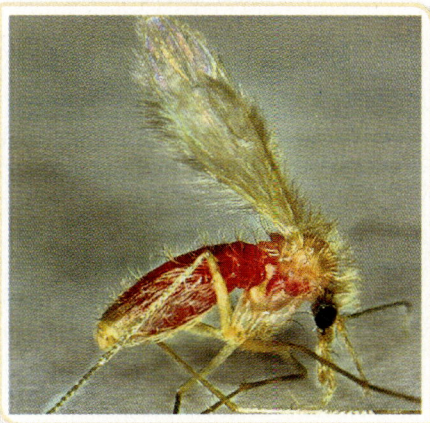

SAND FLY[NEET PG, AIIMS PG]

The leishmaniases are caused by 20 species pathogenic for humans belonging to the genus Leishmania, a protozoa transmitted by the bite of a tiny 2 to 3 millimeter-long insect vector, the phlebotomine sand-fly. Only the female sand-fly transmits the protozoa, infecting itself with the Leishmania parasites contained in the blood it sucks from its human or mammalian host in order to obtain the protein necessary to develop its eggs. The insect vector of leishmaniasis, the phlebotomine sand-fly, is found throughout the world's inter-tropical and temperate regions.

- Body: Brownish, Less than 5 mm length, Hairy body and wings
- Mandibles: well developed in females, absent in males
- Palps: Pendulous, 5 segments
- Long antennae
- Wings: Hairy, venation more or less parallel, held erect above the body
- Most active in night, shade and twilight
- Six genera; New world: Lutzomyia, Brumptomyia, Warileya and Old world: Phlebotomus, Sergentomyia, Chinius
- Transmits[AIIMS PG]: Kala azar, Sand fly fever (3 day fever), Oriental sore, Chandipura virus, Oroya fever (Carrion's disease)

PSM PLATE 7

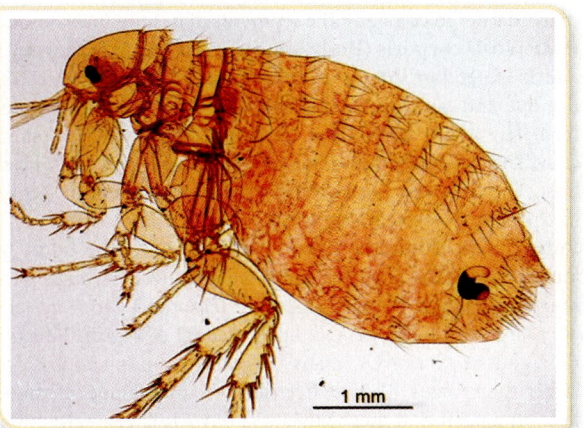

ORIENTAL RAT FLEA

Identification

- The Oriental Rat Flea is brown and has a laterally compressed body (flattened from side to side) body.
- The head does not have the spiky large combs like cat fleas and dog fleas.
- Body length 1.5mm to 4mm.
- The flea's body consists of three regions: head, thorax, and abdomen. The head and the thorax have rows of bristles (called combs) and the abdomen consists of eight visible segments.
- A flea is *wingless* so it cannot fly, but it can jump long distances with the help of small powerful legs. A flea's leg consists of four parts. The part that is closest to the body is the coxa. Next is the femur, tibia and tarsus. A flea can use its legs to jump up to 200 times its own body length (about 20 in or 50 cm).
- The main criteria that are used for species identification in fleas are the presence or absence and shape of the pronotal and genal combs. Adult Xenopsylla cheopis lack both genal and pronotal comb (combs of bristles in the front and back). This characteristic can be used to differentiate the oriental rat flea from the cat flea, dog flea, and other fleas.
- Based on structural differences the fleas that are commonly encountered in the US fall into 3 groups, mainly those which possess a genal and pronotal comb, those that only have a pronotal comb and those that lack both types of combs.
- Males and females are *sexually dimorphic*. Females have dark-colored *spermatheca* that resemble small sacs, a distinguishing characteristic of this species. Males have complex genitalia that are easily distinguishable from the females.

Vector

Oriental rat flea, is best known as the vector for the bacteria **Yersinia pestis** from rats to humans. The primary host of Oriental Rat Flea is rats (**Rattus species**), but it will feed on other mammals including humans. This flea is the vector for transmitting **murine typhus** in Australia and is a primary carrier of **bubonic plague** in Asia, Africa, and South America. *Xenopsylla cheopis* is the flea species that was the main vector for the bubonic plague. Some flea species include:

- Cat flea (*Ctenocephalides felis*)
- Dog flea (*Ctenocephalides canis*)
- Human flea (*Pulex irritans*)
- Moorhen flea (*Dasypsyllus gallinulae*)
- Northern rat flea (*Nosopsyllus fasciatus*)
- Oriental rat flea (*Xenopsylla cheopis*)

Transmission

Adults of both sexes of Xenopsylla cheopis feed on blood. **Xenopsylla cheopis** has mouthparts adapted to cutting through skin and sucking up blood that has pooled. In feeding, it secretes saliva into the wound to prevent the blood from coagulating. Along with the saliva, the flea secretes any bacteria it may have picked up by eating the blood of an infected individual into the host. When **Y. pestis** pathogens enter the gut of the flea, they multiply quickly, blocking food from entering the digestive system. This triggers the hungry flea to bite a new host, further spreading the bacteria.

Control

Application of DDT powder (50-100g/kg, 5-10%) to rodent burrows, runs, living areas of commensal rats and burrows of field rats. Where DDT resistance has developed, organophosphorus compounds should be used. Control measures against fleas must precede rodent control, otherwise the fleas will leave dead rats and bite man more actively.

Key to Common Fleas

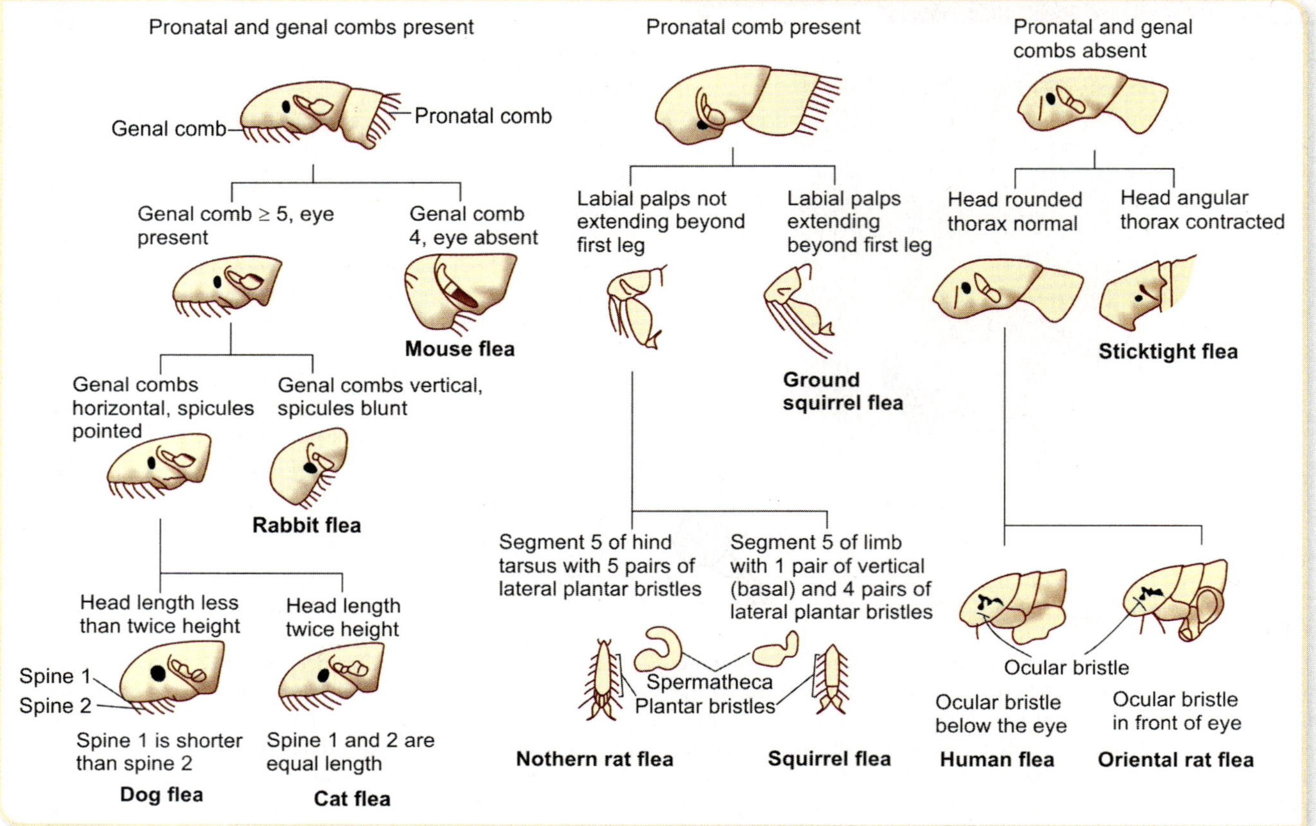

Fig: Key to common fleas

PSM PLATE 8

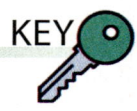 KEY

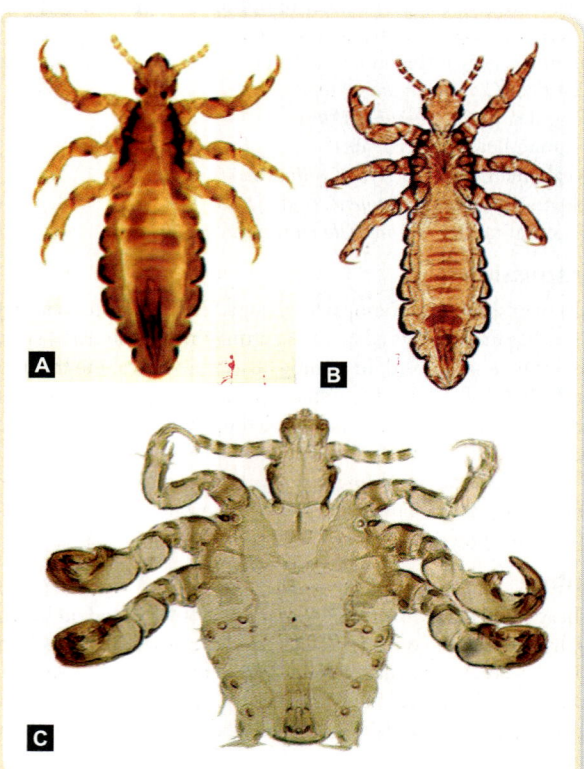

PEDICULOSIS (LICE)

Lice are small wingless ectoparasites of mammals and birds. Pediculosis is caused by sucking lice of the order Anoplura. There are three types of lice, which form the ectoparasitic fauna of man. **Pediculosis humanus** var. capitis, the head louse; **Pediculosis capitis** var. corporis, the body louse; and Phthirus pubis, the pubic louse.

A. **Pediculosis humanus var. capitis (Head Louse):** These are dorsoventrally flattened, wingless insects. The head has a pair of five segmented antennae, and mouth parts adapted for sucking blood. The thorax is small, where all the three segments are fused together. **Pediculosis humanus** var. capitis, the head louse, is slightly smaller (2.4–3.3 mm) when compared with the body louse, darker in color and the segments of its antennae are smaller.

B. **Pediculosis corporis (Body louse):** Is 2 to 4 mm in length and is a little larger, but similar in morphology, to the head louse Body lice live and lay eggs on clothing and only move to the skin to feed. The thorax bears three short legs, each of which ends in a claw. The claws help to hold on to hair and fibers of clothing of the host. The abdomen is relatively large, composed of nine segments of which only seven are apparent.

C. **Pubic louse (Phthirus pubis) (crab louse):** The adult pubic louse resembles a miniature crab when viewed through a strong magnifying glass. Pubic lice have six legs; their two front legs are very large and look like the pincher claws of a crab. This is how they got the nickname "crabs." Females lay nits and are usually larger than males. To live, lice must feed on blood. If the louse falls off a person, it dies within 1–2 days. It is generally found in

the pubic and perineal region. The crab louse has a characteristic body form, and is readily recognized by:
1. its small size and square body
2. head impacted on the thorax
3. the relatively enormous and powerful legs and claws
4. the first pair of legs slenderer than others
5. its extreme inertness.

It does not move very much from the site of its birth. The crab louse is quite distinctive in appearance. Its body is square, and the second and third pairs of legs carry heavy, pincer-like claws. When static, the crab louse uses these huge claws to grip adjacent hairs close to the skin surface.

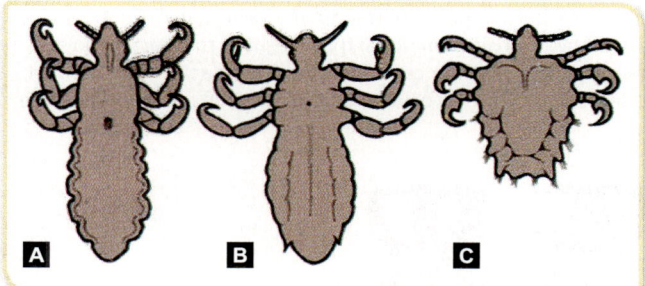

Fig: Common lice in humans: (A) head louse (**Pediculus humanus capitis**), (B) body louse (**Pediculus humanus corporis**), (C) Pubic louse (**Pthirus pubis**-Crab louse)

 **PSM PLATE 9**

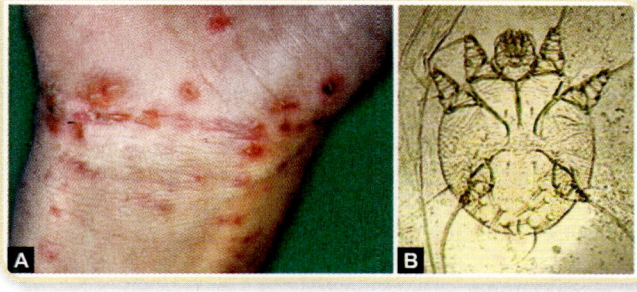

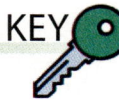 KEY

SCABIES

Scabies is an infestation of the skin by the mite Sarcoptes scabiei.
A. **Classic scabies** typically manifests as an intensely pruritic eruption with a distribution on sides and webs of the fingers, wrists, axillae, areolae, and genitalia are among the common sites of involvement. Crusted scabies, a less common variant that primarily occurs in the setting of reduced cellular immunity and is associated with a heavy mite burden, is characterized by thick scale, crusts, and fissures. Pruritus is the most prominent and common clinical feature of scabies. Host type I and IV hypersensitivity reactions involving multiple cell lines underline the pathophysiology of the scabietic rash and pruritus. The itch is characteristically described as intense, intractable and generalized pruritus that usually spares the scalp. It is worse at night and after a hot shower, but occasionally patients are asymptomatic. The diagnosis of scabies is confirmed through the detection of scabies mites, eggs, or feces with microscopic examination.

B. **Sarcoptes scabiei var. hominis**: Mite identified by light microscopy (100x amplification) in skin scrapings of a burrow (after 10% KOH). It has an ovoid body, flattened dorsoventrally. The adult female = 0.4 x 0.3 mm and Adult male = 0.2 x 0.15 mm. The body is creamy white and is marked by transverse corrugations, and on its dorsal surface by bristles and spines (denticles). There are four pairs of short legs; the anterior two pairs end in elongated peduncles tipped with small suckers. In the female, the rear two pairs of legs end in long bristles (setae), whereas in the male bristles are present on the third pair and peduncles with suckers on the fourth. The mites burrow into the upper layer of the skin but never below the stratum corneum. The burrows appear as tiny raised serpentine lines that are grayish or skin-colored and can be a centimeter or more in length.

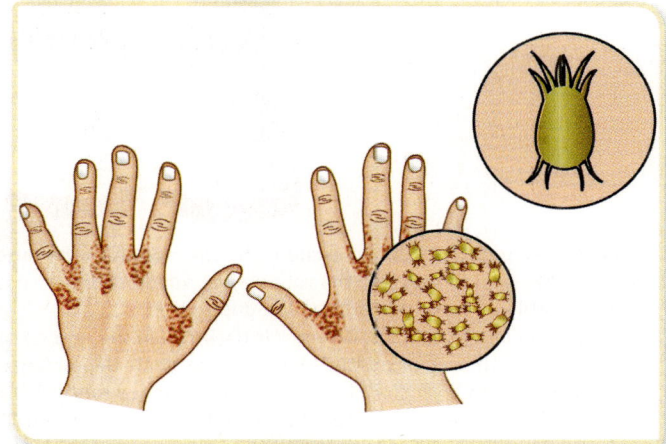

FIG: Scabies itch mite

 **PSM PLATE 10**

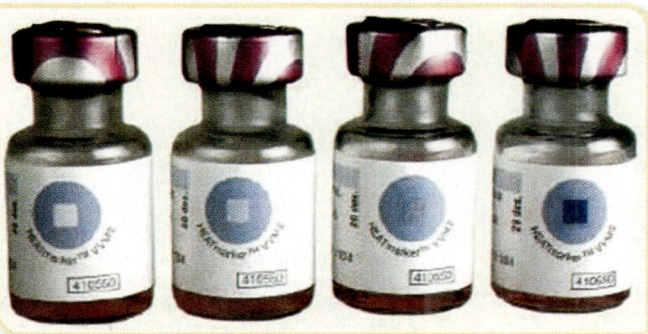

PICTURE MEDEASY

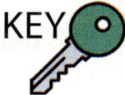 Key

VACCINE VIAL MONITOR

Vaccine Vial Monitor

A vaccine vial monitor (VVM) is a label containing a heat sensitive material, which is placed on a vaccine vial to register cumulative heat exposure over time. The combined effects of time and temperature cause the inner square of the VVM to darken, gradually and irreversibly.

A direct relationship exists between the rate of color change and temperature:
- The lower the temperature, the slower the color change.
- The higher the temperature, the faster the color change.

The VVM is a circle with a small square inside it. It can be printed on a product label, attached to the cap of a vaccine vial or tube, or attached to the neck of an ampoule. The inner square of the VVM is made of heat sensitive material that is light at the starting point and becomes darker with exposure to heat. At the starting point, the inner square is a lighter color than the outer circle. From then on, until the temperature and/or duration of heat reaches a level known to degrade the vaccine beyond acceptable limits, the inner square remains lighter than the outer circle.

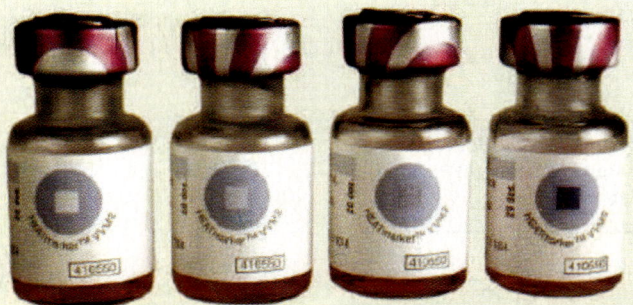

At the discard point, the inner square is the same color as the outer circle. This reflects that the vial has been exposed to an unacceptable level of heat and the vaccine degraded beyond acceptable limits. The inner square will continue to darken with heat exposure until it is much darker than the outer circle.

Whenever the inner square matches or is darker than the outer circle, the vial must be discarded. VVMs are located either on the label or on the top of the cap or on the neck of the ampoule depending on the type of vaccine (liquid or freeze-dried). VVM for liquid type vaccines are placed on custom labels to allow reference to VVM readings even though those vials have been opened and intended to be used in subsequent sessions according to multi-dose vial policy (MDVP). VVM for freeze dried vaccines are placed either on top of the cap (vials) or on the neck of the ampoule so it is discarded by the time of reconstitution. Since freeze-dried vaccines must be discarded within six hours or at the end of the session whichever comes first, VVM can only be referred until the time of reconstitution.

Rule 1: If the inner square is lighter than the outer circle, the vaccine can be used provided that the expiry date has not passed.
Rule 2: If the inner square is the same color or darker than the outer circle, the vaccine must not be used.

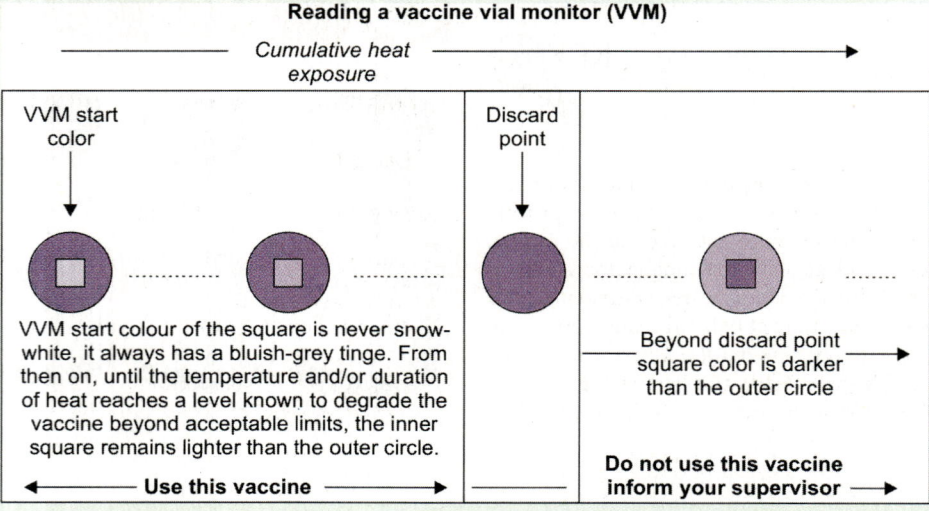

PSM PLATE 11

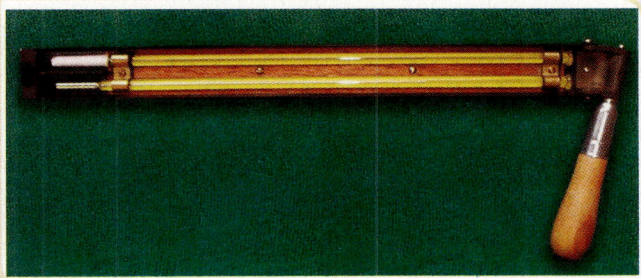

SLING PSYCHROMETERS

Psychrometers measure relative humidity without agitation. They are a type of hygrometer that employs two thermometers (a dry bulb and a wet bulb) and reads humidity based on the difference between the two.

1. **Dry and wet bulb hygrometer**: Contains two thermometers. One dry and other moistened with a wick. If the readings are same between the two, there is 100% humidity. However, if there is a difference, Relative humidity can be calculated by special psychrometric charts. A cotton wick, which is wetted prior to use, covers the bulb of one of the thermometers. This thermometer is referred to as the wet bulb, while the other thermometer is termed the dry bulb. The dry bulb measures room temperature. The thermometers may be graduated in degrees Celsius or degrees Fahrenheit.
2. **Sling psychrometer:** Two thermometers (one dry and one wet) are mounted side by side are mounted on a rotating frame. The speed of this frame is 5 meters per sec (4 revolutions/ sec). It is first rotated for 15 seconds and readings are noted. Again, it is rotated for 10 seconds and readings are noted. A chart is used to measure humidity.

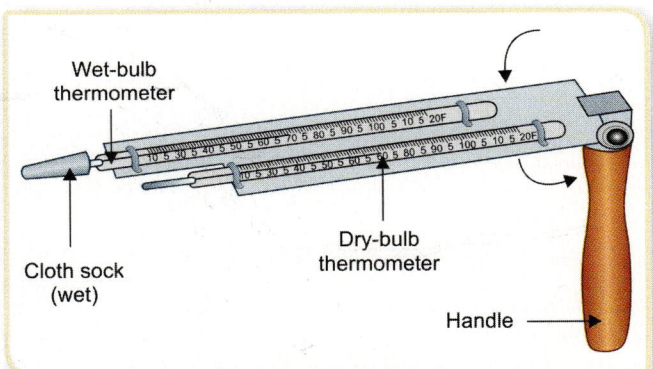

Fig: Sling psychrometer

3. **Assman Psychrometer:** It is a portable device that uses clockwork fan, which aspirates air at a rate of 5 meters per sec.

PSM PLATE 12

KATA THERMOMETER

- Kata thermometer is used to measure **cooling power of air.**
- There are 2 types of Kata thermometer- Dry and Wet. Wet Kata thermometer is covered by a muslin cloth.
- At least four readings are taken of which 1st is discarded.
- A **dry Kata reading of >6** and **wet Kata Reading of >20** are regarded as indices for thermal comfort.

NOTES

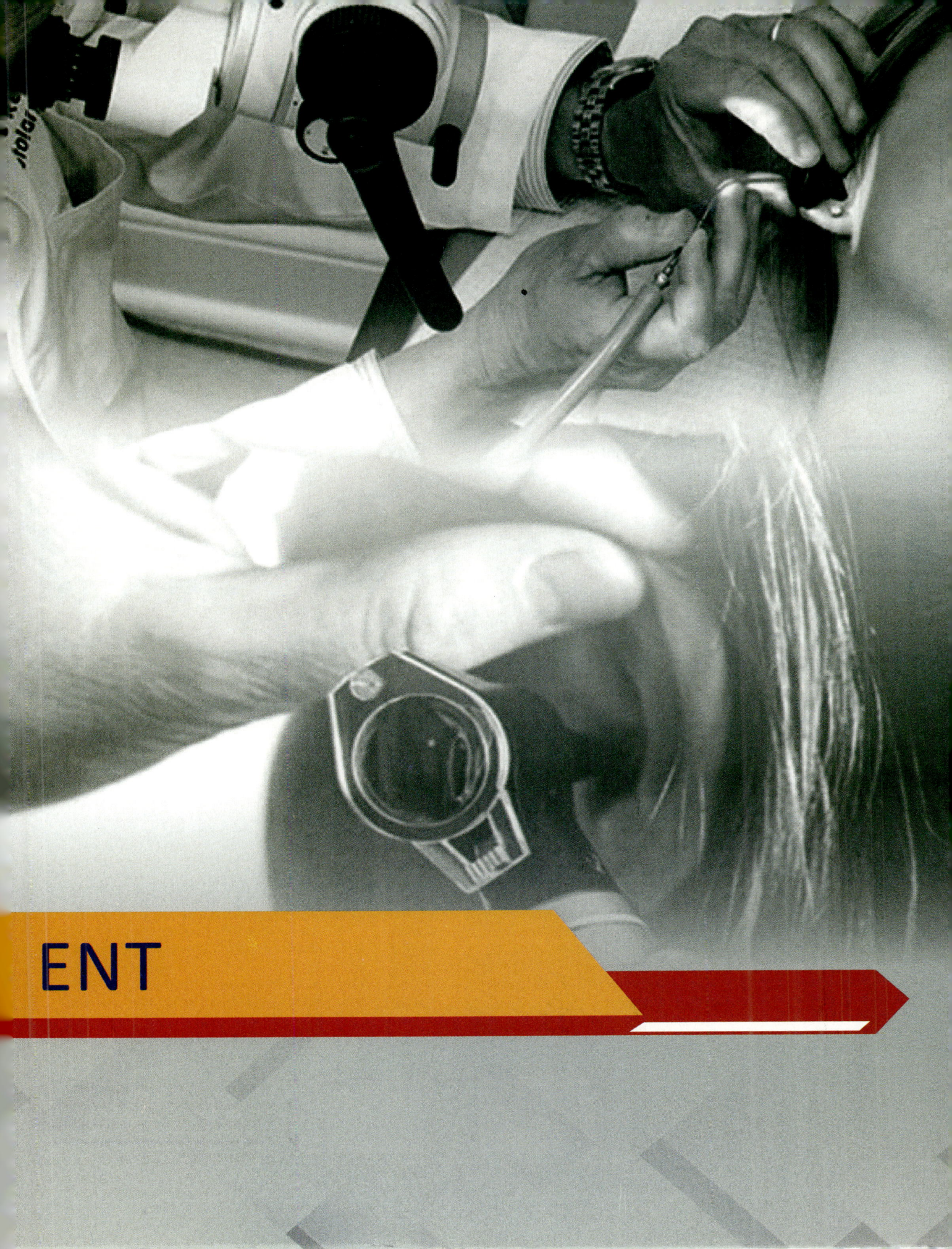

ENT

ENT PLATE 1

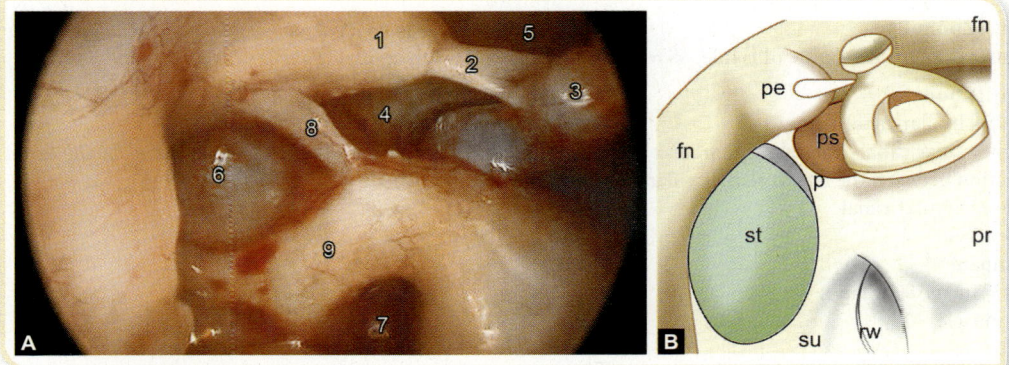

MIDDLE EAR CAVITY

A. Endoscopic view of middle ear cavity
1. Pyramid
2. Stapedius tendon
3. Head of stapes
4. Posterior tympanic sinus
5. Facial recess (area above stapes)
6. Sinus tympani
7. Round window niche
8. Ponticulus
9. Subiculum

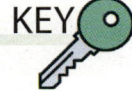 KEY

B. Diagrammatic representation of the Endoscopic view of middle ear

fn = Facial nerve
st = Sinus tympani
rw = Round window
p = Ponticulus
pe = Pyramid
ps = Posterior tympanic sinus

Boundaries of Sinus Tympani

Above: Ponticulus
Below: Subiculum
Laterally: Facial nerve with facial canal
Importance: Cholesteatoma may lie hidden in this space which can be missed during surgery

ENT PLATE 2

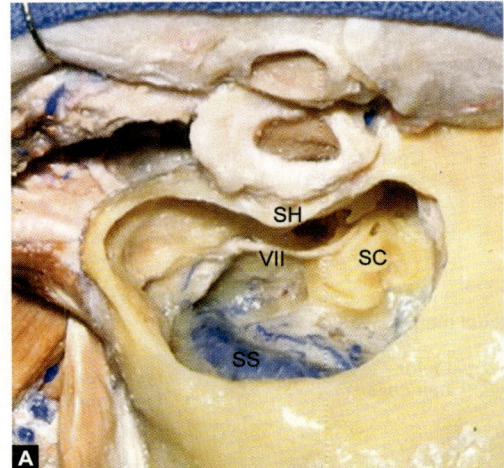
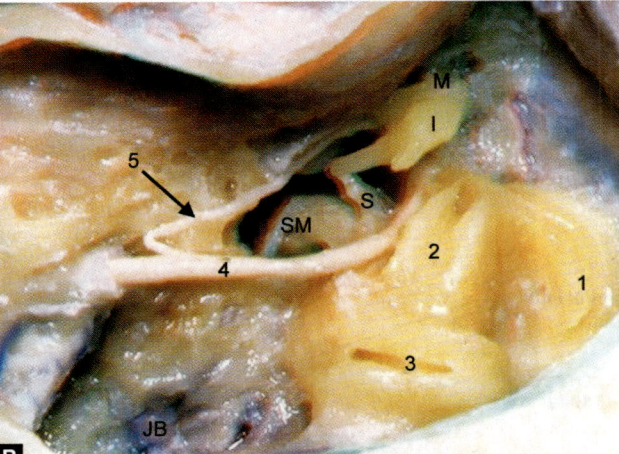

CC 4.0 International http://operativeneurosurgery.com   CC 4.0 International http://operativeneurosurgery.com

MASTOIDECTOMY

A. Mastoidectomy (Zoom Out)
SC = Semicircular canals, SH = Spine of Henle, SS = Sigmoid sinus, VII = 7th cranial (Facial) nerve

B. Mastoidectomy (Zoom in)
1 = Superior semicircular canal
2 = Lateral semicircular canal- Lateral semicircular canal can be identified acute angled from facial nerve, as the facial nerve passes in a dorsal direction between the lateral semicircular canal and the stapes
3 = Posterior semicircular canal
4 = VII cranial nerve
5 = Chorda tympani
M = Malleus, I = Incus, S = Stapes
SM: Stapedius muscle
JB: Jugular bulb

ENT PLATE 3

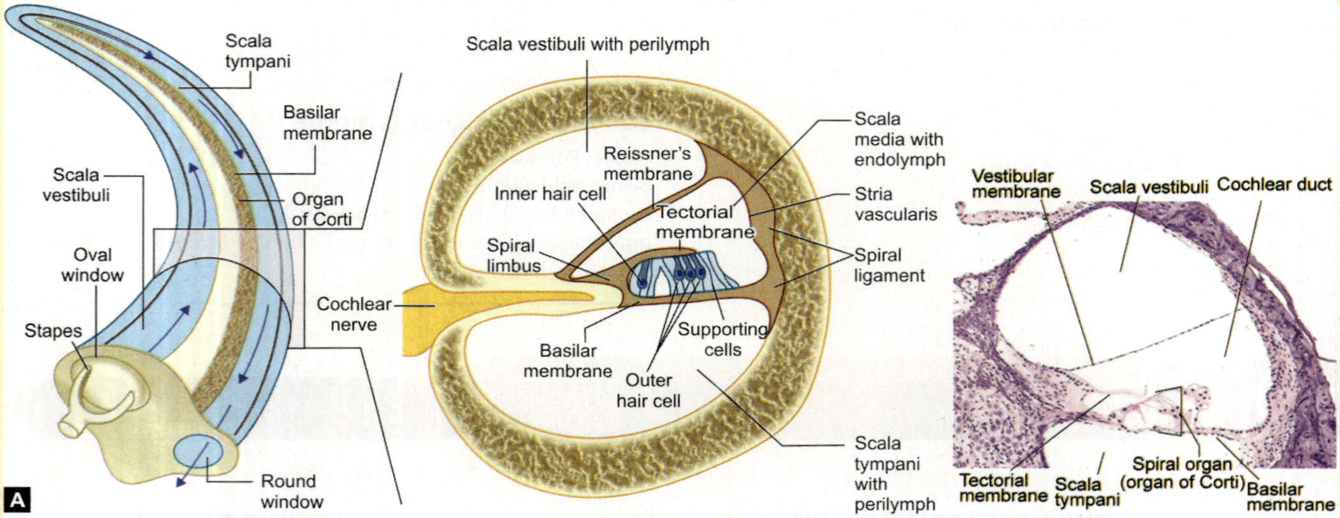

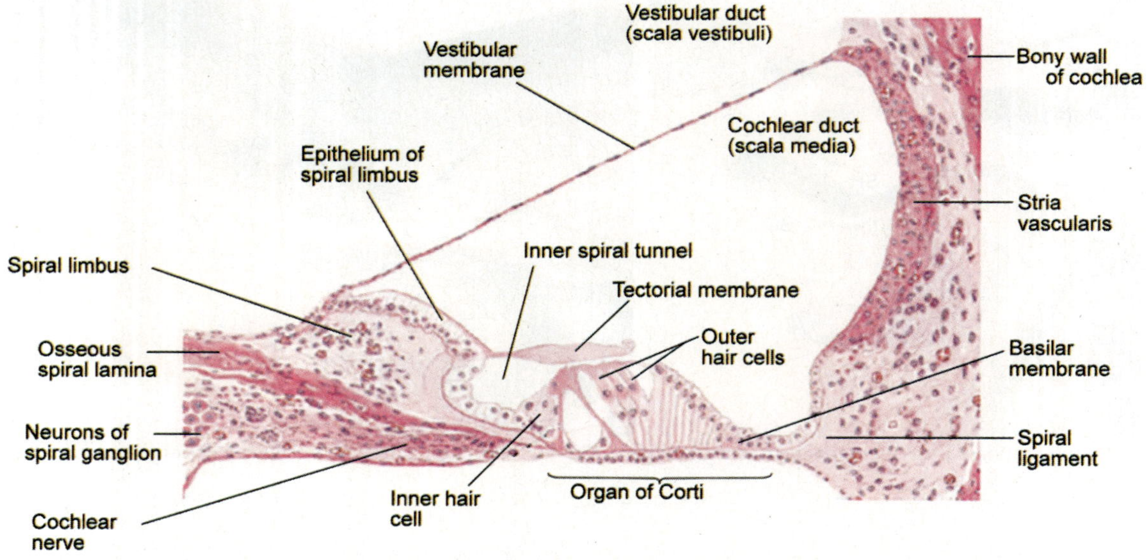

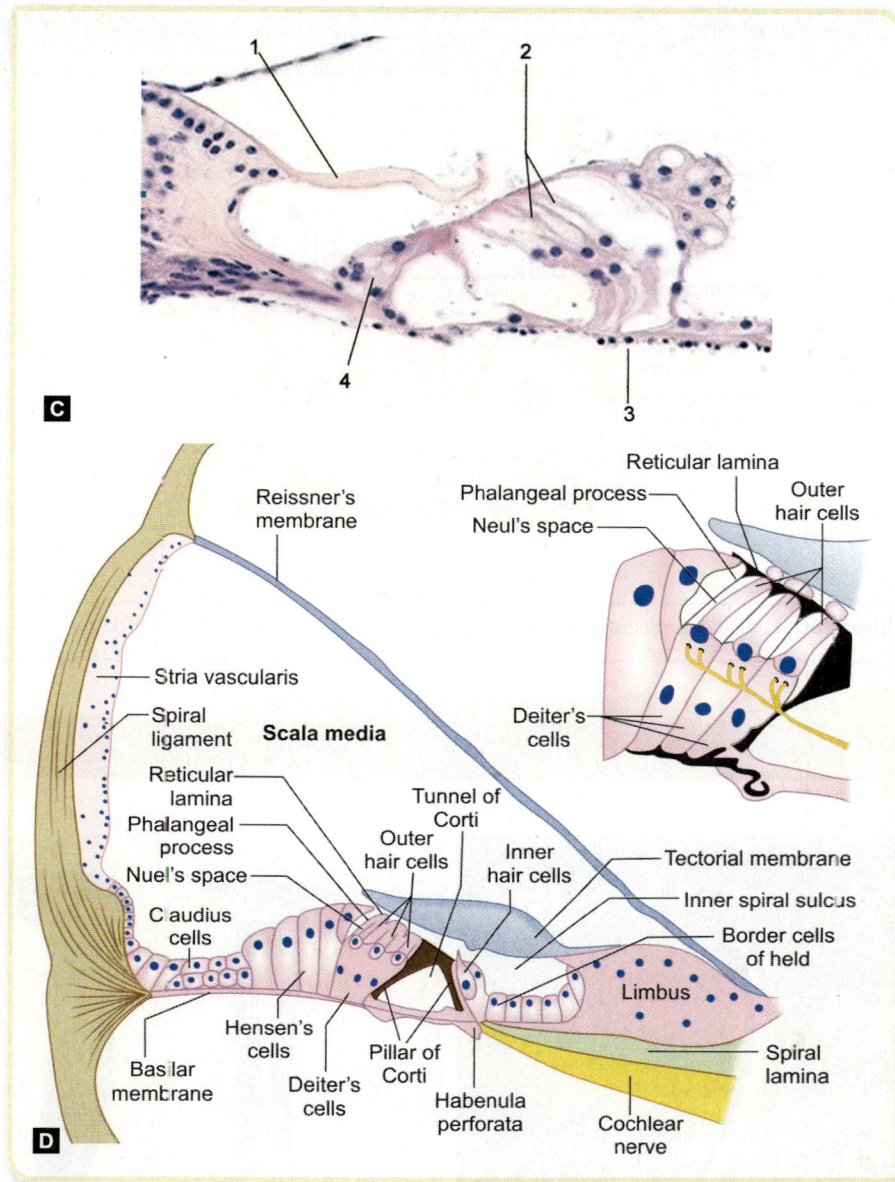

PLATE LEGENDS

A. Cross section of cochlear duct: Representation above, Histological below (with labelling)
B. Cross section of scala media (with labelling)
C. Cross section of Organ of Corti (High power)
   1. Tectorial membrane
   2. Outer hair cell
   3. Basilar membrane
   4. Inner hair cell

Difference Between Outer and Inner Hair Cells		
	Inner hair cells (Type 1)	Outer hair cells (Type 2)
Cell numbers	3500	12000
Number of rows	Single	3-4
Shape	Flask shape	Cylindrical
Development	Early	Late
Nerve supply	Mainly afferent fibers (95% afferent fibers of spiral ganglion)	Mainly efferent fibers (Only 5% afferent fibers of spiral ganglion)
Function	Transmit auditory stimuli	Modulates function of inner hair cell

Contd...

Difference Between Outer and Inner Hair Cells		
	Inner hair cells (Type 1)	Outer hair cells (Type 2)
OAE generation	No	Yes
Ototoxicity	More resistant	More sensitive
High intensity sound	More resistant	More sensitive

D. Cross section of cochlear duct: Detailed diagrammatic representation with all supporting cells labelled

 ENT PLATE 4

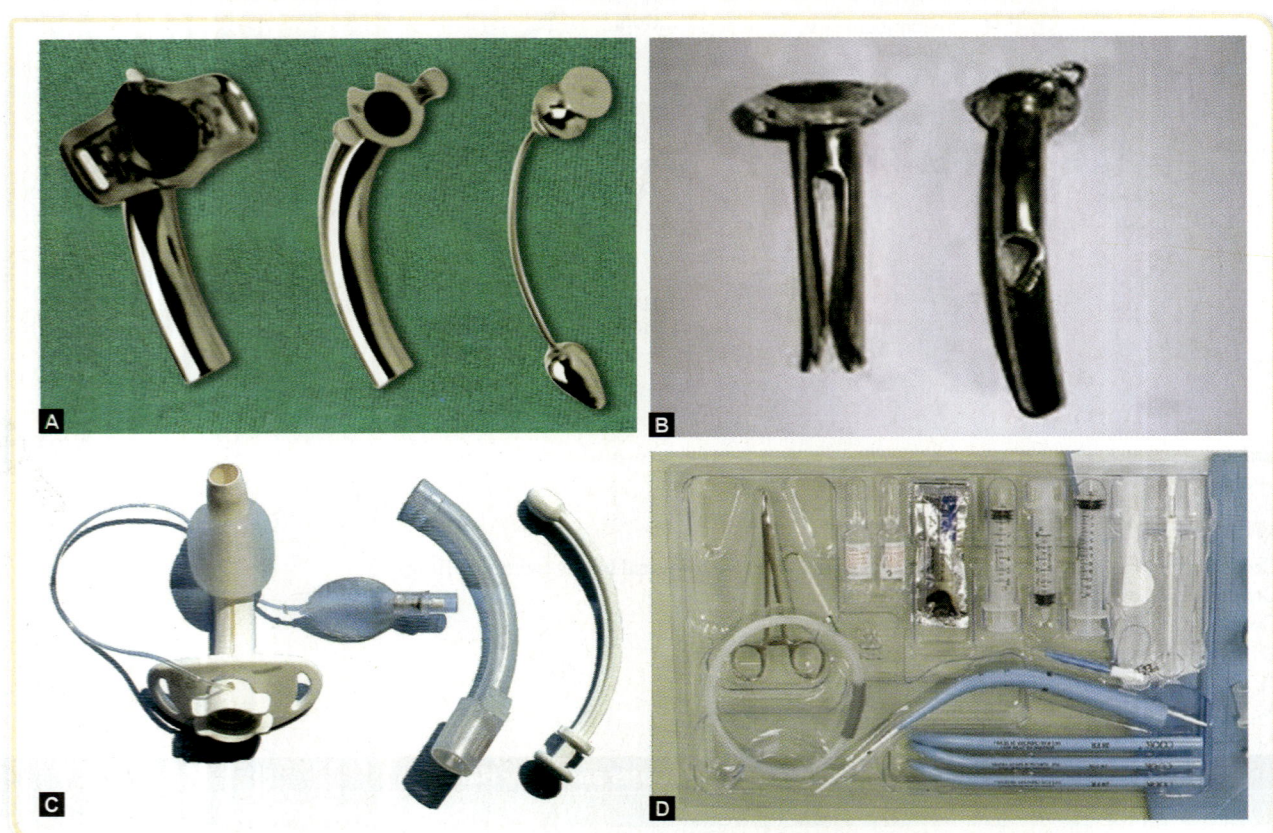

TRACHEOSTOMY TUBES

Tracheostomy tubes can be single lumen (to increase inner caliber), double lumen (easy to remove, clean and replace), cuffed (prevent air leak), uncuffed, fenestration (For better speaking but there is a high risk for granuloma formation at the site of the fenestration).

Material Used

- A tracheostomy tube may be made of an alloy of silver, copper and phosphorus, e.g. Fuller, Negus, Jackson's tube.
- **PVC (polyvinyl chloride):** They are disposable, single use tubes.

- **Silicone:** Bacteria and secretions do not adhere and there is minimum crusting.
- **Siliconised PVC:** It has the properties of both PVC and silicon, i.e. it is thermolabile and adjusts to tracheal wall while silicon prevents crusting.
- **Silastic:** It is soft and non-irritating, and minimizes crusting.
A. **Jackson's tracheostomy tube:** It has three parts: **outer tube, inner tube and an obturator**. Outer tube is not split, inner tube can be fixed to the shield of the outer tube by a lock. The obturator helps in the introduction of tube into the trachea. Tracheostomy tube for adults is selected by size or number of the tube. Larger the number (size) greater is the inner diameter. In adults, tubes of inner diameter varying between 6 and 9 or 10 mm can be used. Sometimes size of tube is expressed in French gauge.
B. **Fuller's tracheostomy tube:** It consists of an *outer tube and an inner tube*, the latter being slightly longer. *Outer tube is made of two blades*, which when pressed together, can be easily introduced into the tracheostomy opening. *Inner tube has a hole in the centre* so that patient can still have a chance to breathe from the larynx even when tube is blocked at its outer end.
C. **Cuffed tracheostomy tube:** With inner tube and obturator which can be disposable or non disposable. Used to obtain a closed circuit for ventilation. When cuff is inflated, it prevents aspiration of pharyngeal secretions into the trachea. It can also *prevent airleak*. It is used when there is danger of aspiration of pharyngeal secretions as in unconscious patient or when patient is put on a respirator. *Cuff should be deflated every 2 hours for 5 minutes to prevent damage to trachea*. Now-a-days, tubes with two cuffs are available and inflation of the cuff can be alternated to avoid pressure of cuff at one point.
D. **Percutaneous Dilatational Tracheostomy (PDT) Set**
   Components:
   1. Ciaglia Blue Rhino G2 percutaneous tracheostomy dilator with preloaded guiding catheter
   2. 0.052 inch diameter wire guide with positioning marks
   3. Tracheostomy tube loading dilator
   4. 15 gage, 5 cm introducer needle
   5. 15 gage, 7 cm FEP sheath needle
   6. 14.0 Fr, 4.5 cm dilator
   7. Disposable #15 scalpel
   8. Disposable syringe

Tonsillectomy	
Absolute indications	**Relative indications**
<ul><li>Recurrent attack of tonsillitis (>6 episodes per year or 3 episodes/year for 2 years or longer)</li><li>**Quincy** (Peritonsillar abscess)</li><li>Tonsillitis causing upper airways obstruction (**sleep apnoea**)</li><li>Suspected malignancy</li><li>Craniofacial growth abnormalities</li><li>**Adenoid- tonsillar hypertrophy** associated with: Cor pulmonale, Failure to thrive, Dysphagia, Speech abnormalities</li><li>Tonsillitis associated with abscessed cervical nodes</li></ul>	<ul><li>Diphtheria carriers who do not response to antibiotics.</li><li>Streptococcus carriers</li><li>Chronic tonsillitis that is unresponsive to medical therapy and is associated with: Halitosis, Persistent sore throat, Tender cervical adenitis</li><li>Recurrent streptococcal tonsillitis with valvular heart disease</li></ul>
Contraindications of tonsillectomy	
<ul><li>Hemoglobin level less than **10 g%**</li><li>Presence of **acute infection** in upper respiratory tract, even acute tonsillitis. Bleeding is more in the presence of acute infection.</li><li>**Children under 3 years** of age. They are at poor surgical risks.</li><li>Overt or submucous **cleft palate**.</li><li>Bleeding disorders, e.g. leukemia, purpura, aplastic anemia, hemophilia.</li><li>**At the time of epidemic of polio**.</li><li>**Uncontrolled systemic disease**, e.g. diabetes, cardiac disease, hypertension or asthma.</li><li>Tonsillectomy is avoided during the period of **menses.**</li></ul>	

Types of Hemorrhages after Tonsillectomy			
	Primary	**Reactionary**	**Secondary**
Time frame	Intraoperative	**Within 24 hours post-op**	**After 24 hrs.** usually seen between the 5th to 10th post-op day
Causes	Injury to blood vessels	Presence of clot preventing clipping of superior constrictor muscle	Sepsis and premature separation of the membrane
Treatment	Pressure, ligation or electrocoagulation	Removal of the clot, application of pressure or vasoconstrictor. Ligation or electrocoagulation under general anaesthesia	Removal of clot, topical application of dilute adrenaline or H_2O_2 with pressure usually suffice. For profuse bleeding, electrocoagulation or ligation under GA. Approximation of pillar with mattress sutures. External carotid ligation Transfusion of blood or plasma, depending on blood loss. **Systemic antibiotics**.

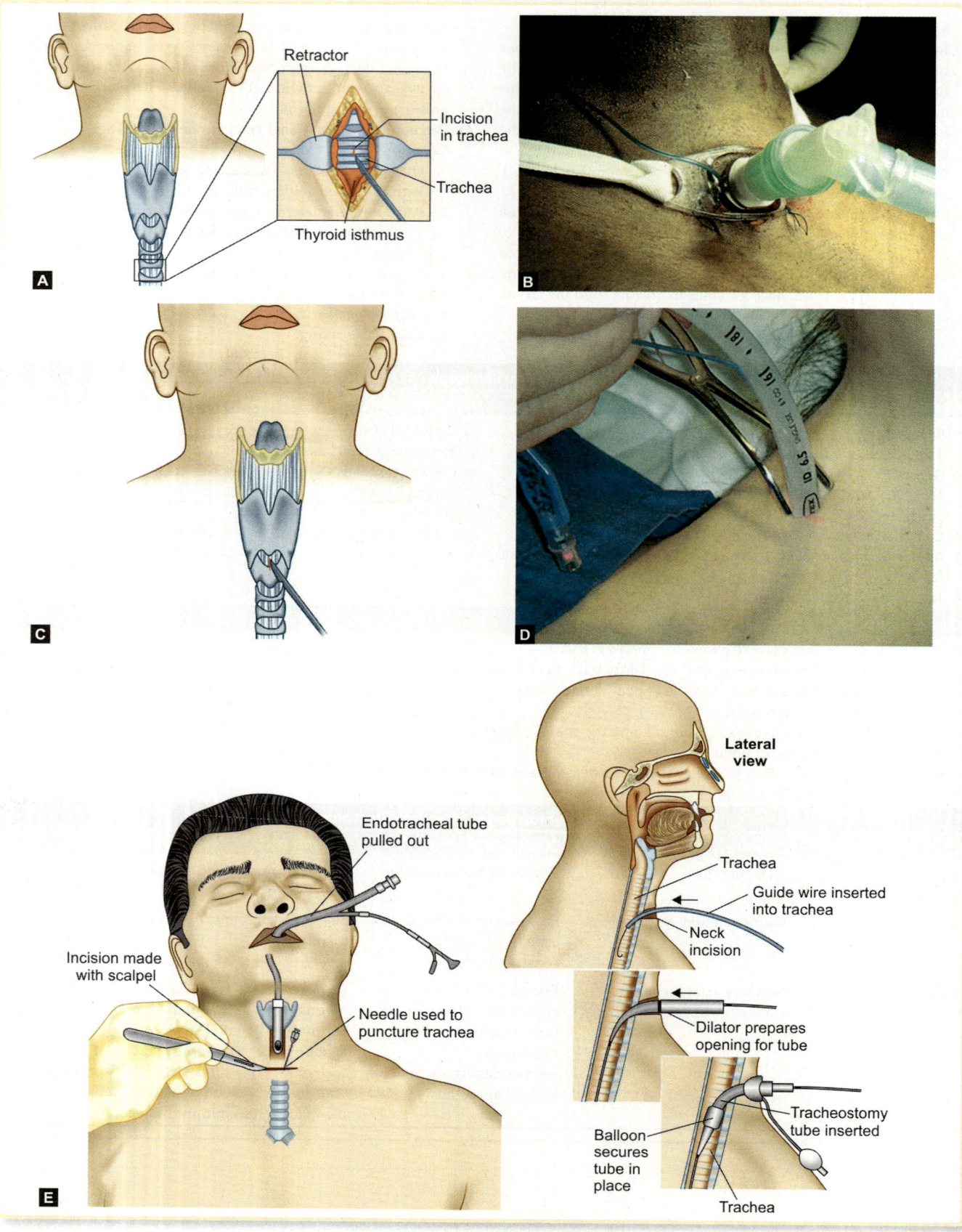

F

G

KEY

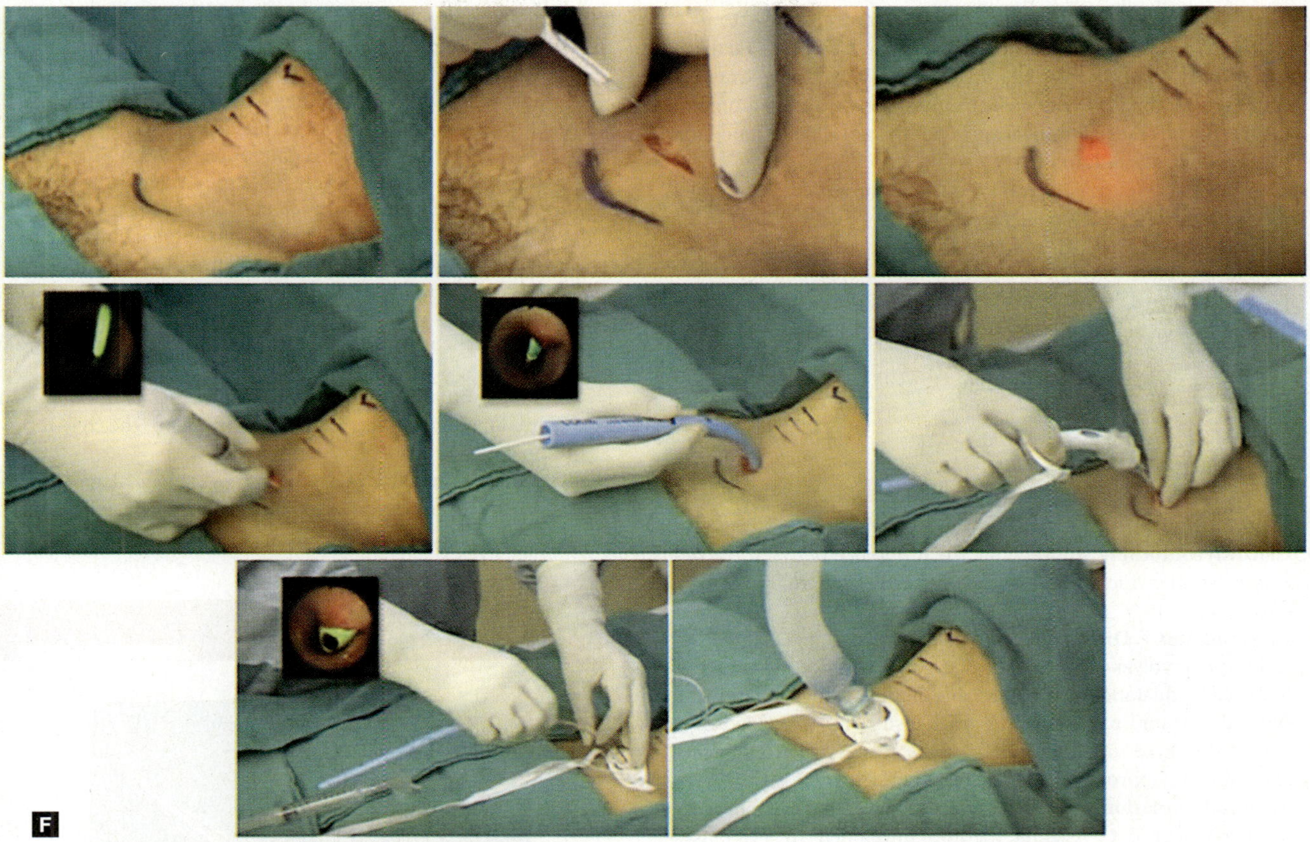

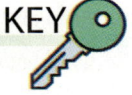

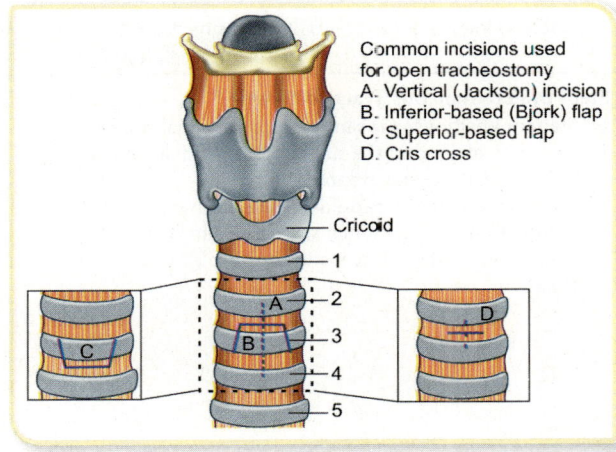

TRACHEOSTOMY PROCEDURE

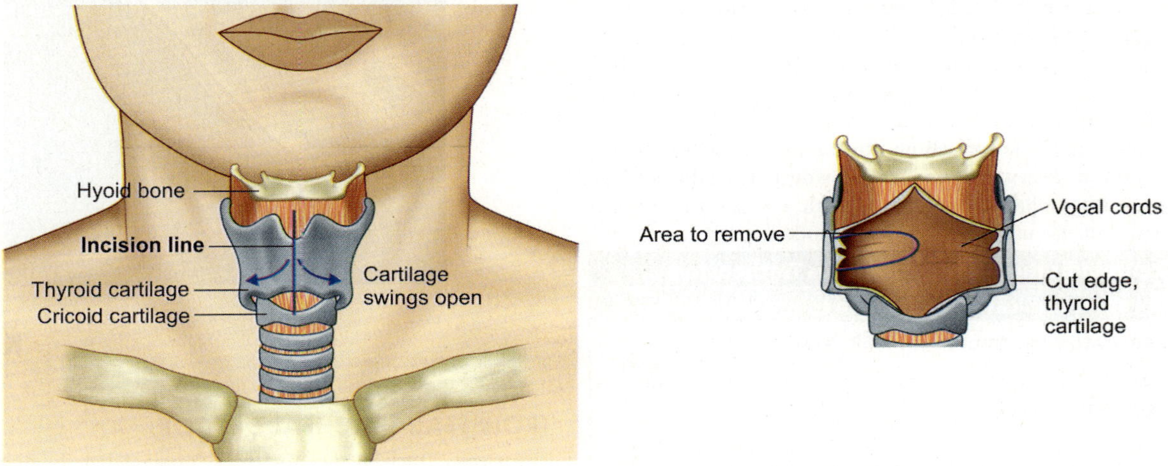

A. **Tracheostomy incision** midway between sternal notch and cicoid cartilage over the 2-3 tracheal ring. Several types of incisions can be made on trachea, but most common are vertical or cruciate.

B. **Tracheostomy stoma:** Note the difference from the cricothyroidotomy stomy which is higher up than the tracheostomy stoma
C. **Cricothyroidotomy incision** between the thyroid cartilage and cricoid cartilage over the cricothyroid membrane. Surgical cricothyroidotomy provides a definitive airway (a cuffed tube in the trachea) if tracheal intubation is not possible. Technique for a surgical cricothyroidotomy is:
   1. Using a scalpel, make a transverse skin incision, then carefully incise through the cricoid membrane.
   2. Enlarge the hole using artery forceps or the handle of the scalpel, rotate through 90 degrees.
   3. Insert a size 6 cuffed tracheal or tracheostomy tube.
   4. Inflate the cuff, check the position and ventilate.

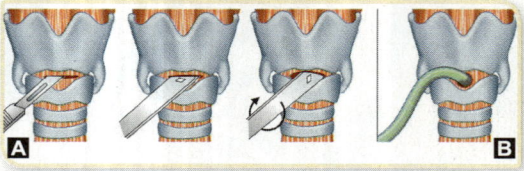

D. **Cricothyroidotomy stoma:** Note the difference between tracheostomy stoma which is lower down compared to Cricothyroidotomy stoma.
E. **Percutaneous Dilatational Tracheostomy (PDT):** PDT technique involves introduction of a guide wire into the trachea followed by dilatation using a variable diameter single dilator (the Blue Rhino) and passage of the tracheostomy tube loaded over one of the three loading dilators. More specifically, the devices allow for two approaches to the dilation of the stoma:
   1. **Serial dilation (Ciaglia Percutaneous Tracheostomy Introducer Set):** Ciaglia method developed in 1985 uses graded dialators. Serial dilation is achieved using numerous progressively larger dilators. Kit contains three soft loading dilators of varying outer diameters (OD), i.e. 21F (7 mm), 24F (8 mm) and 28F (9.3 mm). Cook Ciaglia percutaneous tracheostomy devices are sold sterile for single use.
   2. **Single-stage dilation (Blue Rhino and Blue Rhino G2 Advanced Percutaneous Tracheostomy Introducer Set):** Single-stage dilation is achieved with a single rhino-horn-shaped dilator using an in-and-out motion.

Contraindications of Percutaneous Tracheostomy	
Absolute contraindications	**Relative contraindications**
☐ Emergency tracheostomy	☐ PEEP value > 20
☐ In pediatric (Children younger than 12 years)	☐ Uncorrected coagulopathies
☐ Midline neck mass	☐ Infection near the intended site of tracheostomy
☐ Non intubated patients	☐ Difficult to palpate anatomical landmarks
☐ Unstable spine fracture	☐ Previous neck surgery distorting the anatomy

F. **Steps of Percutaneous Tracheostomy:**
   1. Patient positioning is same as in traditional tracheostomy.
   2. Anatomical landmarks are marked and local anesthetic is infiltrated at the site of incision.
   3. Transverse skin incision is made midway between cricoid cartilage and sternal notch same as traditional tracheostomy.
   4. Curved hemostatic forceps is used for blunt dissection of the tissue.
   5. Bronchoscope is inserted through the ET tube and advanced until the light of the bronchoscope illuminates the incision site.
   6. A 15 gauge introducer needle is inserted at the incision site under direct visualization of the bronchoscope.
   7. Needle is removed and guidewire is introduced through the outer catheter to the level of carina.
   8. The sheath is then removed and replaced by 14 Fr introducer dilator or the Blue Rhino dilator under bronchoscopic visualization depending on which technique is used.
   9. When stoma is enough dilated, the blue rhino dilator is replaced by the Tracheostomy tube mounted over the dilator, through the guidewire catheter, under direct bronchoscopic visualization.
   10. When Tracheostomy tube is at place, the blue dilator, guiding catheter and J wire are removed.
   11. Inner cannula is then inserted and cuff is inflated, and ventilator tubing can be connected. And the ET tube is removed.
G. **Laryngofissure incision:** Given over thyroid cartilage, done for accessing the inner part of larynx like in case of Laryngectomy.

 **ENT PLATE 6**

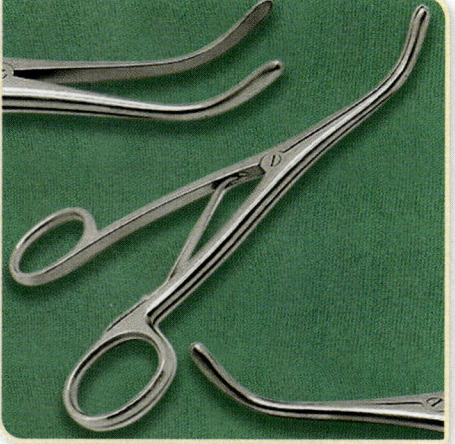

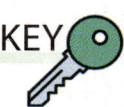 KEY

TROUSSEAU TRACHEAL DILATOR

Trousseau Tracheal Dilator is a non-ratcheted, single spring, finger ring instrument used to widen a tracheal incision to dilate the tracheostoma during or after the tracheostomy to insert the tracheostomy tube. It allows easier introduction of the tracheostomy tube and prevents formation of a false passage.

Feature	Tracheal dilator	Artery Forceps
Pressing the handle of the instrument	Opens the prongs	Closes the prongs
Ratchet	Absent	Present
Inner aspect serrations	Absent	Present

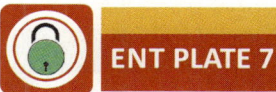

ENT PLATE 7

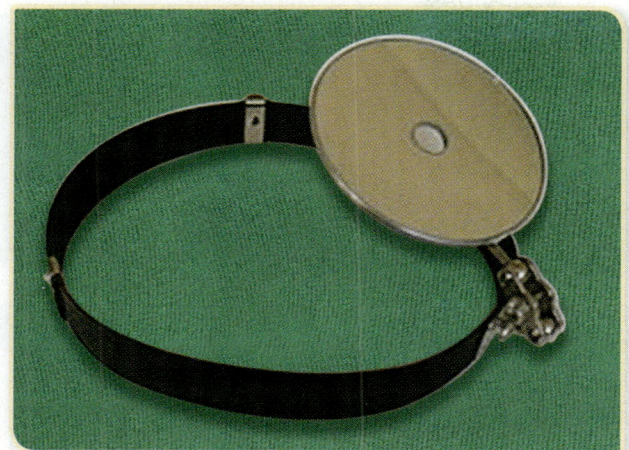

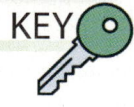

HEAD MIRROR
When parallel rays of light from the Bull's lamp falls on the concave mirror, the light rays converge at the focal point of the mirror. The advantage of wearing this head mirror is that it keeps both hands free for procedures. However, the head has to be kept fixed.

Parts
It consists of a plastic headband to which is attached adjustable concave mirror with a central hole. The diameter of the mirror is 9 cm while that of the central aperture is 2 cm and the focal length of the mirror is approximately 18 cm.

ENT PLATE 8

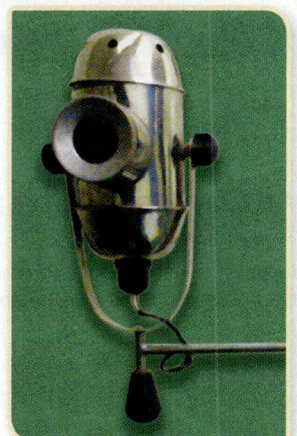

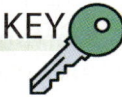

BULL'S LAMP
It consists of a metal box with vents within which is kept a 100 Watt bulb. The light rays come out through a central opening. This opening has a biconvex lens of approximately 30 to 40 cm focal length. The lamp is placed 30 cm behind the left ear of the patient. The lamp can be adjusted to focus the rays on the head mirror.

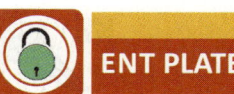

ENT PLATE 9

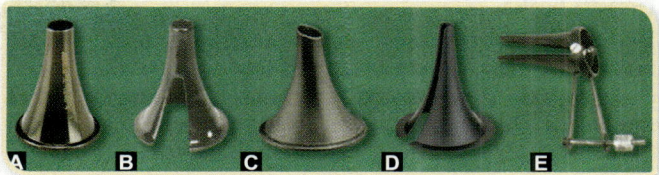

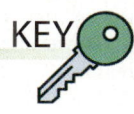

AURAL SPECULUM
A. **Hartmann aural speculum:** This is a funnel shaped speculum that has no slit on the body. The broader end is thickened for better grip.
B. **Rosen aural speculum:** This is an aural speculum with an incomplete slit on its body. The slit is useful for injections on the external canal wall with the speculum in place
C. **Shea aural speculum:** This aural speculum resembles Hartmann aural speculum. However, the narrow end of this speculum is beveled (angled)
D. **Tumarkin aural speculum:** This aural speculum has a complete split on its body to facilitate intra-aural injections into the external canal.
E. **Holmgren adjustable aural speculum-** This is a self-retaining adjustable aural speculum with a screw. Used for examination of ear and ear surgeries.

How to use this Instrument?
The pinna has to be pulled upward, backward and outwards in case of adults. It has to be pulled downwards and outwards in case of children.

Uses
Diagnostic: To examine the external auditory canal and tympanic membrane.
Therapeutic:
- Aural toileting is done through a speculum in case of CSOM.
- Removal of foreign body/wax etc.
- Operative: Used in - a. Myringotomy, b. Myringoplasty, c. Stapedectomy.
- Can be used as dilator in stenosis of external canal.

ENT PLATE 10

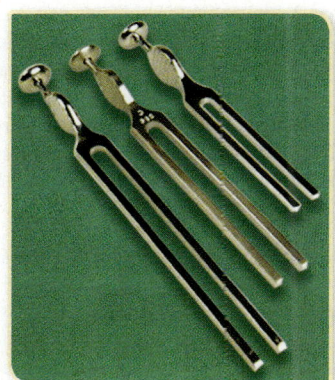

Tuning Forks

Tuning fork test is frequently done to test the type and degree the hearing loss. The tuning fork is struck at the junction of upper one-third and lower two-third of the prongs. The vibrating tuning fork with the prongs is placed at a distance of 2.5 cm from the auricle for air conduction. The vibrating tuning fork is then placed with the base touching the mastoid process for bone conduction. It is available in various frequencies—128, 256, 512 and 1024.

However, 512 Hz tuning fork is commonly used for the following reasons:
- It is present in the mid speech frequency range
- Overtones are minimal
- Sound is more auditory than tactile in nature
- Tone decay is optimal.

ENT PLATE 11

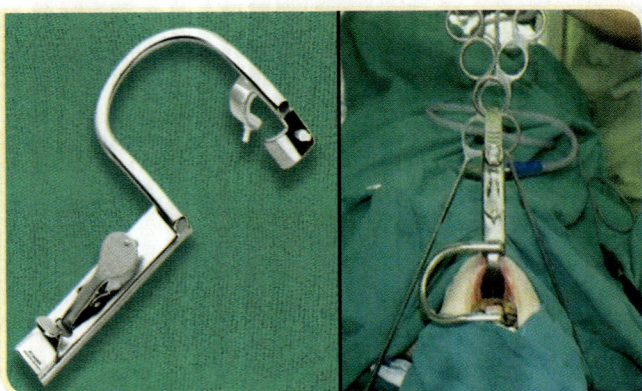

BOYLE-DAVIS MOUTH GAG

History
Griffith Davis started using the mouth gag to perform tonsillectomies. British Anesthesiologist Henry Boyle carried out minor modifications in mouth gag and started using it extensively. Hence the name Boyle -Davis mouth gag.

Parts
The instrument has 2 components i.e. Davis gag, a frame that serves to hold the mouth open and the Boyle tongue depressor to hold the tongue down. It has a set of 3-4 tongue blades of varying sizes. The size of the blade chosen varies from patient to patient. The rough size of the blade should not exceed the distance from the angle of the mandible and the chin of the patient. It can be stabilized using a M jack or Draffin pod allowing the surgeon to have both hands free.

Uses
Tonsillectomy, Adenoidectomy, Pharyngoplasty, Palate surgery.

> **Note**
> It cannot be used in Tongue surgery as it is depressed.

ENT PLATE 12

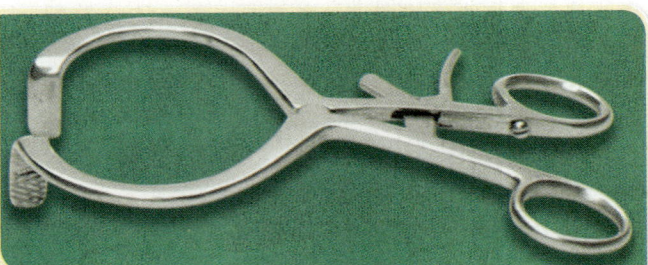

DOYEN MOUTH'S GAG

Used to keep mouth open for intraoral surgery when retraction of the tongue is not required or desirable.

Mostly used for tongue surgery. It is applied on one side of the mouth on molar teeth.

ENT PLATE 13

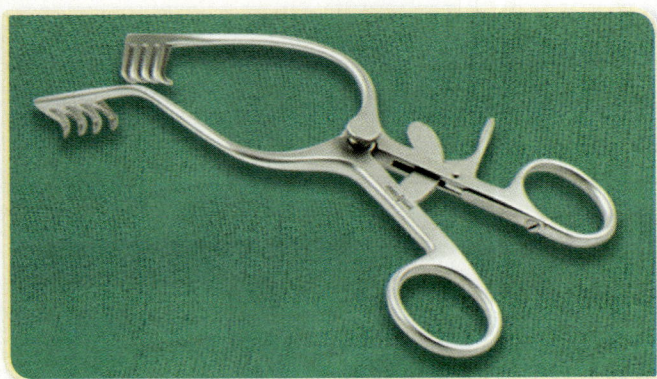

MOLLISON SELF-RETAINING HEMOSTATIC MASTOID RETRACTOR

This is a self-retaining mastoid retractor with two prongs of equal size and on either 4-teeth on each prong. It has a ratchet and mechanism to anchor the prongs in a set position.

Uses
- Harvesting temporalis fascia
- Mastoidectomy, tympanoplasty
- In head and neck surgeries like tracheostomy and laryngofissure

Advantages
- Allows the surgeon to have both hands free.
- Retracts the soft tissue away from the surgical field.
- Has a hemostatic effect because it firmly holds the soft tissue and skin apart.

ENT PLATE 14

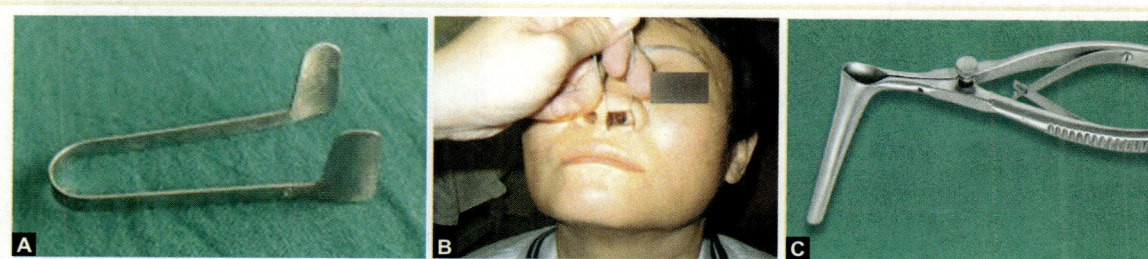

NASAL SPECULUM

A. **Thudicum nassal speculum:** It is a self-retaining nasal speculum.
   Uses: a. Diagnostic: Anterior rhinoscopy—nasal septum, Little's area, lateral wall of nose, nasal cavity b. Therapeutic: removal of foreign bodies, antral wash, nasal packing, surgical procedures inside the nose like polypectomy, SMR, septoplasty.
B. **How to use Thudicum Nasal Speculum:** It is held over the hooked index finger of the non-dominant hand. The blades are then closed by pressing between middle and ring finger and then blades are opened into the nasal cavity.
C. **Killian's Nasal Speculum:** This is a self-retaining nasal speculum and is available with blades of different sizes. The distance between the blades can be adjusted and fixed with a screw. Uses are similar as Thudicum nasal speculum.

ENT PLATE 15

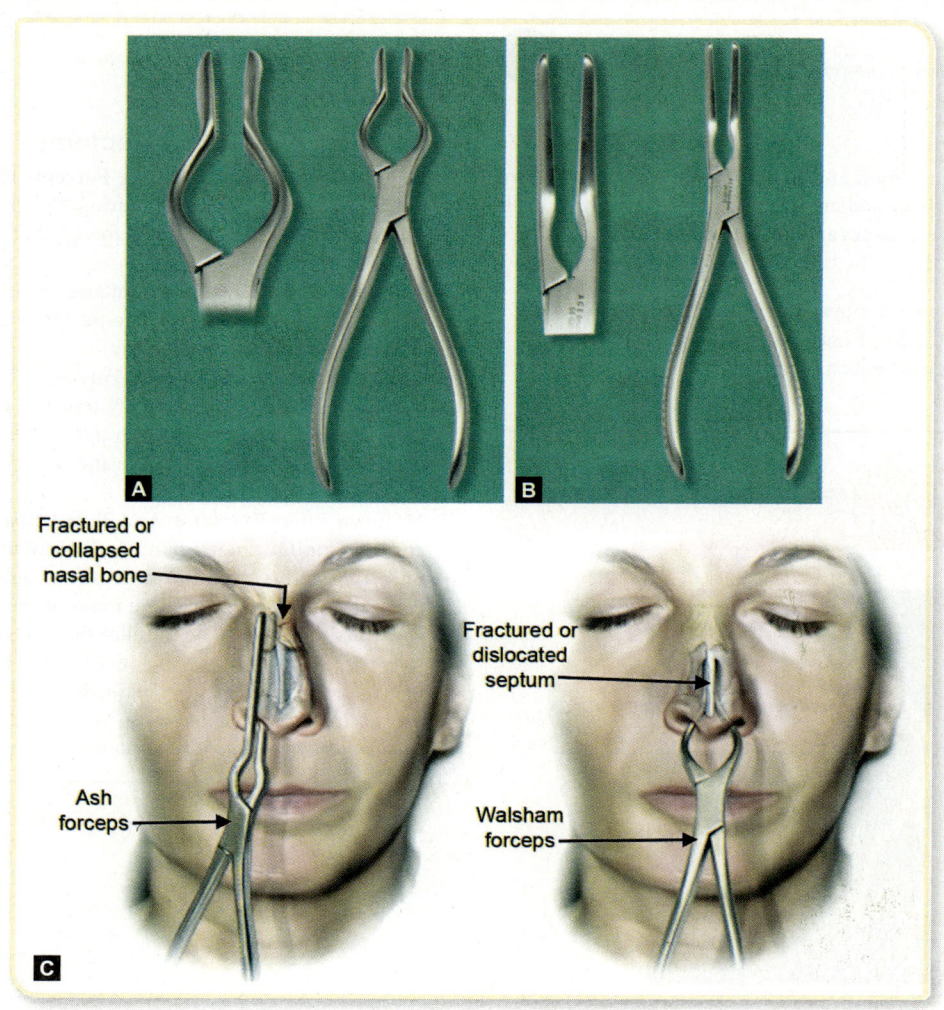

WALSHAM AND ASCH FORCEPS

A. Walsham Septum-Straightening Forceps
B. Asch septum forceps

Asch forceps	Walsham's forceps
Curved blades	Straight blades
Gap seen between prongs on approximation	No gap seen between prongs on approximation
Used to elevate and straighten the septum	Used to refracture and realign the nasal bone

C. Use of both Asch and Walsham forceps

ENT PLATE 16

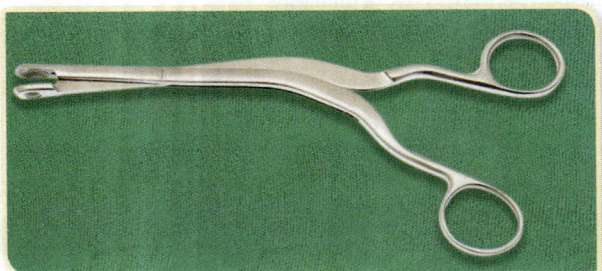

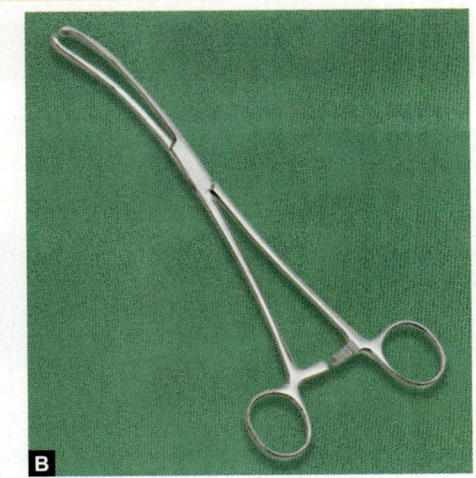

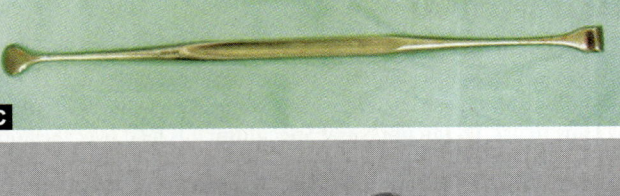

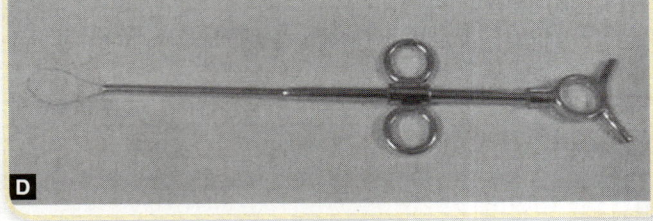

LUC FORCEPS

This forceps has a screw joint and has a fenestrated tip with sharp blades that grasp the tissue and cut it. Hence, this forceps is suitable for biopsy of various soft tissues and delicate bone.

Uses

- SMR or septoplasty for removal of cartilage and bone
- Polypectomy and Caldwell-Luc operation
- Edge biopsy from oral cavity and oropharynx
- Turbinectomy

ENT PLATE 17

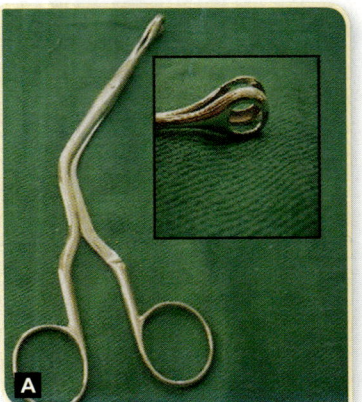

Instruments Used in Tonsillectomy

A. **Dennis Brown Tonsil Holding Forceps:** It is used to hold the tonsil and pull it medially during the process of dissection. This instrument resembles Luc forceps but differs from it in the following:
   - The edges of the jaw are blunt and do not cut tissue.
   - The upper jaw is smaller than the lower jaw.
   - The tip has a box mechanism.
B. **Colver Tonsil Pillar Grasping Forceps:** This instrument is also used to hold the (upper pole of) tonsil to pull it medially prior to dissection. It can be both straight or curved. It is especially useful where the tonsil is friable and the grip cannot be changed repeatedly.
C. **Mollison Pillar Retractor And Tonsil Dissector:** It has a blunt end used for initial non traumatic dissection of tonsil and another retracting end is used to retract the anterior pillar to look for bleeding points and left behind tonsillar tissue.
D. **Eve Tonsillar Snare:** The tonsillar snare has a 28-gauge stainless-steel wire whicvh is usually 3 inches long. It is used to snare the lower pole of the tonsil after dissection. The lower pole is crushed on snaring and thromboplastin is released which is a powerful vasoconstrictor. Hence, it has both cutting and crushing action.

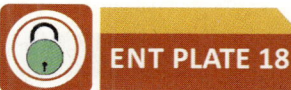

ENT PLATE 18

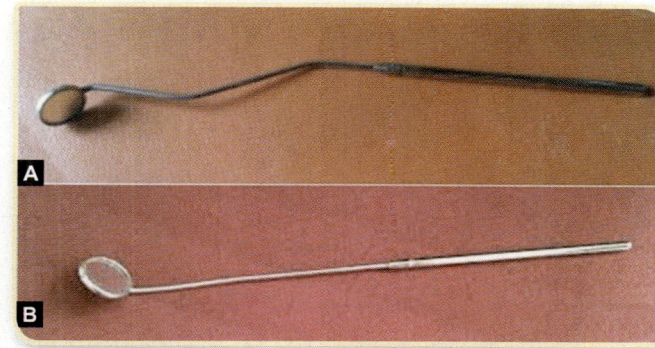

RHINOSCOPY AND LARYNGOSCOPY MIRROR

A. **St. Clair Thompson posterior rhinoscopy mirror:** This instrument has a bayonet shaped, curved handle (hence differs from indirect laryngoscopy mirror) designed so that the examiner's hand does not block his vision. The mirror is available in sizes of 0 to 5. It is a plain mirror and does not magnify the image. The mirror surface is either heated or dipped in Savlon in order to prevent fogging during the procedure. The tongue is depressed gently with a tongue depressor and this mirror is introduced inside like a pen with the mirror facing upwards.

Uses: Posterior rhinoscopy to examine the postnasal space after adenoidectomy to look for remnants if any

B. **Indirect laryngoscopy mirror:** This instrument has a straight handle, shaft and a plain mirror at an angle. The focal length of this mirror is at infinity. The mirror is available in various sizes ranging from 8 mm to 30 mm. The tongue is held with a dry gauze piece with the left hand. The handle of the mirror is held like a pen. The patient is asked to breathe through the mouth. The patient is asked to phonate 'eee' for observing vocal cord adduction and is asked to breathe gently for observing vocal cord abduction.

Uses

- For examination of tongue base, valleculae, glossoepiglottic fold, pharyngoepiglottic fold, arytenoids, aryepiglottic folds, ventricular bands, vocal cords, interarytenoid region, pyriform fossae and posterior pharyngeal wall for inflammatory, benign and neoplastic lesions
- To remove small foreign bodies
- To remove tissue samples for histopathological examination

Structures not Seen in this Procedure:

- Post-cricoid region
- Apex of pyriform fossa
- Ventricles
- Undersurface of vocal cords and adjoining subglottic region
- Laryngeal surface of epiglottis

ENT PLATE 19

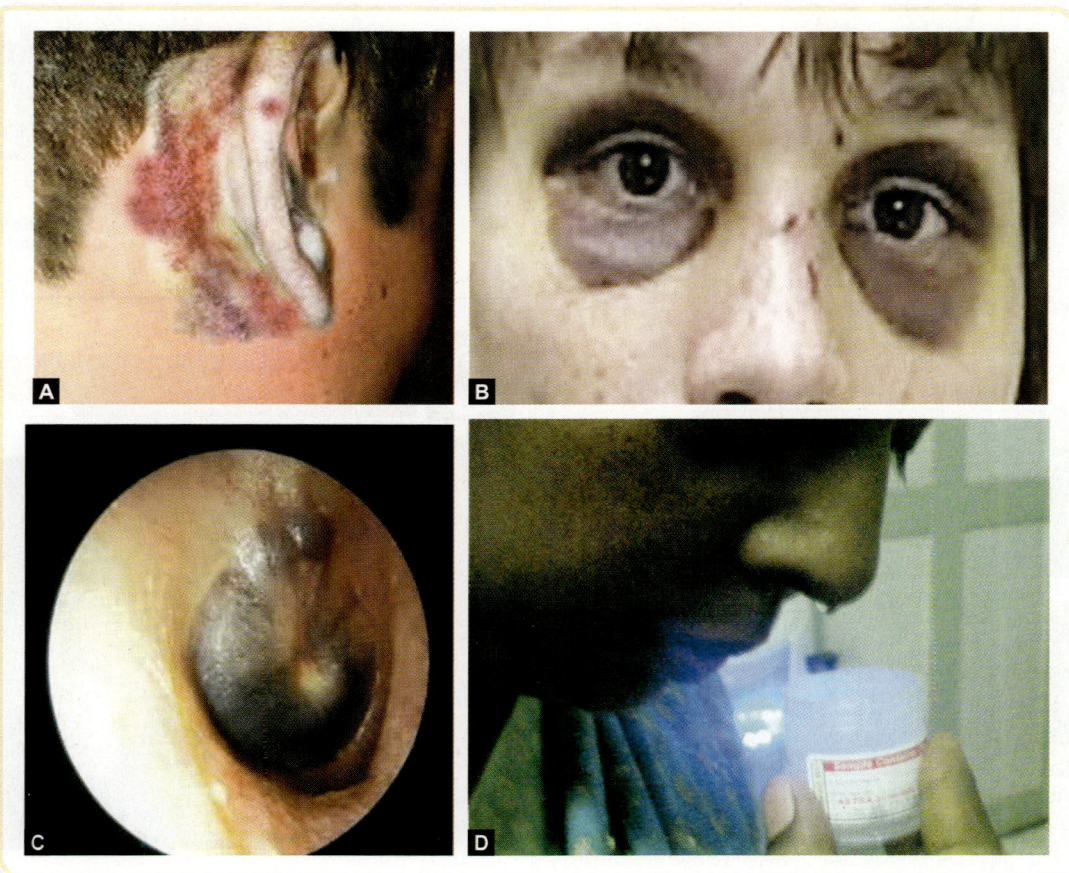

SIGNS OF BASILAR SKULL FRACTURE

Fracture through petrous portion of temporal bone
A. **Battle sign:** Post auricular hematoma[NEETPG]
B. **Raccoon eyes or Panda Bear eyes:** is due to leakage of blood from anterior fossa to the periorbital region. Absence of conjunctival injection helps to differentiate from orbital trauma.
C. **Laugier sign (Hemotympanum):** Blood in the middle ear cavity
D. **CSF Rhinorrhea (Teapot sign):** CSF leak from the nose giving appearance of a teapot. Sphenoid ostium lies anterosuperior to the sphenoid sinus. CSF leak is hence evident when patient bends forward as an increased amount of CSF gains access to the sphenoid ostium (Teapot sign)

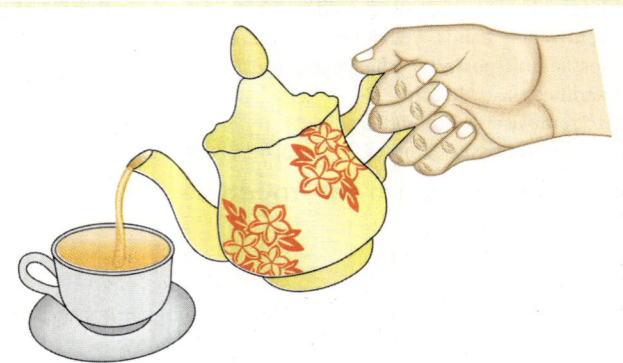

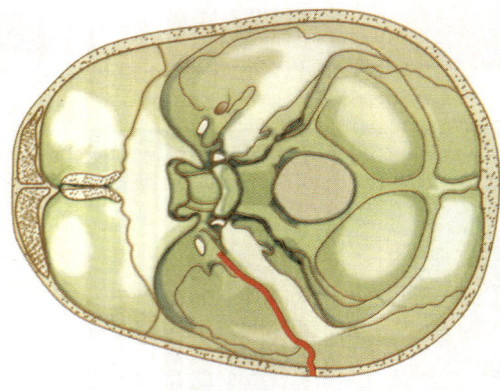

Fracture through petrous portion of temporal bone

Periorbital ecchymosis

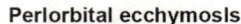

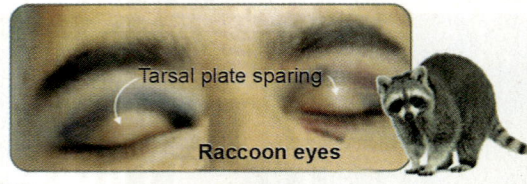

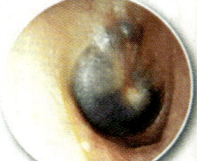
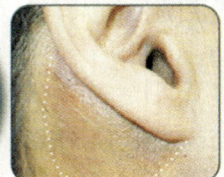
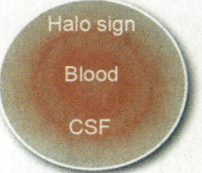

Hemotympanum — **Postauricular ecchymosis (Battle's sign)** — CSF otorrhea

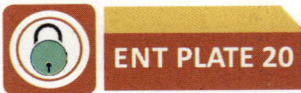

ENT PLATE 20

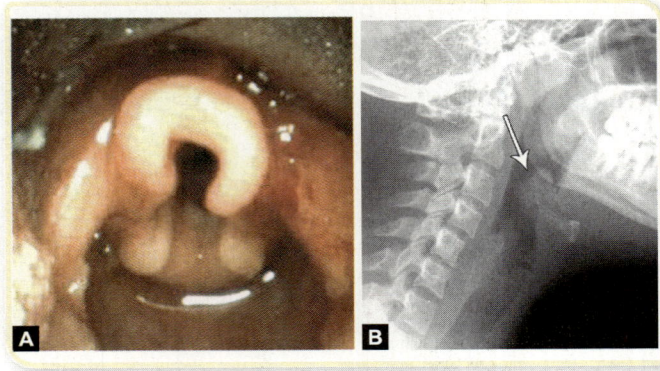

LARYNGOMALACIA

A. **Omega shaped Epiglottis in Laryngomalacia:** Laryngomalacia literally means 'abnormal softening of the larynx. Laryngomalacia may affect the epiglottis, the arytenoid cartilages, or both. It is a dynamic lesion resulting in collapse of the supraglottic structures during inspiration, leading to airway obstruction and stridor. Laryngomalacia is the most common cause of congenital stridor.
B. In Laryngomalacia or Epiglottitis lateral X-ray film, the epiglottis appears thumb shaped (rather than the usual leaf shape)

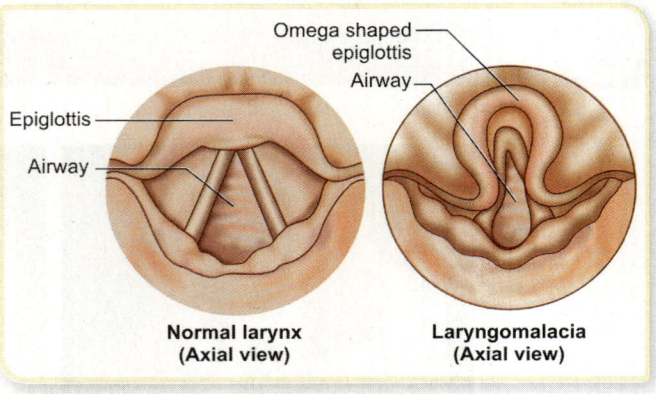

Normal larynx (Axial view) — Laryngomalacia (Axial view)

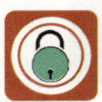

ENT PLATE 21

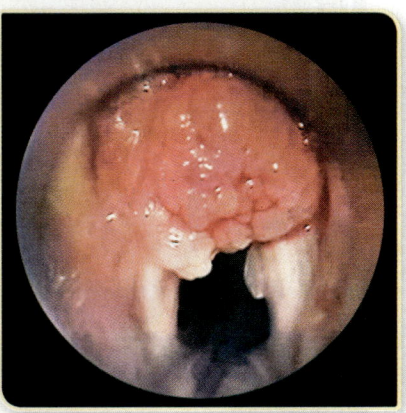

RESPIRATORY PAPILLOMATOSIS

Typical description and image is of ***respiratory papillomatosis.*** History of maternal genital infection or papillomas are frequently mentioned. Exuberant tissue resembling miniature clusters of grapes may be seen, especially on the anterior part of the true vocal folds, the false folds, and the epiglottis.

	Recurrent Respiratory Papillomatosis (RRP)
Definition	Rare condition characterized by recurrent growth of benign papillomas in the respiratory tract, most commonly in the larynx.
Essentials of diagnosis	▫ Hoarse voice ▫ Gradual onset of stridor ▫ Recurrent disease requiring multiple surgical procedures. ▫ Viral etiology
Etiology	Papillomatosis is caused by infection with human papillomavirus (HPV), the most commonly identified subtypes being **HPV-6 and HPV-11** (HPV-11 is more aggressive and more prone to malignant changes). The same HPV subtypes are responsible for genital warts, and there is a recognized association between maternal genital warts and respiratory papillomatosis.
Epidemiology	▫ Mean age ages of 2 and 5 years, but papillomas can present in any age group. ▫ There is no difference in incidence between males and females.
Risk factors	▫ The **first-born, vaginally delivered child** of a teenage mother is associated with an increased chance of developing respiratory papillomatosis. ▫ Genital Condylomas of mother during pregnancy are considered the most important risk factor for acquiring JoRRP by vertical HPV transmission from mother to child. ▫ Cesarean delivery was *not* found to be protective against respiratory papillomatosis ▫ In adults viral transmission may occur during oral sex, but this remains unproven. Re-activation of a latent HPV infection acquired in childhood is another possible cause.
Types	The disease is categorized as juvenile-onset (JoRRP) if it develops before the age of 18, and adult-onset (AoRRP) for cases that develop after the age of 18. ▫ **Juvinile onset:** because of diffuse involvement of the larynx, usually manifests in infancy or childhood as hoarseness and stridor. This form of papillomatosis is often aggressive and rapidly recurrent ▫ **Adult-onset** papillomas are occasionally solitary or at least more localized than juvenile-onset lesions and also less aggressive
Clinical features	The clinical course is highly variable, with frequent relapses, and may be lifelong. ▫ Hoarseness, abnormal cry, or both are the **most common** presenting symptoms of respiratory papillomatosis. ▫ If the disease is untreated, then a gradual progression to dyspnea, stridor, and eventually, complete airway obstruction can occur. ▫ Stridor and airway obstruction are rarely the first symptoms.
Malignant transformation	The malignant transformation from benign nonkeratinizing squamous papillomas to squamous cell carcinoma can occur in children, but is rarely seen. Malignant transformation most commonly occurs in the distal bronchopulmonary tree, and the prognosis is universally poor.
Evaluation	If the diagnosis of respiratory papillomatosis is suspected, then a histopathologic confirmation is required. At microlaryngoscopy, the papillomas are seen to be **firm, irregular, exophytic lesions** that **bleed easily** on manipulation. Examination should include tracheobronchoscopy to determine whether distal spread has occurred.
Treatment	▫ The **primary treatment modality** for respiratory papillomatosis is surgery. The aims of treatment are to maintain an adequate airway while avoiding tracheotomy, preserving the voice, and controlling the papilloma. ▫ The most widely accepted means of surgical ablation of respiratory papilloma is with the **CO2 laser.** Because respiratory papillomatosis typically requires multiple procedures to maintain the airway, there is a significant risk of scarring and web formation due to repeated thermal damage caused by the laser. For this reason, it is advisable to leave small amounts of the papilloma in sites where scarring is likely to occur, such as the anterior commissure. ▫ Other disadvantages of using the laser include destruction of the papilloma, which both precludes histologic examination and exposes the operating room staff to virus particles in the laser plume. ▫ Up to 20% of reported cases of respiratory papillomatosis are severe enough to require **tracheotomy**, although, if possible, a tracheotomy should be avoided because of the increased risk of distal spread. ▫ Several adjuvant systemic therapies are available. The risks and benefits of adjuvant therapy should be carefully considered before use. Adjuvant therapies in use or under investigation include *indole 3-carbinol, diindolymethane,* **alfa interferons, acyclovir,** *photodynamic therapy, ribavirin,* **retinoic acid,** *mumps vaccine injections,* and **cidofovir.** There is still insufficient evidence on the effectiveness of antiviral therapy. The ideal dose, frequency, and duration of cidofovir therapy are yet to be known. ▫ Maximum total dose of cidofovir should not exceed **3 mg/kg.** ▫ Due to high toxicity of cidofovir, analysis of laboratory parameters like morphology with blood smear, urea, creatinine, ALT, AST, and bilirubin levels before the treatment, 1 day and 4 weeks after the injection. All papillomas should be examined histopathologically to exclude any dysplastic features or malignant transformation.

ENT PLATE 22

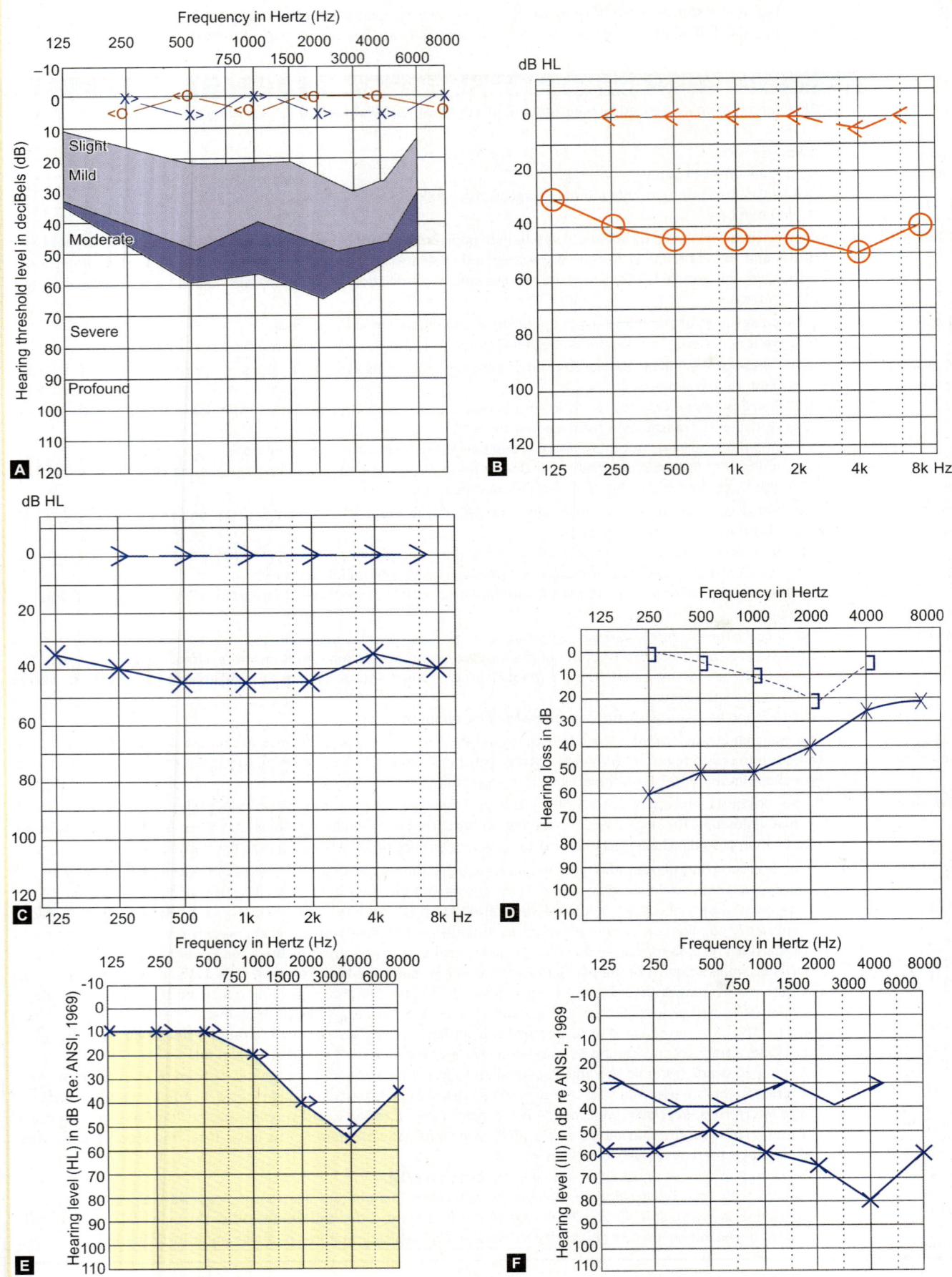

SYMBOLS USED IN AUDIOGRAM

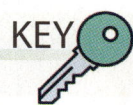

Modality	Ear	
	Right	Left
AC unmasked	○	×
BC unmasked	△	□
AC masked	<	>
BC masked	⌐	⌐
No response	○↘	×↙

Mnemonic

- For 1st and 2nd symbols remember the mnemonic: **Cross the Square from Left side**
- For 3rd and 4th symbols - Note that the Open end of symbols > and] represents the ear side.
- **Red for Right**

A. **Normal Audiogram:** The Air Bone (AB) conduction gap is less than 10-15 dB. The shaded area below the lines represents the imaginary mild moderate Hearing loss. Severe and profound hearing loss are lebelled more lower down in case the audiometric lines lies in that area. See the symbols used in audiogram above.

B. **Conductive hearing loss of Right ear:** Difference between bone conduction and air conduction is more than 20 db which tells it is conductive loss. Red color of lines on the graph and symbols tell it is right side.

C. **Conductive hearing loss of Left ear**

D. **Conductive hearing loss due to Otosclerosis**[AIIMSPG]**:** There is typically an apparent lowering in the bone conduction hearing threshold by about 5 dB at 500 Hz. 10 dB at 1000 Hz, 15-20 dB at 2000 Hz and 5 dB at 4000 Hz. This peculiar configuration in the bone conduction hearing level, most marked (i.e., notched) at 2000 Hz is termed as **CARHART'S NOTCH**. If the notch in the bone conduction level is not duplicated by the air conduction curve, then it is a true Carhart's notch.

Cumming's 5th ed: "This is not a true depression in bone conduction, but rather an artifact caused by a lack of the normal contribution of the mobile ossicular chain to bone conduction. This depression improves after the mobility of the ossicular chain is restored, e.g. after stapedectomy"

E. **Sensory neural hearing loss:** There is no air bone gap and both air conduction and bone conduction have come down. Hence it is sensory neural loss. Blue color and symbols tell it is left side. Carhart's notch must be differentiated from **Boiler's notch** which is due to noise induced hearing loss. Boiler's notch is seen at 4 khz and is seen both in air conduction as well as bone conduction, in contrast to Carhart's notch which is seen at 2 khz and is only seen in bone conduction.

F. **Mixed hearing loss:** There is air bone gap more than 20 dB and bone conduction has also come down. Color and symbols indicate left side.

ENT PLATE 23

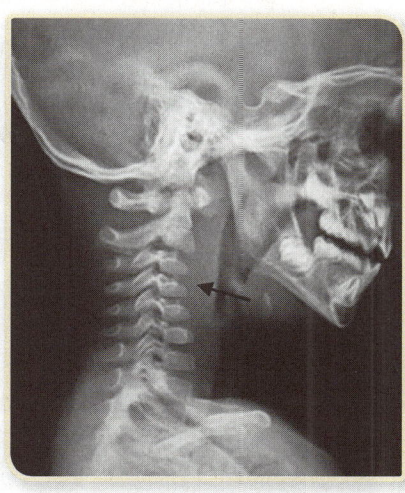

RETROPHARYNGEAL ABSCESS X-RAY

Widening of the prevertebral space and sometimes air fluid levels within. Next flexion and Head extension is the natural position in retropharyngeal abscess with straightening of the cervical spine **(Ramrod's Spine)**

ENT PLATE 24

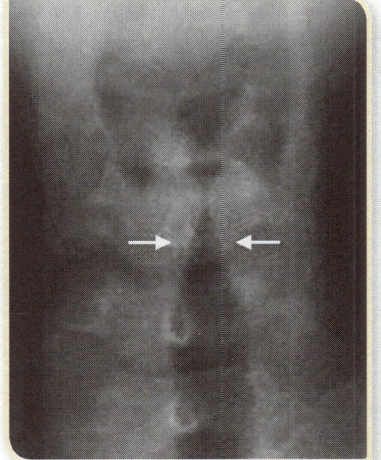

THE STEEPLE SIGN (WINE BOTTLE SIGN)[NEETPG]

Refers to the tapering of the upper trachea on a frontal chest radiograph resembling a church steeple. The appearance is suggestive of laryngotracheobronchitis or croup.

ENT PLATE 25

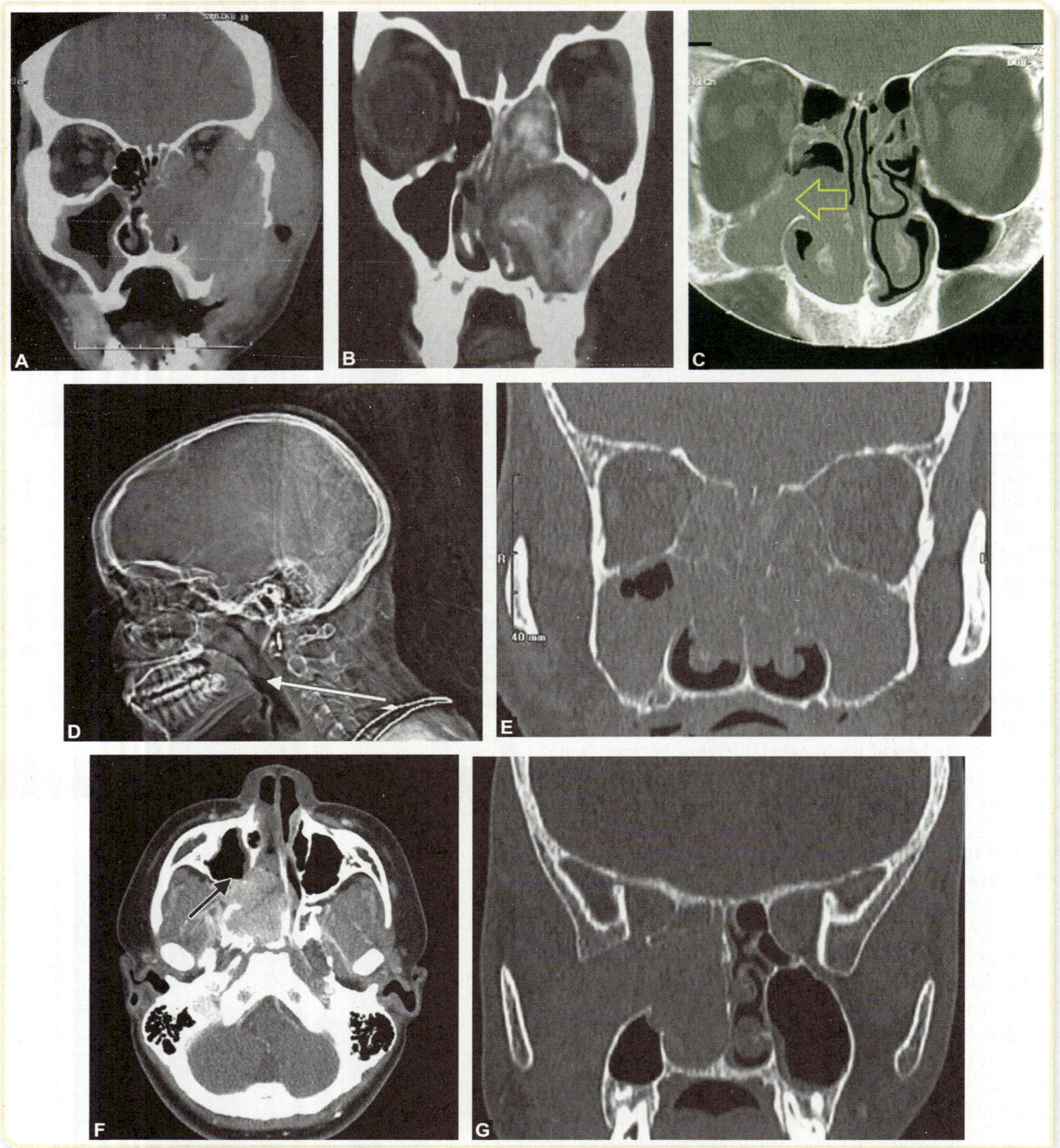

CT SCAN PNS

A. Maxillary Carcinoma will show extensive destruction but the lesion will not be heterogenous, with possible destruction of outer wall. Invasion of orbital cavities and opposite side cavities should be noted. Age, if given is a great help in diagnosis but not confirmatory. If bony destruction is absent carcinoma is essentially ruled out.

B. Fungal sinusitis: Heterogeneous lesion, evidence of destruction present, but not as extensive as in carcinoma. Outer wall of maxilla is usually preserved. Orbital cavities are usually not involved.

C. Ethmoidal polyps: Usually bilateral, homogenous mass, no bone destruction, all sinuses involved.

D. Antrochoanal polyp: Homogenous mass, usually unilateral. Maxillary ostium may be widened (arrow), this is not bone destruction. No evidence of bone destruction. All cavity outlines are well preserved.

E. Dodd/Crescent sign in Antrochoanal polyp: Crescent of air between the mass and posterior pharyngeal wall. This sign is positive in AC polyp but negative in Juvenile Nasopharyngeal Angiofibroma.

F. The Holman-Miller sign (also called the **antral sign**) is seen in juvenile nasopharyngeal angiofibroma; it refers to the anterior bowing of the posterior wall of the maxillary antrum as seen on a lateral skull radiograph or cross-sectional imaging.

G. Hondousa Sign in Juvenile Nasopharyngeal Angiofibroma: JNA with infratemporal involvement shows widening of space between ramus of mandible and maxillary body (Hondousa et al. 1954).

ENT PLATE 26

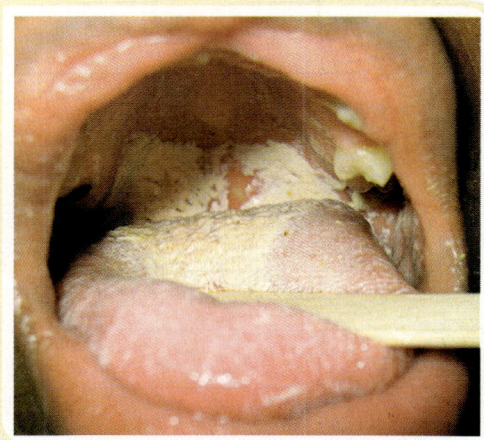

PERITONSILLAR ABSCESS (QUINSY)

Peritonsillar abscess (Quinsy) is a collection of pus in the peritonsillar space. Peritonsillar space lies between the capsule of tonsil and the superior constrictor muscle.
1. The tonsil, pillars and soft palate on the involved side are congested and swollen. Tonsil itself may not appear enlarged as it gets buried in the oedematous pillars
2. Uvula is swollen and oedematous and pushed to the opposite side.
3. Bulging of the soft palate and anterior pillar above the tonsil.
4. Mucous may be seen covering the tonsillar region.
5. Cervical lymphadenopathy is commonly seen. This involves jugulodigastric lymph nodes.

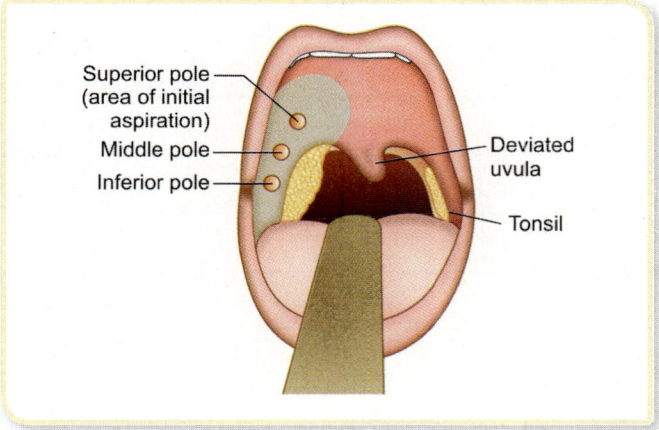

FIG: Illustration of peritonsillar abscess/quinsy

ORAL THRUSH[NEETPG]

Clinical photograph showing typical presentation of oral thrush (white curdy patches in dorsum of tongue). When gently scraped off, these patches reveal inflamed tissue that tends to bleed easily. Beginning on the tongue, the creamy white spots can spread to the gums, palate, tonsils, throat, and elsewhere. The causative organism is the yeast like fungus *Candida albicans*.

ENT PLATE 27

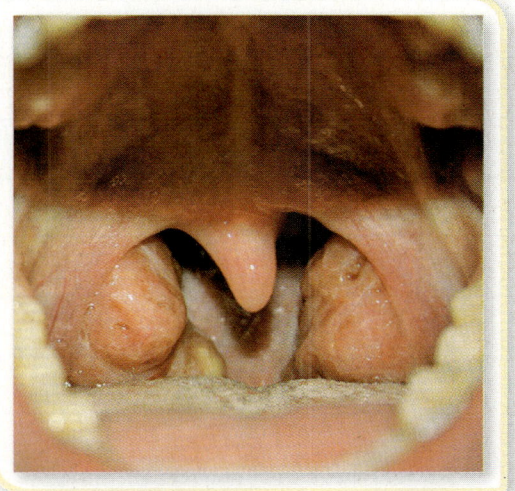

Notes

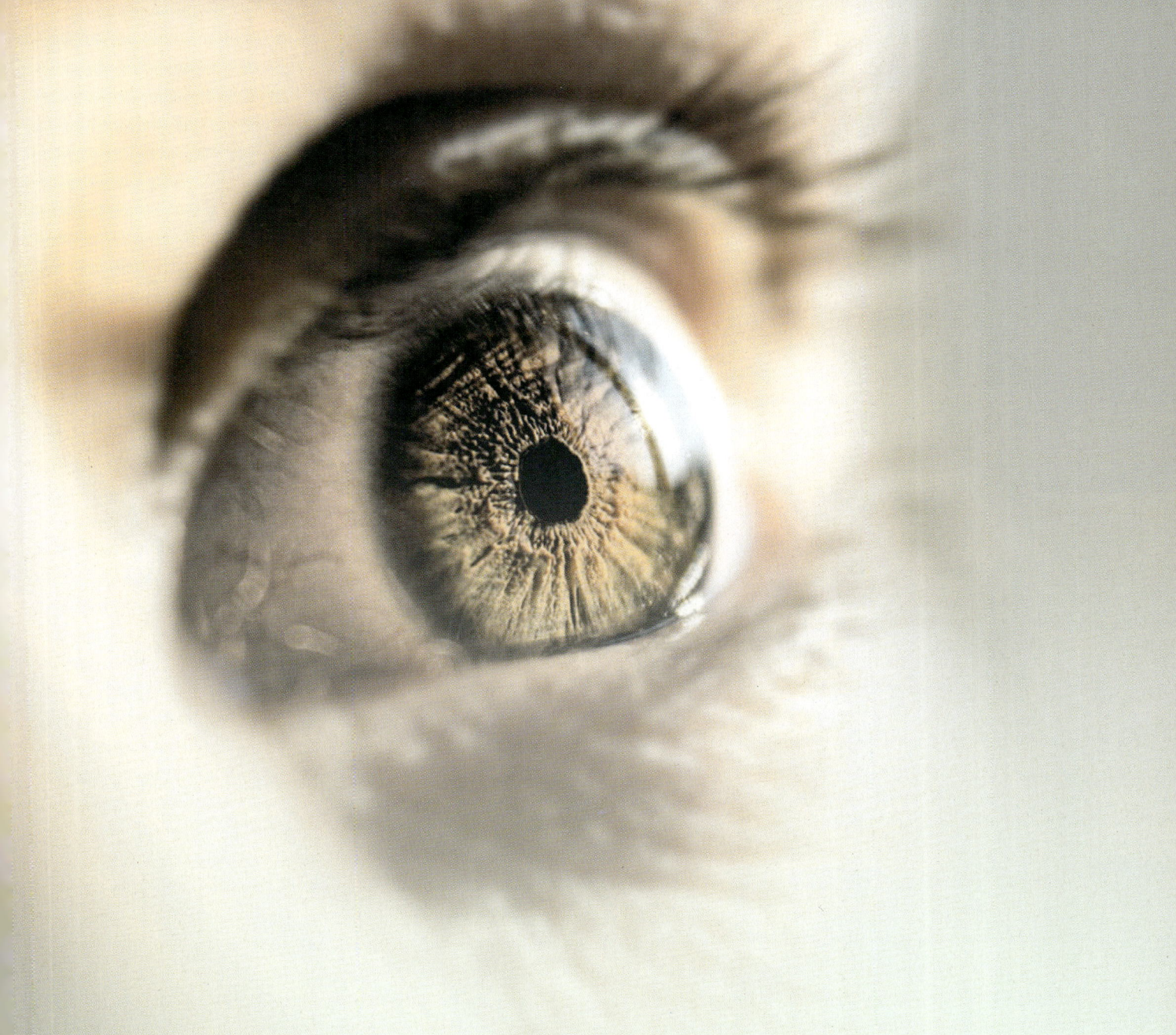

OPHTHALMOLOGY

OPHTHAL PLATE 1

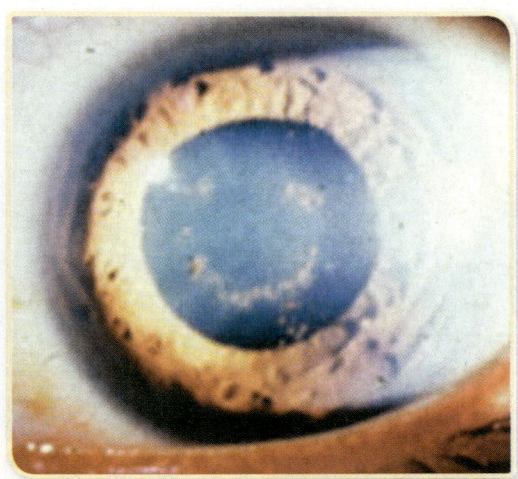

VOSSIUS RING

Vossius ring is deposition of iris pigment on the **anterior lens capsule** when the posterior surface of iris is forced against the anterior lens capsule due to **blunt trauma.** The iris pigment is deposited in a circular fashion.

OPHTHAL PLATE 2

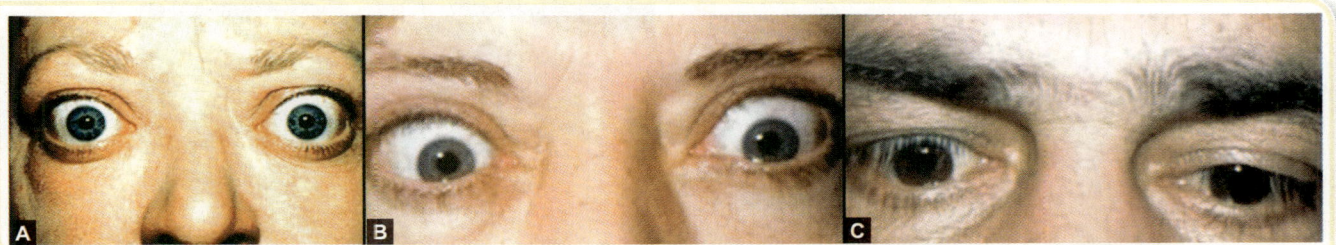

Source: Wikimedia commons-Jonathan Trobe, M.D. – University of Michigan Kellogg Eye Center

LID RETRACTION SIGNS OF GRAVE'S OPHTHALMOPATHY

A. **Dalrymple's sign:** Retraction of the upper/lower lids in primary gaze. Retraction of upper and lower lids occurs in about **50%** of patients with Graves' disease. The upper lid margin normally rests 2 mm below the limbus. Lid retraction is suspected when the margin is either level with or above the superior limbus, allowing sclera to be visible (scleral show) Likewise, the lower eyelid normally rests at the inferior limbus; retraction is suspected when sclera shows below the limbus. Lid retraction may occur in isolation or in association with proptosis, which exaggerates its severity.
B. **Kocher sign:** Describes a staring and frightened appearance of the eyes, which is particularly marked on attentive fixation
C. **Lid lag/von Graefe's sign:** Signifies retarded descent of the upper lid on down gaze. When globe is moved downward, the upper lid lags behind
- Difficulty in eversion of upper lid (**Gifford's sign**)
- **Infrequent blinking (Stellwag's sign)**

OPHTHAL PLATE 3

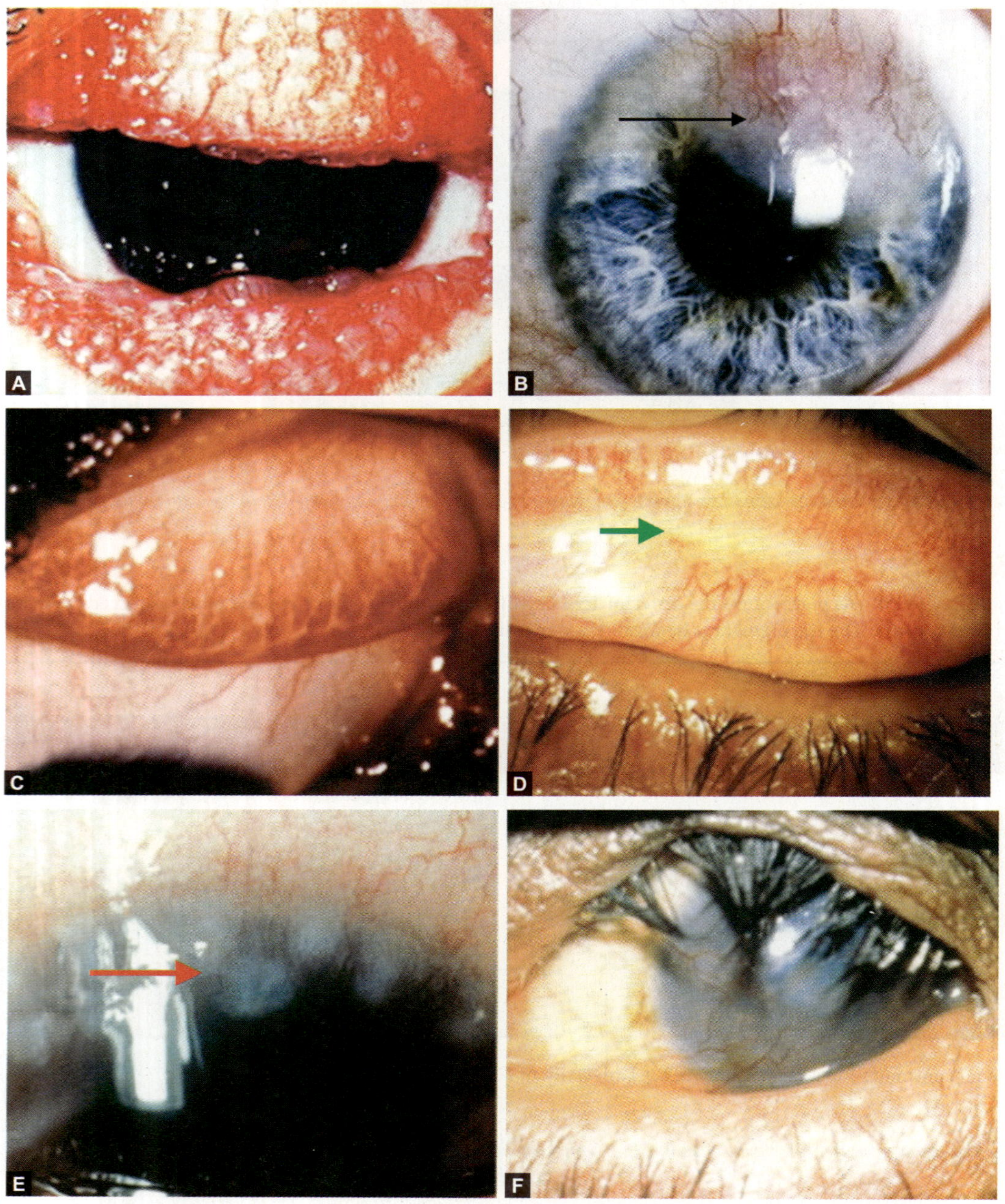

CLINICAL SIGNS OF TRACHOMA
- **A.** Mixed follicular papillary conjunctivitis
- **B.** Severe pannus
- **C.** Linear scars
- **D.** Arlt line
- **E.** Herbert pits
- **F.** Corneal scarring, vascularization and cicastrial entropion

OPHTHAL PLATE 4

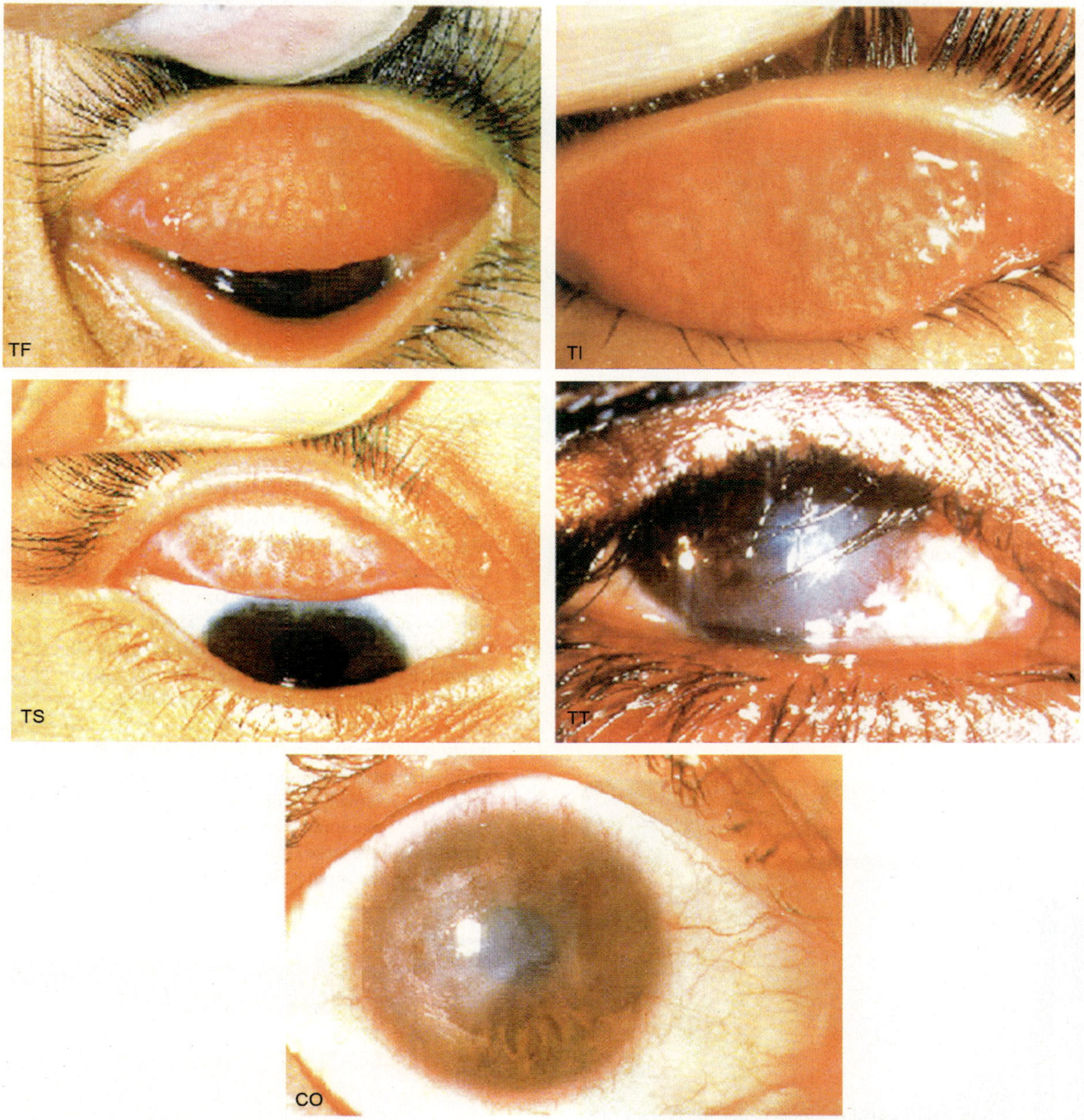

TF

TI

TS

TT

CO

WHO GRADING OF TRACHOMA

WHO Grading of Trachoma
TF = Trachomatous inflammation (*follicular*): Five or more follicles (>0.5 mm) on the superior tarsus
TI = Trachomatous inflammation (*intense*): Diffuse involvement of the tarsal conjunctiva, obscuring 50% or more of the normal deep tarsal vessels; papillae are present
TS = Trachomatous conjunctival *scarring*: Easily visible fibrous white tarsal bands
TT = Trachomatous *trichiasis*: At least one lash touching the globe
CO = Corneal *opacity* sufficient to blur details of at least part of the pupillary margin

OPHTHAL PLATE 5

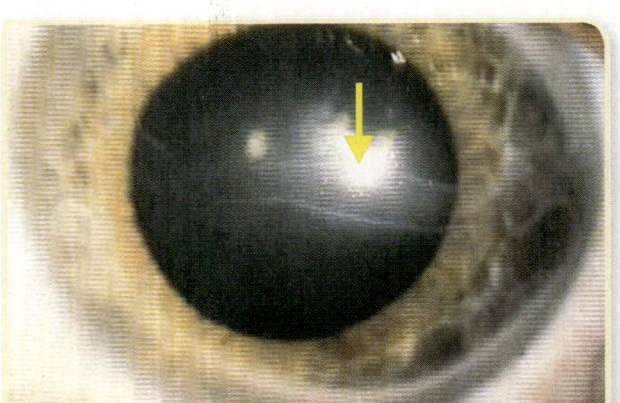

HABB STRIAE

Horizontally oriented lines, caused by endothelialized ruptures of Descemet's membrane in cases of buphthalmus (congenital glaucoma). Differ from vertically oriented lines occurring after forceps delivery.

OPHTHAL PLATE 6

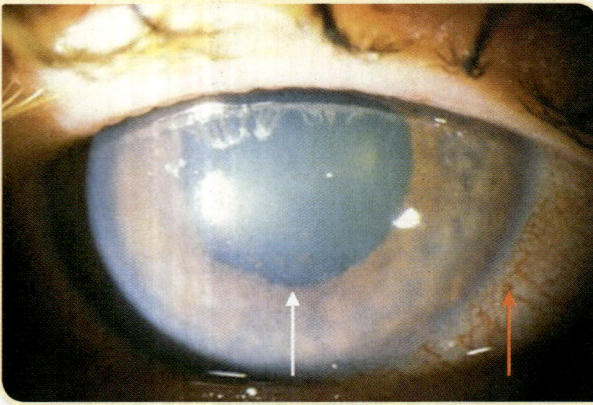

SIGNS OF ACUTE (CONGESTIVE) ANGLE-CLOSURE GLAUCOMA

- VA usually 6/60-HM.
- IOP is usually very high (50–100 mmHg)
- Conjunctival hyperemia with violaceous circumcorneal injection. (Red arrow)
- Anterior chamber is shallow and aqueous flare may be present.
- Corneal epithelial edema (Red arrow)
- Unreactive mid-dilated vertically oval pupil (White arrow)
- Fellow eye generally shows an occludable angle

OPHTHAL PLATE 7

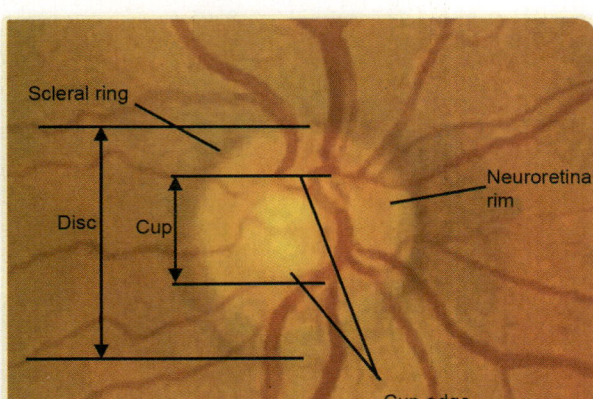

NORMAL OPTIC NERVE HEAD

- The **neuroretinal rim (NRR)** is the tissue between the outer edge of the cup and the optic disc margin. The normal rim has an orange or pink color and a characteristic configuration in most healthy eyes: the inferior rim is the broadest followed by the superior, nasal and temporal **(the 'ISNT' rule).**
- Optic disc size is important in deciding if a **cup-disc (C/D) ratio** is normal. Normal median vertical diameter for non-glaucomatous discs is **1.50 mm** in a Caucasian population
- The C/D ratio indicates the diameter of the cup expressed as a fraction of the diameter of the disc; the vertical rather than the horizontal ratio is generally used in clinical practice. The NRR occupies a relatively similar cross-sectional area in different eyes.
- Small discs have small cups with a median C/D ratio of about 0.35
- Large discs have large cups with a median C/D ratio of about 0.55
- Only 2% of the population have a C/D ratio greater than 0.7.

OPHTHAL PLATE 8

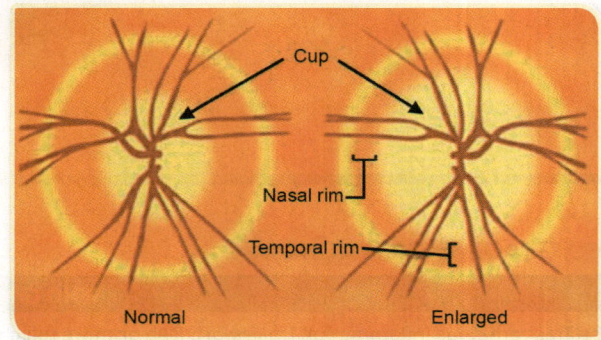

NORMAL VS ENLARGED OPTIC NERVE

Normal vs enlarged optic nerve head compared schematically (See PLATE 7 for details)

OPHTHAL PLATE 9

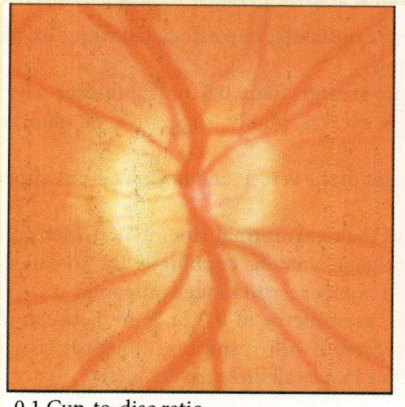

0.1 Cup-to-disc ratio
Normal optic nerve without cupping
Disc margins are sharp
Neural rim is intact

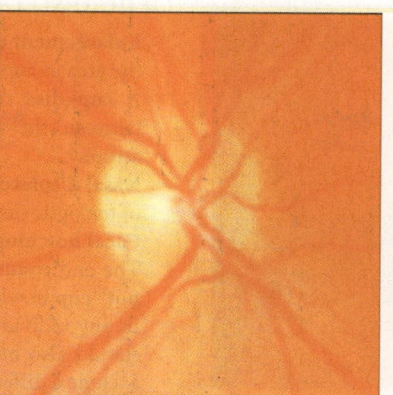

0.2 Cup-to-disc ratio
Normal optic nerve with small cup

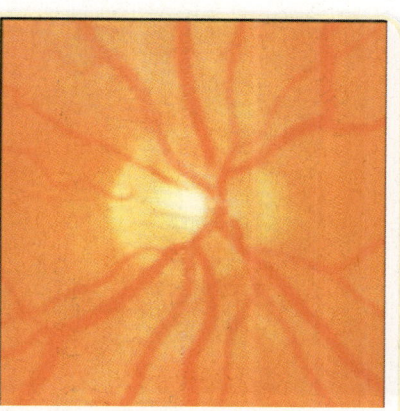

0.3 Cup-to-disc ratio
Normal optic nerve with slightly larger (than #2) cup

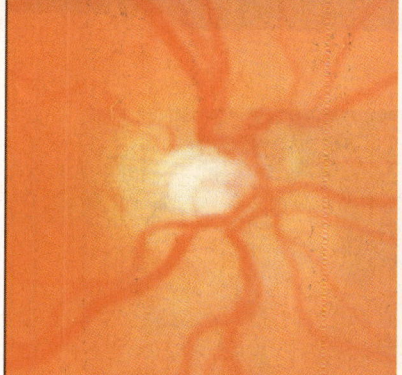

0.4 Cup-to-disc ratio
Early glaucoma
Neural rim is intact

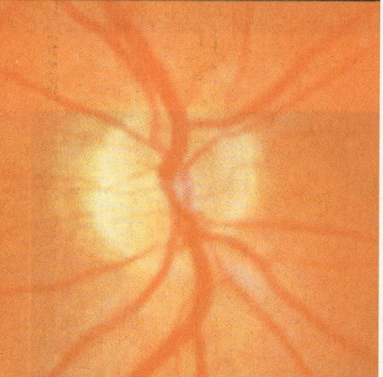

0.5 Cup-to-disc ratio
Glaucoma with moderate cupping
Neural rim is intact

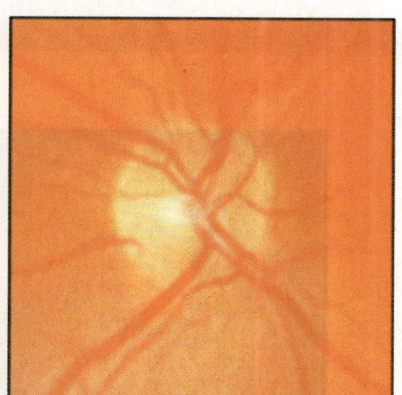

0.6 Cup-to-disc ratio
Glaucoma with moderate cupping
Notch defect at 6:30 where neural rim is absent (Superior visual filed defect corresponds)

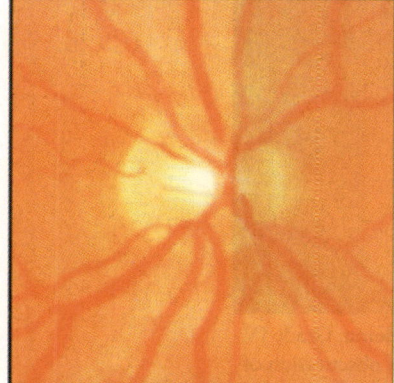

0.7 Cup-to-disc ratio
Glaucoma with advanced cupping
Neural rim is thin

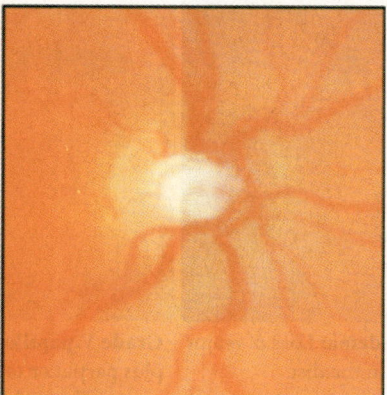

0.8 Cup-to-disc ratio
Glaucoma with advanced cupping
Neural rim absent at 12:00
Disc hemorrhage at 11:00

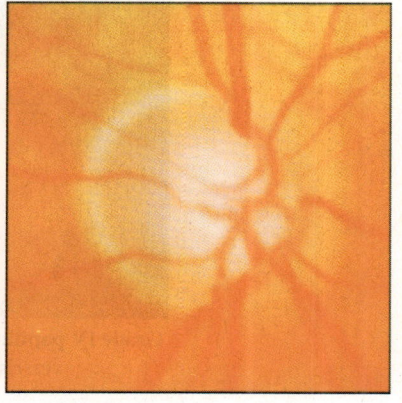

0.9 Cup-to-disc ratio
Glaucoma with advanced cupping and myopia
Sloped loss of temporal neural rim

PROGRESSION OF OPTIC NERVE CUPPING IN GLAUCOMA
Description is given in the plates.

OPHTHAL PLATE 10

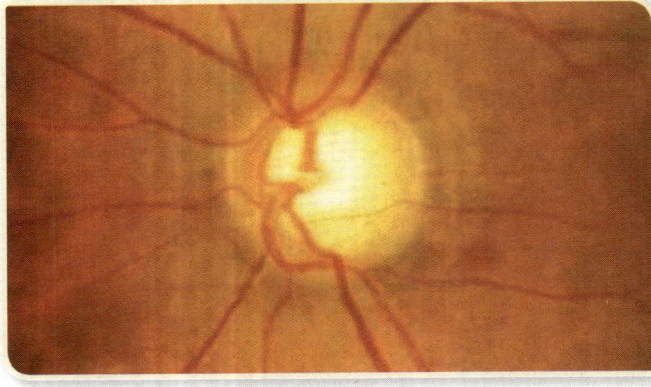

OPTIC DISC CHANGES IN GLAUCOMA

- **Enlargement of the optic disc cup** associated with **disc pallor** in the area of cupping.
- A **cup–disc ratio greater than 0.5** or significant asymmetry between the two eyes is highly suggestive of glaucomatous atrophy.
- **Nasal displacement** of the vessels and **hollowed-out appearance** of the optic disc
- **Focal notching of the neuroretinal rim** (at 6 O' clock position)
- The end result of glaucomatous cupping is the so-called "**bean pot**" **cup** in which no neural rim tissue is apparent
- In any individual, **asymmetry of 0.2** or more between the eyes should also be regarded with suspicion, though it is critical to exclude a difference in overall disc size.

OPHTHAL PLATE 11

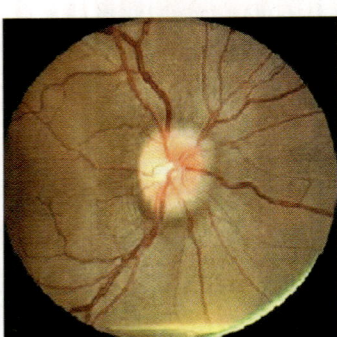 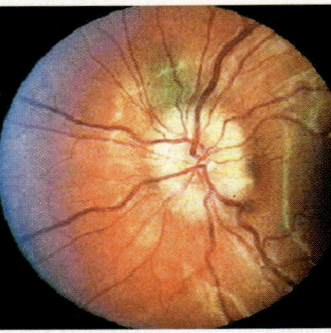 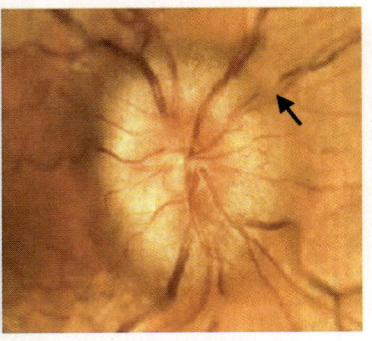

Grade I papilloedema: C-shaped halo with a temporal gap

Grade II papilloedema: The halo becomes circumferential

Grade III papilloedema: Loss of major vessels as they leave the disc (arrow)

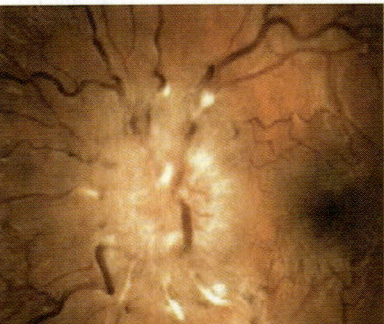 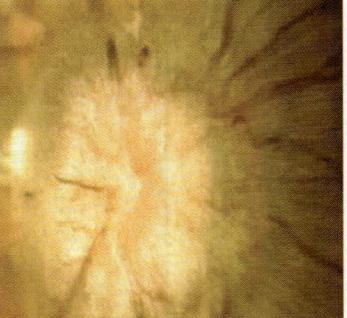

Grade IV papilloedema: Loss of major vessels on the disc

Grade V papilloedema: Grade IV plus partial or total obscuration of all vessels of the disc

GRADES OF PAPILLOEDEMA

Details are given in the plate

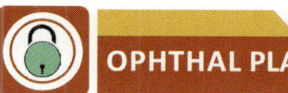
OPHTHAL PLATE 12

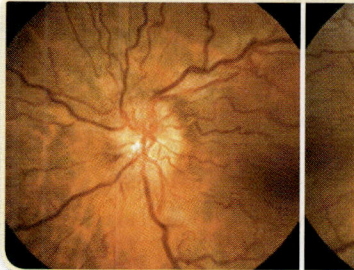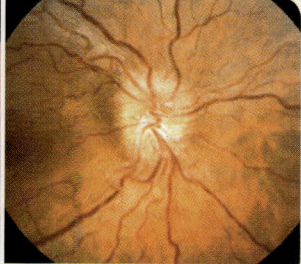

- There may also be **peripapillary edema** (which can extend to the macula), retinal exudates and choroidal folds
- With persistent raised intracranial pressure, the hyperemic elevated disk gradually becomes gray-white as a result of astrocytic gliosis and neural atrophy with secondary constriction of retinal blood vessels, thus leading to the stage of **atrophic papilloedema**
- There may also be **retinochoroidal collaterals** (previously known as opticociliary shunts) linking the central retinal vein and the peripapillary choroidal veins

OPHTHAL PLATE 13

 KEY

BILATERAL PAPILLOEDEMA (RAISED ICT)
Also see PLATE -11
- There, slow and fast axonal transport is blocked, and axonal distention, particularly noticeable at the superior and inferior poles of the optic disk, occurs as the first sign of papilloedema.
- **Hyperemia of the disk with dilated surface capillaries, blurring of the peripapillary disk margin, and loss of spontaneous venous pulsations are the signs of mild papilloedema**.
- Circumferential peripapillary retinal folds (**Paton's lines**) also develop.
- In acute papilloedema, there are **hemorrhages and cotton-wool spots** on and around the optic disk
- In chronic papilloedema, which is likely to be the consequence of prolonged, moderately raised intracranial pressure, a process of compensation appears to limit the optic disk changes such that there are few if any hemorrhages or cotton-wool spots.

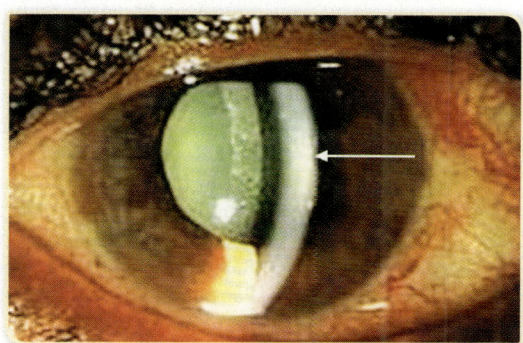

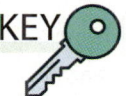 KEY

Acute Angle-Closure Glaucoma Sequelae
Glaucomflecken (White arrow) are small grey white anterior capsular or sub capsular opacities, due to infarction of the lens fibers as a result of High IOP.

OPHTHAL PLATE 14

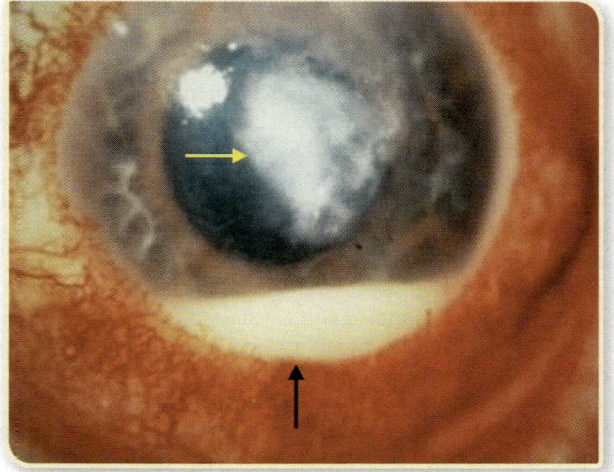

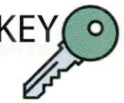 KEY

FUNGAL KERATITIS
Fungal ulcers are indolent and have a gray infiltrate with **irregular edges (Yellow arrow)**, often a **hypopyon (Black arrow)** marked inflammation of the globe, superficial ulceration, and **satellite lesions** (usually infiltrates at sites distant from the main area of ulceration).

	Fungal Keratitis	
Types		▫ **Yeasts** (e.g. genus Candida), ovoid unicellular organisms that reproduce by budding, are responsible for most cases of fungal keratitis in temperate climates. ▫ **Filamentous fungi** (e.g. genera Fusarium and Aspergillus), multicellular organisms that produce tubular projections known as hyphae. They are the most common pathogens in tropical climates. Aspergillus is the commonest in India.
Predisposing factors		▫ Common predisposing factors are chronic ocular surface disease, long-term use of topical steroids (often in conjunction with prior corneal transplantation), contact lens wear, systemic immunosuppression and diabetes. ▫ Filamentary keratitis may be associated with trauma, often relatively minor, involving plant matter or gardening/agricultural tools.

Clinical features		The diagnosis is often delayed unless there is a high index of suspicion, and often infection will initially have been presumed to be bacterial.
		▫ Presentation is with a gradual onset of pain, grittiness, photophobia, blurred vision and watery or mucopurulent discharge. **Symptoms are in general less than in bacterial ulcer of same size.**
		▫ **Signs**
		  • **Candida keratitis**
		    ♦ Yellow-white densely suppurative infiltrate
		    ♦ A collar-stud/ button morphology may be seen in case of Yeast
		  • **Filamentous keratitis**
		    ♦ A grey or yellow-white stromal infiltrate with indistinct **fluffy margins.**
		    ♦ Progressive infiltration, often with satellite lesions.
		    ♦ Feathery branch-like extensions or a ring-shaped infiltrate may develop.
		    ♦ Rapid progression with necrosis and thinning can occur.
		    ♦ Penetration of an intact Descemet membrane may occur and lead to endophthalmitis without evident perforation.
		  • An epithelial defect is not invariable and is sometimes small when present.
		  • Other features include anterior uveitis, hypopyon, endothelial plaque, raised IOP, scleritis and sterile or infective endophthalmitis.

Diagnosis		Samples for laboratory examination should be acquired before commencing antifungal therapy
		▫ **Staining**
		  • Gram and Giemsa staining are both about 50% sensitive.
		  • Periodic acid-Schiff (PAS) and Grocott–Gömöri methenamine-silver (GMS) stains may also be used, but are more commonly performed on histological sections.
		▫ **Culture:** Corneal scrapes should be placed on Sabouraud dextrose agar, although most fungi will also grow on blood agar or in enrichment media. If applicable, contact lenses and cases should be sent for culture.
		▫ **Corneal biopsy** is indicated in the absence of clinical improvement after 3–4 days and if no growth develops from scrapings after a week. A 2–3 mm block should be taken, using a technique similar to the scleral block excision during trabeculectomy. The excised block is sent for culture and histopathological analysis.
		▫ **Confocal microscopy** is rarely available, but may permit identification of organisms in vivo.

Management		▫ **General measures**
		  • Hospital admission should be considered for patients who are not likely to comply or are unable to self-administer treatment. Hospital admission is usually required.
		  • It should also be considered for aggressive disease particularly if involving an only eye.
		  • Discontinuation of contact lens wear is mandatory.
		  • A clear plastic eye shield should be worn between eye drop instillation if significant thinning (or perforation) is present. Removal of the epithelium over the lesion may enhance penetration of antifungal agents. It may also be helpful to regularly remove mucus and necrotic tissue with a spatula.
		▫ **Topical treatment** should initially be given hourly for 48 hours and then reduced as signs permit. Because most antifungals are only fungistatic, treatment should be continued for at least 12 weeks. **Natamycin 5%** drops (especially for filamentous fungi) or amphotericin B 0.15% drops (especially for Candida), initially q1–2h around the clock, then taper over 4 to 6 weeks
		▫ A broad-spectrum antibiotic should also be considered to address or prevent bacterial co-infection.
		▫ Cycloplegia: (cyclopentolate 1%, homatropine 2% or atropine 1%) are used to prevent the formation of posterior synechiae and to reduce pain
		▫ **Subconjunctival fluconazole** may be used in severe cases.
		▫ **Systemic antifungals** may be given in severe cases, when lesions are near the limbus, or for suspected endophthalmitis. Options include voriconazole 400 mg b.d. for one day then 200 mg b.d., itraconazole 200 mg daily, reduced to 100 mg daily, or fluconazole 200 mg b.d.
		▫ **Tetracycline** (e.g. doxycycline 100 mg b.d.) may be given for its anticollagenase effect when there is significant thinning.
		▫ IOP should be monitored using a Tono-Pen.
		▫ Superficial keratectomy can be effective to de-bulk the lesion.
		▫ Therapeutic keratoplasty (penetrating or deep anterior lamellar) is considered when medical therapy is ineffective or following perforation.

Contd...

	Fungal Keratitis
Penetrating Keratoplasty	☐ Inspite of Intensive Antifungal Therapy If : • Increasing Hypopyon • Central To Peripheral Corneal Involvement • Impending/Frank Perforation • Scleral Involvement ☐ Therapeutic PK With/Without Scleral Graft with Amphotericin B wash ☐ Use • Debulk Fungal Load • Reestablish Integrity of Globe • Absolute Diagnosis of Fungal Etiology ☐ Optical PK for corneal opacity in healed corneal ulcer

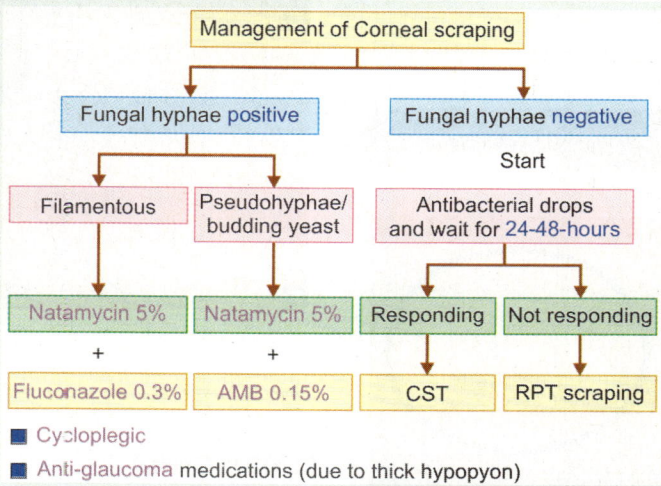

■ Cycloplegic
■ Anti-glaucoma medications (due to thick hypopyon)

OPHTHAL PLATE 15

Clinical Features

☐ **Indolent retinitis** frequently starts in the periphery and progresses slowly. It is characterized by a mild granular opacification which may be associated with a few punctate hemorrhages, but vasculitis is absent.

☐ **Fulminating retinitis**
- Mild vitritis
- Vasculitis with perivascular sheathing and retinal opacification.
- Dense, white, well-demarcated, geographical areas of confluent opacification often associated with retinal hemorrhages
- Slow but relentless **'brushfire-like'** extension along the course of the retinal vascular arcades that may involve the optic nerve head.
- Retinal detachment associated with large posterior breaks may occur in uncontrolled disease and require vitreoretinal surgery and the use of silicone oil tamponade.

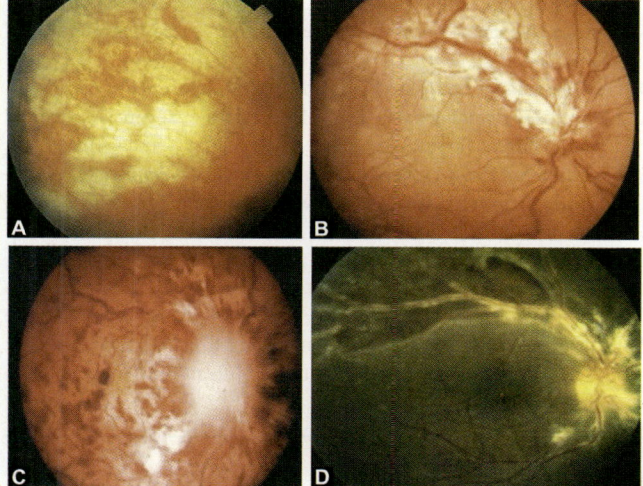

 KEY

CYTOMEGALOVIRUS RETINITIS

A. Indolent retinitis
B. Fulminating disease
C. Advanced disease involving the optic nerve head
D. Large posterior retinal tear with shallow localized detachment

OPHTHAL PLATE 16

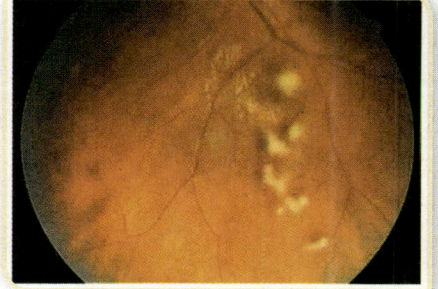

INTERMEDIATE UVEITIS (PARS PLANITIS)

Clumps of inflammatory cells (snowballs) in the vitreous of a patient with pars planitis.
- **Slit-lamp examination** may show mild aqueous flare, and fine KPs at the back of cornea. Anterior vitreous may show cells.
- **Fundus examination** with indirect ophthalmoscope reveals the whitish exudates present near the ora serrata in the inferior quadrant. These typical exudates are referred as **snow ball opacities**. These may coalesce to form a grey white plaque called **snow banking**.

OPHTHAL PLATE 17

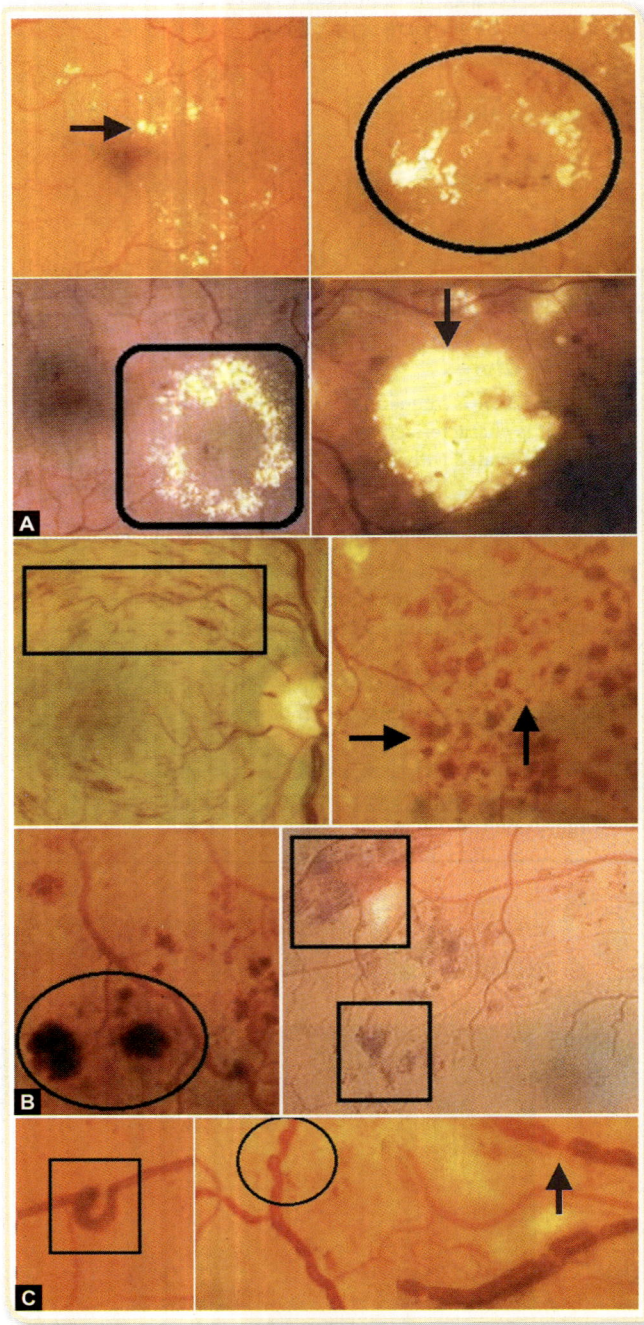

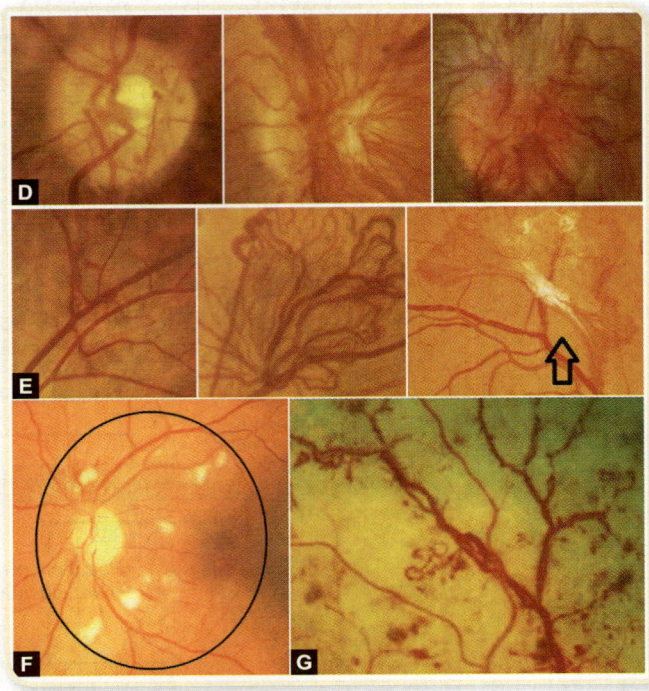

PLATE LEGENDS

A. **Exudates (Hard Exudates)** (small exudates- side arrow, incomplete ring exudate- circle, Ring exudate- Square and Plaque of exudate- down arrow)
   Note: Cotton wool spots are soft exudates
B. **Rentnal hemorrhage:** retinal nerve fiber layer hemorrhages- rectangle, Dot hemorrhage- small arrow, Blot hemorrhages- Large arrow, Deep dark hemorrhages – circle, Flame hemorrhage – square.
C. **Venous changes:** Looping- square, Beading- circle, Segmentation- arrow
D. **New vessels on the disc (NVD);** Mild, moderate and severe
E. **New vessel elsewhere (NVE);** Mild-moderate, Severe; Associated with fibrosis (arrow)
F. **Cotton wool spots (soft exudates);** Superficial white, pale yellow-white or grayish-white areas with ill-defined (feathery) edges, frequently showing striations
G. **Intraretinal microvascular abnormalities (IRMA)** are arteriolar-venular shunts that run from retinal arterioles to venules, thus bypassing the capillary bed and are therefore often seen adjacent to areas of marked capillary hypoperfusion. They are fine, irregular, tortuous, red intraretinal lines that run from arterioles to venules.

OPHTHAL PLATE 18

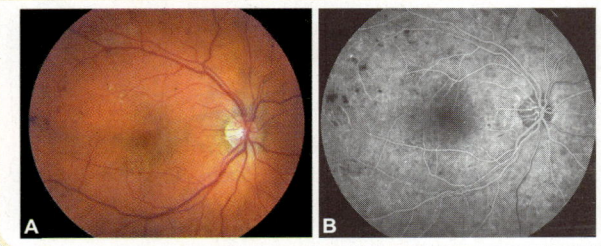

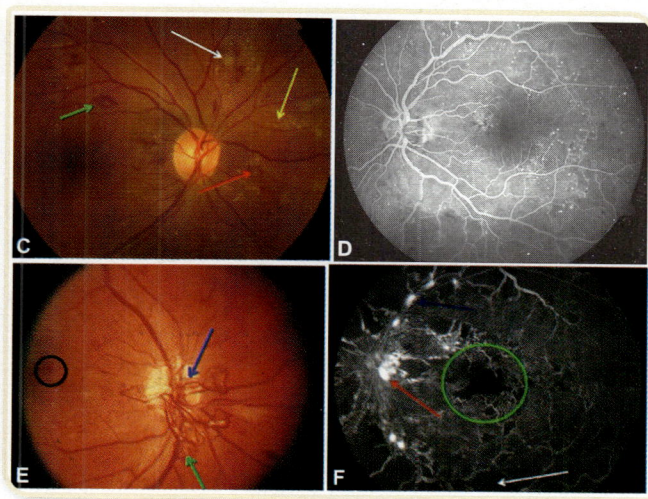

B. Mild Non proliferative Diabetic retinopathy (NPDR): Fluorescein Angiogram
C. Non proliferative Diabetic retinopathy (Moderate): Fundus with exudate (yellow arrow), microaneurysms (red arrow), cotton wool spot (white arrow), nerve fiber layer hemorrhage (green arrow)
D. Non proliferative Diabetic retinopathy (Moderate): Fluorescein Angiogram showing microaneurysms
E. Proliferative Diabetic retinopathy: Fundus with new vessels on the optic disc (Blue arrow), new vessels elsewhere (Green arrow), dot and blot haemorrhage (Circle). In cases of neovascularization, these are new vessels that are leaky so initially they are small in size than progressively they get bigger in size and intensity.
F. Proliferative Diabetic retinopathy: Fluorescein angiogram in proliferative diabetic retinopathy with macular ischemia: macular ischemia (green circle), capillary non-perfusion (white arrow), optic disc new vessels (red arrow), venous beading (blue arrow)

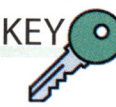

Early treatment Diabetic Retinopathy Study classification of diabetic retinopathy can be classified into nonproliferative retinopathy, maculopathy, and proliferative retinopathy.

DIABETIC RETINOPATHY

A. Mild Non proliferative Diabetic retinopathy (NPDR): Fundus

Nonproliferative Retinopathy/Background Diabetic Retinopathy (BDR)		
The capillaries develop tiny dot-like out pouching called **microaneurysms**. **Flame-shaped hemorrhages** are so shaped because of their location within the horizontally oriented nerve fiber layer.		
Stage	**Description**	**Management**
Non Proliferative Diabetic Retinopathy (NPDR) - Mild	At least one dot hemorrhage or microaneurysm with or without hard exudates	Review range 6–12 months, depending on severity of signs, stability, systemic factors, and patient's personal circumstances
Non Proliferative Diabetic Retinopathy (NPDR) - Moderate	Any one of the following: ☐ Four or more blot hemorrhages per quadrant in one to three quadrants ☐ Venous beading in one quadrant only ☐ Cotton wool spots in one or more quadrants	Review in approximately 6 months PDR in up to 26%, high-risk PDR in up to 8% within a year
Non Proliferative Diabetic Retinopathy (NPDR) - Severe	The 4-2-1 rule; one or more of: ☐ Severe hemorrhages in all 4 quadrants ☐ Significant venous beading in 2 or more quadrants ☐ Moderate IRMA (intraretinal microvascular abnormalities) in 1 or more quadrants	Review in 4 months PDR in up to 50%, high-risk PDR in up to 15% within a year
Non Proliferative Diabetic Retinopathy (NPDR) - Very severe	The presence of any two categories for BDR – severe	Review in 2–3 months High-risk PDR in up to 45% within a year

\# Microaneurysms are the first ophthalmoscopically detectable change in diabetic retinopathy

Diabetic Maculopathy		
Diabetic maculopathy manifests as focal or diffuse retinal thickening or edema, caused primarily by a breakdown of the inner blood–retinal barrier at the level of the retinal capillary endothelium, which allows leakage of fluid and plasma constituents into the surrounding retina. Diabetic maculopathy (foveal edema, exudates or ischemia) is the _most common cause of visual impairment in diabetic patients_, particularly type 2. The fluid is initially located between the outer plexiform and inner nuclear layers; later it may also involve the inner plexiform and nerve fiber layers, until eventually the entire thickness of the retina becomes edematous.		
Stage	**Description**	**Management**
Diabetic maculopathy early (M1)	Microaneurysms, hemorrhages or exudates within a radius of ≥ 1 but < 2 disc diameters of the centre of the fovea	Treatment once it becomes **clinically significant**, which is defined as any retinal thickening within 500 microns of the fovea, hard exudates within 500 microns of the fovea associated with retinal thickening, or retinal thickening greater than one disc diameter in size, of which any part lies within one disc diameter of the fovea.
Diabetic maculopathy observable (M2)	Circinate or groups of hard exudates within a radius of > 1 but < 2 disc diameters of the centre of the fovea	

Contd...

Diabetic Maculopathy

	Diabetic Maculopathy	
Diabetic maculopathy referable (M3)	Microaneurysms or dot hemorrhages within a radius of 1 disc diameter of the centre of the fovea Blot hemorrhages within a radius of 1 disc diameter of the centre of the fovea Any hard exudates within a radius of 1 disc diameter of the centre of the fovea	

Proliferative Diabetic Retinopathy

Stage	Description	Management
Proliferative diabetic retinopathy (PDR) Mild to moderate	New vessels on the disc (NVD) or new vessels elsewhere (NVE), but extent insufficient to meet the high-risk criteria	Treatment considered according to severity of signs, stability, systemic factors, and patient's personal circumstances such as reliability of attendance for review. If not treated, review in up to 2 months
PDR - High risk	New vessels on the disc (NVD) greater than about 1/3 disc area Any NVD with vitreous or preretinal hemorrhage NVE greater than 1/2 disc area with vitreous or preretinal hemorrhage (or hemorrhage with presumed obscured NVD/E)	Treatment advised – see below Should be performed immediately when possible, and certainly same day if symptomatic presentation with good retinal view
Advanced diabetic eye disease	Any of the following: ☐ Vitreous hemorrhage ☐ Rubeosis Iridis ☐ Retinal detachment	Pars plana vitrectomy may be required

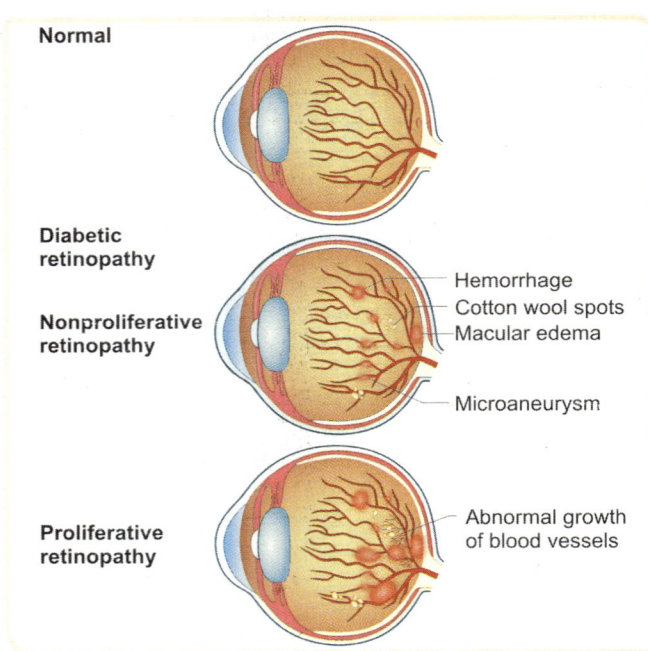

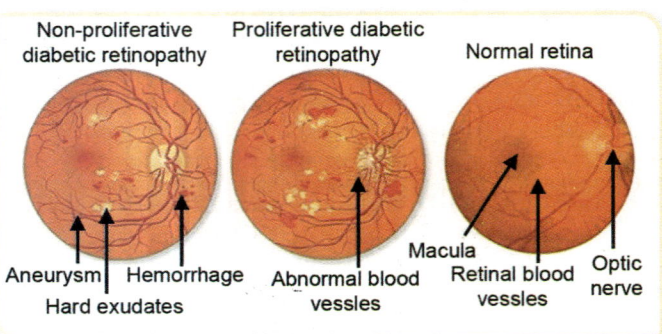

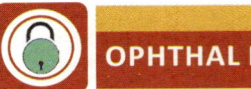

OPHTHAL PLATE 19

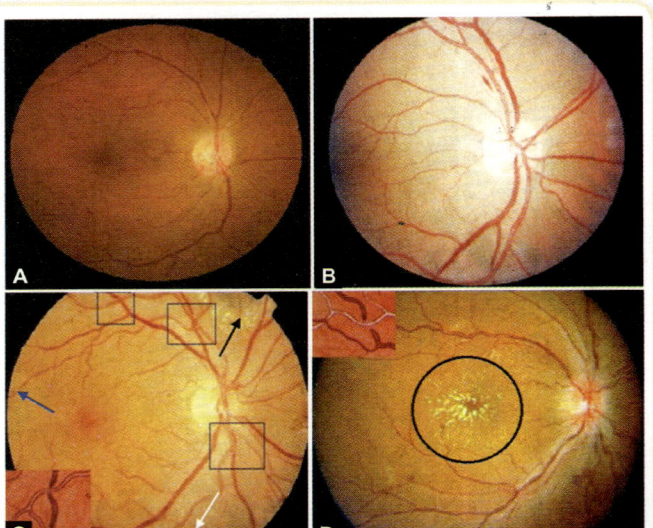

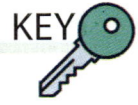

KEY

HYPERTENSIVE RETINOPATHY

The appearance of the fundus in hypertensive retinopathy is determined by the degree of elevation of the blood pressure and the state of the retinal arterioles. In mild to moderate systemic hypertension, the retinal signs may be subtle. Focal attenuation of a major retinal arteriole is one of the earliest signs.

Keith and Wegner Classification of Hypertensive Retinopathy

Stage	Description	Hemorrhage	Exudate	Disc edema
Grade I (A)	Subtle broadening of the arteriolar light reflex, mild generalized arteriolar attenuation, particularly of small branches, and vein concealment.			
Grade II (B)	It comprises marked generalized narrowing and focal attenuation of arterioles (increased light reflection) associated with deflection of veins at arteriovenous crossings (**Salus' sign**- in boxes).	+		
Grade III (C)	This consists of Grade II changes **plus copper-wiring** (insat) of arterioles, banking of veins distal to arteriovenous crossings (**Bonnet sign**), tapering of veins on either side of the crossings (**Gunn sign**) and right-angle deflection of veins (**Salus sign**). Flame-shaped hemorrhages (white arrow), dot blot hemorrhages (blue arrow), and hard exudates (black arrow) may be present	+	+	
Grade IV (D)	This consists of all changes of Grade III and papilloedema. Plus **silver-wiring** of arterioles can be seen (insat). Sometimes star shaped hard exudate around macula (**macular star** in circle)	+	+	+

OPHTHAL PLATE 20

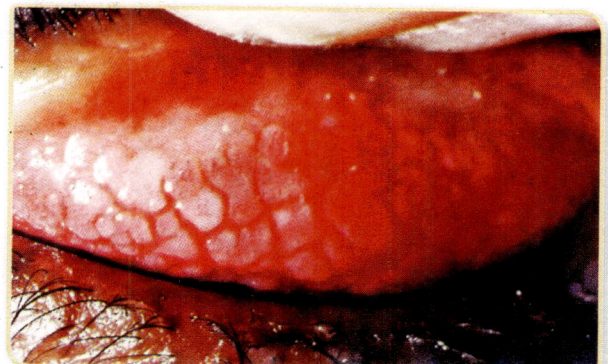

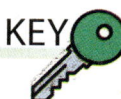
KEY

VERNAL KERATOCONJUNCTIVITIS

Vernal keratoconjunctivitis is characterized by giant papillae (diameter > 1 mm) on the superior tarsal conjunctiva, giving a **cobblestone appearance.** The papillae causing cobblestones in vernal keratoconjunctivitis have **eosinophil.** More common in summer; hence the name **spring catarrh** looks a misnomer. Recently it is being labelled as '**Warm weather conjunctivitis.**'

Palpebral Form	Bulbar Form
The typical lesion is characterized by the presence of hard, flat topped, papillae arranged in a '**cobble-stone**' or '**pavement stone**', fashion	Common in dark skin individuals (Africans/ Indians) Dusky red triangular congestion of bulbar conjunctiva in palpebral area Gelatinous thickened accumulation of tissue around the limbus; and Presence of discrete whitish raised dots along the limbus (**Horner Tranta's spots**)

- Treatment is purely symptomatic.
- VKC is a chronic bilateral inflammation of the conjunctiva, commonly associated with a personal and/or family history of atopy. More than 90% of patients with VKC exhibit one or more atopic conditions, such as asthma, eczema, or seasonal allergic rhinitis.
- *Type I hypersensitivity*
- Itching is the most important and most common symptom. Other commonly reported symptoms are photophobia, foreign body sensation, tearing, and blepharospasm.
- Ocular signs of VKC commonly are seen in the cornea and conjunctiva. In contrast to atopic keratoconjunctivitis (AKC), the eyelid skin usually is not involved.
- A *ropy mucous discharge* may be present. Large numbers of eosinophils are seen in discharge.
- While corneal vascularization is rare, the cornea may be affected in a variety of ways. **Punctate epithelial keratopathy (PEK)** may result from the toxic effect of inflammatory mediators released from the conjunctiva. The appearance of PEK may be a precursor for **the characteristic shield ulcer**, which is **pathognomonic of VKC.** PEK can coalesce, resulting in frank epithelial erosion and forming into a shield ulcer, which is typically shallow with white irregular epithelial borders.
- Although the pathogenesis of a shield ulcer is not well understood, the major factor in promoting development may be chronic mechanical irritation from the giant tarsal papillae. Some evidence suggests that the major basic protein released from eosinophils may also promote ulceration.
- Another type of corneal involvement is vernal **pseudogerontoxon,** which is a degenerative lesion in the peripheral cornea resembling corneal arcus. Keratoconus may be seen in chronic cases, which may be associated with chronic eye rubbing.
- Conjunctival scrapings of the superior tarsal conjunctiva show an abundance of eosinophils. Conjunctival biopsy reveals that there are a large number of mast cells within the substantia propria
- The irritation is best relieved by cold compresses, antihistaminic eye drops and the **topical instillation of steroid drops 4-6 hrly.**
- After a few days, the acute irritation usually subsides and thereafter, a maintenance dose 3 or 4 times a day along with topical mast cell stabilizing agents during the seasonal period of activity generally keeps the symptoms in check.
- Mast cell stabilizers such as sodium cromoglycate (2%) drops 4-5 times a day are quite effective in controlling VKC, especially atopic cases. Olopatadine is a new mast cell stabilizer that is prescribed twice daily.
- Subtarsal injection of triamnicolone in severe cases may be helpful. As the symptoms and signs subside, topical steroids can be tapered off and discontinued, and mast cell stabilizers continued.
- Chronic steroid usage may lead to the patient silently developing steroid-induced glaucoma, or bacterial or fungal corneal superinfections, which are all potentially blinding conditions.

Hence, steroids should be always for short periods, and hence should always be under the guidance of the ophthalmologist.
- **Antibiotics are likely to cause an allergic reaction.** Acetyl cysteine 20% can be used for the treatment of sticky mucus production. Cold compresses and tinted glasses are of help.
- Cryotherapy of lesions may be considered.

OPHTHAL PLATE 21

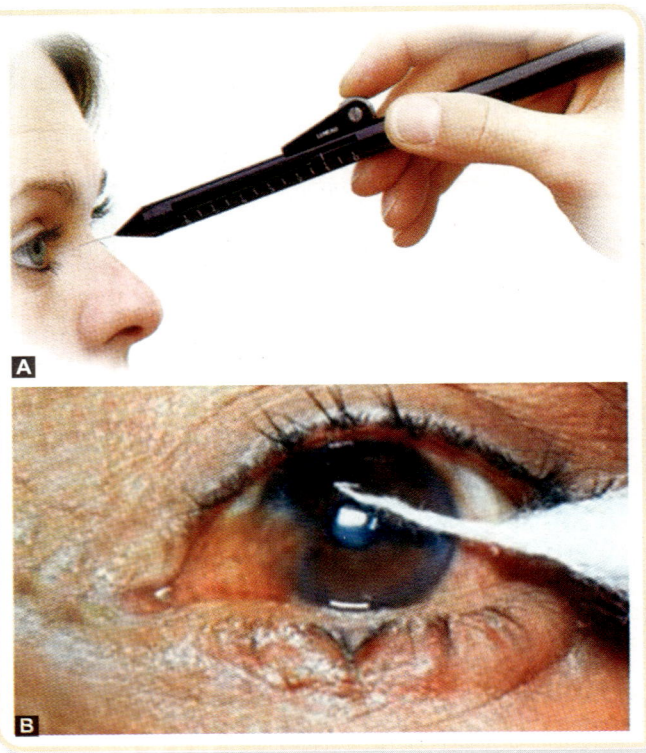

TESTING CORNEAL SENSATIONS

A. **The most common quantitative method is the handheld esthesiometer (Cochet-Bonnet).** It tests only A delta fibers and not C and temperature fibres. Noncontact corneal aesthesiometer (uses air puff technique) is another method. The advantage of NCCA over the Cochet–Bonnet aesthesiometer is that a large, continuous range of stimulus intensities can be produced. Furthermore, the stimulus is more precise and sensory-specific, testing is less variable than with use of a filament, there is no corneal microtrauma is prevented. Patient apprehension is also lesser, and lower stimulus thresholds can be detected. However, it is not commercially available and is less portable.

B. To test the corneal sensations, patient is asked to look ahead; the examiner touches the corneal surface with a **fine twisted cotton** (which is brought from the side to avoid menace reflex) and observes the blinking response. Normally, there is a brisk reflex closure of lids. Always compare the effect with that on the opposite side. **The exact quantitative measurement of corneal sensations is made with the help of an aesthesiometer.**

OPHTHAL PLATE 22

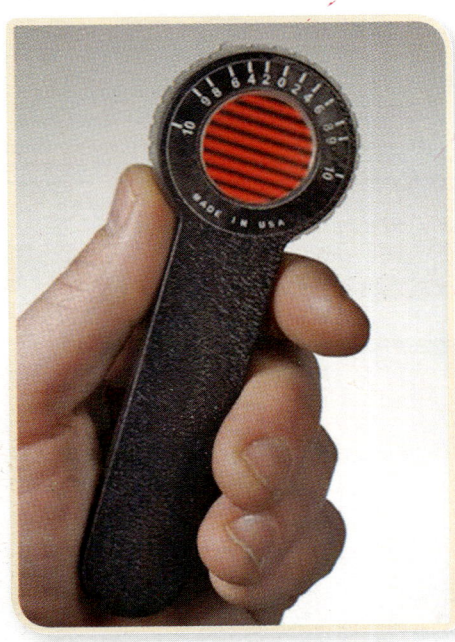

MADDOX ROD

The Maddox rod consists of a series of fused cylindrical red glass rods which convert the appearance of a white spot of light into a red streak. The optical properties of the rods cause the streak of light to be at an angle of 90° with the long axis of the rods; when the glass rods are held horizontally, the streak will be vertical and vice versa. The test is performed as follows:
1. The rod is placed in front of the right eye. This dissociates the two eyes because the red streak seen by the right eye cannot be fused with the unaltered white spot of light seen by the left eye.
2. The amount of dissociation is measured by the superimposition of the two images using prisms. The base of the prism is placed in the position opposite to the direction of the deviation.
3. Both vertical and horizontal deviations can be measured in this way but the test cannot differentiate phoria from tropia.

OPHTHAL PLATE 23

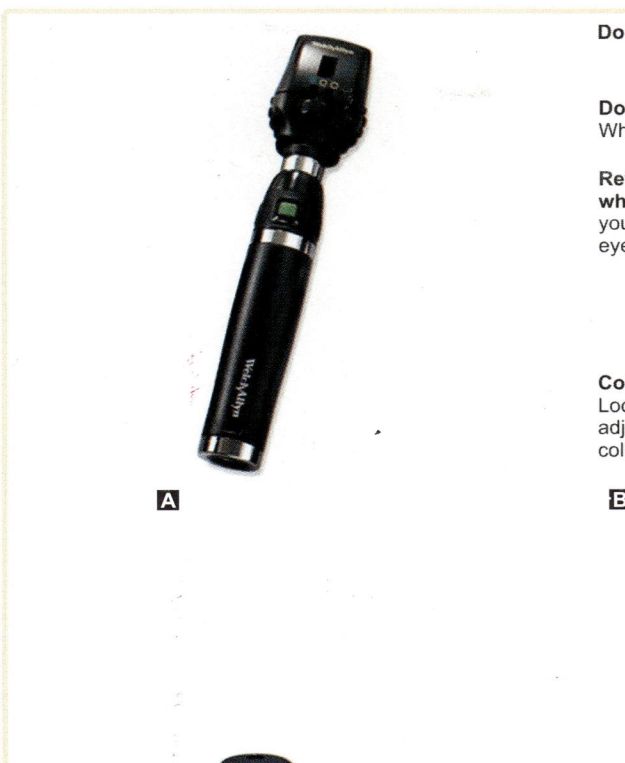

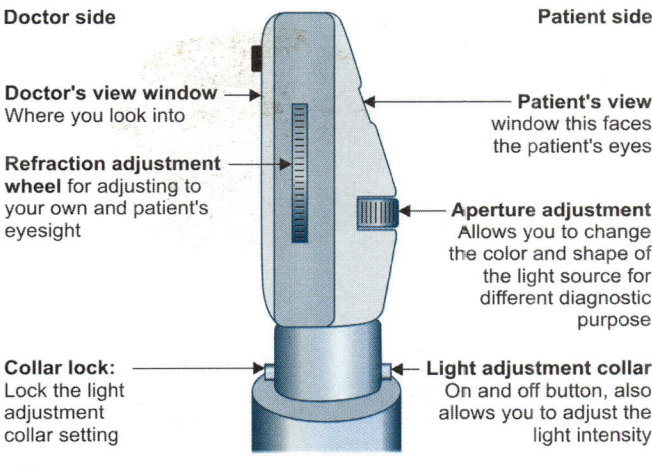

Doctor side — **Patient side**

- **Doctor's view window** Where you look into
- **Refraction adjustment wheel** for adjusting to your own and patient's eyesight
- **Collar lock:** Lock the light adjustment collar setting
- **Patient's view window** this faces the patient's eyes
- **Aperture adjustment** Allows you to change the color and shape of the light source for different diagnostic purpose
- **Light adjustment collar** On and off button, also allows you to adjust the light intensity

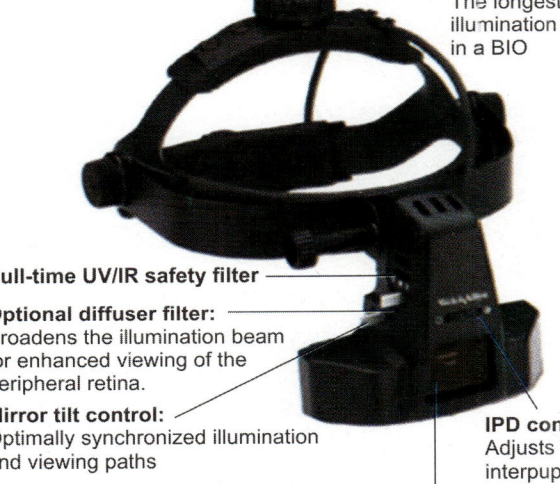

- **Halogen light source:** The longest-lasting illumination available in a BIO
- **Full-time UV/IR safety filter**
- **Optional diffuser filter:** Broadens the illumination beam for enhanced viewing of the peripheral retina.
- **Mirror tilt control:** Optimally synchronized illumination and viewing paths
- **Ergonomically designed controls:** Convenient and durable for simple operation and protection against accidental drops
- **IPD control:** Adjusts to handle interpupillary distances of 49 mm to 74 mm – ideal for people with close-set eyes
- **Sealed optics:** For enhanced viewing and durability

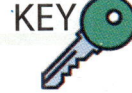
KEY

OPHTHALMOSCOPE

A. Direct Ophthalmoscope (Unlabeled)
B. Direct Ophthalmoscope (Labeled)
C. Indirect Ophthalmoscope (Unlabeled)
D. Indirect Ophthalmoscope (Unlabeled)

Ophthalmoscopy		
	Direct Ophthalmoscopy	**Indirect ophthalmoscopy**
Magnification	About 15 times	3 times if 20 D lens is used and 4 times if 14 D condensing lens is used 5 times when a +13D condensing lens is used
Condensing lens	Not required	Required
Illumination	Not so bright, so not useful in hazy media	Bright, so useful in hazy media
Examination distance	As close to the patient's eye as possible	At an Arm's length

Contd...

	Ophthalmoscopy	
	Direct Ophthalmoscopy	**Indirect ophthalmoscopy**
Diameter of the field of observation view	Smaller (about 10° in diameter) About 2 disc diopters (DD)	Wider (about 37° in diameter) About 8 disc diopters (DD)
Brightness	There is relatively low brightness	There is relatively greater brightness
Structures seen	Central retina only	Peripheral retina seen *(by using a scleral depressor in addition to the indirect ophthalmoscopy itself)*
Image of the fundus that is seen	Virtual and erect image	Real and inverted image
Stereopsis	Image formed is not stereoscopic	Binocular indirect ophthalmoscopy provides better stereopsis
Retina anterior to the equator	Not well seen (seen with difficulty)	Seen better
Scleral indentation	Difficult	Can be easily done in binocular indirect ophthalmoscopy
Visualization in hazy media	Poor	Better
Other comments	Image brightness: 1/2 =4 watts Working distance: 1-2cm Area seen: 50-70% Stereopsis: None	Investigation of choice to diagnose retinal detachment, ROP, peripheral retinal degenerations - Done in dilated pupil
Optics	Optical principle of the simplest form of direct ophthalmoscope (O, observer's eye; P, patient's eye; M, semi-silvered mirror)	The light source mounted above and between the examiner's eyes illuminates the condenser, which images the source at the periphery of the patient's pupil. The illumination does not overlap the observation beam. The condenser lens is handheld; it forms an inverted aerial image of the retina

OPHTHAL PLATE 24

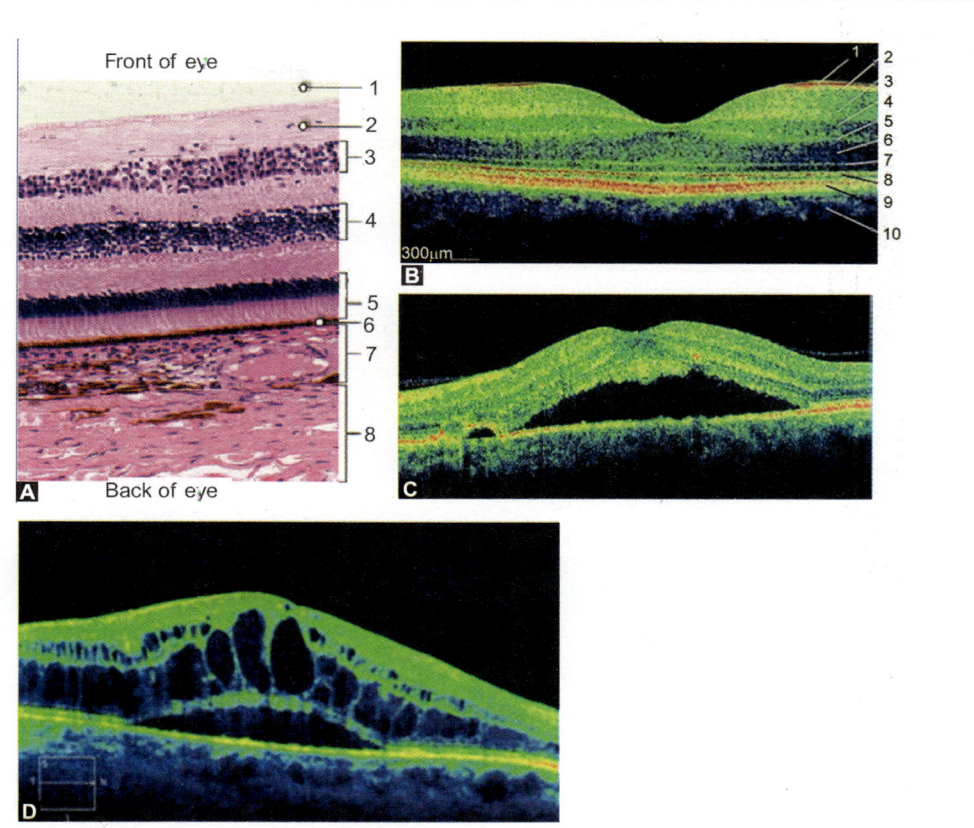

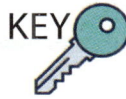

PLATE LEGENDS

A. Retinal layers histology

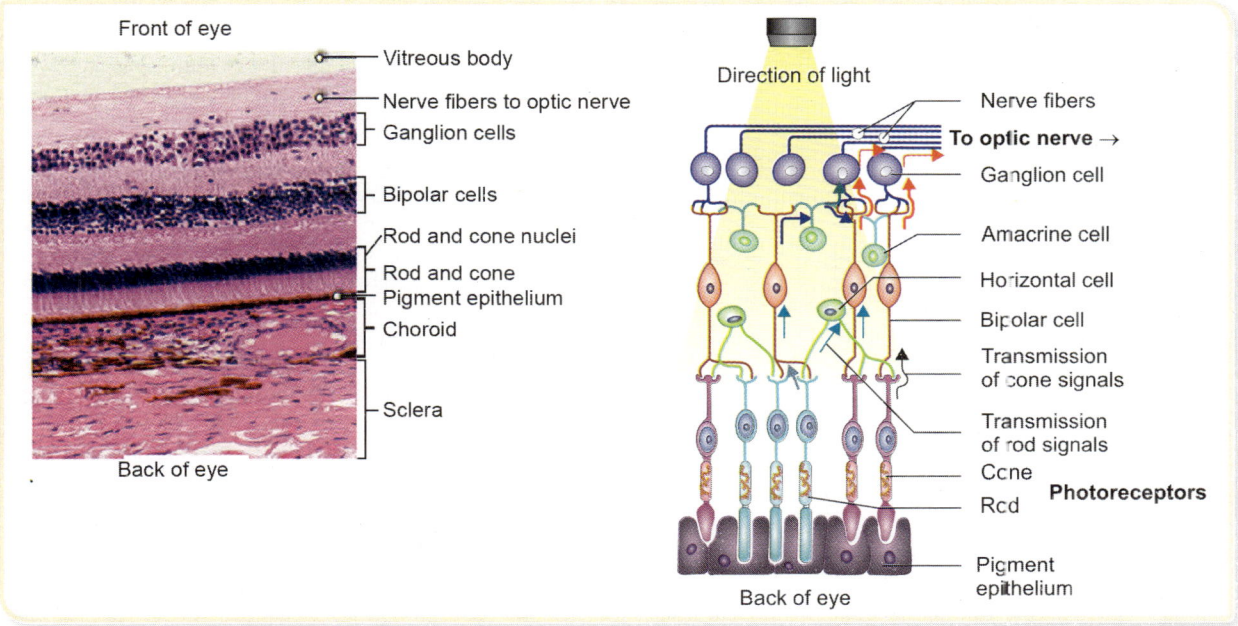

Fig: Retinal layers histology

Layers of Retina

#	Layer	Description
1	Inner limiting membrane	Innermost layer of retina and is essentially a basement membrane. It separates the retina from vitreous and is formed by the union of terminal expansions of the Muller's fibres
2	Nerve fiber layer (Stratum Opticum)	Consists of axons of the ganglion cells, which pass through the lamina cribrosa to form the optic nerve.
3	Ganglion cell layer	Consists of cell bodies of ganglion cells (2nd order neurons of visual pathway). There are two types of ganglion cells. • **Midget ganglion cells** are present in the macular region and the dendrite of each such cell synapses with the axon of single bipolar cell. • **Polysynaptic ganglion cells** lie mainly in the peripheral retina and each cell may synapse with up to a hundred bipolar cells.
4	Inner Plexiform layer [AIIMS PG]	Consists of connections between the axons of bipolar cells and dendrites of the ganglion cells, and processes of amacrine cells.
5	Inner Nuclear Layer	Contains cell bodies of bipolar cells (majorly), cell bodies of horizontal amacrine and Muller's cells and capillaries of central artery of retina. *The bipolar cells is the 1st order neurons of visual pathway.*
6	Outer Plexiform Layer [AIIMS PG]	Consists of connections of rod spherules and cone pedicles with the dendrites of bipolar cells and horizontal cells.
7	Outer Nuclear Layer	Contains nuclei of rods and cones
8	External Limiting membrane	Fenestrated membrane, through which passes the processes of rods and cones.
9	Inner/ outer segment Junction (Photoreceptor layer- Rods and Cones)	Rods and cones (photoreceptors) arranged in a palisade manner.
10	Retinal Pigment Epithelium	Outermost layer of retina. Consists of a single layer of pigment cells. Firmly adherent to the underlying basal lamina (Bruch's membrane) of choroid

Photoreceptors

	Rods	Cones
Number	120 millions	6.5 millions.
Photosensitive substance	Rhodopsin	Photopsin
Responsible for	Peripheral vision and vision of low illumination (scotopic vision).	Central vision (photopic vision) and colour vision.

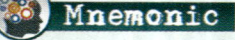 **Mnemonic** = = In New Generation Improved Interns Opt Only Externship to Rule PGME

In (Inner limiting) New (Nerve fiber layer) Generation (Ganglion layer) Improved (Inner plexiform) Interns (Inner Nuclear) Opt (Outer Plexiform) Only (Outer Nuclear) Externship (External limiting) to Rule (Rods and Cones) PGME (Pigment epithelium layer)

B. Normal Optical Coherence Tomography
1. Nerve fiber layer
2. Ganglion cell layer
3. Inner Plexiform layer
4. Inner Nuclear Layer
5. Outer Plexiform Layer
6. Outer Nuclear Layer
7. External Limiting membrane
8. Inner/outer segment Junction
9. Retinal Pigment Epithelium
10. Larger Choroidal vessels

C. Detached Retinal pigment epithelium: Optical coherence tomography (OCT) is a safe, non-invasive, fast, reliable test that provides high resolution, cross-sectional images of the retina and vitreoretinal interface. It is an increasingly important tool for the diagnosis and monitoring of a wide range of vitreoretinal conditions. Current commercial OCT machines use a near infrared broadband light source (not a laser) to illuminate the retina. Familiarity with the appearance of a normal macular OCT scan is important to confidently identify pathological changes.

D. OCT Picture of cystoid macular edema: Multiple cysts are seen in the region of macula which are fluid filled and multiple pockets are there due to disruption of blood retinal barrier primarily in outer plexiform layer.

FAQ Retinal Layers

- **Microaneurysms** are present mainly in **inner nuclear layer.**
- **Cotton wool spots** are present in **nerve fiber layer.** It is seen more commonly in hypertensive retinopathy
- Normal retinal vasculature is found in **between outer plexiform and inner nuclear layer.**
- Soft exudates or Cotton wool spots are small yellowish type, irregular margins, due to axonal debris. It's due to axonal transport blockage.
- Hard exudates are slightly large, sharp margins, due to lipid deposits. Hard exudates are mostly in outer plexiform layer

OPHTHAL PLATE 25

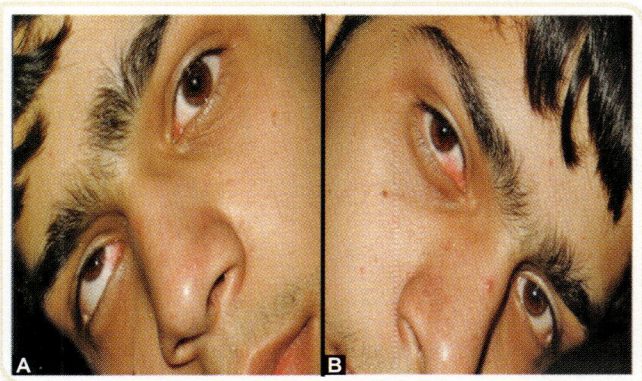

Source: Dr Vineet Sehgal

Right Trochlear Nerve Palsy- Superior Oblique Palsy

- Superior Oblique action is Intorsion, Depression in adduction, better Intorter on Abduction.
- Patients complain of diplopia – vertical, diagonal or torsional
- If the principal complaint is torsion - B\L palsy should be suspected
- Compensatory head posture
- Facial Asymmetry
- Chin down in bilateral palsies
- Combination of Elevation, Extorsion, Esotropia (**Since SO does Depression, Intorsion, Abduction**)
- Diagnosis is based on either Head tilt or Park three step test.

OPHTHAL PLATE 26

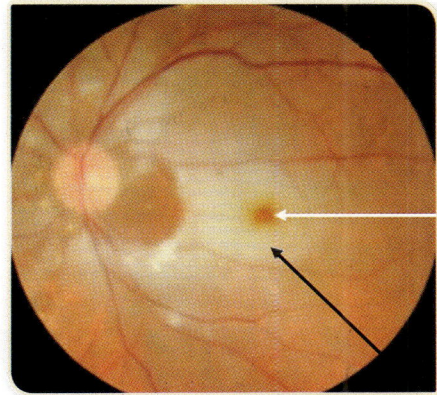

KEY

RIGHT SUPERIOR OBLIQUE PALSY

A. On right head tilt there is elevation and slight esotropia (**Fig. A**)

Mnemonic- **WOOG** = worse on opposite gaze, that is not there on left head tilt (**Fig. B**).

So patient would like to have left head tilt. So remember **mnemonic BOOT**- Better on opposite tilt

BERLIN'S EDEMA OR COMMOTIO RETINA

It follows post blunt trauma, and manifests as pale retina due to retinal edema (Black arrow), with a Cherry Red Spot in the central foveal region (White arrow).

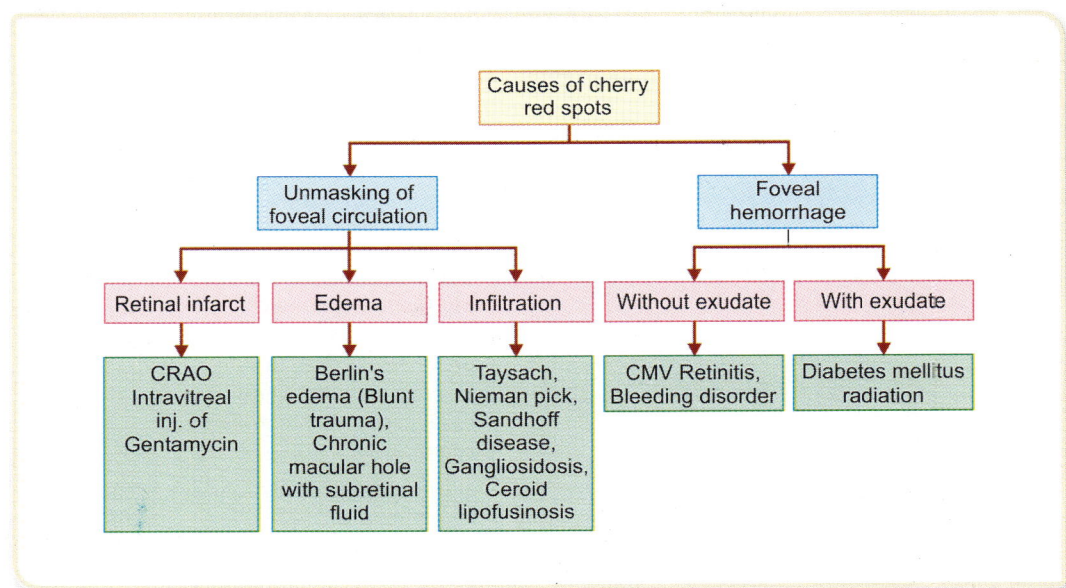

245

OPHTHAL PLATE 27

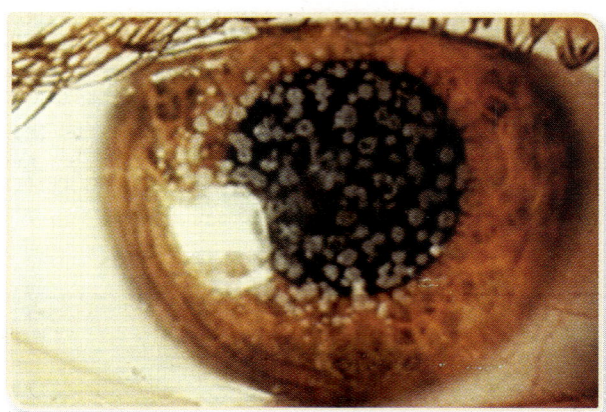

GRANULAR DYSTROPHY

B/L Small, discrete, sharply demarcated, grayish-white opacities, DROP, CRUMB, RING shaped may resemble *'snowflakes'*, can take form of *'Christmas tree'* and often described as *'popcorn'* type.
- Initially stroma is clear between lesion while periphery remain free.
- Vision not affected early and impairment, is rare before 5th decade
- Light Microscope: Eosinophilic, hyaline deposits in stroma and beneath epithelium; stains bright red with MASSON'S TRICHROME.

	Corneal Dystrophies				
	Inheritance	Age of onset	Pattern	Comments	Treatment
Epithelium					
Epithelial basement membrane dystrophy (AKA; Cogan's microcystic dystrophy)	AD	Variable	Map, Dot, Fingerprints	**Most common** of all corneal dystrophies seen in working age adults. Most cases are asymptomatic. 10% develop recurrent corneal erosions and severe disabling pain.	Bandage Soft contact lens, Hypertonics, Cuettage, Phototherapeutic keratotomy, Anterior stromal puncture
Meesmann's (Juvenile epithelial dystrophy)	AD	1st decade	Epithelial microcytes	In most cases, condition is asymptomatic and does not require treatment.	Bandage Soft contact lens, Keratoplasty
Bowman's					
Reis Buckler	AD	1st decade	Ring shaped dystrophy	Progressive recurrent corneal erosions that usually result in diffuse anterior scarring.	Bandage Soft contact lens, Keratoplasty
Stromal					
Macular	AS	1st decade	Dense grey opacity in the central cornea	Due to accumulation of **mucopolysaccharides** owing to a local enzyme deficiency. Marked defective vision in early life, which usually requires penetrating keratoplasty.	Bandage Soft contact lens, Keratoplasty
Granular	AD	1st or 2nd decade	Milky granular Hyaline, Drop/ring shaped deposits with clear stroma in between	Slowly progressive and usually asymptomatic	Bandage Soft contact lens, Keratoplasty

Contd...

Corneal Dystrophies

	Inheritance	Age of onset	Pattern	Comments	Treatment
Lattice (AKA; **Biber-Haab-Dimmer** dystrophy)	AD	1st decade	Branching spider-like **amyloid** deposits, sparing the periphery	It appears at the age of 2 years, but the occurrence of recurrent erosions and progressive clouding of central cornea is apparent by the age of 20 years. Soon, visual acuity is impaired. Usually penetrating keratoplasty is required by the age of 30-40 years.	Bandage Soft contact lens, Keratoplasty
Posterior (Endothelium and Descemet Membrane)					
Posterior Polymorphous Corneal Dystrophy (PPMD)	AD	1st decade	Variable lesion; vesicles, curvilinear lines or geographical opacities at Descemet membrane	Very slowly progressive and thus usually asymptomatic	Bandage Soft contact lens, Hypertonics, Keratoplasty
Fuchs' epithelial endothelial dystrophy (late hereditary endothelial dystrophy).	AD	4-5th decade (F> M)	Guttata / corneal edema	Slowly progressive, Bilateral I. **Stage of cornea guttata:** beaten-metal' appearance. Asymptomatic stage II. **Edematous stage** or stage of endothelial decompensation: stromal edema, blurring vision III. **Stage of bullous keratopathy:** Epithelial Edema with formation of bullae, which when rupture cause pain, decreased visual acuity. IV. **Stage of scarring:** Epithelial bullae are replaced by scar tissue and cornea becomes opaque and vascularized.	Bandage Soft contact lens, Hypertonics, Keratoplasty, DSAEK- Descement's automated endothelial keratoplasty
Cornea Guttata of Vogt	AD	Old age (F> M)	Drop like excrescences involving the entire posterior surface of Descemet's membrane.	Cornea guttata may occur independently or as a part of early stage of Fuch's dystrophy.	It rarely affects the vision and hence treatment is usually not required.

Footnote:
Most important Corneal Dystrophies to remember are Stromal Dystrophies, which can be remembered by

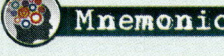 Mnemonic

- **M**arilyn—**M**acular Dystrophy
- **M**onroe—**M**ucopolysaccharide
- **A**lways—**A**lcian Blue stain
- **G**ets—**G**ranular Dystrophy
- **H**er—**H**yaline
- **M**an in—**M**asson Trichrome stain
- **L**os—**L**attice Dystrophy
- **A**ngeles—**A**myloid
- **C**alifornia—**C**ongo Red

Contd...

Corneal Dystrophies

	Inheritance	Age of onset	Pattern	Comments	Treatment
Stains used and patterns for histopathological diagnosis of the stromal corneal dystrophies					

Technique	Granular	Lattice	Macular
PAS (Periodic acid Schiff)		+	+
Alcian blue			+
Trichrome Masson	+	+	
Congo red (under polarization)		+	

Note: Lattice Dystrophy- Shows green birefringence with polarizing microscope

Footnote:
- Macular dystrophy is least found but most severe
- It is the only dystrophy with AR inheritance pattern.
- Cogan map print dot is most common corneal dystrophy
- Granular dystrophy is most common stromal dystrophy

OPHTHAL PLATE 28

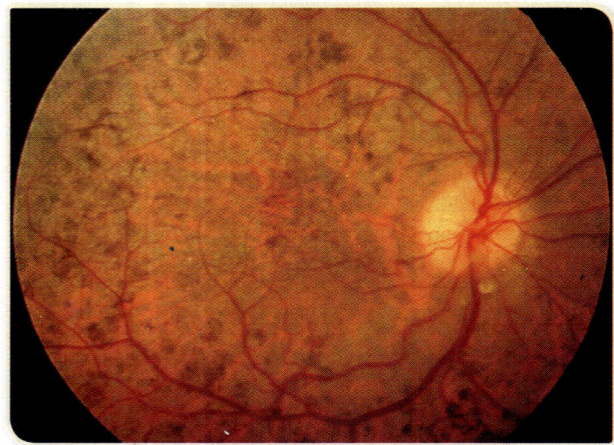

SALT AND PEPPER APPEARANCE OF FUNDUS/RETINA

Causes of Salt and Pepper Retinopathy
- Retinitis Pigmentosa
- Congenital rubella (Ocular defects in Congenital Rubella is congenital cataract, salt and pepper retinopathy and microphthalmos)
- Perinatal Influenza
- Congenital Syphilis
- Thioridazine toxicity (involving the mid-periphery and posterior pole)
- Fundus flavimaculatur (Stargardt macular dystrophy)
- Kearns–Sayre syndrome (Salt-and-pepper pigmentary degeneration of the retina)
- Choroderemia
- Varicella
- Mumps

OPHTHAL PLATE 29

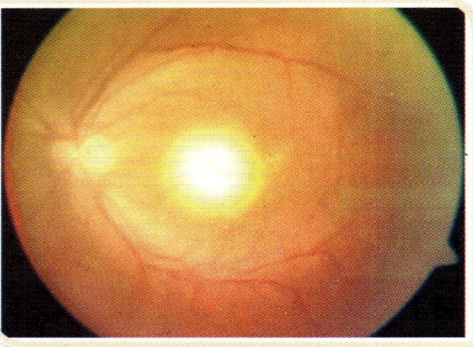

Credit: Sudharshan S, Ganesh SK, Biswas J

NECROTIZING RETINOCHOROIDITIS

Fundus picture showing a typical **"headlight in the fog appearance"** of a focal necrotizing retinochoroiditis with overlying vitritis in a patient with **acquired toxoplasmosis**. Classically, the initial lesion starts in the superficial retina, gradually involving the full-thickness retina, adjacent choroid, vitreous, and even sclera. A yellowish white or grey exudative lesion is seen with ill-defined borders because of the surrounding area of retinal edema.

Ocular Toxoplasmosis	
Congenital	• The most common manifestation of congenital toxoplasmosis is **retinochoroiditis.** Chorioretinal scars, often bilateral, are seen in about 80% of patients with congenital toxoplasmosis.
	• There is a moderate predilection for macular involvement, which may relate to fetal vascular patterns. The retinal inflammation in congenital toxoplasmosis tends to be self-limited, and the lesions may already be healed at birth or may develop months or years after birth.
	• Other ocular manifestations include microcornea, microphthalmos, nystagmus, and strabismus.

Contd...

	Ocular Toxoplasmosis
Acquired	▫ Active ocular infection with toxoplasmosis typically manifests as a localized necrotizing retinitis. The classic lesion is a **gray-white focus of retinal necrosis at the edge of a pigmented chorioretinal scar.** ▫ An adjacent choroiditis, retinal vasculitis, vitritis, iritis, and papillitis may also be seen. There is an overlying vitritis that can be so dense as to prohibit an adequate view of the posterior segment. When the white retinal lesion can just be seen through a dense vitritis, it has been described as a **"headlight in the fog."** ▫ The patient may present with floaters (vitritis), decreased vision (vitritis, papillitis, retinal necrosis, macular edema, choroidal neovascular membranes, vascular occlusions, retinal detachment), pain, redness, and photophobia (iritis). Complications that can result in permanent loss of vision include macular inflammation resulting in a scar, choroidal neovascular membranes, vascular occlusions, optic nerve involvement, and retinal detachment. ▫ Ocular toxoplasmosis in individuals who have AIDS may be unilateral or bilateral, with single or multiple lesions, and it is often chronic or recurrent, requiring prolonged therapy. ▫ The retinitis may be slowly progressive or very aggressive, with large areas of full-thickness retinal necrosis and severe vitritis. Patients who have AIDS have been reported to have unusual forms of ocular toxoplasmosis. Ocular toxoplasmosis presenting as an iridocyclitis without retinal involvement was confirmed by polymerase chain reaction techniques in an AIDS patient who had retinitis in the fellow eye. ▫ Panophthalmitis with a presumed secondary orbititis has also been reported
Primary Prophylaxis	▫ Patients with AIDS should be treated for acute toxoplasmosis; in immunocompromised patients, toxoplasmosis is rapidly fatal if untreated. ▫ **Drug of choice**: Pyrimethamine Plus Sulfadiazine ▫ Alternative: Trimethoprim Sulfamethoxazole (TMP-SMX), Dapsone Pyrimethamine, Atovaquone with or without pyrimethamine
Treatment	▫ Patients with **ocular toxoplasmosis** are usually treated for 1 month with **pyrimethamine plus either sulfadiazine or clindamycin** and sometimes with prednisone ▫ No treatment required for punched out lesion ▫ Spiramycin can be given in pregnancy

OPHTHAL PLATE 30

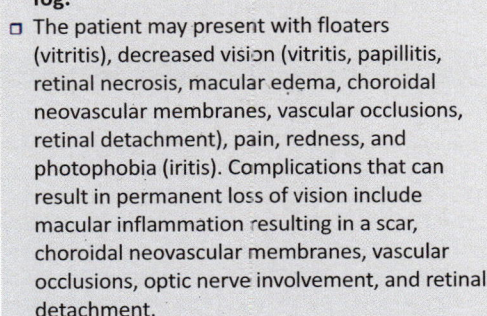

CORNEAL ULCER
Corneal ulcer with perforation on superionasal area

OPHTHAL PLATE 31

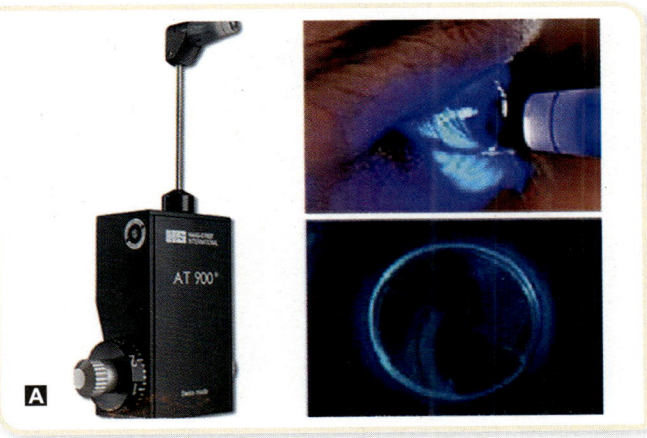

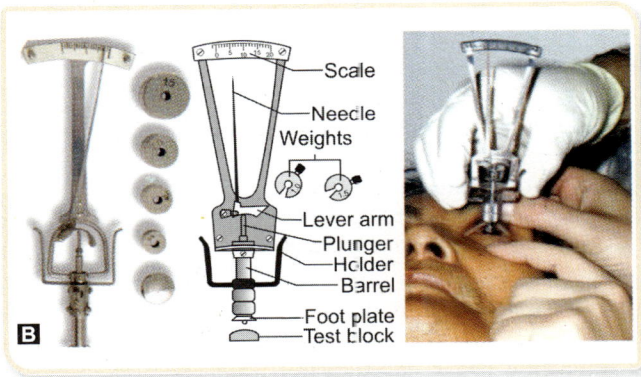

KEY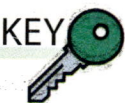

TONOMETER

A. Goldmann tonometer and its application
Goldmann applanation tonometer technique
- Most commonly used tonometer
- Consists of a double prism mounted on a slit lamp
- The prism applanates the cornea for surface area of diameter 3.06 mm
- The eye is anesthetized and tear film is stained with fluorescein
- Patient is made to sit in front of the slit lamp
- Cornea and biprisms are illuminated by cobalt light from slit lamp
- The biprism is advanced until such a time it touches the cornea
- The applanation force is provided until inner ends of two semicircles meet
- This is the end point
- IOP is measured by multiplying dial readings by 10

B. Schiotz tonometer and its application
Technique of using a schizont tonometer
- The cornea is anesthetized
- Patient is asked to fix his eye on a target
- The foot plate is kept on the cornea
- It is customary to start with weight of 5.5 gms
- The reading is noted on a scale
- A conversion table is needed to convert the readings

Advantages of schizont tonometry is that it is cheap, easy to use and handy.

Disadvantages are that it gives false readings when there is scleral rigidity as in high myopes or after scleral surgery.

Tonometer

The intraocular pressure (IOP) is measured with the help of an instrument called tonometer

A tonometer uses certain physical principles to measure pressure within the globe. Basically, the force necessary to deform a globe is directly related to the pressure within that globe. Three styles of tonometer currently are in use. Indentation, or high-displacement, tonometers utilize a plunger to indent the cornea by a variable amount. This indentation displaces a significant volume of intraocular fluid at the time of corneal deformation and results in a near doubling of the IOP. Conversion tables, in turn, estimate the original IOP from the indentation tonometric value obtained. Applanation, or low-displacement, tonometers raise IOP negligibly, because they subject the eye to sufficient force only to flatten the cornea. The amount of force required to achieve a constant degree of corneal flattening is converted into IOP values. Noncontact tonometers flatten the cornea using a puff of air, and the time required to flatten the cornea is correlated to estimated IOP. Each form of tonometer has a place in the examination of eyes

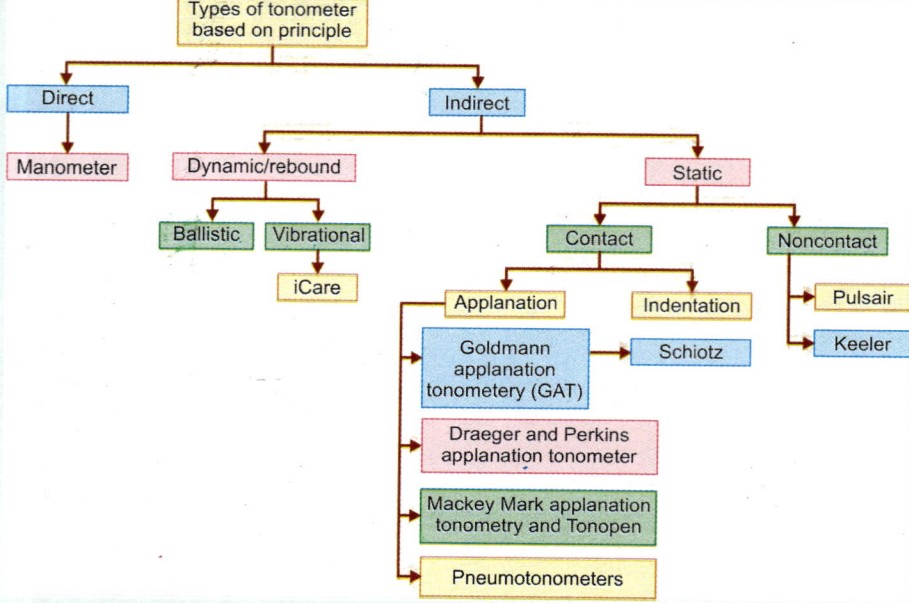

Footnote:
- **Goldmann applanation tonometry (GAT)** is a **Gold standard** Tonometer and is based on **Imbert–Fick principle,** which states that for an ideal, dry, thin-walled sphere, the pressure (P) inside the sphere equals the force (F) necessary to flatten its surface divided by the area (A) of flattening (i.e. P = F/A)
- **Pneumotonometers** are also based on the principle of applanation but, instead of using a prism, the central part of the cornea is flattened by a jet of air. Contact is not made with the subject's eye and topical anesthesia is not required, so it is particularly useful for screening in the community. Pneumotonometer may be used to estimate IOP in eyes that have scarred and irregular corneas
- **Perkins** applanation tonometer uses a Goldmann prism adapted to a small light source
- **Schiotz tonometer** uses the principle of indentation tonometry, in which the extent of corneal indentation by a plunger of known weight is measured; it is now seldom used in clinical practice
- **Rebound/dynamic tonometry** (e.g. **iCare**) involves a 1.8 mm plastic ball attached to a wire; deceleration of the probe upon contact with the cornea is proportional to IOP. Because only a very small force is applied to the cornea a topical anesthetic is not required. The instrument can be used for **self-monitoring** and screening in the community.
- **Drager and Perkins** are type of Goldman that can be used **without slit lamp**.
- In LASIK **Dynamic Contour Tonometer** is the application of choice.
- **Tonopen is a hand held tonometer** used for measuring IOP in diseased cornea and in children. Reichert tonopen based on Mackay Marg principle. It can measure extremes of IOP as well as in scarred or irregular corneas.
- **Mackay Marg/tonopen** used for **irregular corneas**

OPHTHAL PLATE 32

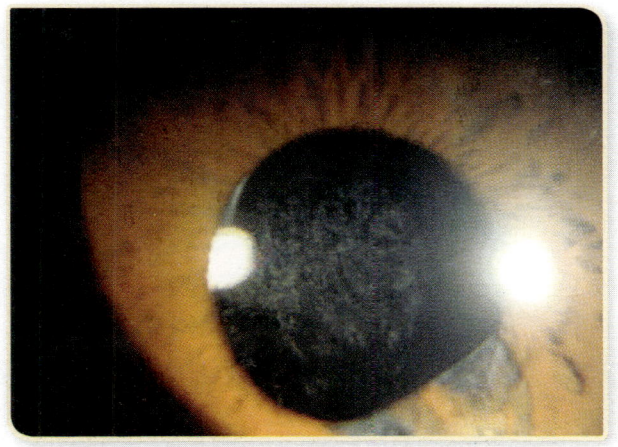

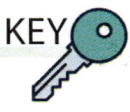

AFTER CATARACT

This is after cataract. This picture shows a cluster of Elschnig pearls that have formed behind the lens after cataract surgery. These grape-like clusters form from residual lens epithelial cells that migrate along the remaining capsular bag. They can be seen with a microscope and are usually visually insignificant.

After Cataract can be of two types:
a. Anterior capsular opacification
b. Posterior Capsular opacification: Posterior capsular opacification can be of two types: Soemeering Ring and Elsching pearls

Prevention:
a. Polishing of posterior capsule intra-operatively
b. Using of square edge design IOL

Treatment : NdYAG lASER

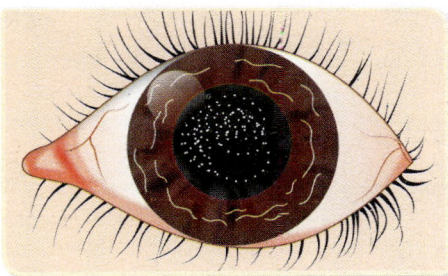

Fig: Elschnig Pearls results from proliferation of lens epithelium on the posterior capsule several months post cataract extraction

OPHTHAL PLATE 33

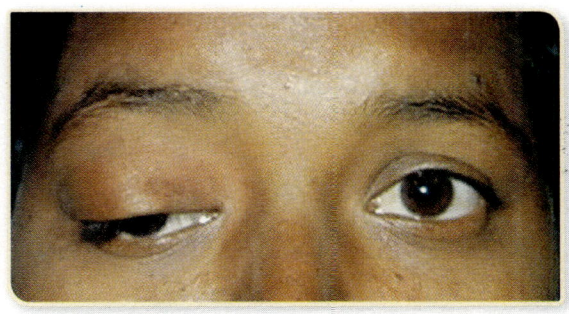

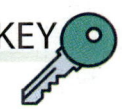

PTOSIS
- Ptosis is Drooping of eyelid.
- Ectropion is eversion and entropion is inversion of eyelid
- Lagophthalmos is inability to close the eyelid seen in facial nerve palsy or tumors

Differential diagnosis: Lugophthalmos, Ectropion, Entropion
Remember: Lagophthalmos is tested when the patient looks down, Ptosis is seen as drooping in primary position

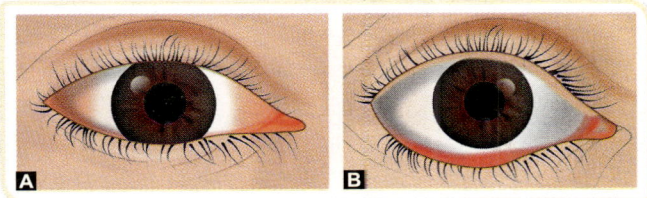

Fig: A. Entropion – eyelid turned in; B. Ectropion – eyelid turned out

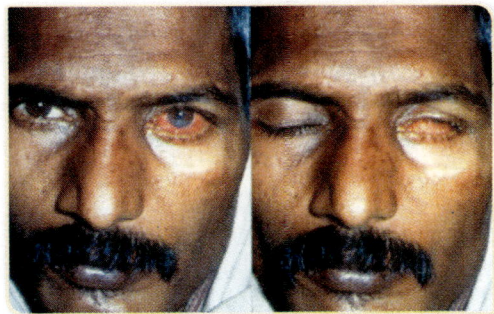

Fig: Classically you can observe that in left side image when the patient tries to close the eye, he is not able to close it fully. That is called Lagophthalmos

OPHTHAL PLATE 34

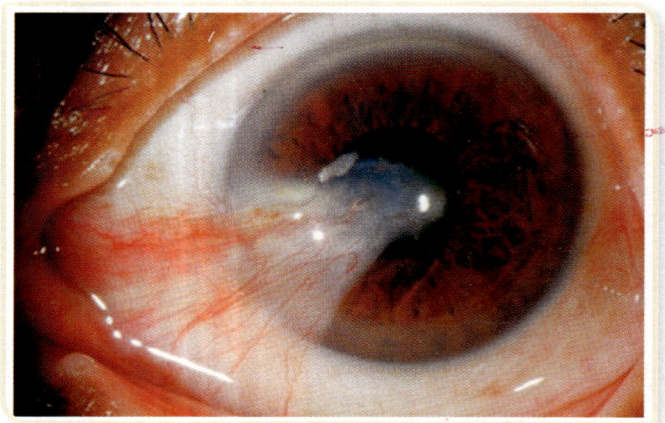

© JM Varas (Creative Commons)

PTERYGIUM

- Pterygium is a growth onto the cornea, usually nasally, of fibrovascular tissue that is continuous with the conjunctiva. It occurs in the palpebral fissure area, more often nasally than temporally, although either or both ("double" pterygium) may occur.
- It is a degenerative lesion.
- Pterygium is associated with UV radiation not infrared.
- Infrared causes more of glass blowers cataract.
- Pterygium excision is associated with **high rate of recurrence such upto 30-80%**. To avoid recurrence autograft of conjunctiva, mitomycin c, 5- fluorouracil can be used.
- Probe can't pass underneath pterygium, can be passed through pseudopterygium though.
- The histopathology of pterygium is characterized by elastotic degeneration with hyalinization of the conjunctival stroma, collection of basophilic elastic fibers, and granular deposits. Bowman's membrane is destroyed within the corneal component.

Treatment

- Bare sclera technique (30-80 % recurrence rate)
- Conjunctival graft (Autograft/ Allograft)
- Use of mitomycin (for prevention)
- Amniotic membrane graft (For prevention)
- Partial Lamellar keratoplasty (For prevention)

Pterygium	Pseudopterygium
Stromal tissue degeneration	Inflammatory adhesion to cornea
More common nasally	Can occur anywhere
Probe can be passed through	Probe can't be passed through
Mostly at 3 O' clock -9 O' clock position	Can occur anywhere
History of old age or UV exposure	History of chemical, thermal injury

OPHTHAL PLATE 35

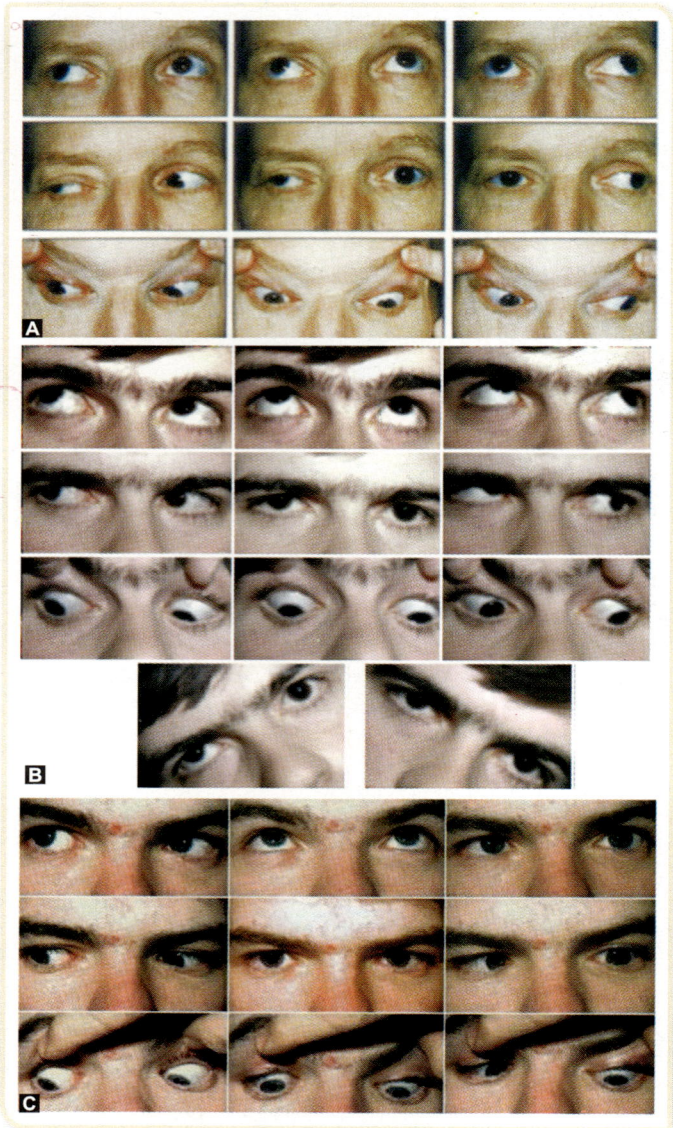

PLATE LEGENDS

A. **Right 3rd (Oculomotor) nerve palsy:**

B. **Right superior oblique muscle (6th-Trochlear nerve) palsy:** There is a right hypertropia in primary position that increases in left gaze and with head tilt to the right. **Mnemonic- WOOG** = worse on opposite gaze, that is not there on left head tilt. So patient would like to have left head tilt. So remember **mnemonic BOOT**- Better on opposite tilt

C. **Right 6th (Abducent) CN nerve palsy:** Extraocular movements in 9 cardinal positions of gaze. Restriction of right eye in lateral gaze suggestive of the right lateral rectus palsy (6th nerve). In primary gaze the right eye is medial, hence Lateral rectus (6th nerve) palsy.

3rd, 4th and 6th Cranial Nerve Palsy

	3rd (Oculomotor) nerve palsy	Superior oblique muscle (6th-Trochlear nerve) palsy	6th cranial nerve (abducent) palsy
Causes	Posterior circulation aneurysm Brainstem lesions Microvascular ischemia Cavernous sinus disease	Posterior circulation aneurysm Brainstem lesions Microvascular ischemia Cavernous sinus disease	Posterior circulation aneurysm, Brainstem lesions, Microvascular ischemia, Cavernous sinus disease, Elevated intracranial pressure, Superior orbital fissure syndrome
Clinical features	▫ Diplopia: Horizontal and vertical ▫ Abduction and depression in primary position: due to unopposed action of the lateral rectus and superior oblique muscles. The intact superior oblique muscle also causes intorsion of the eye at rest, which increases on attempted downgaze. ▫ Normal abduction as lateral rectus is intact. ▫ Limited adduction due to medial rectus weakness. ▫ Limited elevation due to weakness of the superior rectus and inferior oblique. ▫ Limited depression due to weakness of inferior rectus ▫ Varying degree of ptosis ▫ In complete 3rd nerve involvement, dilated pupil and defective accommodation due to parasympathetic palsy	▫ Diplopia- oblique/ tortional diplopia worse on downward gaze ▫ Combination of Elevation, Extorsion, Esotropia (Since Superior oblique does Depression, Intorsion, Abduction) ▫ Ipsilateral hypertropia ▫ The hypertropia is greater when they look to the opposite side. ▫ Hypertropia is greater when they tilt their head toward the same side. ▫ Spontaneous tilt of head to the contralateral side to compensate for diplopia. ▫ Diagnosis is based on either Head tilt or Parks Bielschowsky three step test	▫ Diplopia (uncrossed, horizontal diplopia) on lateral gaze to the ipsilateral side worse at distance. ▫ Head turn towards the paralyzed side ▫ Esotropia (one or both eyes turns inward) i.e. convergent squint in long standing LR Palsy ▫ Headache vomiting pain if a/w lesions causing raised Intracranial tension

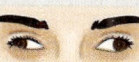

Ptosis
Pupillary dilatation
Downwad outward

Extosion on downward gaze

Lateral gaze palsy

Cranial nerve palsy	Exam finding - evidence of incomitance		
	← Direction of gaze	Primary Position	Direction of Gaze →
Right 3rd nerve palsy	Smaller angle of horizontal squint	Right eye turns downwards and outwards	Unable to adduct right eye Larger angle of squint Double vision further apart
Right 4th nerve palsy	No obvious squint	Right eye turns upwards and outwards	Right eye elevates more as it moves medially Double vision further apart
Right 6th nerve palsy	Unable to adduct right eye Larger angle of squint Double vision further apart	Right eye turns medially	Able to adduct right eye No obvious squint

Interpretation of incomitance (that is, angle of squint varies with direction of gaze)

Mnemonic In primary gaze see the deviation of eye DUM; Downward and Outward= 3rd nerve, Upward and Outward= 4th nerve, Medially= 6th nerve

> **Note**
>
> Hypertropia is an ocular disorder characterized by either constant or intermittent upwards deviation of one eye in comparison to the other eye. On the other hand, hypotropia involves downward deviation of one eye compared to the other.

Parks-Bielschowsky Three-Step Test

The three-step test, also known as the Parks-Bielschowsky three-step test or the Parks-Helveston three-step test, is a diagnostic test used to identify which muscle is paretic in the case of an acquired hypertropia. This test is most useful in diagnosing superior oblique palsies in clinical practice.

The three-step test may also be used to diagnose the less common inferior oblique or vertical rectus muscle palsy. It is designed for the diagnosis of a single paretic vertical muscle and is unreliable when there are multiple paretic muscles. This test may also help in identifying if a superior rectus palsy is true or simulated in a patient with an inhibitional palsy of the contralateral antagonist.

- The first step in the three-step test is to determine which eye is hypertropic in primary position.
- The second step is to determine whether the hypertropia increases on right or left gaze.
- The third step is determination if the hypertropia increases upon left head tilt or right head tilt.

OPHTHAL PLATE 36

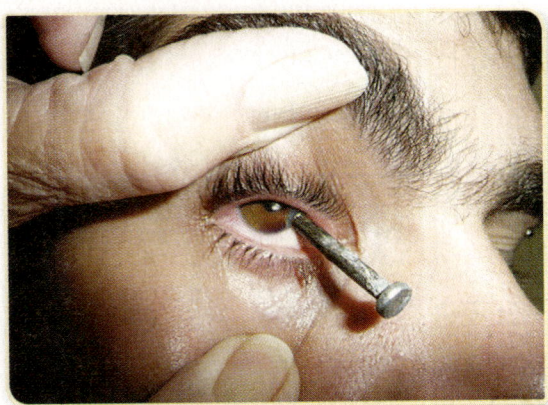

METALLIC FOREIGN BODY (NAIL) IN EYE^AIIMSPG

- Penetrating injury refers to a single full-thickness wound, usually caused by a sharp object, without an exit wound. A penetrating injury may be associated with intraocular retention of a foreign body.
- MRI is contraindicated in metallic foreign body of eye
- CT scan is the investigation of choice in metallic foreign body of eye
- **Seidel test** is done to localize the entry wound in penetrating injury of eye by using fluorescein dye
- Magnetic removal of ferrous metallic foreign bodies involves the creation of a sclerotomy adjacent to the foreign body, with application of a magnet.
- Forceps removal may be used for non-magnetic foreign bodies and magnetic foreign bodies that cannot be safely removed with a magnet.
- Prophylaxis against infection: Antibiotics.

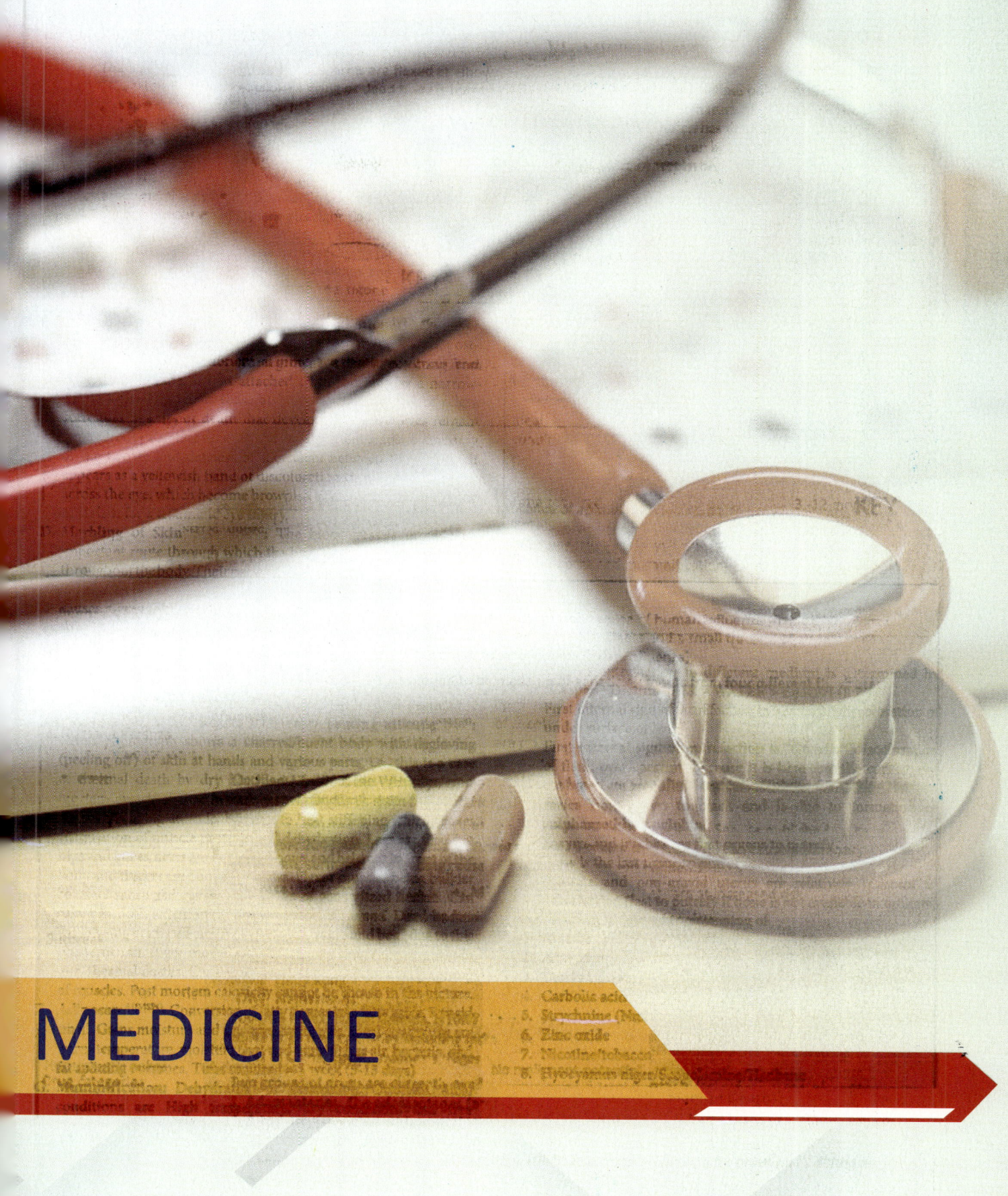

MEDICINE

MEDICINE PLATE 1

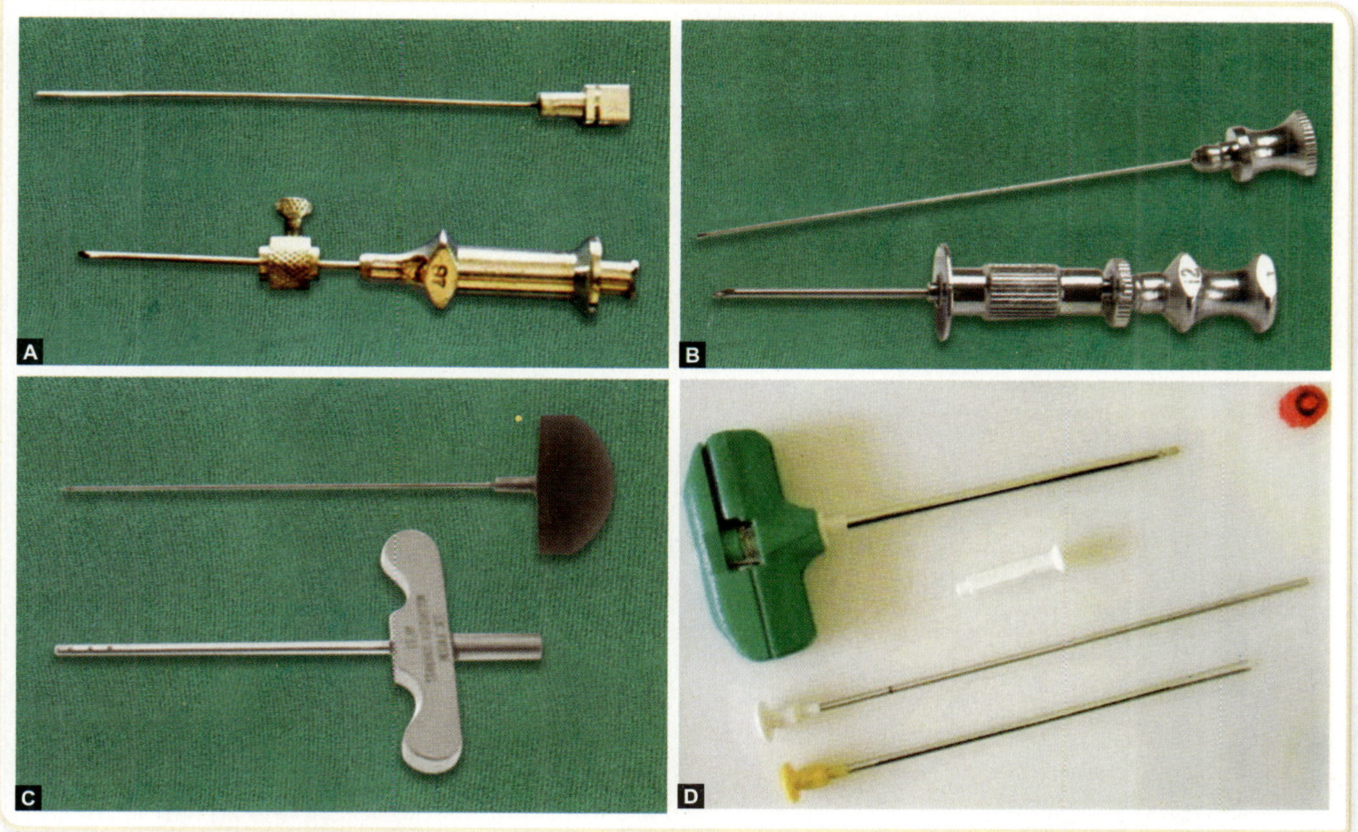

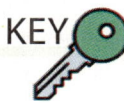

BONE MARROW BIOPSY NEEDLES

There are 3 types of needles that can be used. They have a stylet and the length of the needle to be inserted into the marrow cavity can be adjusted with the use of a guard.

A. Salah's needle; with side screw
B. Klima needle; with central screw, mostly used for sternal puncture
C. Islam Bone marrow aspiration/ trephine needle: Dome shaped handle and T bar for stability and control
D. Modern Jamshidi bone aspiration/ trephine needle

Trephine Biopsy

Simpler than aspiration
Can be done in outpatient or bedside
Valuable in case of previous dry tap

Bone Marrow Biopsy	
Indications ▫ Aplastic anemia and myelosclerosis ▫ Megaloblastic anemia ▫ Leukemia ▫ Storage diseases ▫ Tumors – primary/secondaries ▫ Multiple myeloma ▫ Parasitic diseases, e.g. Malaria, Leishmania ▫ Iron content study ▫ Bone marrow transplantation	**Contraindications** ▫ Deep penetration of bone leading to injury to aorta ▫ Hemorrhage ▫ Infection ▫ Shock **Complications** Bone marrow aspiration is usually without any risk. However if platelet count is < 20,000/mm^3 sternal puncture is avoided.

Contd...

Bone Marrow Biopsy

Site: The procedure can be done at any one of the following sites.
- Sternal body or manubrium
- Posterior iliac crest
- Tibia (medial aspect just below the tibial tubercle)
- Spinous process of vertebra
- Site of bone infiltration or tumor.

Note: The posterior iliac crest and tibia are the preferred sites in children.

Procedure: Under strict aseptic precautions.
- Local anesthesia is infiltrated from the skin up to the periosteum
- **Position:** For iliac crest both lateral and prone (face down) position can be done
  - First the guard of the needle is adjusted so that only a further 5 mm can be advanced into the marrow. The bone marrow needle is then pushed into the skin – subcutaneous tissues up to the periosteum.
  - The needle is advanced into the periosteum at right angles and a clockwise counter clock wise motion until a sensation of decreased resistance is felt when the marrow cavity is entered. The stylet is removed, a 10 or 20 ml syringe is attached to the needle, and with sharp suction up to 0.5 ml of marrow is aspirated into the syringe to avoid mixing with peripheral blood. While aspirating, patient experiences an intense suction pain indicating the needle is in the marrow.
  - A drop of aspirate is placed on the slides to get a pure bone marrow smear.

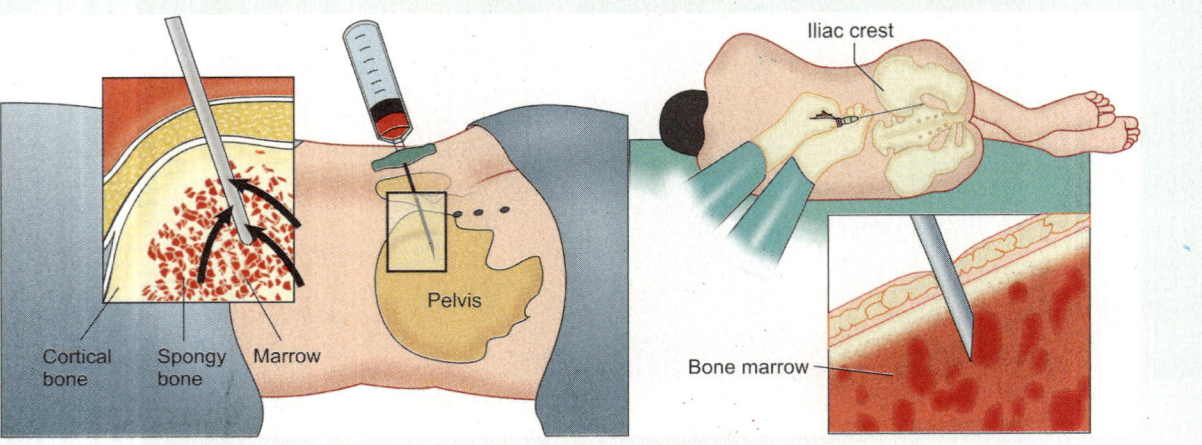

Note

Dry Tap
- Faulty technique
- Hypoplasia and aplasia of bone marrow
- Tightly packed marrow
- Myelofibrosis

MEDICINE PLATE 2

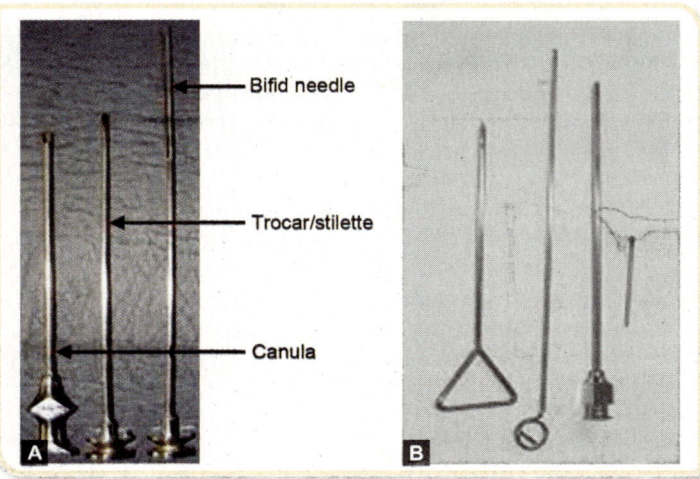

LIVER BIOPSY NEEDLES

Different types of needle are used:
A. **Vim Silverman Needle:** Points of Identification: It is steel needle, with stellate and Bifid needle with length of 15–18 cms.
B. **Menghini Needle:** When using Menghini, after making a track with the track maker, the needle is fitted with a 2 ml syringe containing normal saline and introduced. The needle is first flushed and then applying a suction force it is advanced further and quickly withdrawn. The specimen is then flushed out of the needle.

Indications	Contraindications
▫ Differentiating different types of Jaundice.	▫ Hydatid cyst
▫ Diagnosis of Cirrhosis	▫ Cavernous hemangioma
▫ Tumours of Liver – Primary, secondaries	▫ Bleeding diseases
▫ Parasitic infestations, e.g. Amebiasis	**Complications**
▫ Storage diseases	▫ Bleeding into liver
▫ Wilson's disease	▫ Bile leakage
▫ Hemochromatosis	▫ Infections
▫ Granulomatous diseases, e.g. Tuberculosis	
▫ Unexplained hepatomegaly	

MEDICINE PLATE 3

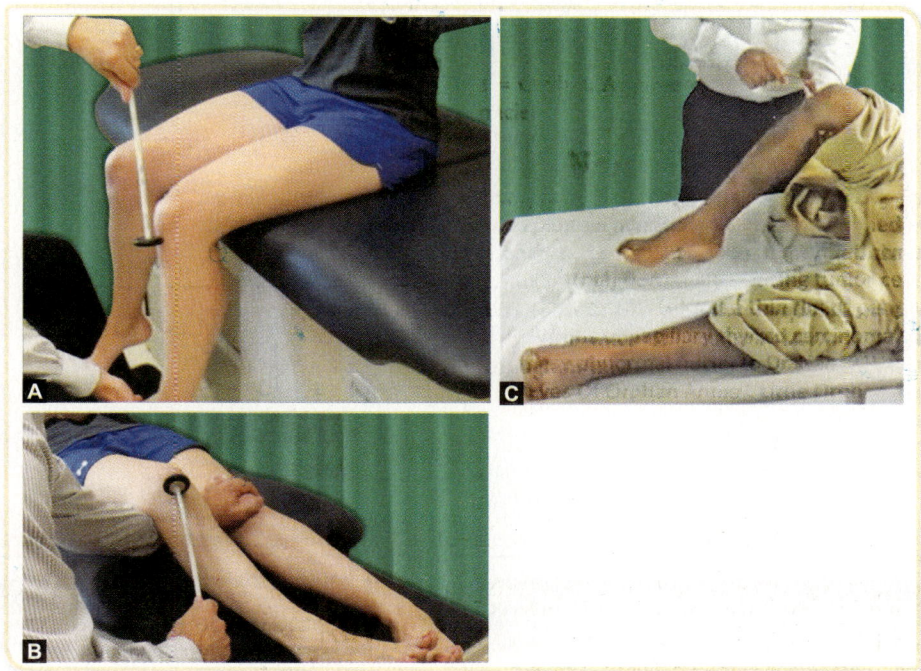

KNEE JERK

The patellar reflex is contraction of the quadriceps femoris muscle, with resulting extension of the knee, in response to percussion of the patellar tendon. A firm tap on the tendon draws the patella down, stretching the quadriceps and provoking reflex contraction. If the reflex is brisk, the contraction is strong and the amplitude of the movement is large. If the examiner places one hand over the muscle, and with the other hand taps the patellar tendon just below the patella, He/she can palpate the contraction as well as observe the rapidity and range of response. Palpation helps in judging the latency between the time of the stimulus and the resulting response.

The knee jerk can be elicited in various ways.
A. The patient may sit in a chair with the knees slightly extended and the heels resting on the floor or sit on an examination table with the legs dangling. If the patient is lying in bed, the examiner should partially flex the knee by placing one hand beneath it and then tap the tendon. The responses on the two sides can be compared by lifting both knees simultaneously, supporting them on one forearm as the patient's heels rest lightly on the bed, before tapping the tendons. If the patient is wearing loose pajamas, the examiner can suspend both legs by holding the pajamas, as he/she uses the other hand to strike the tendon.

B. Another technique is having the patient sit with one leg crossed over the other and tapping the patellar tendon of the uppermost leg, but this method does not facilitate side-to-side comparison.
C. Incorrect method of doing Knee jerk. As quadriceps (Thigh) should have been exposed completely.

Reflexes

Reflex	The group of reflex	Muscles	Nerves (N)	Segments
Sub eyesbrow	Deep, periosteal reflex	Orbicularis oculi	N trigeminus (V) – N.facialis (VII)	Medulla oblongata and pons
Corneal (lid)	Superficial, from mucous membrane	Orbicularis oculi	N trigeminus (V) – N.facialis (VII)	Medulla oblongata and pons
Jaw Jerk (mandibular, chin, masseter) reflex (Bechterev's)	Deep, periosteal reflex	Masseter	N trigeminus (V) – N mandibularis (sensory and motor)	Medulla oblongata and pons
Pharyngeal	Superficial, from mucous membrane	Constrictor pharyngis and others	N glosso-pharyngeus, N vagus (sensory and motor), 9th and 10th pair of CCN	Medulla oblongata
Palatal (palatine)	Superficial, from mucous membrane	Levatores velli palatini	N glosso-pharyngeus, N vagus (sensory and motor)	Medulla oblongata
Biceps	Deep, stretch reflex	Biceps brachii	N musculo-cutaneus	C5-C6
Triceps	Deep, stretch reflex	Triceps brachii	N radialis	C7-C8
Radial (carporadial, brachioradial)	Deep, periosteal reflex	Pronator flexor, digitorum, brachioradialis, biceps	N medianus, N. radialis, N musculo-cutaneus	C5-C8
Scapulo-humeral (scapuloperiosteal) reflex (Bechterew's)	Deep, periosteal reflex	Teres major, subscapularis	N subscapularis	C5-C6
Upper superficial abdominal	Superficial, dermal	obliquus, rectus abdominis	N intercostales	D7-D8
Middle superficial abdominal	Superficial, dermal	Transversus, obliquus, rectus abdominis	N intercostales	D9-D10
Lower superficial abdominal	Superficial, dermal	Transversus, obliquus, rectus abdominis	N intercostales	D11-D12
Cremasteric	Superficial, dermal	Cremaster	N genitofemoralis	L1-L2
Knee jerk, or patellar reflex (quadriceps stretch reflex)	Deep, stretch reflex	Quadriceps femoris	N femoralis	L3-L4
Achilles (ankle jerk)	Deep, stretch reflex	Triceps surae	N tibialis (N ischiadicus)	S1-S2
Plantar (sole)	Superficial, dermal	Flexor digitorum pedis and others	N ischiadicus	L5-S1
Anal	Superficial, dermal	Sphincter ani externus	N anococcygeal	S4-S5

Reflex Pattern with Different Neurological Disorders

Site or type of lesion	Muscle stretch reflex	Superficial reflex	Pathological reflex	Associated movements
Neuromuscular junction	N or ↓	Normal	Absent	Normal
Muscle	Usually N, May be ↓	Normal	Absent	Normal
Peripheral nerve	↓ Or Absent	N, ↓ or Absent in the distribution of nerve	Absent	Normal
Corticospinal tract (Upper motor neuron)	Hyperactive (↑)	↓ Or Absent	Present	Pathological associated movement present
Extrapyramidal	Usually normal	N or Slightly ↑	Absent	Normal associated movement absent
Cerebellum	Pendular	Normal	Absent	Normal
Psychogenic	N or ↑ especially in range of response	N or ↑	Absent	Normal or Bizarre

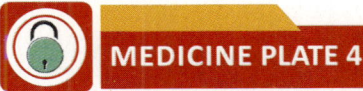

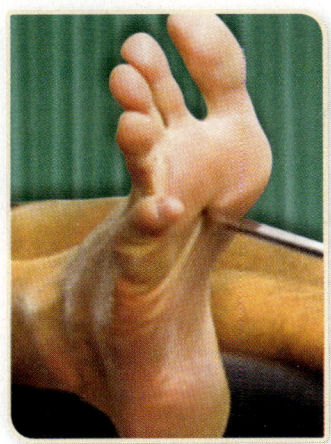

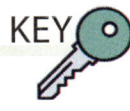

KEY

BABINSKI SIGN

Positive Babinski's sign (extensor plantar response) is seen with lesions of the corticospinal tract (pyramidal tract). That is on eliciting the plantar response, there is dorsiflexion of the great toe, along with extension and fanning out of the other toes. Babinski's sign can be elicited only by stroking the lateral aspect of the dorsum of the foot in presence of minimal pyramidal tract lesion. When test is repeated the plantar response may become fatigued, and the extensor plantar response may not be elicited.

MEDICINE PLATE 5

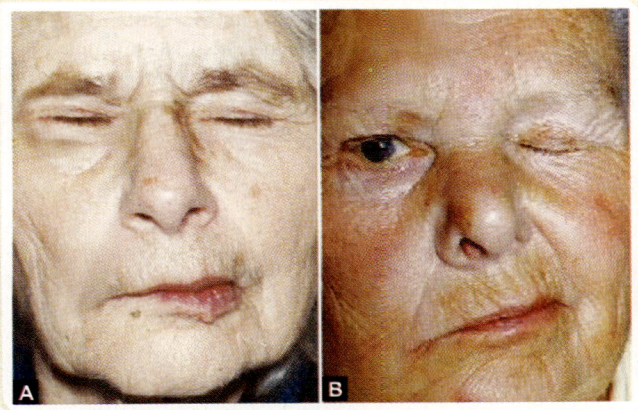

KEY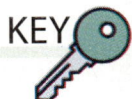

TYPES OF FACIAL NERVE PALSY

A. Upper motor neuron type facial nerve palsy
B. Lower motor neuron type facial nerve palsy

Types of Facial Nerve Palsy		
	Upper motor neuron (UMN)	Lower motor neuron (LMN)
AKA	Supranuclear palsy	Nuclear and Infranuclear palsy Bell's palsy
Lesion	Above the facial nerve nucleus	At or after the facial nerve nucleus
Side affected	Contralateral	Ipsilateral
Weakness of	Lower face weakness but much less weakness of the upper face.	Both upper and lower face weakness, Hyperacusis (nerve to stapedius) Metallic taste (chorda tympani) Reduced lacrimation (greater petrosal nerve)
Taste	Not affected	Loss of taste sensation

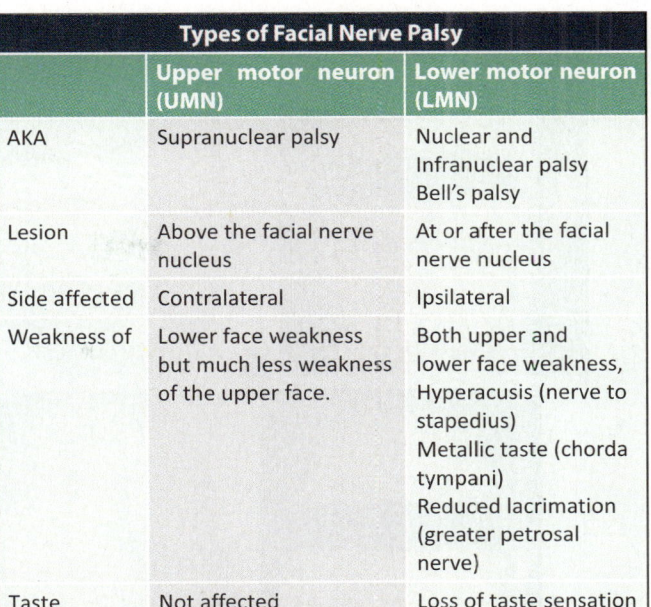

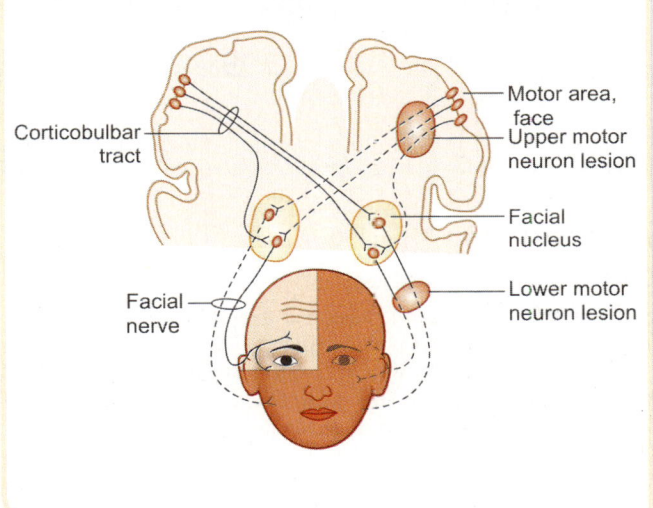

MEDICINE PLATE 6

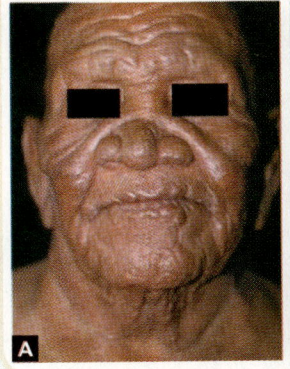
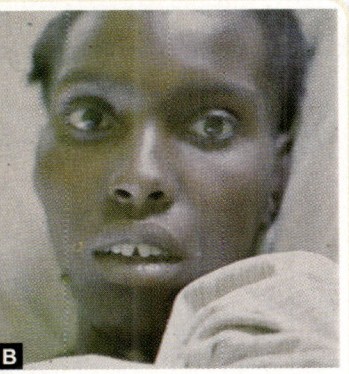

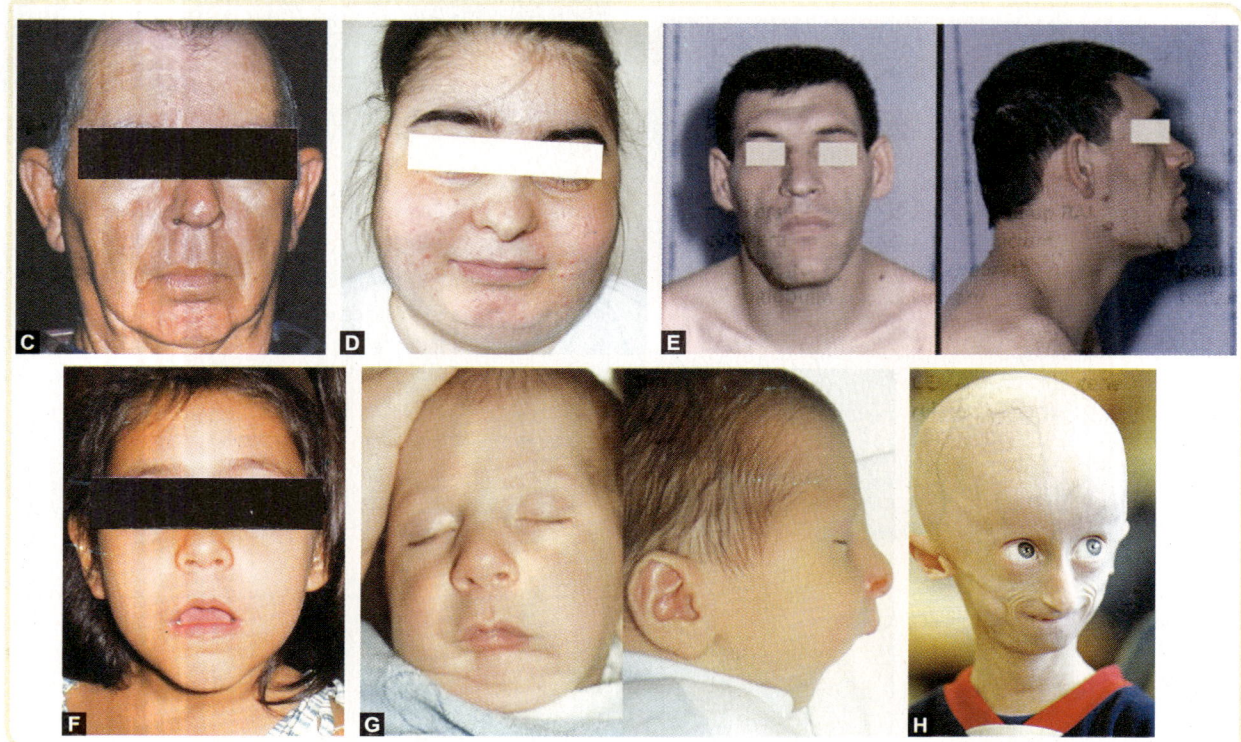

PLATE LEGENDS

Different Types of Faces

A. **Leonine faces:** Seen in leprosy, and shows thickening of the skin and ear lobes, flattened nasal bridge and loss of hair over the lateral aspect of eyebrows and eyelashes (madarosis).
B. **Hippocratic faces:** Pale and pinched face, sunken eyes and hollow cheeks seen in impending death or chronic illness.
C. **Mask like faces** seen in Parkinson's disease: Immobile, fixed and expressionless face with infrequent blinking of the eyes (< 10 per minute) (Normal rate of blinking is about 20 per minute), fluttering of the eyelids is seen (blepharoclonus). It is also seen in *Scleroderma*.
D. **Moon faces** seen in Cushing's syndrome or steroid treatment. Rounded 'moon face' and puffy face with excessive hair growth.
E. **Acromegalic faces** Prominent lower jaw, coarse features, large widened nose, thick lips, prominent ears, prominent cheekbones and widespread teeth, facial lines are marked. The forehead and overlying skin is thickened, sometimes leading to frontal bossing.
F. **Adenoid faces,** also known as the long face syndrome, refers to the long, open mouth face of a child with adenoid hypertrophy.
G. **Bird faces:** Seen in Pierre Robin syndrome. It gives rise to three problem, a very small lower jaw, a slit like hole in the palate of mouth (called cleft palate) and retroglossoptosis (tongue appears to fall into the throat)
H. **Progeric faces** This is seen in Hutchinson Guilford progeria syndrome showing disproportionately small face in comparison to the head, micrognathia, prominent eyes, both upper eyelids' retraction, beaked nose, thin lips, Prominent scalp veins, alopecia with grey and sparse hairs, and protruding ears with absence of earlobe.

MEDICINE PLATE 7

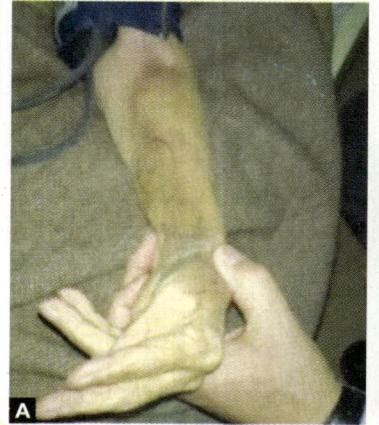
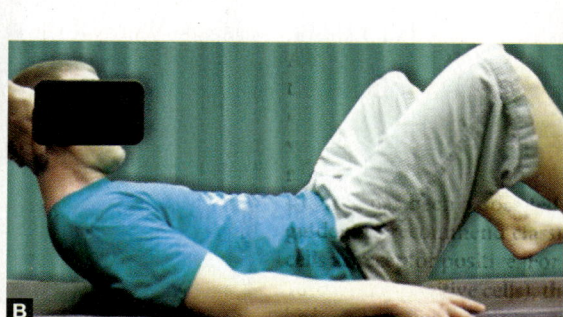
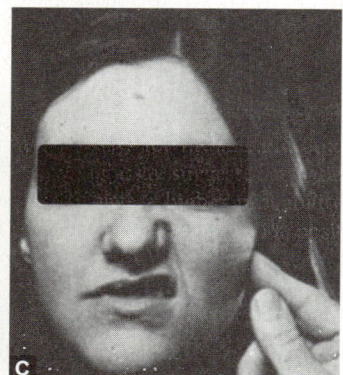

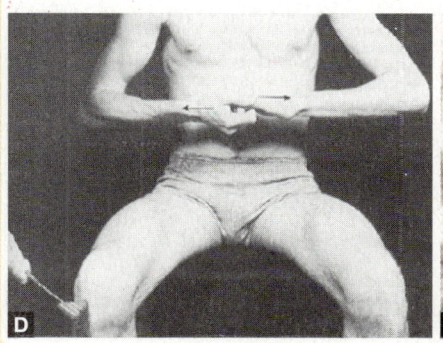 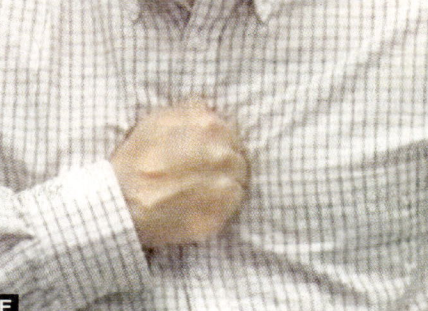 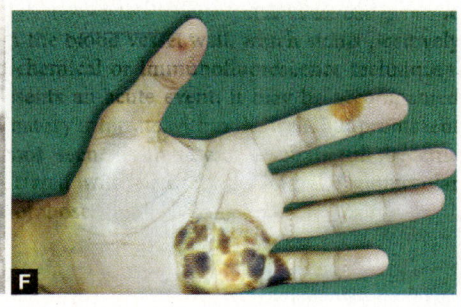

Credits: Roberto J. Galindo

NAMED SIGNS IN MEDICINE

A. **Trousseau's sign** is carpopedal spasm caused by inflating the blood-pressure cuff to a level above systolic pressure for 3 minutes. It is a sign of hypocalcemia.
B. **Brudzinski sign:** This sign is present in meningeal irritation. The patient's hips and knees flex during passive neck flexion due to severe neck stiffness.
C. **Chvostek's sign** is the twitching of the facial muscles in response to tapping over the area of the facial nerve. It is seen in hypocalcemia.
D. **Jendrassik maneuver:** This is a reinforcement maneuver used to amplify lower limb reflexes. The patient is asked to hook together the flexed fingers of both hands and pull.
E. **Levine's sign:** A clenched fist held over the central area of the anterior chest wall to describe ischemic cardiac chest pain.
F. **Osler's nodules:** This is a cutaneous manifestation of bacterial infective endocarditis.

MEDICINE PLATE 9

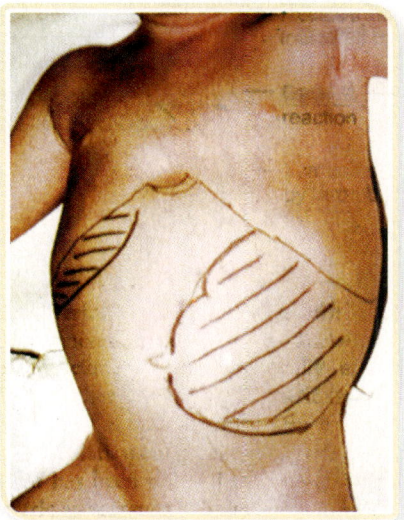

MASSIVE SPLENOMEGALY

This figure indicates massive splenomegaly with hepatomegaly.
Massive splenomegaly: The spleen extends greater than 8 cm below left costal margin and/or weighs more than 1000 g.

Diseases Associated with Massive Splenomegaly	
Chronic myeloid leukemia	Gaucher's disease
Lymphomas (Non-Hodgkin's)	Chronic lymphocytic leukemia
Hairy cell leukemia	Sarcoidosis
Myelofibrosis with myeloid metaplasia	Autoimmune hemolytic anemia
Portal hypertension Polycythemia vera	Diffuse splenic hemangiomatosis Kala azar Chronic Malaria

MEDICINE PLATE 8

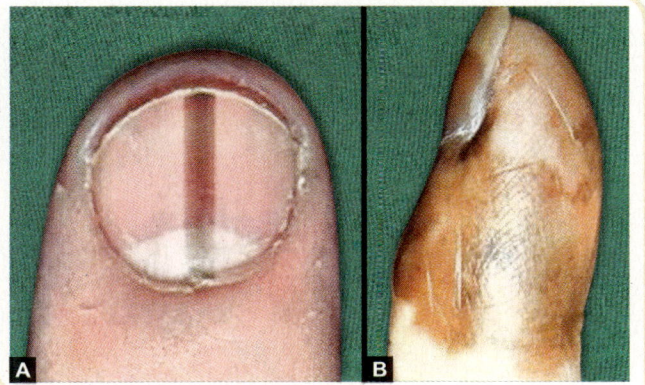

ACRAL LENTIGINOUS MELANOMA

Pigmented band starting at proximal nail fold (Fig A) is called Hutchinson's nail sign. It can have periungual spread (Fig B)

However not given in the original table of Harrison but text says that, Malaria is conventionally described to cause **Tropical splenomegaly syndrome**, also known as **hyper reactive malarial splenomegaly**, due immunological over-stimulation to repeated attacks of malarial infection over a long period of time. Condition is usually seen in malaria-endemic areas like Africa and Indian subcontinent.

Causes of Hepatosplenomegaly	
Infections	Malaria Kala azar Typhoid fever Infectious mononucleosis Disseminated tuberculosis
Hepatic diseases	Viral hepatitis Cirrhosis Non cirrhotic portal fibrosis
Hemolytic anemias	Thalassemias Hereditary spherocytosis G6PD deficiency
Hematological malignancy	ALL, AML CML Hodgkin's lymphoma Non Hodgkin's lymphoma
Miscellaneous	Glycogen storage disorder Mucopolysaccharidosis Collagen vascular disease

Abbreviations: ALL, Acute Lymphocytic Leukemia; AML, Aute Myeloid Leukemia; CML, Chronic Myclogenous Leukemia.

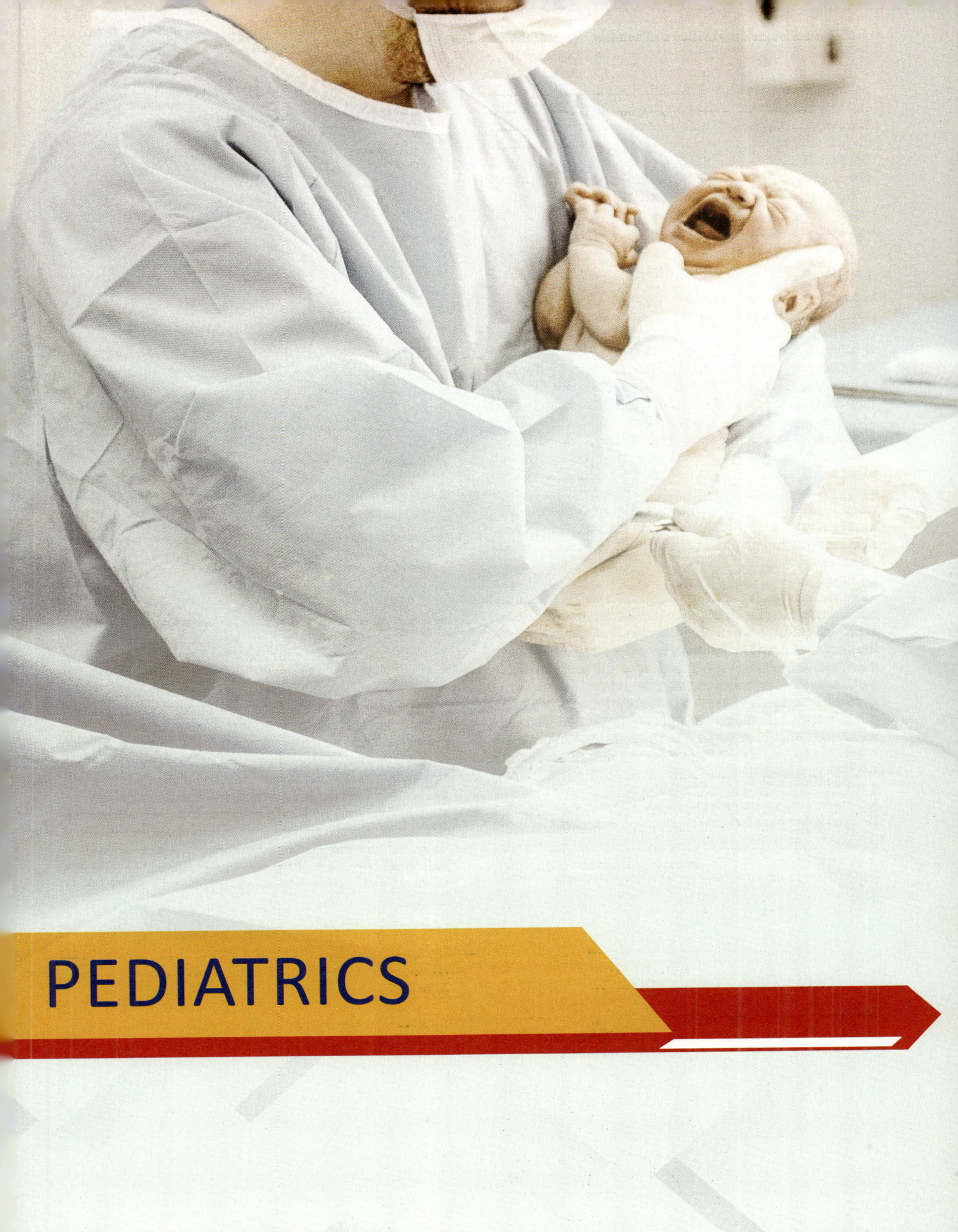
PEDIATRICS

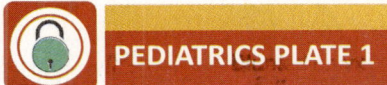

PEDIATRICS PLATE 1

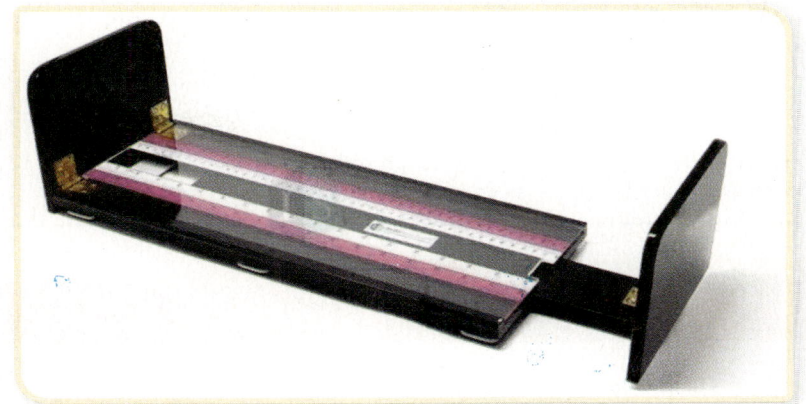

INFANTOMETER
The infantometer method of measuring length of child. The standing height can be measured for children more than 2 years, while for younger children, the recumbent length should be measured using the infantometer.

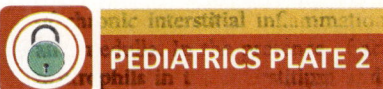

PEDIATRICS PLATE 2

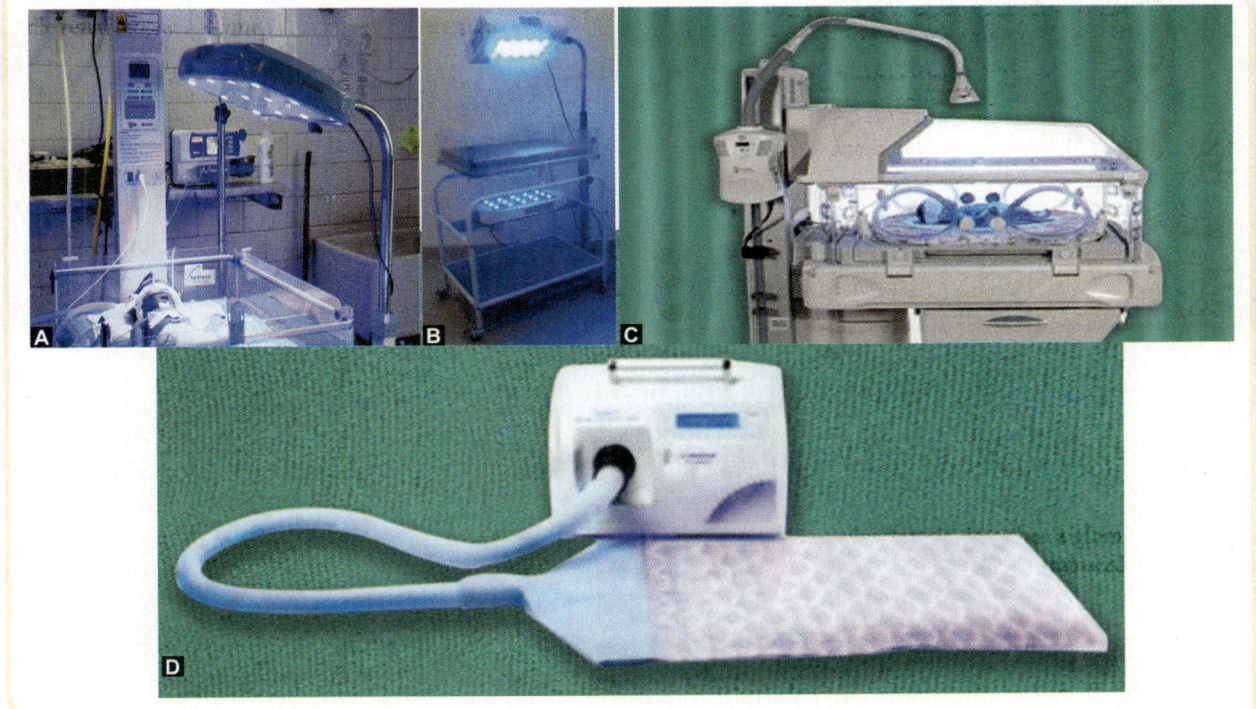

PHOTOTHERAPY UNITS/SYSTEM
A. Single surface Phototherapy unit (from above)
B. Double surface Phototherapy unit (both from above and below)

C. Halogen spotlight Phototherapy system
D. Fiberoptic blanket Phototherapy system

Phototherapy or exposure to light is known to cause photoisomerization of unconjugated bilirubin to more polar, water soluble, harmless compounds, which are readily excreted. Blue green light is most effective for phototherapy as it both penetrates the skin and is absorbed by bilirubin to have the photochemical effect. Note eyes are effectively covered to prevent retinal damage.

Commercially available light source for phototherapy are:
- **Fluorescent tubes**
- **Halogen spot lights**
- **Fiberoptic blankets**
- **The gallium nitride LED** is one of the most recent innovations in phototherapy.

These devices provide high irradiance in the blue to blue green spectrum without excessive heat generation.

PEDIATRICS PLATE 3

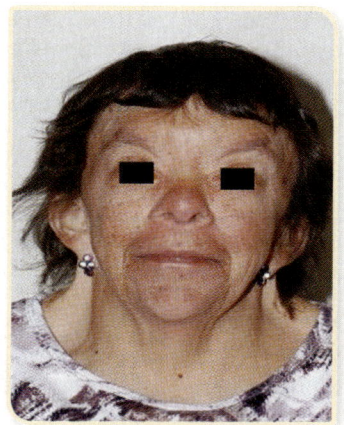

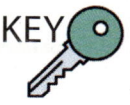

TURNER'S SYNDROME

Turner syndrome or **Ullrich-Turner syndrome** (also known as "Gonadal dysgenesis") encompasses several conditions in human females, of which monosomy X (absence of an entire sex chromosome, the Barr body) is most common. It is a chromosomal abnormality in which all or part of one of the sex chromosomes is absent.

Karyotype: 45,XO or 45,XO/46,XX Mossaic	Rudimentary ovaries gonadal streak (underdeveloped gonadal structures that later become fibrosed)	External genitalia: Female phenotype	Internal genitalia: Hypoplastic female phenotype	Breast: Immature female phenotype
Clinical Features				
Infancy	Lymphedema of hands & foot, web neck, Broad chest (shield chest) and widely spaced nipples, Low hairline, Low-set ears, cardiac defects and coarctation of the aorta, urinary tract malformations and horseshoe kidney			
Childhood	Short stature, cubitus valgus, short neck, short 4th metacarpals, hypoplastic nails, palmar crease, micrognathia, scoliosis, otitis media and sensorineural hearing loss, ptosis and amblyopia, multiple nevi and keloid formation, autoimmune thyroid disease, visuospatial learning difficulties			
Adulthood	Pubertal failure and primary amenorrhea, hypertension, obesity, dyslipidemia, impaired glucose tolerance and insulin resistance, autoimmune thyroid disease, cardiovascular disease, aortic root dilation, osteoporosis, inflammatory bowel disease, chronic hepatic dysfunction, increased risk of colon cancer, hearing loss			

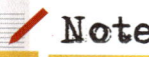

- Most common cardiac manifestation is isolated nonstenotic **bicuspid aortic valves** (in one third to one-half of patients). In later life, bicuspid aortic valve disease can progress to dilatation of the aortic root. Less frequent defects include aortic coarctation (20%), aortic stenosis, mitral valve prolapse, and anomalous pulmonary venous drainage
- Antithyroid antibodies, thyroid peroxidase, or thyroglobulin antibodies occur in 30–50% of patients.
- Recurrent bilateral otitis media develops in about 75% of patients. Sensorineural hearing deficits are common, and the frequency increases with age
- Turner's syndrome patients have **normal intelligence** (Kaplan & Sadock Psychiatry 10th ed page 16)

PEDIATRICS PLATE 4

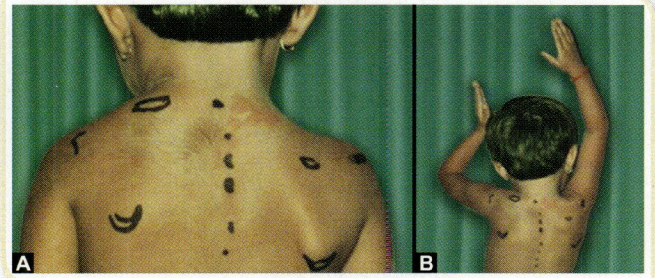

(*Source*: Kadavkolan AS, Bhatia DN, Dasgupta B, Bhosale PB - Int J Shoulder Surg 2011)

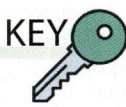
KEY

SPRENGEL DEFORMITY

A. Cosmetic aspect of Sprengel's deformity is shown. The landmarks show marked elevation of the left scapula as compared with the right.
B. Functional aspect of Sprengel's deformity is shown. Marked restriction of abduction on the left side is seen as compared to the right.

The functional aspect of the deformity has been attributed to:
- A forward curvature of the superior angle of the scapula over the apex of the thorax.
- Abutment of the medial scapular border against the spinous processes of adjacent vertebrae.
- The omovertebral bone.

Sprengel deformity, or congenital elevation of the scapula, is a disorder of development that involves a high scapula and limited scapulothoracic motion. The scapula originates in early embryogenesis at a level posterior to the 4th cervical vertebra, but descends during development to below the 7th cervical vertebra. Failure of this descent, either unilateral or bilateral, is the Sprengel deformity. The severity of the deformity depends on the location of the scapula and associated anomalies. The scapula in mild cases is simply rotated, with a palpable or visible bump corresponding to the superomedial corner of the scapula in the region of the trapezius muscle. Function is generally good. In moderate cases, the scapula is higher on the neck and connected to the spine with an abnormal omovertebral ligament or even bone. Shoulder motion, particularly abduction, is limited. In severe cases, the scapula is small and positioned on the posterior neck, and the neck may be webbed. The majority of patients have associated anomalies of the musculoskeletal system, especially in the spine (including Klippel-Feil anomaly with congenital cervical vertebral fusions making spinal evaluation important.

Syndromes associated with Sprengel's deformity include teratological conditions such as **inencephaly** (a triad of occipital defect, spina bifida of cervical vertebrae, and fixed retroflexion of the head) and the **Klippel-Feil syndrome.**

| The Cavendish Grade of Sprengel's Deformity ||
Grade	Indications
1	Very mild, shoulder level and deformity invisible when dressed
2	Mild, shoulders almost level, lump visible in web of the neck when dressed
3	Moderate, shoulder elevated 2 to 5 cm. Deformity easily visible.
4	Severe, superior angle of scapula near occiput, with or without neck webbing

Treatment

In mild cases, treatment is generally unnecessary, although a prominent and unsightly superomedial corner of the scapula can be excised. In more severe cases, surgical repositioning of the scapula with rebalancing of parascapular muscles can significantly improve both function and appearance.

PEDIATRICS PLATE 5

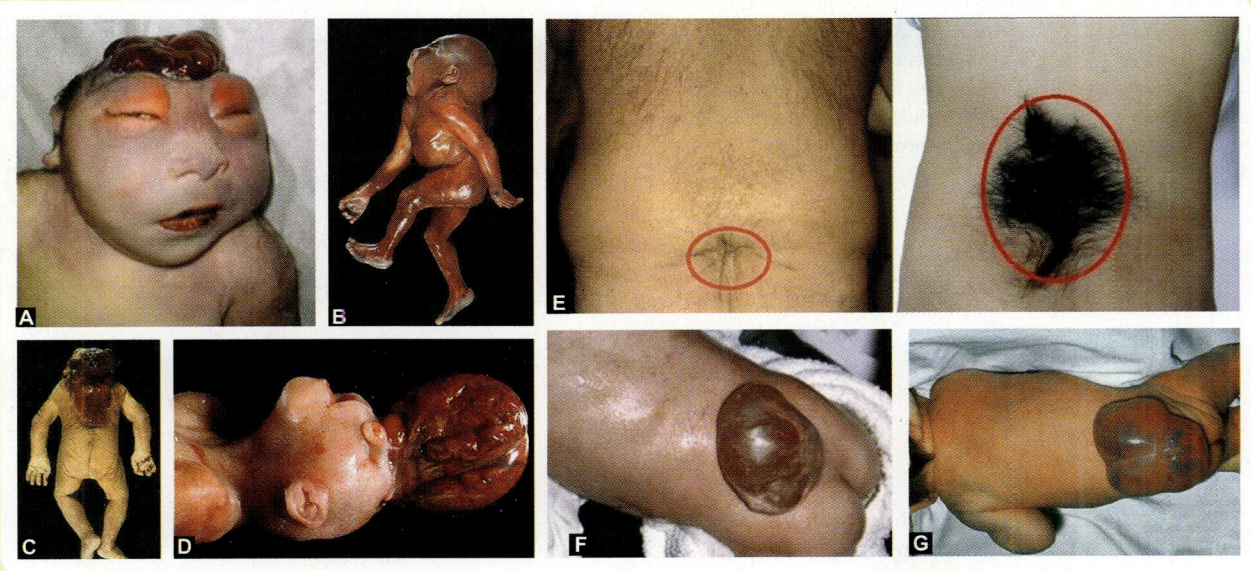

NEURAL TUBE DEFECTS

A. **Anencephaly:** Defect of cranial vault, frontoparietal region: partially degenerated brain tissue visible within the cranial bone defect. Severe swelling of palpebral and large appearing nose is seen.

B. **Iniencephaly:** Imperfect formation of the base of the skull, with rachischisis and exaggerated lordosis of the spine. This is iniencephaly. The key features are: (1) imperfect formation of the base of the skull, (2) rachischisis, and (3) exaggerated lordosis of the vertebral column.

C. **Complete/ total rachischisis** is demonstrated here in a case of iniencephaly. Craniospinal rachischisis is the failure of closure of most or all the neuraxis resulting in an absence/exposure of major portions of the brain and spinal cord.

D. **Exencephaly:** The cranial vault is not completely present, but a brain is present, because it was not completely exposed to amniotic fluid. Such an event is very rare. It may be part of craniofacial clefts with limb-body wall complex.

E. **Spina bifida occulta** is the simplest form of the spina bifida in which only the bony defect is present but no protrusion of meninges (protective layers covering the spinal cord) and the spinal cord. On right a dimple is shown on the lower back in the midline. A red circle is made around the dimple. It is also a common sign of spina bifida occulta. Due to a bony defect on the posterior side of vertebra, a space develops and skin is depressed at that point making a dimple on the skin. On left a tuft of hair on the lower back is one of the typical signs of spina bifida occulta. A red circle is made around the hair tuft on this picture.

F. **Meningocele:** Protrusion of the membranes that cover the spine and part of the spinal cord through a bone defect in the vertebral column containing CSF and lacks nervous tissue.

G. **Myelomeningocele:** A fluctuant midline mass that may transilluminate occurs along the vertebral column, usually in the lumbar region of a newborn baby with myelomeningocele. The skin is intact, and the placode-containing remnants of nervous tissue can be observed over the lesion, which is filled with cerebrospinal fluid.

Neural Tube Defects

NEURAL TUBE DEFECTS (DYSRAPHISM): This group of congenital anomalies of the CNS results from failure of the neural tube to close spontaneously. NTD are the most common malformations accounting for 0.5-1.3 cases/1000 live births with multifactorial etiology. Neural tube defects (NTDs) are a group of severe congenital abnormalities resulting from the failure of neurulation of multifactorial etiology around the 28th day of conception.

Contd...

Neural Tube Defects		
Cranial NTD	**Spinal NTD**	**Craniospinal NTDS**
Exencephaly	Spina bifida occulta	Craniospinal rachischisis
Anencephaly	Lumbra dermal sinus	
Cranial meningocele	Spina bifida aperta (spina bifida cystica) +/- posterior meningocele or myelomeningocele rachischisis	
Cranial myelomeningocele		
Encephalocele (myeloencephalocele)	Anterior meningocele / myelomeningocele	
Spinal meningocele	Lateral meningocele/ myelomeningocele	
	Iniencephaly	

Open NTDs	Closed NTDs (skin covered)
Anencephaly	Lipomyeloschisis
Myelomeningocele (spina bifida)	Lipomyelomeningocele
Myeloschisis	Meningocele
Hemimyelomeningocele	Myelocystocele
Hemimyelocele	
Craniorachischis	

Types of Spina Bifida

	Spina bifida occulta	Meningocele	Myelomeningocele
Incidence	5% of population	Most common type of spina bifida per 5000 live births	Most common type of spina bifida 1 per 800 live births
Location	Lumbosacral area is the most common location	Present along the length of spinal cord and skull. Lumbosacral area is the most common location	Present along the length of spinal cord, but not seen in skull. Lumbosacral area is the most common location
Clinical features	A mild form of Spina Bilda. Mostly asymptomatic & detected on X-ray. But may have a patch of hair, a lipoma or pigmentation of the low back	Cystic swelling in the skull or along the backbone. Content of meningocele do not contain the spinal cord. Neurological deficits are rare.	Cystic swelling in the lower back. Sac consists of both meninges and spinal cord contents. Most common and most severe form of spina bifida. If not treated leads to irreversible neurological deficit.

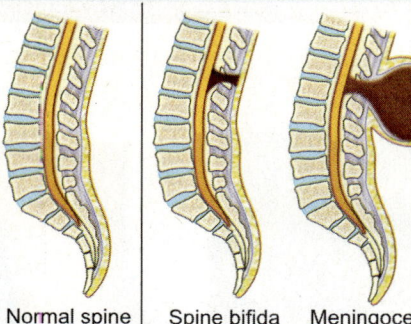

Normal spine | Spine bifida occulta | Meningocele | Myelomeningocele

Footnote:
- Before surgical correction of the defect, the patient must be thoroughly examined with the use of plain roentgenograms, ultrasonography, and MRI to determine the extent of neural tissue involvement, if any, and associated anomalies, including diastematomyelia, tethered spinal cord, and lipoma.
- **Urologic evaluation,** usually including cystometrogram (CMG), will identify those children with neurogenic bladder who are at risk for renal deterioration.
- Those patients with leaking cerebrospinal fluid (CSF) or a thin skin covering should undergo immediate surgical treatment to prevent meningitis.
- A CT scan of the head is recommended for children with a meningocele because of the association with hydrocephalus in some cases.
- An **anterior meningocele** projects into the pelvis through a defect in the sacrum. Symptoms of constipation and bladder dysfunction develop due to the increasing size of the lesion.
- Female patients may have associated anomalies of the genital tract, including a rectovaginal fistula and vaginal septa. Plain roentgenograms demonstrate a defect in the sacrum, and CT scanning or MRI outlines the extent of the meningocele.

PEDIATRICS PLATE 6

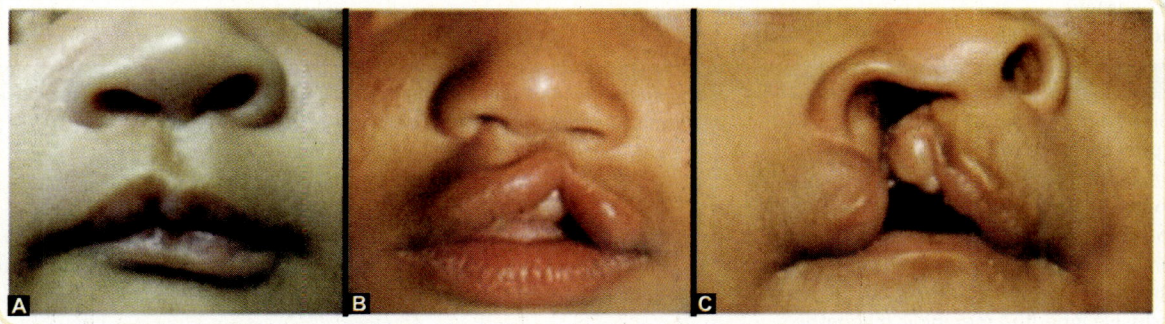

Credit: Shkoukani MA, Chen M, Vong A

UNILATERAL CLEFT LIP

A. Microform type
B. Incomplete type
C. Complete type

CLP is traditionally classified by phenotype, which can have variable expression ranging from microform to complete clefting, and may involve the alveolar ridge and palate. Phenotypes have been correlated with specific genetic linkage patterns, suggesting a possible correlation. CLP and CP are embryologically distinct processes from disruption at different stages of development and possess unique epidemiologic and genetic features.

PEDIATRICS PLATE 7

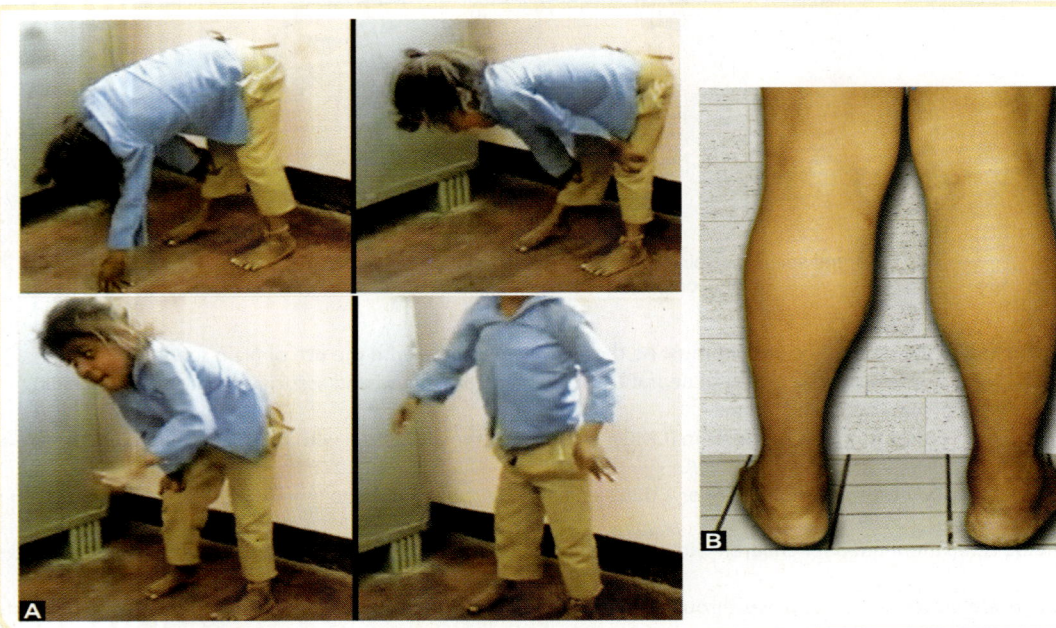

Credit: Senanayake HM, Dedigama AD, De Alwis RP, Thirumavalavan K

A. **Gower's sign**: Gowers' sign is pathognomonic in patients with Duchenne muscular dystrophy.
These patients, when rising, 'climb up' their thighs using their hands in order to overcome the weakness of the pelvic girdle and paravertebral muscles. Gowers' sign is a screening test for muscle weakness, typically seen in Duchenne muscular dystrophy but also seen in numerous other conditions.
B. **Pseudohypertrophy of calf.**

Muscular Dystrophy
A muscular dystrophy is distinguished from all other neuromuscular diseases by four obligatory criteria: 1. It is a primary myopathy 2. It has a genetic basis 3. The course is progressive 4. Degeneration and death of muscle fibers occur at some stage in the disease. This definition excludes neurogenic diseases such as spinal muscular atrophy, nonhereditary myopathies such as dermatomyositis, nonprogressive and non-necrotizing congenital myopathies such as congenital muscle fiber–type disproportion (CMFTD), and nonprogressive inherited metabolic myopathies. **Duchene Muscular Dystrophy (DMD)** is the most common hereditary neuromuscular disease affecting all races and ethnic groups. Duchene recognized most of the characteristic clinical features in 1861: hypertrophy of the calves, progressive weakness, intellectual impairment, and proliferation of connective tissue in muscle

Contd...

Muscular Dystrophy	
Incidence	1 : 3,600 liveborn infant boys
Inheritance	X-linked recessive trait. The abnormal gene is on the **X chromosome** at the Xp21 locus and is one of the largest genes identified
Deficiency	**Dystrophin deficiency:** Dystrophin is expressed in brain and retina, as well as in striated and cardiac muscle, though the level, is lower in brain than in muscle. This distribution may explain some of the CNS manifestations.
Clinical features	☐ **Gower's sign** positive: A maneuver performed by a patient with weak knee and thigh flexors on changing from the sitting to the standing position. It consists of first flexing the trunk at the hips, then placing the hands on the knees, and then extending the trunk by using the hands to walk up the legs. Evident by age 3 yr and is fully expressed by age 5-6 yr. ☐ **Intellectual impairment** occurs in all patients, although only 20–30% have an IQ <70. ☐ **Cardiomyopathy,** including persistent tachycardia and myocardiac failure, is seen in 50–80% of patients. with this disease. The severity of cardiac involvement does not necessarily correlate with the degree of skeletal muscle weakness. ☐ Enlargement of the calves **(pseudohypertrophy)** and wasting of thigh muscles are classic features. After the calves, the next most common site of muscular **hypertrophy is the tongue**, followed by muscles of the forearm. Fasciculation of the tongue do not occur. ☐ Progressive muscle weakness. Proximal muscles and neck flexors are involved more. Leg involvement is more severe than arm. ☐ Contractures of heels and illiotibial tract by 6 years of age ☐ Progressive scoliosis and chest deformity ☐ Death occurs usually at about 18–20 yr of age
Becker muscular dystrophy	Becker muscular dystrophy is the same DMD, with a genetic defect at the same locus, but clinically it follows a milder course. In Becker muscular dystrophy, boys remain ambulatory until late adolescence or early adult life. Calf pseudohypertrophy, cardiomyopathy, and elevated serum levels of creatine kinase (CK) are similar to those of patients with Duchene dystrophy. Learning disabilities are less frequent. The onset of weakness is later in Becker than in Duchene dystrophy. Death often occurs in the mid to late 20s; fewer than half of patients are still alive by age 40 yr. These survivors are severely disabled.

PEDIATRICS PLATE 8

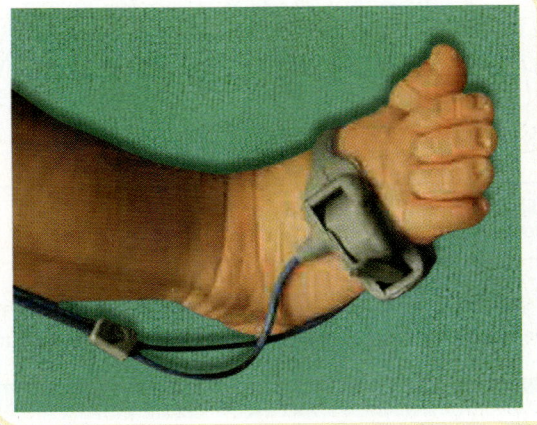

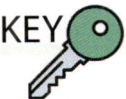

REUSABLE NEONATAL SPO₂ WRAPS SENSOR

Reusable neonatal SPO_2 wraps sensor[AT,MSPG] (Pulse oximeter) for hand or foot of patients weighing 1 - 4 kg. It is manufactured without latex. Pulse oximeters determine oxygen saturation noninvasively through absorption spectrophotometry. The Neonatal Resuscitation Program (NRP) guidelines advocate the use of pulse oximetry during resuscitation, especially when there is a need for providing positive pressure ventilation or supplemental oxygen.

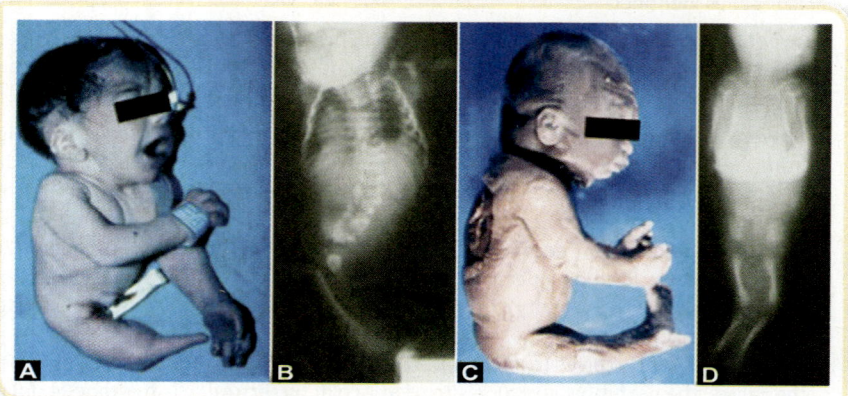

SIRENOMELIA^{NEETPG}

(A,B) Photograph and corresponding radiograph of a newborn with Type VII sirenomelia.
(C,D) Photograph and corresponding radiograph of a stillborn with Type I sirenomelia.
Sirenomelia, also known as sirenomelia sequence or mermaid syndrome, is a severe malformation of the lower limb characterized by fusion of the legs and a variable combination of severe urogenital and gastrointestinal malformations. The first hypothesis, based on the aberrant abdominal and umbilical vascular pattern of affected individuals, postulates a primary vascular defect that leaves the caudal part of the embryo hypoperfused. The second hypothesis, based on the overall malformation of the caudal body, postulates a primary defect in the generation of the mesoderm.

Fig: Schematic digram depicting the seven types of sirenomelia. Stocker and Heifetz classification. F = femur; Fi = fibula; T = tibia.

Type	Characteristics
I	All thigh and leg bones are present
II	Single fibula
III	Absent fibula
IV	Partially fused femurs, fused fibulae
V	Partially fused femurs
VI	Single femur, single tibia
VII	Single femur, absent tibia

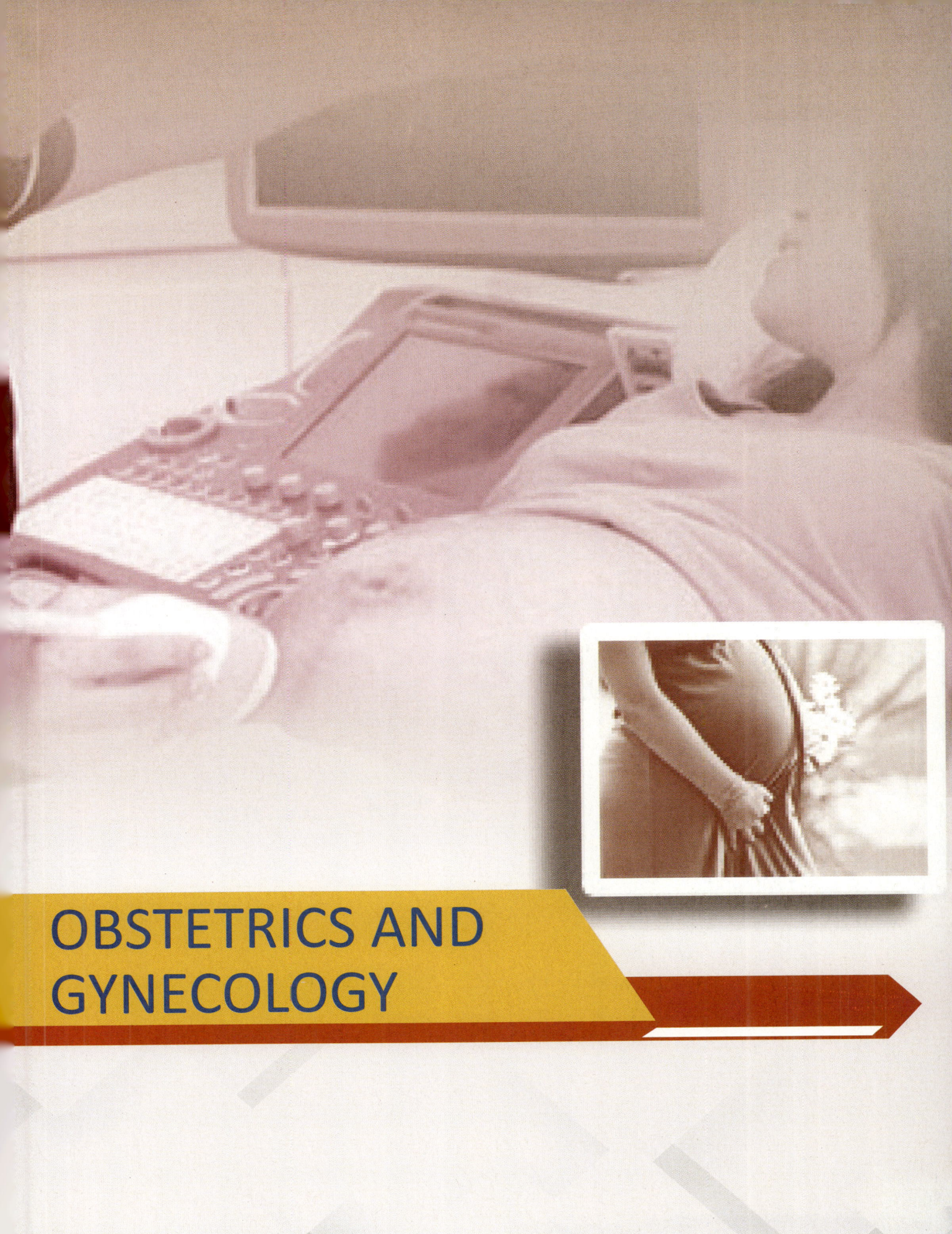

OBSTETRICS AND GYNECOLOGY

OBG PLATE 1

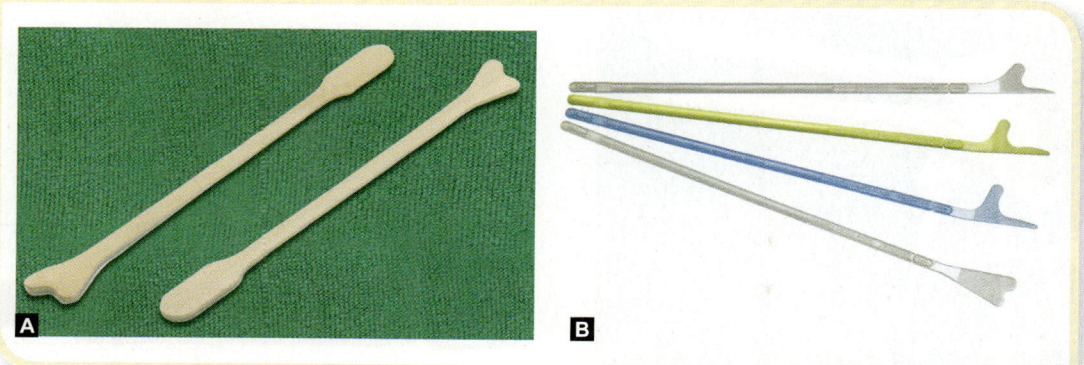

PAP SMEAR COLLECTING DEVICES

A. **Ayre:** Traditional wooden spatula with U shape broad surface on one side and a flat narrow surface on another. The broad end is for vaginal sample collection and the narrow end is for cervical sample collection.
B. **Szalay:** Long tipped plastic spatula. Szalay spatula has a tapered tip that permits safe penetration into the endocervix. Szalay Cyto Spatula, is introduced into the cervical canal until the shoulder of the spatula comes to rest on the surface of ectocervix. The spatula is rotated once or twice in one direction to collect cells.

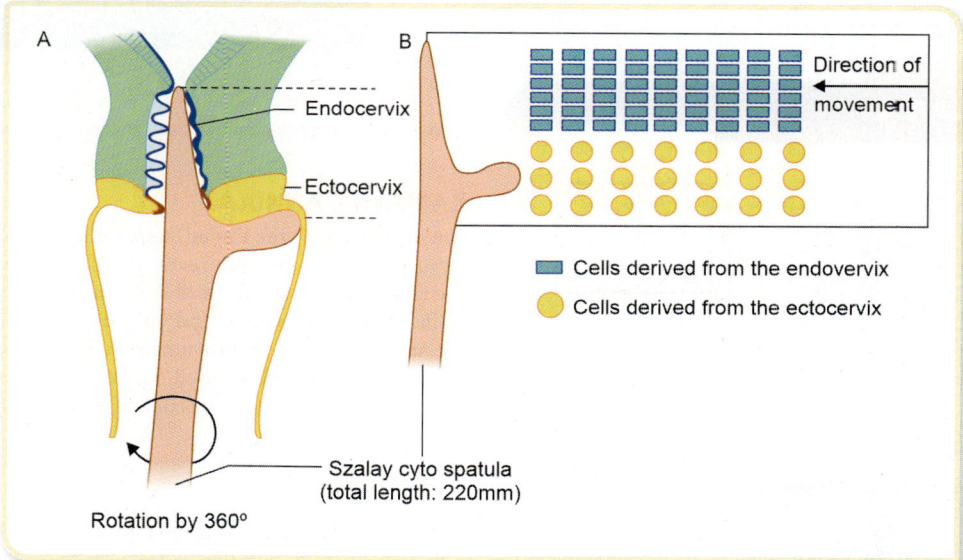

OBG PLATE 2

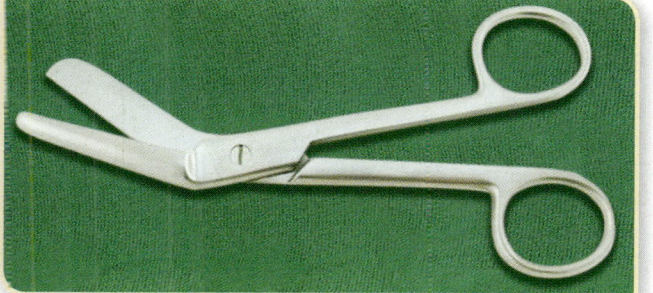

EPISIOTOMY SCISSOR

Angulation in the scissor: To prevent extension of pelvic tears in to the anal margins, obstetric anal sphincter injuries/complete perineal tear.

Structures Cut in Episiotomy

1. Vaginal mucosa
2. Superficial and deep transverse perineal muscles, bulbospongiosus, levator ani muscles.
3. Internal pudendal blood vessels
4. Subcutaneous tissue
5. Perineal skin

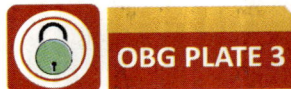

OBG PLATE 3

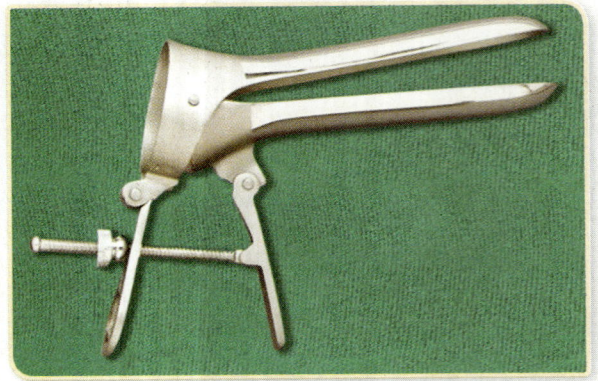

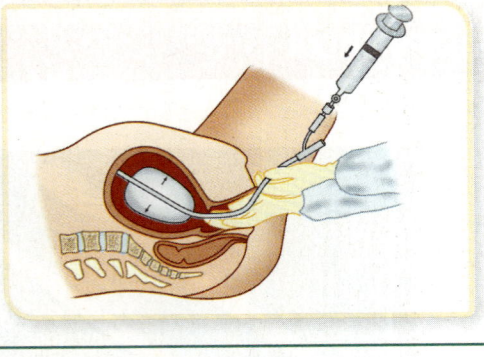

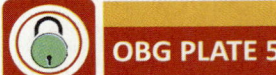

OBG PLATE 5

CUSCO'S SPECULUM
Bivalved self retaining speculum. Its advantage over Sim's speculum is that no assistance is required to hold it in place. Hence, minor procedures like papsmear, IUCD insertions can be performed independently. Its disadvantage is the limited visualization of vagina walls.

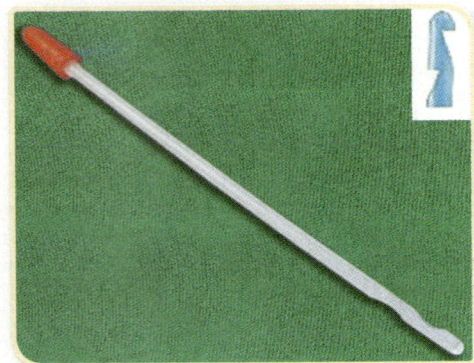

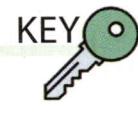

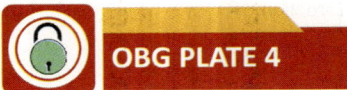

OBG PLATE 4

KARMAN CANNULA
Harvey Karman in the United States refined the technique of Vacuum or suction aspiration in the early 1970s with the development of the Karman cannula, a soft, flexible cannula that avoided the need for initial cervical dilatation and so reduced the risks of puncturing the uterus. The given instrument is Karman cannula that comes in various sizes mainly used for termination of pregnancy. The diameters of 4-6 are used for endometrial biopsy.

Material: Polypropylene

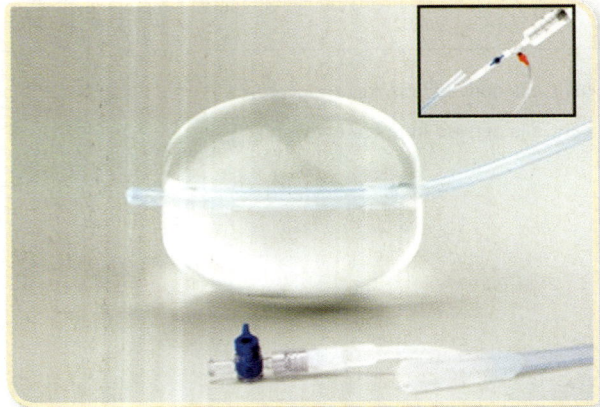

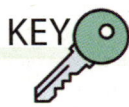

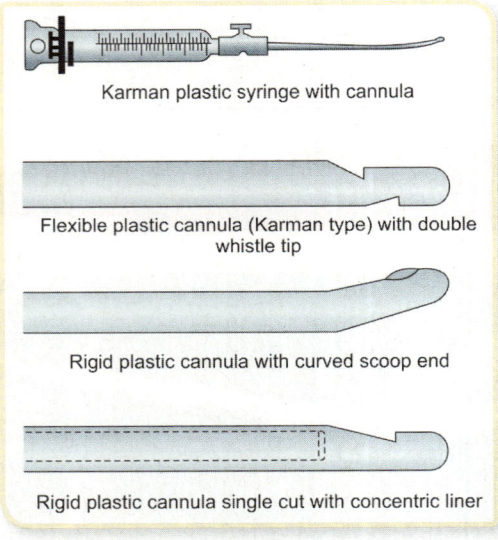

Fig: Sets of Manual Vacuum Aspiration

BAKRI POSTPARTUM BALLOON
A Bakri Postpartum Balloon works on the principle of *tamponade (for uterine atony)* to stop bleeding. *Success rate* is approximately 85 percent.

Procedure: Insertion requires two or three team members. The first performs abdominal sonography during the procedure. The second places the deflated balloon into the uterus and stabilizes it. The third member instills fluid to inflate the balloon, rapidly infusing *at least 150 mL* followed by further instillation over a few minutes for a total of *300 to 500 mL* to arrest hemorrhage.

Advantage: There is continuous drainage hence the risk of infection is reduced.

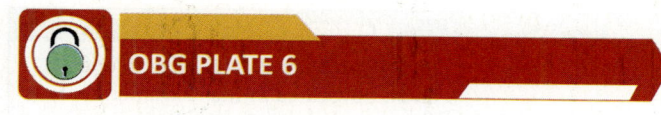

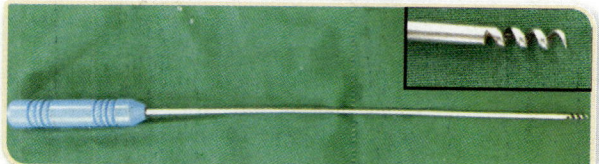

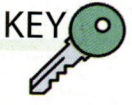

MYOMA SCREW

The myoma screw is a corkscrew-type instrument that is available in 5 or 10 mm size. The myoma screw (single or multiple) is inserted in the center of the leiomyoma and is used to fix or stabilize the leiomyoma during the performance of a myomectomy.

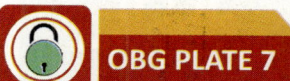

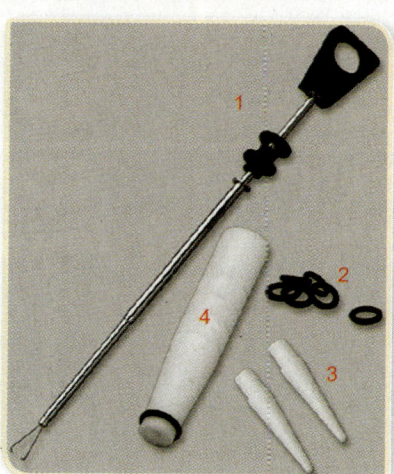

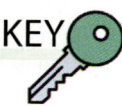

FALOPE RING APPLICATOR

1. Falope ring applicator
2. Falope rings
3. Ring mounting cone
4. Ring mounting screw

Check this video for details

The Silastic ring is an inert, radio opaque silicone band that is simply applied to a looped section of the fallopian tube with the Silastic Ring Applicator. The Silastic Ring Applicator contains forceps to grasp the fallopian tube 3 to 4 cm from the corneal area. The fallopian tube is gently drawn into the inner cylinder of the instrument, forming a knuckle. The Silastic Ring located on the inner cylinder is released onto the knuckle, occluding the base. This procedure is repeated on the second fallopian tube. Once in place, the Silastic Ring will not slip.

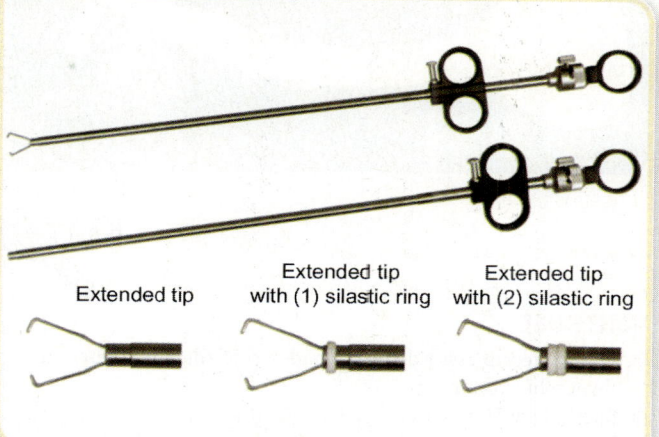

Fig: Falope ring applicators with extended tip

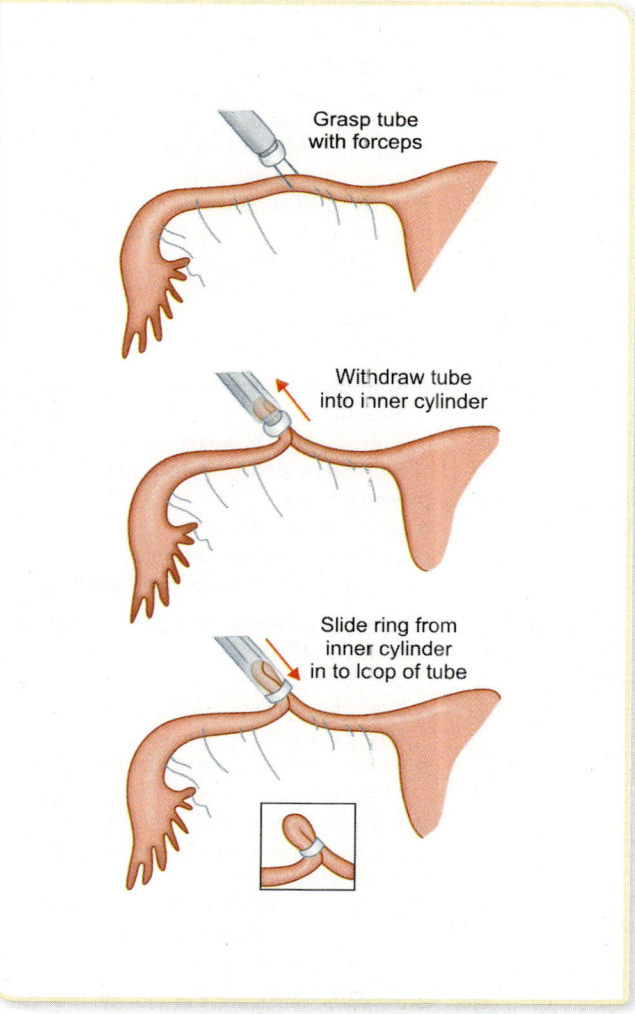

Fig: Falope ring applicator steps illustration

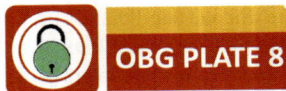

OBG PLATE 8

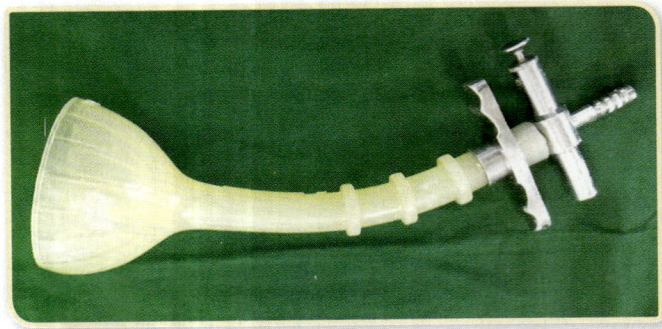

Ventouse

- Reduced maternal pelvic floor injuries and is advocated as the instrument of first choice.
- Perineal injury (3rd and 4th degree tears) are less compared to forceps
- Postpartum maternal discomfort (pain) are less compared to forceps
- Easier to learn comparing to forceps
- Simplicity of use in delivery makes it convenient to the operator (suitable for trained midwives)

 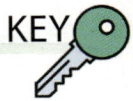

OBG PLATE 9

VENTOUSE

- Designated to assist delivery, made up of silicone rubber cup or disposable plastic cup.
- Suction cup 4 sizes (30, 40, 50 & 60 mm)
- Pulling force is applied to drag the cranium (0.2 - 0.8 kPa).

	Ventouse

Indications	- DTA with adequate pelvis (e.g. POP)
	- Delay in descent of high head in case of 2nd baby of twins
	- Delay in late 1st stage (uterine inertia/ cervical dystocia)
	- Applied after Cx dilatation >7 cm (in contrast to forceps which are applied only in fully dilated Cervix i.e. 10 cm)
	- Alternative to forceps, **Except**-
	  • Face presentation
	  • After coming head of breech ⎫ Forceps
	  • Fetal distress ⎬ are best
	  • Prematurity ⎭

Contraindications	- Non vertex presentation (face, brow & breech) - Prematurity (<34 weeks)- chances of scalp avulsion or subaponeurotic hemorrahage. - Fetal distress - Fetal bleeding disorder - Suspected fetal macrosomia - Following recent scalp blood sampling
Advantages of Ventouse Over Forceps	- It can be used in unrotated or malrotated head (OP, OT position). It helps in autorotation - It is not a space occupying device like the forceps blades - Traction force is less (10 kg) compared to forceps - It is comfortable and has lower rates of maternal trauma and genital tract lacerations - Analgesia need is less. Pudendal block with perineal infiltration is adequate but for forceps regional or general anesthesia is often needed

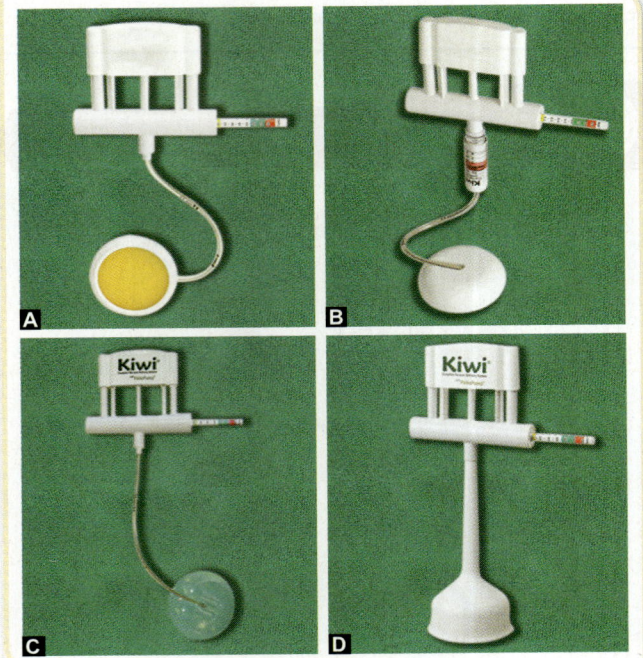

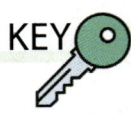

NEW GENERATION VENTOUSE

A. Kiwi Omni Cup: This is a new generation of 'hand-help' vacuum extractors. These are single-use and do not need the cumbersome external source of suction. But, they have higher failure rate than the conventional ventouse likely because of poor technique and emphasizes the need for training.

B. Kiwi Omni MT: The Omni-MT has the same great features as the OmniCup with the addition of the Traction Force Indicator.

C. Kiwi Omni C: The Omni-C is designed specifically for the confined abdominal space of C-section deliveries. The Omni-C's even slimmer cup profile, finger grooves and baffle filter on the inside make it the only vacuum designed specifically for use during C-section. Its use contributes to less blood loss, fewer extensions of the uterine incision, and fewer cervical lacerations.

D. Kiwi ProCup: The ProCup offers a soft flexible cup which expands and molds to the fetal head. Specifically, for use with low occiput anterior and outlet presentations, if the clinician prefer a rigid stem over a flexible stem.

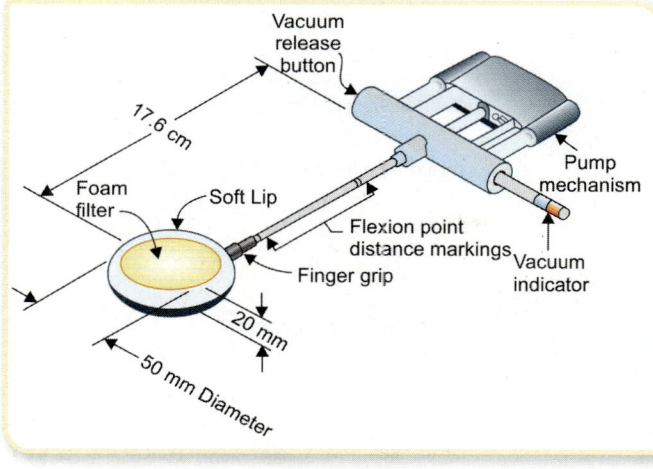

Fig: Omni cup

OBG PLATE 10

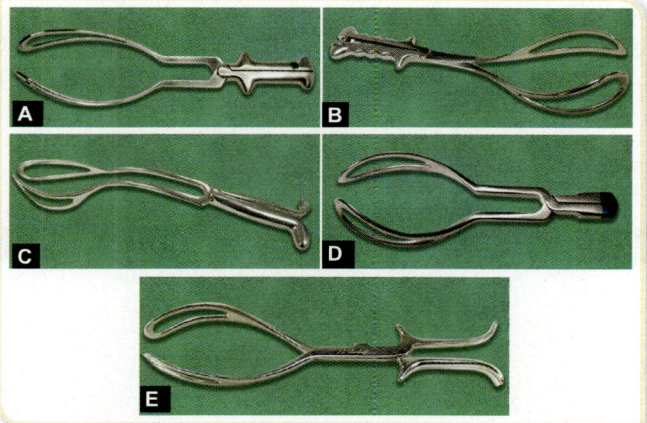

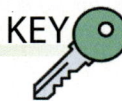 **KEY**

COMMONLY USED OBSTETRICS FORCEPS

A. Simpson forceps
- Most commonly used forceps.
- Used to extract after coming head in breech delivery.
- Fenestrated blades, parallel shanks, English lock and finger guard
- Have both pelvic and cephalic curve
- Parallel shanks are better for multipara

B. Elliott forceps:
- Similar to Simpson forceps but with an adjustable pin at the end of the handle which is used to adjust pressure. Shanks are overlapping
- Have both Pelvic and cephalic curve
- Overlapping shanks – better for nullipara
- More rounded cephalic curve – less ideal for very molded head

C. Piper's forceps
- Fenestrated blades, have a perineal curve to allow application to the after-coming head in breech delivery.
- Longest of all obstetric forceps.

D. Wrigley's forceps
- Used in low or outlet delivery when the maximum diameter is about 2.5 cm above the vulva.
- Fenestrated blades, parallel shank, Short length results in low chances of uterine rupture
- Similar to Simpson forceps except that it is short and without finger guard
- Now a day these forceps are most commonly used in cesarean section delivery where manual traction is proving difficult.

E. Kielland's forceps
- Have small pelvic curve (Almost straight), sliding lock, Both Shanks overlaps to each other and a knob on each Handle
- Sliding lock is helpful in Asynclitic presentation of the baby. An asynclitic presentation is when your baby's head is "tilted" to one side as he moves down through your pelvis during labor.
- Kielland's forceps lack traction because of almost no pelvic curve.
- Used for O.P position
- Most commonly used forceps for rotation.

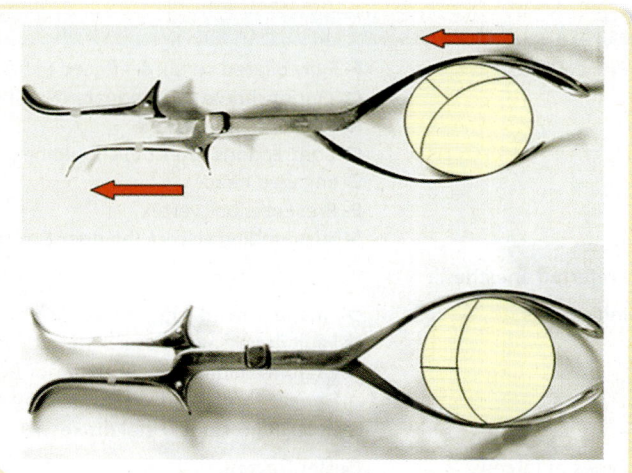

Fig: Correction of Asynclitic position through Kielland's forceps

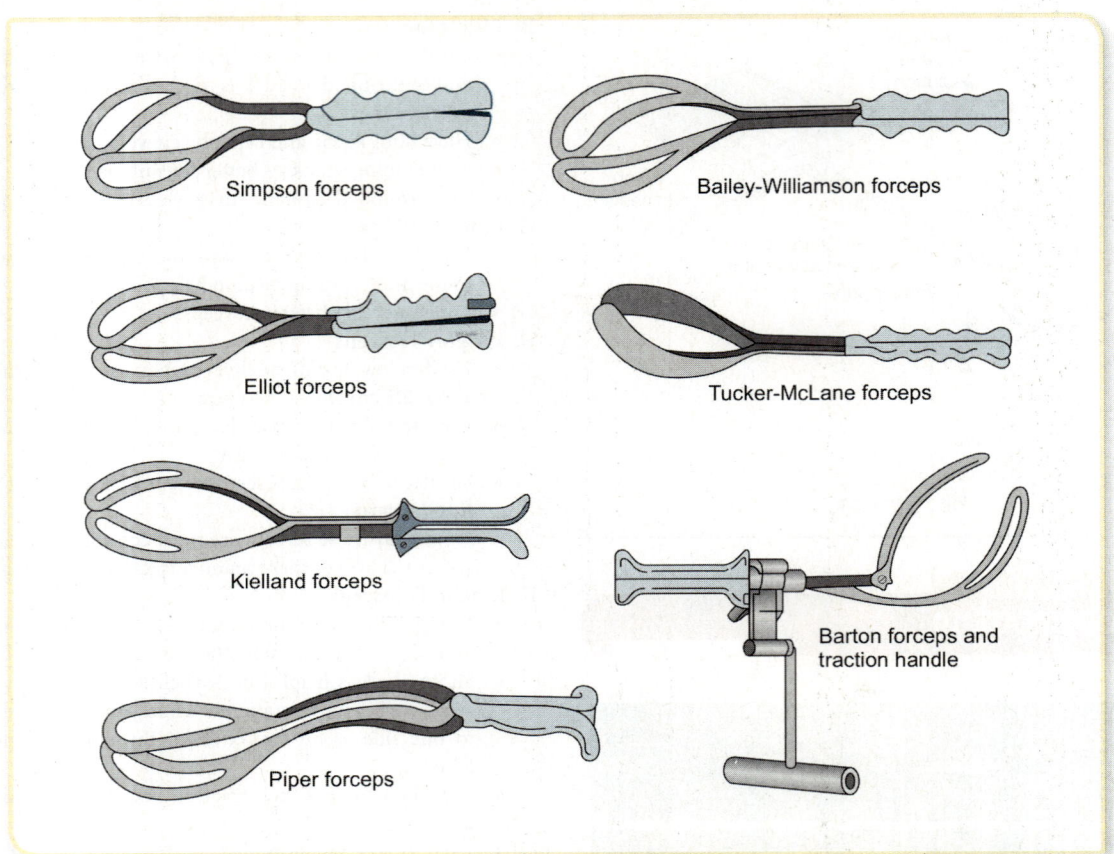

Fig: Diagrammatic representation of Obstetric forceps

	Forceps Delivery		
Prerequisite	**F-** Fully dilated cervix & effaced (≈10cm) **O-** Outlet should be adequate (No CPD) **R-** Ruptured membrane **C-** Contractions (uterine) should be present **E-** Engaged head **P-** Presentation- vertex **S-** Surrounding viscera (bladder & rectum) empty & baby should be alive		
Preferred anesthesia	Pudendal block		
Indications	▫ Fault in forced (Uterine inertia) ▫ Fault in passage (Tissues inelastic in elderly primi) ▫ Fault in child (Occipito-posterior position, After coming head of breech) ▫ Danger threatening the wellbeing of mother (PIH, Heart disease) ▫ Fetal indications (Fetal distress)		
Types of forceps	**Outlet forceps**	**Low or Mid cavity forceps**	**Rotational forceps**
	e.g. Wrigley's forceps	e.g. Neville Barnes, Andersons, Simpsons.	e.g. Kielland's forceps, Braton forceps, Tucker McLane forceps
	Outlet forceps are used when: ▫ Fetal scalp is visible without separating labia ▫ Fetal skull has reached the pelvic floor ▫ Sagittal suture is in the antero posterior diameter or right or left occiput anterior or posterior position (rotation does not exceed 45°) ▫ Fetal head is at, or on, the perineum	Low or mid-cavity forceps are used when: ▫ Fetal head is one-fifth palpable per abdomen ▫ Leading point of the skull is above station plus 2 cm but not above the ischial spines ▫ Rotation of 45° or less.	Rotational forceps are used when the rotation is more than 45°

Contd...

Forceps Delivery	
Advantages of Forceps Over Ventouse	❑ In cases, where moderate traction is required, forceps will be more effective compared to ventouse ❑ Forceps operation can quickly expedite the delivery in case of fetal distress where ventouse will be unsuitable as it takes longer time ❑ It is safer in premature baby. The fetal head remains inside the protective cage ❑ It can be employed in anterior face or in after-coming head of breech presentation, where ventouse is contraindicated ❑ Lesser neonatal scalp trauma, retinal hemorrhage, jaundice or cephalohematoma compared to ventouse ❑ Higher rate of successful vaginal delivery as ventouse has got higher failure rates than forceps ❑ Cup detachment ("Pop-off") occurs when the vacuum is not maintained in ventouse. No such problems once forceps blades are correctly applied ❑ Number of types of forceps are available for outlet, mid cavity or rotational delivery. Traction force is more (about 20 kg for a primary and about 13 kg in a multi)

 OBG PLATE 11

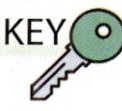 KEY

HEGAR'S DILATOR

❑ These are double ended solid rods curved and tapering near the tip with size 1/2 mm to 23/24 mm, hence a set of 12 dilators
❑ 1/2 labelled rod can dilate the cervical canal up to 1 mm from one end and up to 2 mm from other end.
❑ Length of uterus is measured by a uterine sound before inserting the Hegar's dilator otherwise there are chances of perforation.
❑ Maximum diameter should be more than the internal os diameter.
❑ **Uses:** Cervical stenosis, D&C, Hysteroscopy, drainage of pyometra and hematometra, Before amputation of cervix in Fothergill's operation

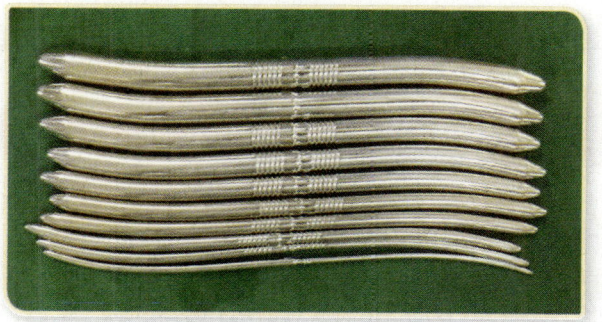

 OBG PLATE 12

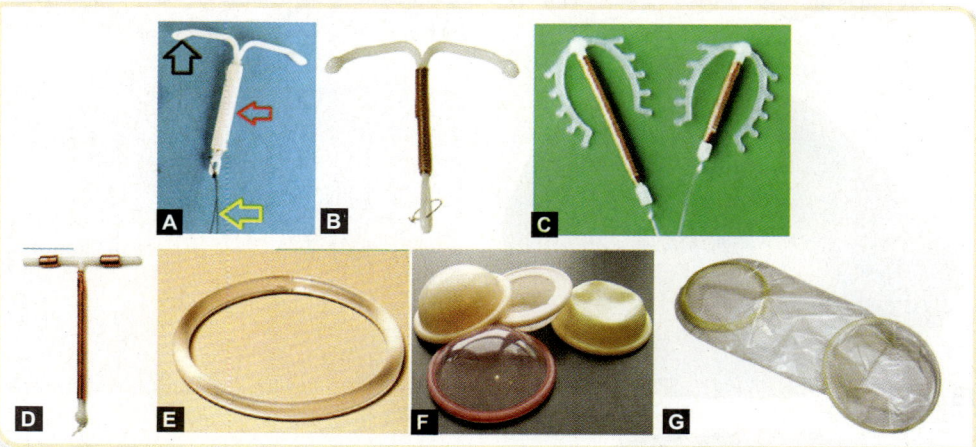

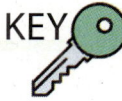 KEY

INTRAUTERINE DEVICES

A. Mirena
- Hormonal IUD Mirena with T shaped polyethylene frame impregnated with barium sulfate for visibility during X-rays (black arrow), hormone cylinder (red arrow) and removal thread (yellow arrow)

B. Nova T 380
- T-shaped polyethylene frame impregnated with barium sulfate for visibility during X-rays
- $380mm^2$ surface area copper, in the form of copper wire with a silver core, wrapped around the vertical stem of the T
- Two removal threads pigmented with iron oxide
- Suffix number of the device signifies the amount of copper

C. Multiload Cu 250/375
- Flexible curved arms
- Copper wrapped around the polyethylene frame impregnated with barium sulphate for visibility during X-rays
- Two nylon thread
- Suffix number of the device signifies the amount of copper

D. Copper T 380 A
- T-shaped polyethylene frame impregnated with barium sulfate for visibility during X-rays
- Suffix number of the device signifies the amount of copper
- 380mm² surface area copper, in the form of copper wire with a silver core, wrapped around the vertical stem of the T and also the arms of the "T" hence the Suffix "a"

E. Nuva Ring
- Combined hormonal contraceptive vaginal ring
- It is a flexible plastic (ethylene-vinyl acetate copolymer) ring that releases a low dose of a progestin and estrogen over three weeks.
- The exact position of NuvaRing is not important for it to be effective

F. Diaphragm
- It is an intravaginal device made of latex with flexible metal or spring ring at the margin.
- Inserted up to 3 hrs before intercourse and is to be kept for at least 6 hours after the last coital act.
- Increase the risk of UTI's and cervical erosion
- Requires help of a doctor or paramedical person to measure the size required.
- Diaphragm should completely cover the cervix.
- It cannot effectively prevent ascent of the sperms alongside the margin of the device; hence a chemical spermicidal agent should be placed on the superior surface of the device during insertion

G. Female condom (Femidom)[NEETPG]
- Barrier method with typical failure rate 21% and perfect use failure rate 5%
- It is a 17 cm length pouch made of polyurethane which lines the vagina and external genitalia with one flexible polyurethane ring at each end.
- Unlike male condom Multiple uses can be made with washing, drying and with lubrication.

OBG PLATE 13

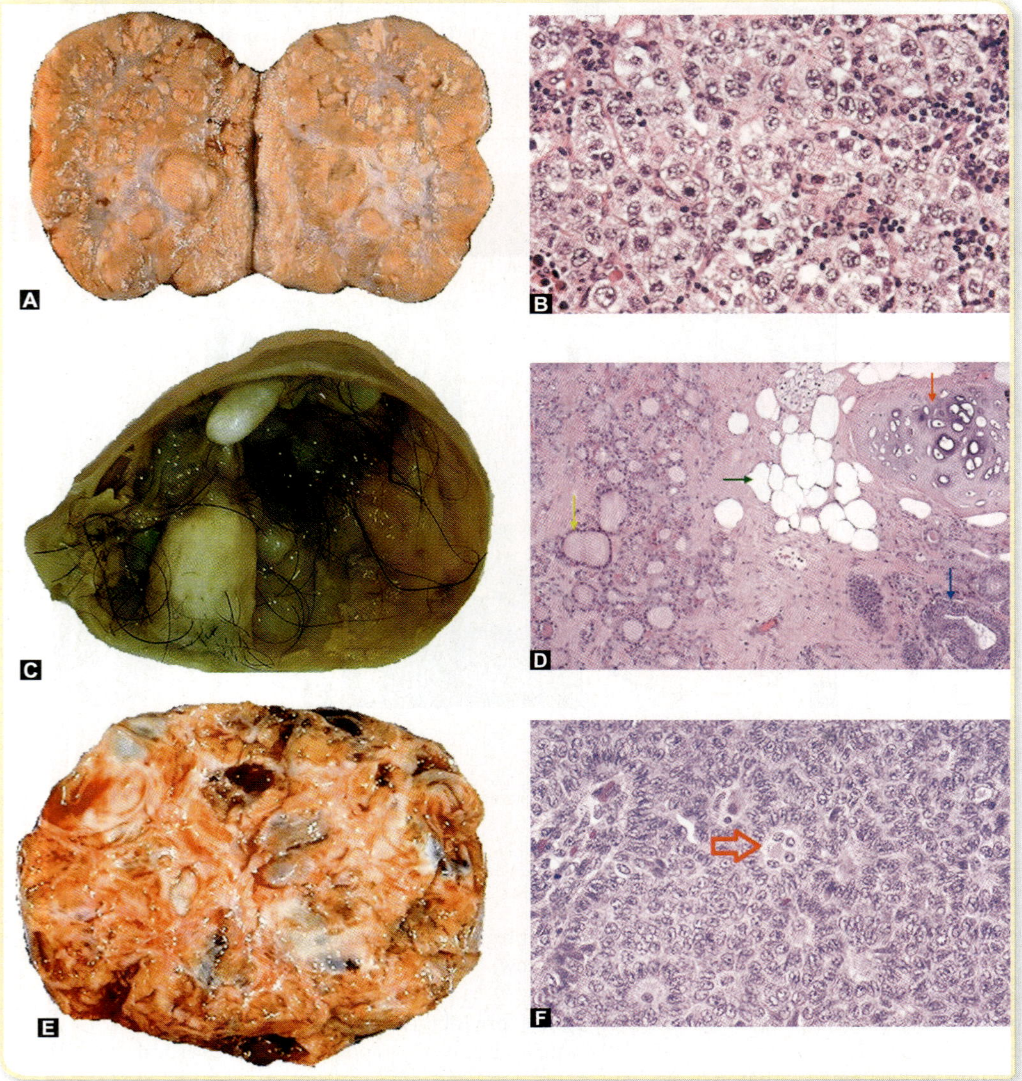

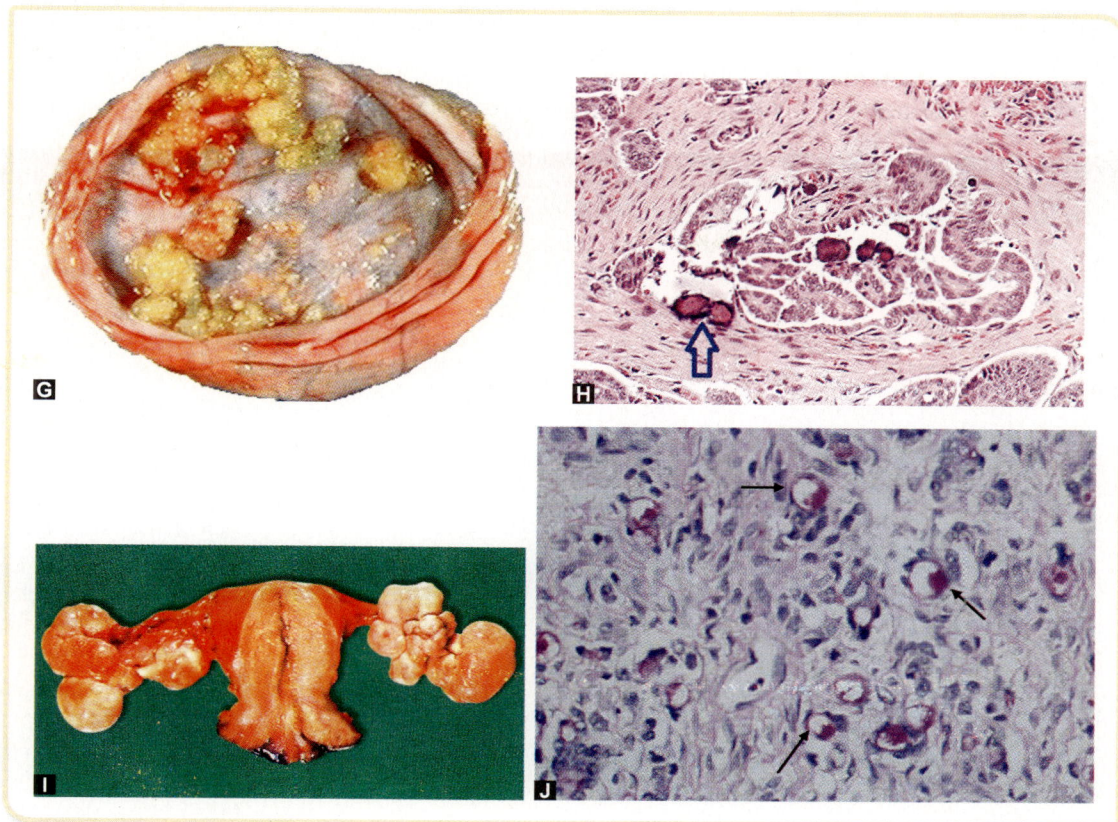

KEY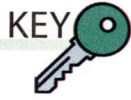

PLATE LEGENDS

A. Dysgerminoma Gross: The size of dysgerminomas varies widely, but they are usually 5 to 15 cm in diameter. Ovarian dysgerminoma that has been sectioned into two halves. Firm and encapsulated. The cut surface of the tumor is solid with some cystic areas and necrosis, fleshy, lobulated and a yellow-white to gray-pink appearance.

B. Dysgerminoma Microscopy: Histopathology of the biopsy specimen: Sheet or cords of Round, polygonal large uniform tumor cells with vesicular nuclei and clear or finely granular cytoplasm that is eosinophilic, separated by scanty **fibrous septa, which are often extensively infiltrated with lymphocytes, plasma cells, and granulomas with epithelioid cells and multinucleated giant cells. Mitotic figures are seen in varying numbers, although they are usually numerous**

C. Mature/Benign Teratoma Gross: Characteristically they are unilocular cysts containing hair and cheesy sebaceous material. On section, they reveal a thin wall lined by an opaque, gray-white, wrinkled epidermis. From this epidermis, hair shafts frequently protrude. Within the wall, it is common to find tooth structures and areas of calcification. A variety of mature, well-differentiated tissue elements may be found from all three embryologic germ layers (ectoderm, mesoderm, endoderm). These tumors are often called "dermoid cysts" because they are mostly cystic and mostly contain ectodermal elements. The most common tissue element of these teratomas is skin, so large amounts of hair and sebum are produced, leading to a challenging cleanup problem in surgical pathology following dissection of these tumors. If these tumors are mostly solid, then they are often "immature" teratomas with less differentiated tissue and may behave more aggressively.

Note

Immature Malignant teratoma Gross: The tumors are bulky and have a smooth external surface. On section they have a solid (or predominantly solid) structure. There are areas of necrosis and hemorrhage. Hair, sebaceous material, cartilage, bone, and calcification may be present.

D. Mature teratoma Microscopy: Cyst wall is composed of stratified squamous epithelium and within there is cartilage (Red arrow) as well as adipose tissue (Green arrow) and even intestinal glands (Blue arrow) at the right, while at the left are a lot of thyroid follicles (Yellow arrow). The presence of abundant thyroid tissue within a mature teratoma can be termed struma ovarii.

E. Granulosa cell tumor gross: A variegated cut surface. These tumors are derived from the ovarian stroma and often have a component of thecoma. They are often hormonally active and can produce large amounts of estrogen such that the patient may initially present with bleeding from endometrial hyperplasia.

F. Granulosa cell tumor Microscopy: At higher magnification, an ovarian granulosa cell tumor has nests of cells which are forming primitive follicles (red arrow) called Call Exner bodies.

G. Papillary serous cystadenocarcinoma gross: Note the many papillations on the inner surface which sometimes are visible on the outer surface also. These neoplasms characteristically spread by "seeding" along peritoneal surfaces. Between benign cystadenomas and malignant cystadenocarcinomas lies the grey zone of "borderline" lesions that are not clearly malignant, but are treated as though they could be.

Note

A benign cystadenoma has multiloculation in the inner surface but is smooth and with only a solitary papillation within one loculation

H. **Papillary serous cystadenocarcinoma gross:** Contain small concretions called **psammomma bodies** (purplish rounded and laminated). They are essentially just a form of dystrophic calcification in neoplasms.
I. **Krukenberg tumor gross:** Asymmetrical enlargement, lobular multinodular contour, and either solid (mostly) or cystic consistency (30%).
J. **Krukenberg tumor Microscopy:** Diffuse infiltration by **signet ring cells** containing abundant neutral and acidic (sialo) mucin vacuoles pushing the nucleus to one side. Tumor emboli are found in over 50% of the cases.

Major Histopathologic Categories of Ovarian Cancer

Group	Type	%	Laterality	Also know
Epithelial Neoplasms (60% of all ovarian neoplasms) (mainly in post menopausal females)	Serous cystadenocarcinoma	75–80% of all epithelial cancers	Bilateral in 40–60% of cases	Most common malignant tumor of the ovary, **Psammoma bodies**,
	Mucinous neoplasms	10% of all epithelial ovarian tumors	Bilateral in less than 10% of cases.	Pseudomyxoma peritonei,
	Endometrioid neoplasms	10% of epithelial tumors	Bilateral in 30–50% of cases	Resembles endometrial adenocarcinoma
	Clear cell carcinoma (meso nephroid carcinoma)	less than 1% of epithelial ovarian cancers		Two cell types; "clear cell" & "hobnail cell" Associated with hyperpyrexia and hypercalcemia
	Brenner carcinoma AKA- Transitional cell carcinoma (Essentially benign)	< 1% of epithelial cancers		**Walthard cell rests** of transitional cells, **Coffee bean nuclei**, **Puffed wheat appearance**, Causes **PseudoMeig** syndrome
	Undifferentiated carcinoma	< 10% of epithelial neoplasms.		Absence of any distinguishing microscopic features
Germ Cell Neoplasms (Common in young women)	Dysgerminoma (MC malignant germ cell tumor, MC malignant tumor diagnosed during pregnancy)	30–40% of germ cell tumors	Unilateral in 85–90% of cases	Female counterpart of the seminoma Most radiosensitive (but surgery is the preferred treatment) Tumor with lymphocytic infiltration LDH +ve ALP +ve
	Endodermal sinus tumor (yolk sac tumor)	3RD most common germ cell neoplasm	Unilateral in nearly 100% of cases	**Schiller-Duval body** AFP + Most rapidly growing, deadly tumor
	Immature teratoma	2ND most common germ cell malignancy	Bilateral in less than 5% of cases	AFP +
	Mature teratoma or dermoid	MC benign tumor of the ovary, MC germ cell tumor		MC neoplasm diagnosed during pregnancy (serous cystadenoma is MC but undiagnosed) MC to undergoes torsion during pregnancy during end of 1st trimester
	Embryonal carcinoma	very rare		HCG+ AFP+
	Choriocarcinoma	Rare		AFP – HCG+
	Gonadoblastoma	Rare		Rt ovary> left ovary, Associated with presence of Y chromosome
	Mixed germ cell tumors	10% of germ cell neoplasms		Dysgerminoma + endodermal sinus tumor (most common)
	Polyembryoma	extremely rare		**Embryoid bodies** AFP and HCG +

Contd...

Major Histopathologic Categories of Ovarian Cancer

Group	Type	%	Laterality	Also know
Sex cord-stromal tumors (5-8% of all ovarian tumors)	Granulosa cell tumors	70% of sex cord stromal tumors		**Call-Exner bodies** **MC to involve opposite ovary by metastasis** Causes **PseudoMeig** syndrome Produces estrogen thus asso. with endometrial hyperplasia & Ca
	Thecoma		Exclusively unilateral	Exclusively benign Causes **PseudoMeig** syndrome
	Arrhenoblastoma (Sertoli-Leydig cell tumors)	Rare	Rarely bilateral	Virilising tumor
	Gynandroblastoma	Rare		Both ovarian (granulosa/theca) & testicular (Sertoli/Leydig) cells, Virilising tumor
Metastatic (5–6% of all ovarian malignancies)	**KRUKENBERG TUMOR** eponym is used to denote any GI carcinoma metastatic to the ovary, mostly stomach carcinoma. **Signet cell appearance** on microscopy The primary ovarian tumor stain positive for cytokeratin 7 (CK7+) & negative for CK20. While metastatic lesion is CK7 negative, CK20 positive).			

OBG PLATE 14

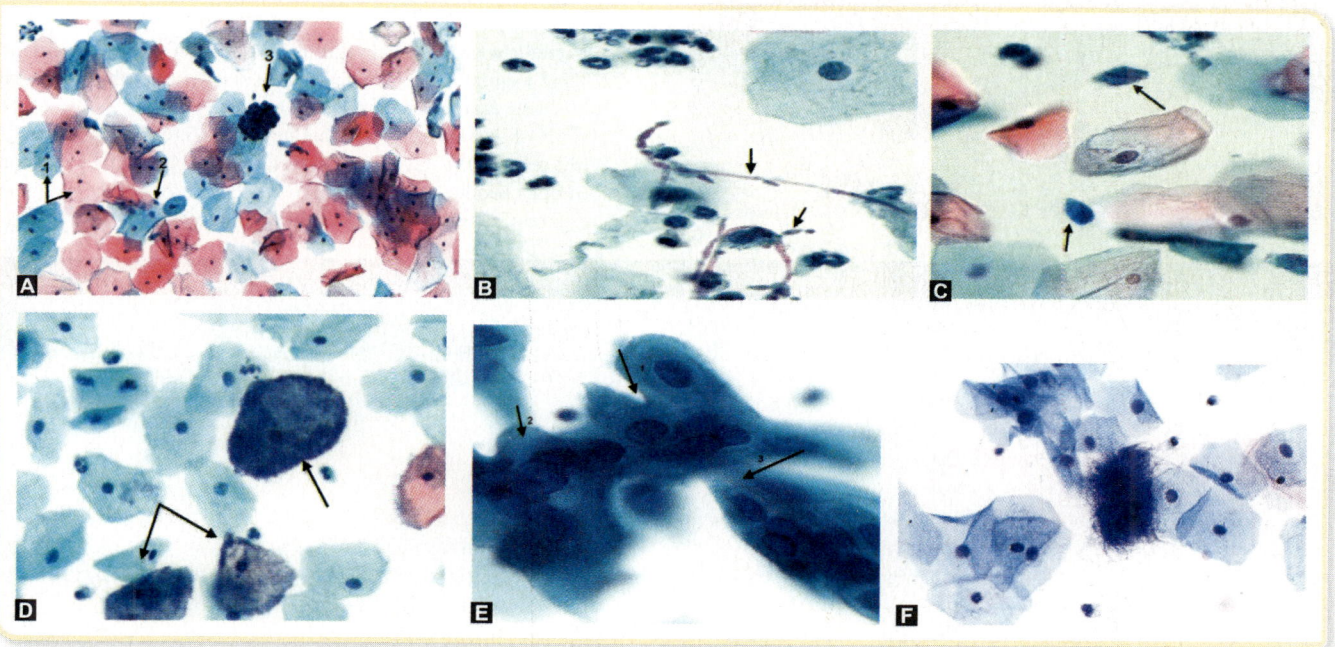

 KEY

VAGINAL INFECTIONS

A. Normal Cervical PAP Smear: Negative for intraepithelial lesion or malignancy
  1. Superficial squamous epithelial cells;
  2. Intermediate squamous epithelial cells;
  3. Endocervical (glandular) epithelial cells.

The presence of infective agents and conditions such as Trichomonas, Herpes simplex virus, Candida and bacterial vaginosis may be detected in cervical samples.

B. Candida is recognized by the presence of fungal hyphae (arrow) and spores.

C. Trichomonas vaginalis: The presence of pale inflammatory haloes around squamous cell nuclei can be a clue to the presence of Trichomonas. Trichomonas organisms may be seen in groups. 3 dimensional clusters of neutrophils ("polyballs") may be seen in the background

- Blue-green stained Pear-shaped, oval, or round cyanophilic organisms, 15 - 30 microns
- Eosinophilic cytoplasmic granules are often evident
- Small oval Nucleus which is pale, vesicular, and eccentrically located
- Flagella are sometimes observed

D. **Bacterial vaginosis (BV):** Indicator cells also known as **"Clue Cells"** form the characteristic picture of BV. Note the presence of multiple microorganisms, which are attached to a single squamous epithelial cell.

E. **Herpes simplex infection:** Darkly-staining viral inclusions may be seen in some nuclei.
   Cellular changes consistent with HSV infection are
   1. Milk glass nuclei
   2. Multinucleated cells; fused nuclei and ground glass chromatin
   3. Nuclear chromatin is present only close to the nuclear membrane.

F. **Actinomyces** forms aggregates of long filamentous organisms (Cotton ball cluster) and perinuclear halo and is usually associated with intra-uterine contraceptive devices.

OBG PLATE 15

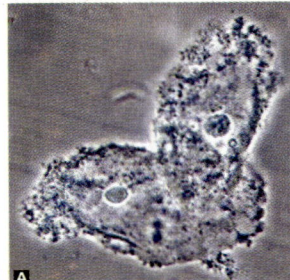
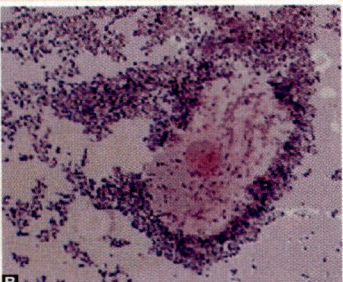

BACTERIAL VAGINOSIS

A. Normal saline wet mount showing two **clue cells** (original magnification ×400)[AIIMS PG].

Note

The ability of *G. vaginalis* to adhere to vaginal and urinary epithelial cells at a pH of 5 to 6 is thought to contribute to its role in the pathogenesis of BV and urinary tract infections.[AIIMS PG]

B. Gram stain vaginal smear demonstrating how coccobacilli on the surfaces of vaginal epithelial cells create the characteristic **granular** appearance and indistinct borders of clue cells. Free floating clumps of Gardnerella are seen.

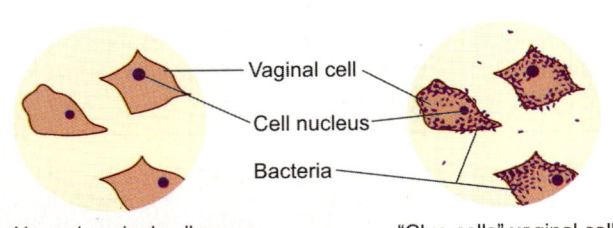

Normal vaginal cells seen under a microscope — "Clue cells" vaginal cells with bacteria stuck to them

Amsel's criteria for bacterial vaginosis: (3 out of 4 should be present)
1. A fishy vaginal odor, which is particularly noticeable following coitus, and vaginal discharge are present.
2. The pH of these secretions is higher than 4.5 (usually 4.7 to 5.7).
3. Whiff test / amine test positive (addition of 10% KOH to vaginal secretions produces fishy odor)
4. Presence of clue cells (> 20% of epithelial cells)

Vaginitis and Bacterial Vaginosis

	Normal vagina	Bacterial vaginosis	*Trichomonas vaginalis* vaginitis	*Candida albicans* vulvovaginitis
Microorganism	Lactobacilli	Gardenella vaginalis, Hemophillus vaginosis, Ureplasma ureolyticum, Mycoplasma hominis, Mobilincus	Trichomonas vaginalis	Candida albicans
Primary symptoms	None	Discharge with fishy odor, may have itching	Discharge, bad odor, may have itching, **Strawberry vagina**	Discharge; itching and burning of vulvar skin
Vaginal discharge	Slight, white, flocculent	Slightly increased, thin, homogeneous, white, gray, adherent with fishy odor	Profuse, yellow, green, frothy, adherent; cervical petechiae often present, with fishy odor (±)	Increased, white, curdy like **cottage cheese**
Inflammation of vulvar or vaginal epithelium	None	None (Hence vaginosis not vaginitis)	Erythema of vaginal and vulvar epithelium; colpitis macularis	Erythema of vaginal epithelium, introitus; vulvar dermatitis, fissures common
pH	< 4.5	> 4.5	> 4.5	≤ 4.5
Amine ("fishy") odor with 10% KOH (Whiff test)	None	Present	May be present	None
Microscopy	Epithelial cells with lactobacilli	**Clue cells**; few leukocytes; no lactobacilli or only a few outnumbered by profuse mixed microbiota, nearly always including *G. vaginalis* plus anaerobic species on Gram's stain (Nugent's score ≥7)	By **hanging drop technique**, Leukocytes; motile trichomonads seen in 80–90% of symptomatic patients, less often in the absence of symptoms	KOH preparation showing budding yeasts and pseudohyphae in up to 80% of *C. Albicans* culture positive persons with typical symptoms

Contd...

		Vaginitis and Bacterial Vaginosis		
Treatment	None	DOC- **Metronidazole** 500 mg PO bid for 7 days Metronidazole gel, 0.75%, one applicator (5 g) intravaginally once daily for 5 days, Clindamycin 2% cream, one full applicator vaginally each night for 7 days	Metronidazole or tinidazole, 2 g orally (single dose) or Metronidazole, 500 mg PO bid for 7 days. If recurrence is there take metronidazole 2 gm po for 5 days. If refractory culture sensitivity for metronidazole and tinidazole	Azole cream, tablet, or suppository—e.g., miconazole (100-mg vaginal suppository) or clotrimazole (100-mg vaginal tablet) once daily for 7 days Fluconazole, 150 mg orally (single dose)
Usual management of sexual partner	None	None	Examination for STD; treatment with metronidazole, 2 g PO (single dose)	None; topical treatment if candidal dermatitis of penis is detected

OBG PLATE 16

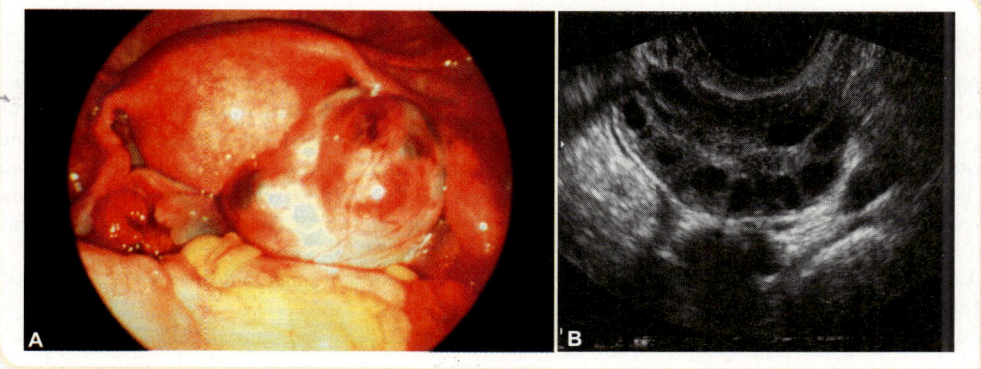

POLYCYSTIC OVARY (LAPAROSCOPIC AND USG VIEW)

A. **Polycystic ovary in laparoscopic view:** PCOS is the commonest cause of anovulatory infertility. Gross specimen shows presence of multiple antral follicles measuring approximately 2-8 mm in diameter and suggest arrest of follicle development prior to preovulatory phase. It can present with heavy, irregular periods, persistent acne or hirsutism, infertility

B. **Polycystic ovary USG image:** Showing bulky ovary with multiple peripherally placed follicles (Necklace sign) and echogenic stroma

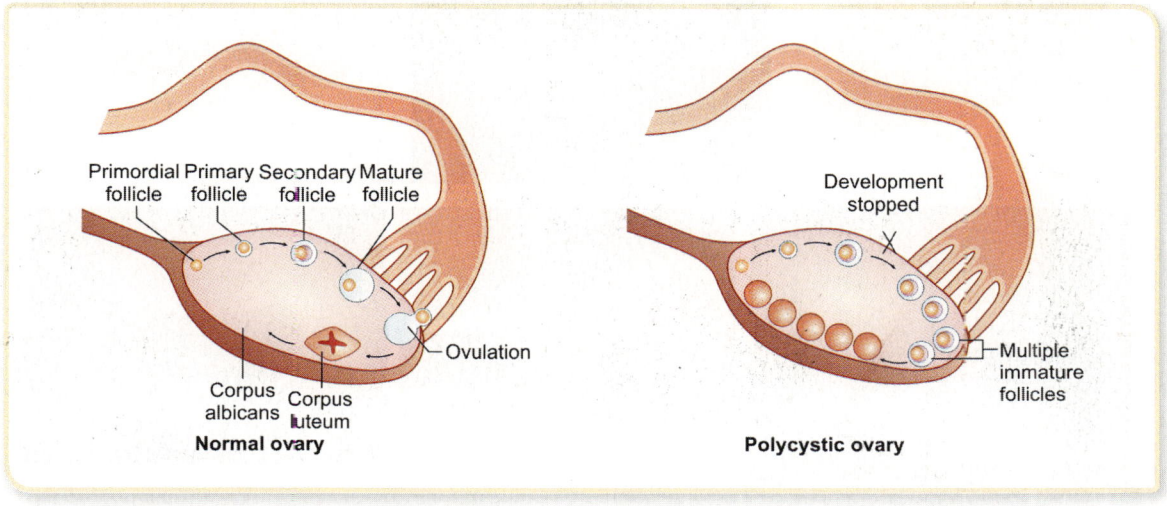

OBG PLATE 17

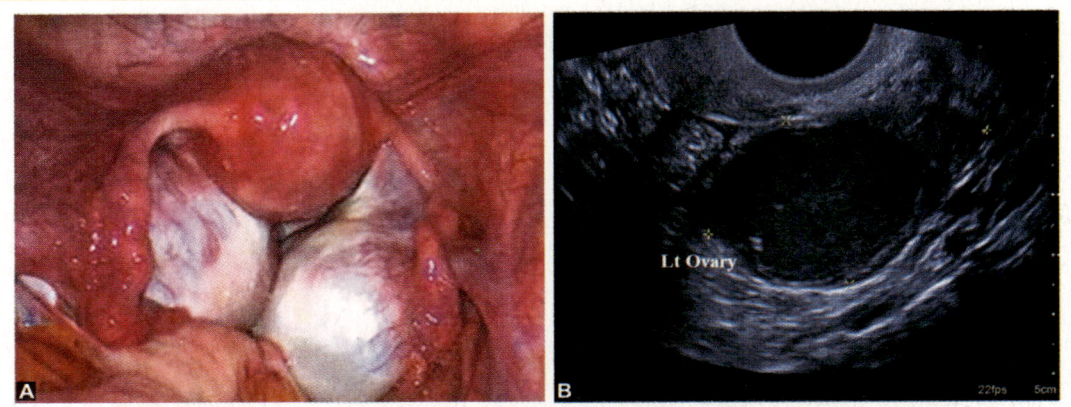

©Dr Sapna Bharat

ENDOMETRIOMA

A. **Endometrioma/chocolate cyst** of ovary is a word used to describe endometriotic cyst of ovary. This is a laparoscopic picture showing bilateral endometrioma in the typical picture showing what is known as **kissing ovaries**. Larger ovarian endometriotic cysts (endometrioma) are usually located on the anterior surface of the ovary and are associated with retraction, pigmentation, and adhesions to the posterior peritoneum. These ovarian endometriotic cysts often contain a thick, viscous dark brown fluid (**Chocolate fluid**) composed of **hemosiderin** derived from previous intraovarian hemorrhage. Because this fluid may also be found in other conditions, such as in hemorrhagic corpus luteum cysts or neoplastic cysts, biopsy and preferably removal of the ovarian cyst for histologic confirmation are necessary for the diagnosis

B. **Endometrioma Ultrasound image** of the left adnexa reveals a mass within the left ovary with diffuse low level internal echoes with small bright foci near the wall of the mass.

OBG PLATE 18

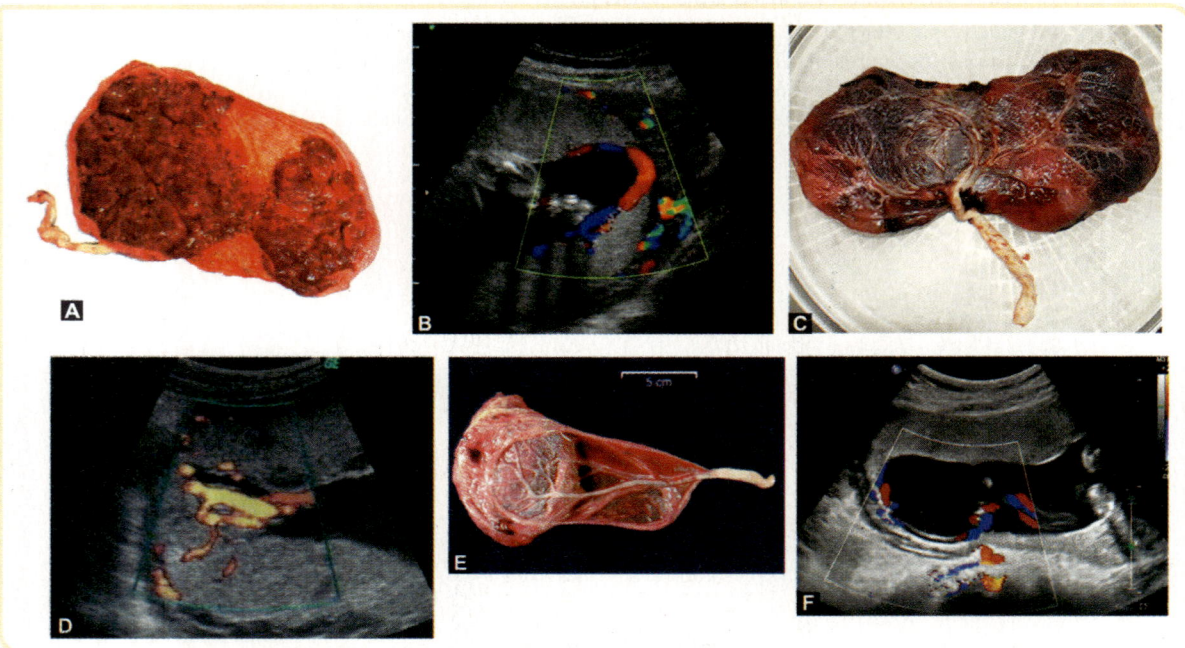

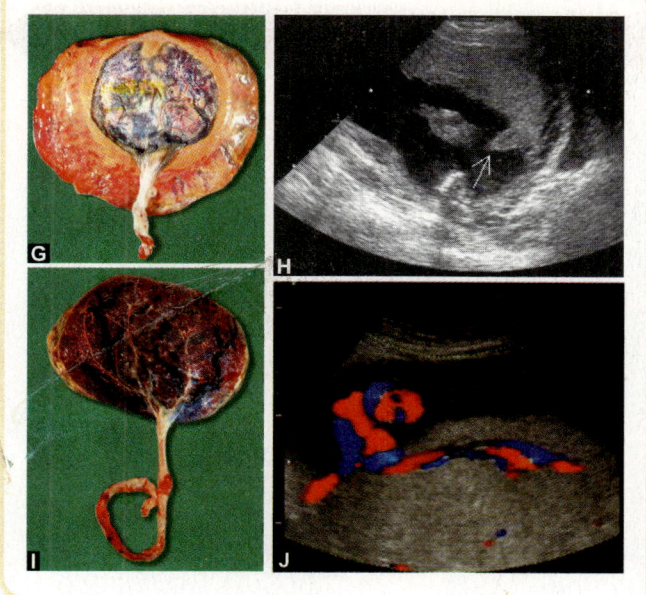

E. **Velamentous insertion of Cord Gross:** The major umbilical vessels separate in the fetal membranes before reaching the placental disk. It is of no major consequence in utero, but could lead to a greater chance for cord trauma with bleeding during delivery.

F. **Velamentous insertion of Cord:** Ultrasound and color Doppler images show the umbilical cord inserting into the placental membranes in the posterior wall before reaching the placental tissue proper superiorly to enter the fundal edge of the anterior placenta.

G. **Circumvallate placenta gross:** Insertion of the membranes away from the peripheral margin due to a folding/rolling of the chorion on itself. Portion of extrachorial disc is present at the edge. Firm ridge at the site of insertion is usually present. If cysts and other gross aberrations present, may be associated with fetal and maternal abnormalities. It is called as complete circumvallate placenta if 100 % (360°) of placental circumference involved. If it is less than that it is called as partial circumvallate placenta. Complete type shows higher risk of complications like placental abruption, preterm labor, IUGR.

H. **Circumvallate placenta USG:** placental edges appear folded and curled in all 4 quadrants (if complete- 360°).

I. **Battledore/ Marginal placenta gross:** umbilical cord insertion site located at or near the placental disc described as marginal or "battledore" (resembling a badminton racket). Fetal IUGR and the presence of a single umbilical artery (two vessel umbilical cord) are slightly increased with marginal insertions. Marginal vessels are prone to undergo twisting, occlusion or thrombosis.

J. **Battledore/ Marginal placenta USG:** Showing marginal insertion of the cord at the placenta.

 KEY

PLACENTAL VARIATIONS

A. **Succenturiate Lobe of placenta gross:** When two or more lobes of placenta of unequal sizes are attached to each other with marginal insertion of the umbilical cord it is known as succenturiate lobe. One or more small accessory lobes—succenturiate lobes—may develop in the membranes at a distance from the main placenta. These lobes have vessels that course through the membranes. If these vessels overlie the cervix to create a vasa previa, they can cause dangerous fetal hemorrhage if torn. An accessory lobe may also be retained in the uterus after delivery.

B. **The succenturiate lobe of placenta USG:** The image shows main lobe of placenta on the posterior wall and small lobe on the anterior wall of the uterus and it is connected by a string of blood vessels.

C. **Bilobate placenta gross:** If both the lobes of such placenta are nearly similar in size it is known as *bilobate placenta, bipartite placenta* or *placenta duplex* and cause postpartum uterine atony and hemorrhage. Placental lobes appear as two well defined masses connected by a thin bridge of chorionic tissue. Cord is usually attached at this bridge of tissue. Usually of no clinical significance, but may be associated with velamentous insertion of the cord (which must be looked for and excluded prior to the onset of labor)

D. **Bilobate placenta USG:** Showing two equal sized lobes with single cord attached at the bridge of the two lobes.

	Bilobed Placenta	Succenturiate Placenta
Placental lobes	Equal size	Different size
Cord attachment	Central	Eccentric velamentous
Placenta lobes attached by	Placental / chorionic tissue	Membranes
Complications	Occasionally velamentous cord insertion	Retained products Velamentous attachment Vasa previa Hemorrhage from vessels

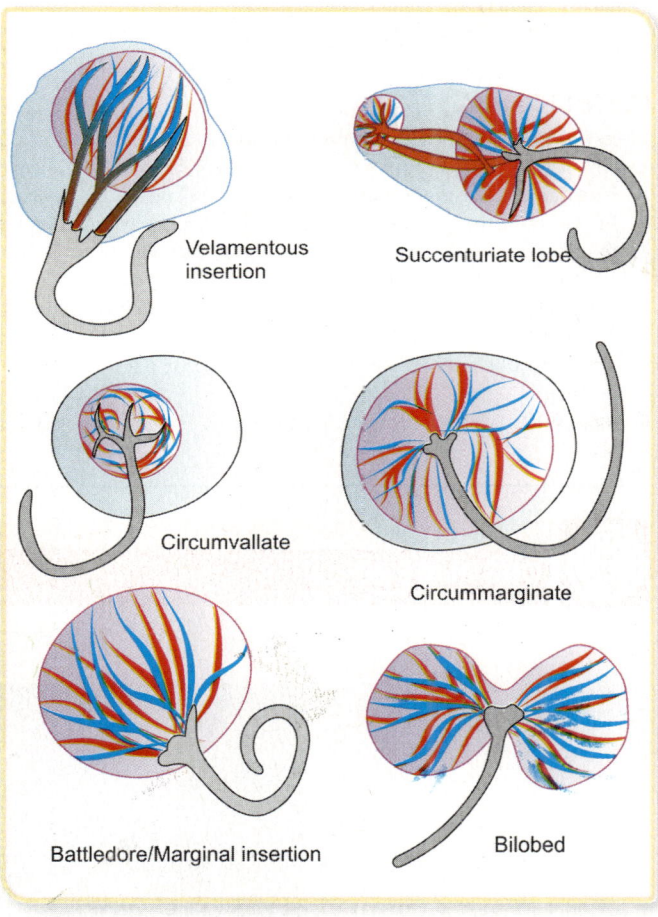

Fig: Placental variations (illustration)

OBG PLATE 19

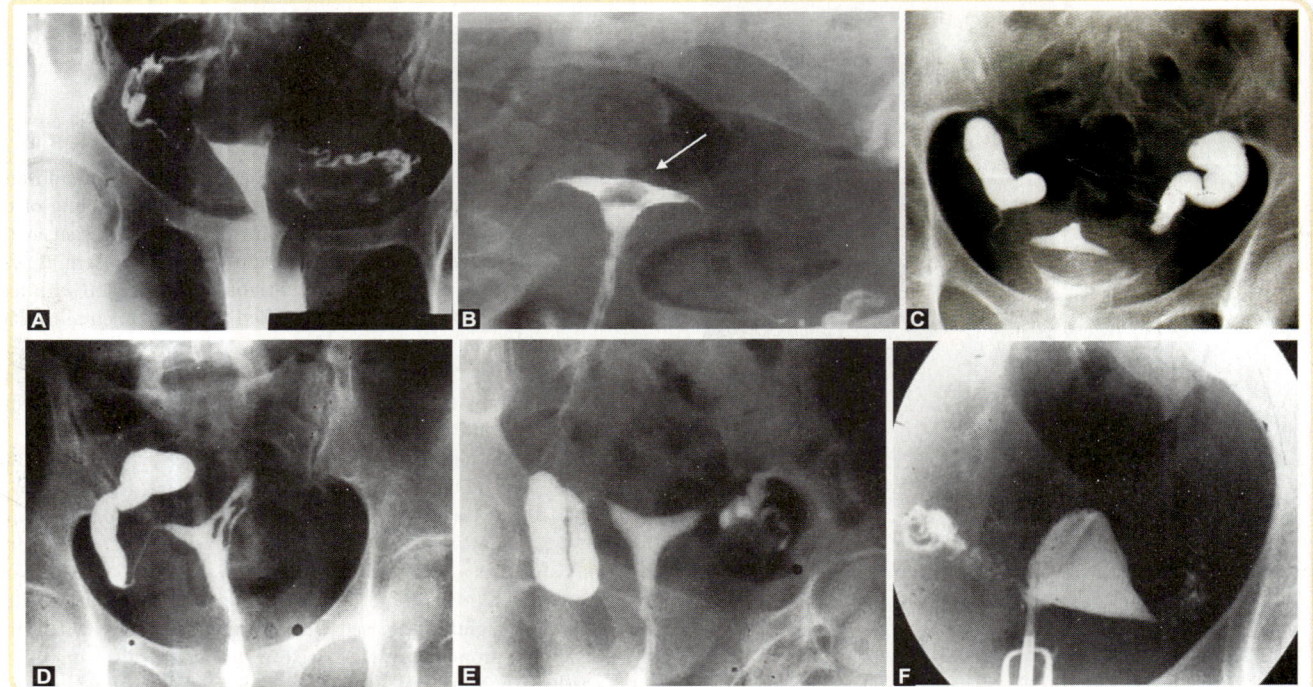

PLATE LEGENDS

Hysterosalpingography is an important tool in the evaluation of infertility. It provides information regarding the shape of the uterine cavity and the patency of the tubes. Tubal factors, many of which follow from sexually transmitted diseases, are an important cause of infertility.

A. **Normal hysterosalpingogram:** shows normal filling and spillage of contrast media.
B. **Endometrial polyps** are seen as filling defects of various size at the level of uterine cavity. This HSG shows a rounded fundal polyp.
C. Displays **bilateral hydrosalpinx**[NEETPG] and clubbing of the tubes with no evidence of any spillage into the peritoneal cavity. The uterine cavity in this HSG is normal.
D. In the figure there is unilateral hydrosalpinx and evidence of adhesions within the uterine cavity consistent with **Asherman syndrome**. There is no filling of the other tube.
E. One tube fills and has unilateral hydrosalpinx; the other shows loculation and minimal fluid accumulation. The uterine cavity here is normal.
F. **Salpingitis isthmica nodosa**: characteristic "salt-and pepper" pattern of tubal filling and evidence of a diverticulum of the tube on one side.

OBG PLATE 20

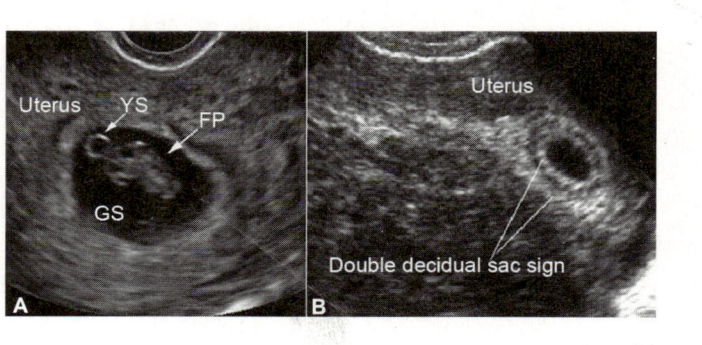

PLATE LEGENDS

A. **Normal early pregnancy on USG:**
   Yolk sac (YC) and fetal pole (FP in Gestational sac (GS)
B. **Double decidual sac sign (DDSS)** is a useful feature on early pregnancy ultrasound in distinguishing between an early intrauterine pregnancy (IUP) and a pseudogestational sac. It consists of the decidua parietalis (that lining the uterine cavity) and decidua capsularis (lining the gestational sac) and is seen as two concentirc rings surrounding an anechoic gestational sac.

OBG PLATE 21

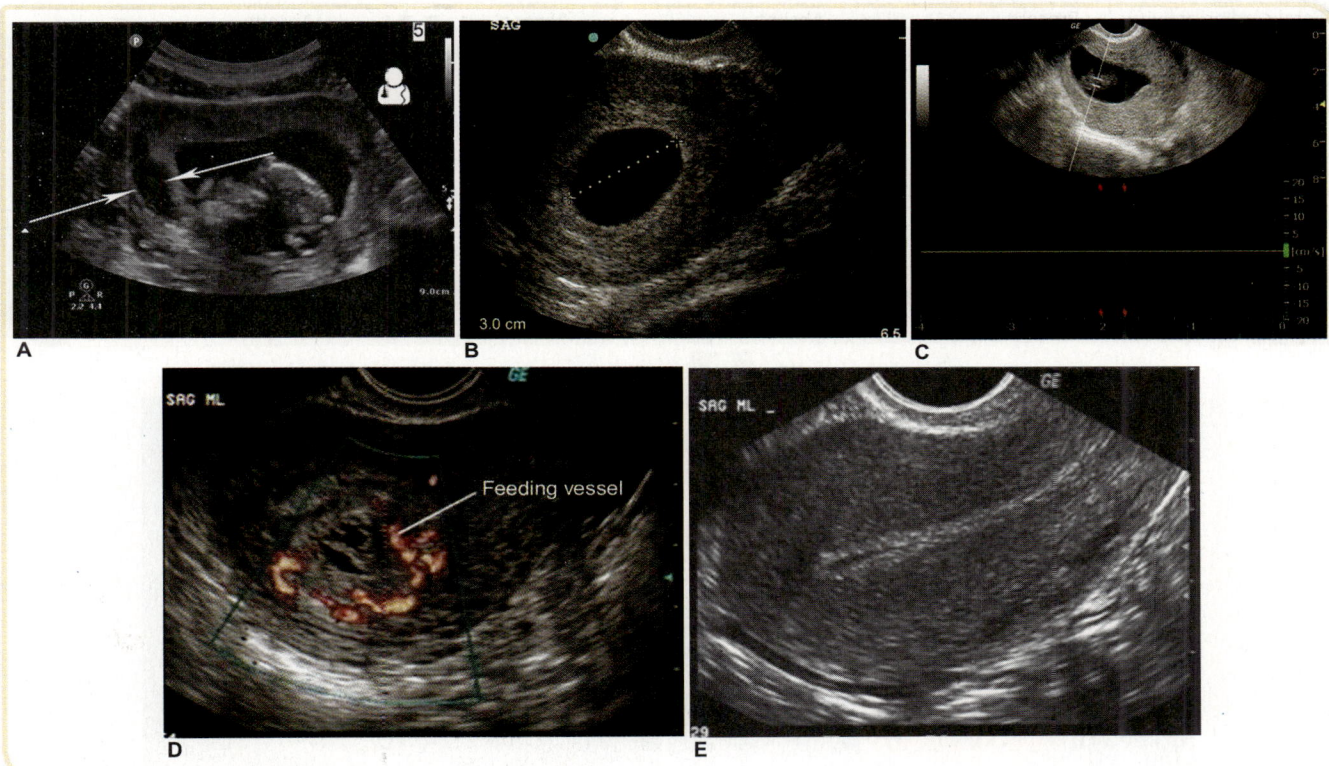

TYPES OF ABORTION

Abortion is the termination of pregnancy, either spontaneously or intentionally, before the fetus develops sufficiently to survive. By convention, abortion is usually defined as pregnancy termination prior to 20 weeks' gestation or less than 500-g birth weight.

Hemorrhage into the decidua basalis, followed by necrosis of tissues adjacent to the bleeding, usually accompanies abortion. If early, the ovum detaches, stimulating uterine contractions that result in its expulsion. When a gestational sac is opened, fluid is commonly found surrounding a small macerated fetus, or alternatively no fetus is visible—the so-called blighted ovum.

Miscarriage is classified as threatened, missed, incomplete and complete based on the ultrasound findings.

A. **Threatened abortion** is usually diagnosed in women with a history of vaginal bleeding and in whom a live embryo can be visualized on the scan. In 15% of these women the pregnancy will be lost. Threatened abortion shows other signs like sub-chorionic or perigestational hemorrhage. This transabdominal pelvic ultrasound demonstrates a single, live Intrauterine pregnancy with a fetal heart rate of 146 and subchorionic hemorrhage.
B. The terms **'blighted ovum'** and **'anembryonic pregnancy'** have been used to describe a gestational sac without a detectable fetal pole in a gestational sac that measures 8 weeks.

> **Note**
> An **anembryonic gestation** (also known as a **blighted ovum**) is a pregnancy in which initially pregnancy appears normal on an ultrasound scan, but as the pregnancy progresses a visible embryo never develops. See absent fetal pole with irregular gestational sac (asterix)

C. **Missed abortion** is defined as the retention of a gestational sac within the uterus following embryonic or early fetal death. The diagnosis is usually based on the absence of cardiac activity within the fetal pole. The absence of cardiac activity in an embryo of crown–rump length (CRL) > 6 mm, or the absence of a yolk sac or embryo in a gestation sac of mean diameter > 20 mm **(blighted ovum)**, enables conclusive diagnosis of a missed abortion. In pregnancies, in which the embryo and sac are smaller than 6 mm or 20 mm, respectively, a repeat ultrasound examination 1 week later is necessary to clarify the diagnosis.
D. **Incomplete abortion:** Endometrial thickness vary between 5 and 15 mm, retained products are usually seen as a well-defined area of hyperechoic tissue within the uterine cavity as opposed to blood clots that are more irregular.
E. **Complete abortion** is usually diagnosed when the endometrium is very thin and regular with no retained products. The ultrasound appearances are therefore comparable to those of the non-pregnant uterus in the early proliferative phase.

USG Diagnosis of Abortion				
	Threatened abortion	Missed abortion	Incomplete abortion	Complete abortion
History	No bleeding	No bleeding	Bleeding PV, Cramps	Bleeding PV, Cramps
Fetal pole	Present	Present	Absent	Absent
Fetal cardiac activity	Present	Absent	Absent	Absent
Endometrium	Thick, Sub chorionic bleed etc	Thick, Sub chorionic bleed etc	Thickness between 5 -15 mm	Thin and regular
Retained products of conception (RPOC)	NA	NA	Well defined hyperechoic area	Not seen
Management	Expectant management	Expectant management	Evacuation required	Evacuation not required

OBG PLATE 22

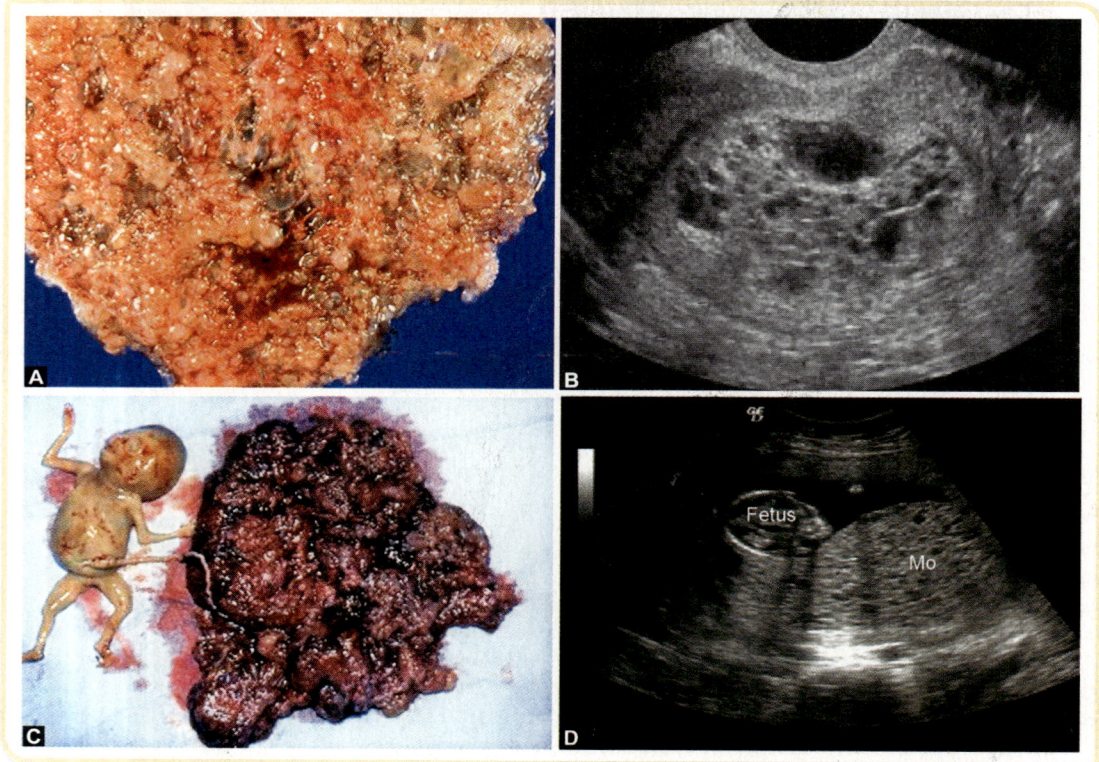

GESTATIONAL TROPHOBLASTIC DISEASE
A. **Complete hydatidiform mole gross:** It occurs when the ovum is lacking a maternal complement of chromosomes and is fertilized by a haploid sperm, usually containing an X chromosome. No fetus develops, but there is an abnormal placenta consisting of a mass of tissue with grape-like, swollen chorionic villi.
B. **Complete Hydatidiform mole USG:** Characteristic **Snowstorm appearance** or bunch of grape appearance without any fetal part characteristic of complete Hydatidiform mole.

C. **Partial Hydatidiform mole gross:** Since a maternal set of chromosomes is present, a fetus develops, but it is malformed, and the pregnancy rarely goes to term. Only some of the villi are grape-like.
D. **Partial Hydatidiform mole USG:** Showing minimal Snowstorm appearance and malformed fetus indicating partial mole.

Complete and Partial Hydatidiform Moles		
Feature	**Partial hydatidiform mole**	**Complete hydatidiform mole**
Karyotype	69XXY, Triploid, paternal and maternal origin	46XX, Diploid, mostly paternal origin
Immunohistochemistry		
HCG	Weak	>2.5 multiples of the Median
Placental alkaline phosphatase	Strong	Weak
HPL	Variable	Weak
Pathology		
Fetus or amnion, fetal vessels	Present	Absent
Hydropic villi	Variable, often focal	Pronounced, generalized
Trophoblastic proliferation	Focal	Variable, often marked
Villous scalloping	Marked	Absent
Clinical		
Mole clinical diagnosis	Rare	Common
Uterus large for dates	Rare	30%-50%
Malignant sequelae	<5%	6%-36%
Persistent disease	20%	<5%
USG		
Theca lutein cysts	Uncommon	Common
	Focal swelling of the villous tissue and focal trophoblastic hyperplasia in the presence of embryonic or fetal tissue. Increase in transverse diameter of gestational sac	Generalized swelling of the villous tissue and diffuse trophoblastic hyperplasia in the absence of embryonic or fetal tissue. Multiple hypoechoic areas corresponding to hydropic villi, at times described as a **"snowstorm" pattern**
$P^{57}kip^2$ ($P^{57}kip^2$ is a paternally imprinted gene which is maternally expressed. It is used in an immunostaining method to differentiate between complete and partial mole)	Positive	Negative

NOTES

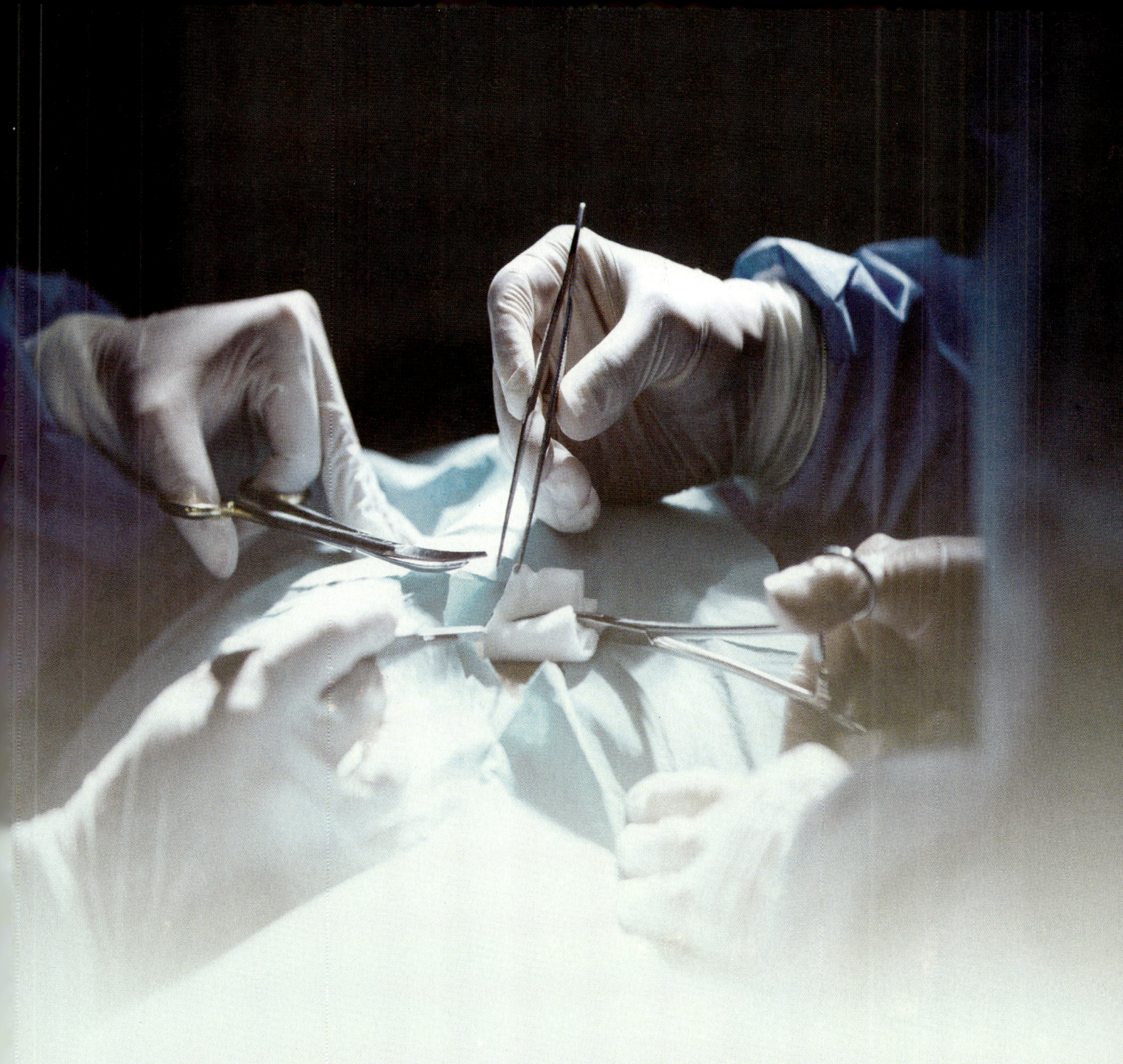

SURGERY

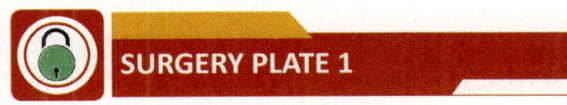

SURGERY PLATE 1

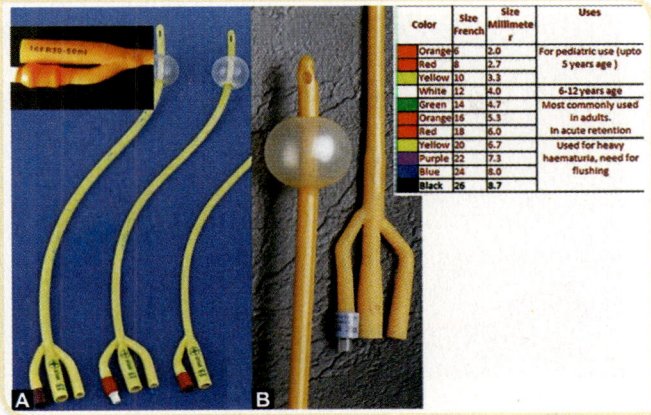

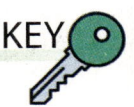

 KEY

FOLEY'S CATHETER

The name comes from the designer, **Frederic Foley**, a surgeon working in Boston, Massachusetts in the 1930s. The French scale or French gauge system is commonly used to measure the size (outside diameter) of a catheter). It is most often abbreviated as Fr, but can often abbreviated as FR or F. The outer diameter of the catheter in millimeters can be determined by dividing the French size by 3; that is **1 F= 1/3 mm outer diameter**. The standard male catheter length of **41-45 cm** can be used for males and females, but a shorter female length of **25 cm** can be more comfortable and discrete for some women.

Change frequency:
- Latex Foley catheter: 4 weekly change
- Silicone Foley catheter: 8 – 12 week change

A. Two Way Foley's Catheter

It is a flexible self-retaining indwelling catheter that is often passed through the urethra and into the bladder. Side channel is used to inflate the balloon so that it is kept indwelling and main channel is to hook the drainage bag. Balloon capacity is typically 5-50 ml (5 ml for retaining catheter, 30-50 ml for hemostasis)

B. Three-Way Catheters

Also called haemostatic catheters, these are generally thicker catheters with an extra channel to be used to flush the bladder. Through this tube, it is possible to inject water (i.e. NaCl 0.9%) into the bladder to flush it continuously in order to clean the bladder of blood clots or other debris, for instance after prostate surgery. These catheters are often of a larger diameter (20-24 Fr.) to allow for large chunks of debris to pass through it.
- Following a transurethral resection of the prostate, a large (24 Fr.) three-way Foley catheter with 30 cc balloon is used to maintain hemostasis.
- Used for bladder irrigation/lavage and clot removal.

Indications for Urethral Catheterization
- Acute and chronic urinary retention
- Maintain a continuous outflow of urine for patients with voiding difficulties, as a result of neurological disorders that cause paralysis or loss of sensation affecting urination
- Need for accurate measurements of urinary output in critically ill patients
- Perioperative use for selected surgical procedures.
- Patients undergoing urological surgery or other surgery on contiguous structures of the genitourinary tract
- Anticipated prolonged duration of surgery
- Need for intra-operative monitoring of urinary output
- To assist in healing of open sacral or perineal wounds in incontinent patients
- Patient requires prolonged immobilization (e.g., potentially unstable thoracic or lumbar spine, multiple traumatic injuries such as pelvic fractures)
- To allow bladder irrigation/lavage. (3-way catheter)
- To facilitate continence and maintain skin integrity (when conservative treatment methods have been unsuccessful)
- To improve comfort for end of life care, if needed
- Management of intractable incontinence

Contraindications for Urethral Catheterization
- Acute prostatitis
- Suspicion of urethral trauma

SURGERY PLATE 2

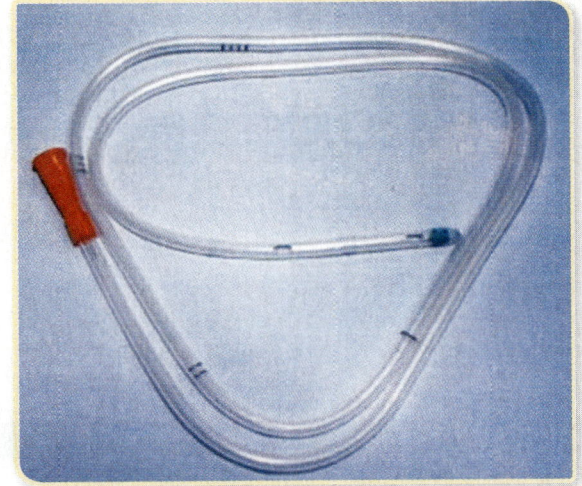

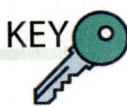 KEY

NASOGASTRIC TUBE (RYLES)
Indications/Uses
- To decompress stomach during upper abdominal surgeries
- To decompress stomach in intestinal obstruction
- To decompress stomach postoperative
- For gastric lavage (14-18 French Catheter is typically used for suction, while enteral feeding tubes may be smaller 8 French).
- For administration of medications or enteral feeding - when the patient is unable to swallow (8 French)
- To monitor gastric bleeding

Contraindications
- Skull base fractures
- Facial fractures
- Obstructed airway
- Esophageal varices
- Clotting disorder

Technique

- Estimate the length of the tube to be inserted. Do this by measuring the NG tube from the tip of the nose, to the earlobe and then to the xiphisternum
- Lubricate the tip of the tube and begin to insert through one of the nostrils. If any resistance is encountered change to the other nostril.
- Ask the patient to take a mouthful of water and as they swallow advance the tube to the desired length.

Positioning: Place patient in sitting position with neck flexed slightly and head of bed elevated to 45°. Flexion of the neck may facilitate passage of the tube into the esophagus and avoid endotracheal insertion.

How to Confirm its Placement in Stomach?

- Greenish grey fluid on aspiration confirms that the tube is in stomach
- Inject 50 ml of air into the tube and listen for gurgling sound in the epigastrium
- pH readings should be between 1 and 5.5 for feeding to commence safely
- Chest X-ray confirmation of placement is mandatory prior to instilling material such as medications or tube feedings down an NG tube

Size

- *NG tube (for adult patients)* - 14-18 French
- *NG tube (for pediatric patients)* - In pediatric patients, the correct tube size varies with the patient's age; to find the correct size (in French), add 16 to the patient's age in years and then divide by 2, so that for an 8-year-old child, for example, the correct size is 12 French ([8 + 16]/2 = 12)

Length: 105-120 cm

Parts: Manufactured from Non-toxic, Non-irritant medical grade PVC.

- Four lateral eyes (to avoid blockage)
- Tip of the tube contains lead or stainless steel shots to make it radiopaque and heavier for easy introduction
- Some tube with radio-opaque line, marked at 40, 50, 60 and 70 cm from the tip for accurate placement

Marking	At	Corresponds to
First marking	40 cm	Gastroesophageal junction
2nd marking	50 cm	Body of the stomach
3rd marking	60 cm	Pyloric region of stomach
4th marking	70 cm	Duodenum

Size in FR	Color Code
8	Blue
10	Black
12	White
14	Green
16	Orange
18	Red
20	Yellow

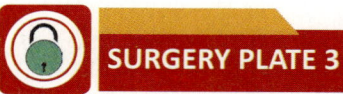

SURGERY PLATE 3

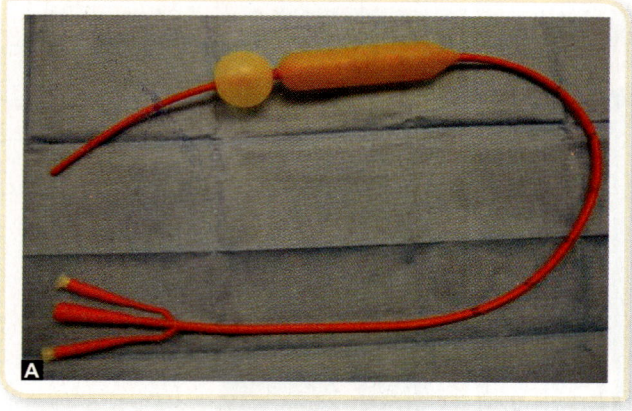

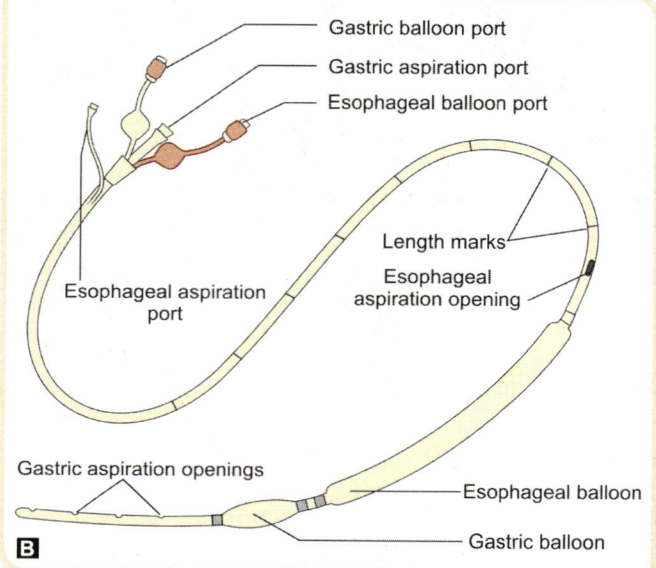

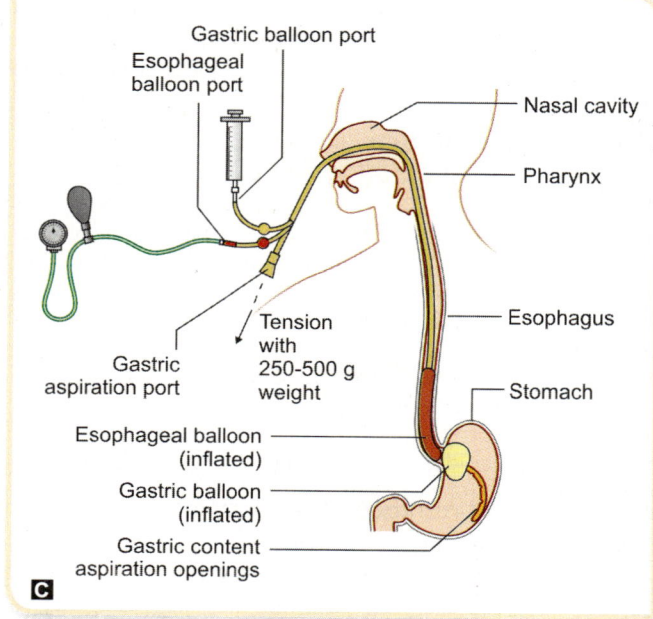

PLATE LEGENDS
A. Sengstaken Blakemore tube original
B. Sengstaken Blakemore tube illustration with labelling
C. Sengstaken Blakemore tube illustration (placement)

Sengstaken–Blakemore Tube
A double-balloon tamponade system was developed by Sengstaken and Blakemore for Balloon tamponade of bleeding esophageal varices.

Indications
- Acute life-threatening bleeding from esophageal or gastric varices that does not respond to medical therapy (including endoscopic hemostasis and vasoconstrictor therapy).
- Acute life-threatening bleeding from esophageal or gastric varices when endoscopic hemostasis and vasoconstrictor therapy are unavailable.

Contraindications
- Recent surgery that involved the esophagogastric junction
- Known esophageal stricture

Clinical Pearls
- In most cases, the esophageal balloon is not inflated during the initial placement of the tube. Never inflate the esophageal balloon before the gastric balloon.
- Keep a pair of scissors near the patient at all times in case the balloons migrate superiorly and obstruct the airway. The whole tube can be cut and removed.
- Direct pressure from the tube can cause mucosal ulceration. Perform frequent examinations to ensure that the tube is not placing excessive force on any given surface.
- Generally, the esophageal tamponade tube is a temporizing measure and should not be left in place for more than 24 hours.

Complications
- Aspiration is probably the most frequent major complication. The greatest risk of aspiration occurs during insertion. The risk of aspiration can be minimized by evacuating the stomach prior to tube placement
- Asphyxiation is caused by proximal migration of the tube and can be prevented with endotracheal intubation. If tube migration results in airway obstruction, cutting across all the tube lumens just distal to the points of bifurcation allows immediate extraction of the entire tube.
- Esophageal perforation or rupture can occur with inflation of a gastric balloon that is inadvertently placed in the esophagus or can be secondary to esophageal mucosal necrosis that results from excessive or prolonged inflation of the esophageal balloon.
- Minor complications include pain, pharyngeal and gastroesophageal erosions and ulcers caused by local pressure effects, pressure necrosis of the nose, lips, tongue, and hiccups.

SURGERY PLATE 4

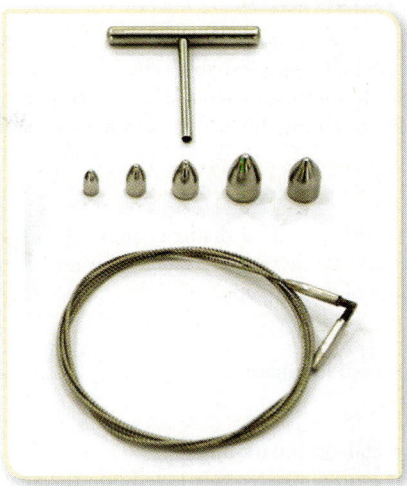

MYER'S VEIN STRIPPER
Varicose vein stripper is used for stripping varicose veins of long and short saphenous system

Parts
- 1 meter long flexible wire with detachable heads
- Fixed or detachable handle on one end
- Various sized detachable Olive on other end

Sterilization
By autoclaving

Uses
Stripping varicose veins of long and short saphenous system secondary to ligation and division of saphenofemoral or saphenopopliteal junction.

SURGERY PLATE 5

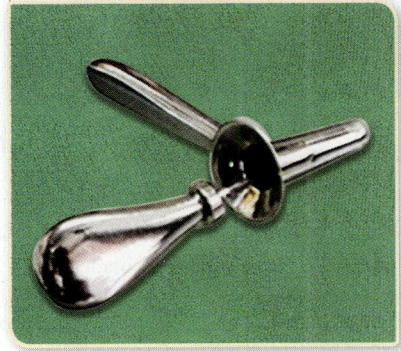

KELLY'S PROCTOSCOPE

Indication
- Diagnostic: Piles, Polyps, Strictures etc.
- Therapeutic: To inject sclerosant in prolapsed piles, Cryotherapy for piles, Polypectomy, Biopsy for carcinoma rectum and anal canal

Parts
Conican shape with proximal diameter more than distal, so as to illuminate the light at the required site. Obturator is the inner part for easy insertion of proctoscope

Types
Illuminating or nonilluminating

Technique
- Do digital rectal examination first
- Proctoscope with obturator is inserted into the anal canal in the direction towards the umblicus.
- Obturator is removed and proctoscope is withdrawn.
- During the course of withdrawal, any pathology is looked for.

Contraindication
Fissure in ano.

SURGERY PLATE 6

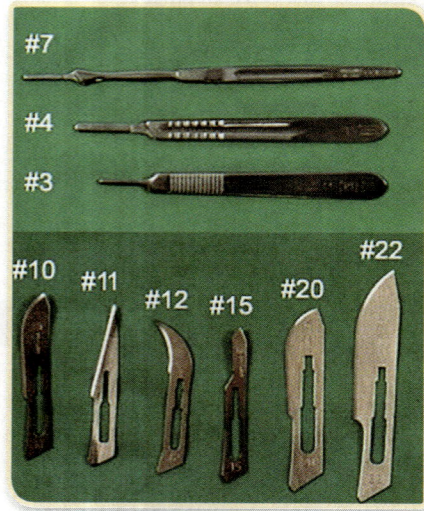

BARD PARKER'S HANDLE AND SURGICAL BLADES
- BP Handle one end is narrow to attach blades
- Handle shaft is grooved or serrated for better grip
- Number of handle written on shaft (say **3, 4, 5, 7**) to attach with different sized of blades
- BP handle is reusable and sterilized by Autoclaving
- Surgical blades are detachable and disposable
- Blade No. **10, 11, 12, 15** fits to BP handle number 3 and 5
- Blade number 18, 19, **20**, 21, **22**, 23, 24 fits to BP handle No. 4
- Surgical blades No. 20 to 24 have wide shaft, and are used to make larger incisions for laparotomy, mastectomy etc. or for sharp dissections to raise skin flaps
- Surgical **blade No. 15** has narrow shaft and is used to make smaller skin incisions and excisions of sebaceous cyst and lipoma, venesection etc.
- Surgical **blade No. 11** has oblique edge with sharp pointed tip (AKA Stab knife), used commonly for abscess drainage, drain insertion etc.

SURGERY PLATE 7

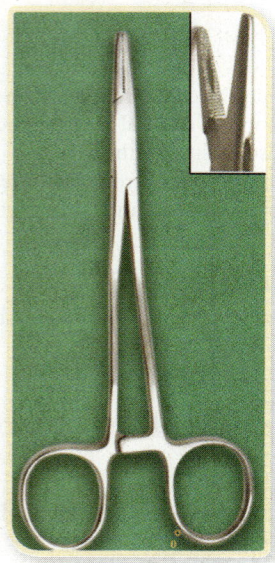

NEEDLE HOLDING FORCEPS
- Blades having criss cross or transverse serrations for needle holding
- Blade length is smaller than hemostatic forceps
- Blade have a central groove unlike hemostatic forceps
- Modified box joint

SURGERY PLATE 8

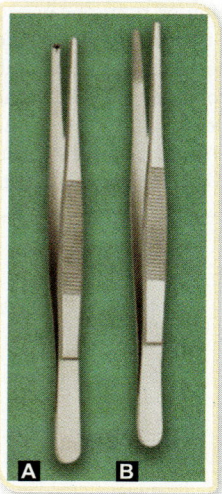

DISSECTING/THUMB FORCEPS

A. Toothed dissecting forceps for holding skin margins, Fascia, Aponeurosis etc.
B. Non toothed dissecting forceps for holding delicate soft tissue.

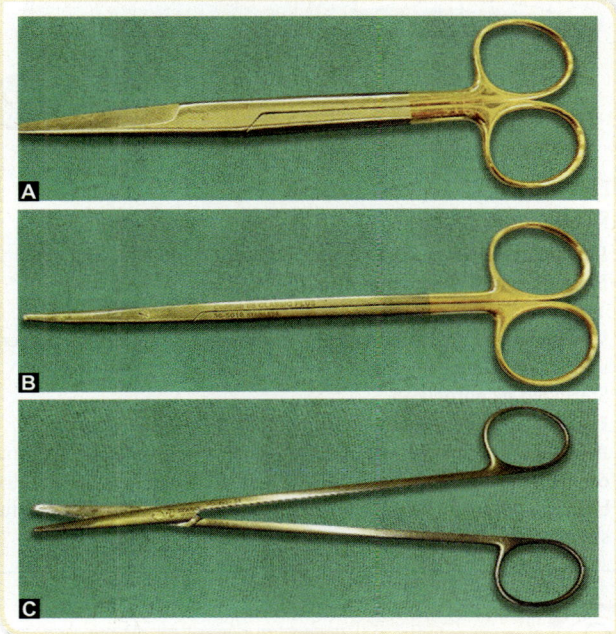

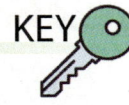

PLATE LEGENDS

A. Mayo's Scissors
- AKA- **Suture cutting scissors**
- Hemi blunt ends (tips), a feature that differentiates it from other surgical scissors
- Straight blade Mayo's scissors are used in suture cutting
- Curved blade Mayo's scissor is used for cutting tough body structures like rectus sheath, linea alba, aponeurosis etc.
- During appendectomy curved Mayo's scissors are used to split internal oblique and transverse abdominis
- Rarely used for dissection of tissues

B. Metzenbaum Scissors
- Longer shaft and shorter blades (straight of curved)
- Used in fine tissue dissection and cutting delicate structures
- Used in opening peritoneum during laparotomy & to dissect hernial sac
- To raise skin flaps in thyroidectomy, MRM, Neck dissection & incisional hernias
- To cut pedicles in nephrectomy, splenectomy, cholecystectomy
- To cut intestine in resection and anastomosis

C. Mcindoe's Scissors
- Same as Metzenbaum scissors, except that blades are smaller and shaft is longer
- Uses are also same as Metzenbaum scissors.

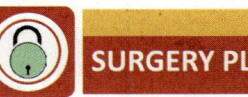

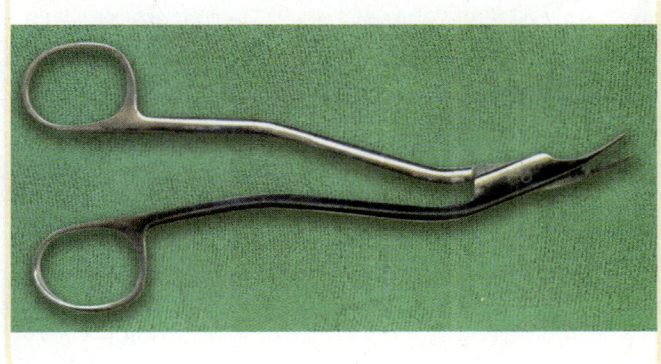

HEATH'S SUTURE CUTTING SCISSORS

- Fine scissors curved at an angle
- Small blades with serrations to grip sutures while cutting
- Used to cut skin sutures after wound healing.

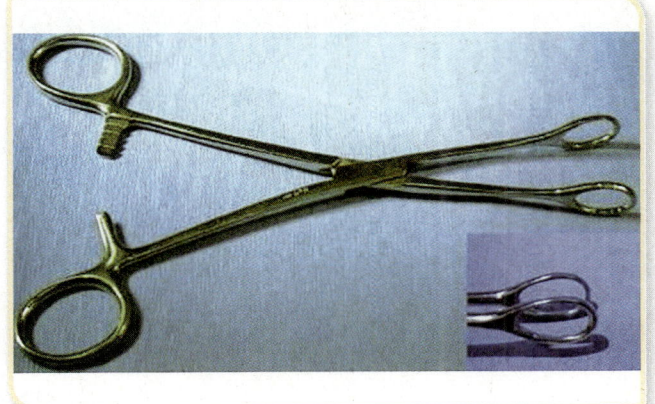

RAMPLEY'S SWAB (SPONGE) HOLDING FORCEPS

- Long instrument (9 and 1/2-inch-long) with finger bows, long shaft with catch, box joint, and a pair of blades
- Tip of blades are oval and **fenestrated with transverse serrations** on inner aspect, to hold swab firmly without slipping.
- Long instrument helps to clean operative area without touching the unsterile area (no touch technique)
- Sterilized by autoclaving
- Used for preoperative **cleaning (scrubbing)** of skin of operative area with aseptic solutions
- Additionally, can be used in **holding fundus of gall bladder, tongue, cervix and for removing laminated daughter cysts during hydatid cyst removal**

303

SURGERY PLATE 12

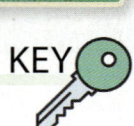 KEY

JONES/DOYEN'S/MAYO'S TOWEL CLIP
- Pincer like instrument, on pressing the shaft the blades opens and on releasing the blades close and tip of the two blades meet the catch the towel/drape
- Sterilization by autoclaving.

SURGERY PLATE 13

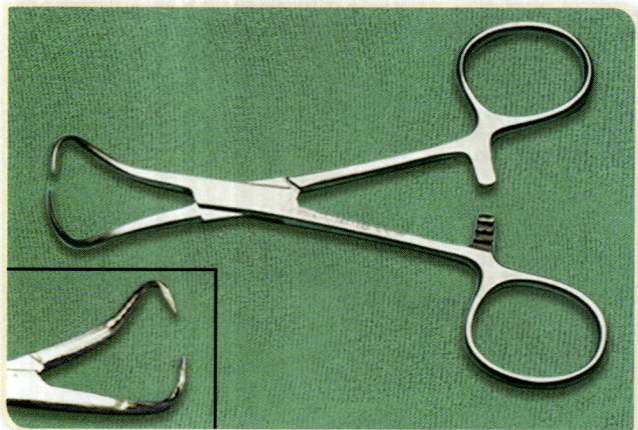

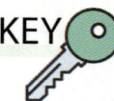 KEY

BACKHAUS TOWEL CLIP
- Blades and tip same as Jones towel clip but do not have spring/ pincer action
- In place it has shaft, finger bows and catch similar to hemostatic forceps
- Used in fixing of drapes
- Additionally, can be used in fixing diathermy cable, suction tubes cables of camera etc.
- Also used to give traction to fractured small long bones, and to fix ribs in Flail chest.

SURGERY PLATE 14

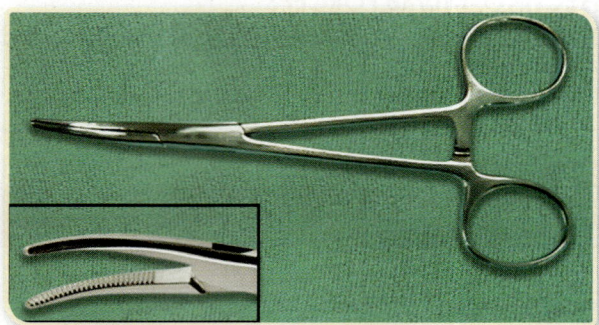

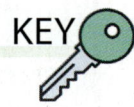 KEY

SPENCER WELL'S HEMOSTATIC FORCEPS (ARTERY FORCEPS)
- **Parts:** Finger bows, shaft, blades (straight or curves) and catch
- Blades are half the length of shaft
- Tips of blades are conical
- Whole length of **inner side of blades are serrated** to prevent slipping of tissue
- Sterilized by autoclave
- Used to catch and hold bleeding vessels to stop bleeding
- Additionally can be used in appendectomy to split internal oblique/ transverse abdominis, to crush the base of appendix, blunt dissection, as a pedicle clamp, to hold cut margins of rectus sheath, peritoneum, aponeurosis.

SURGERY PLATE 15

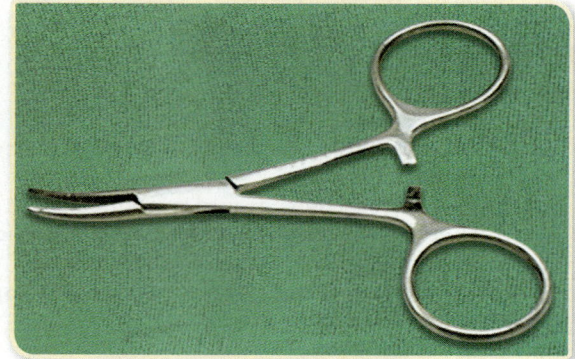

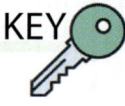 KEY

HALSTED'S HEMOSTATIC FORCEPS (MOSQUITO FORCEPS)
- Similar to Spencer Well's hemostatic forceps except that it is very light, smaller and having pointed tip
- Blades may be straight or curved

- Holds small and fine bleeding vessels
- Additionally, during appendectomy mesoappendix is poked with curved mosquito forceps to tie ligature, lip and palate surgery, pediatric surgeries (routinely), and during circumcision to separate adhesions.

SURGERY PLATE 16

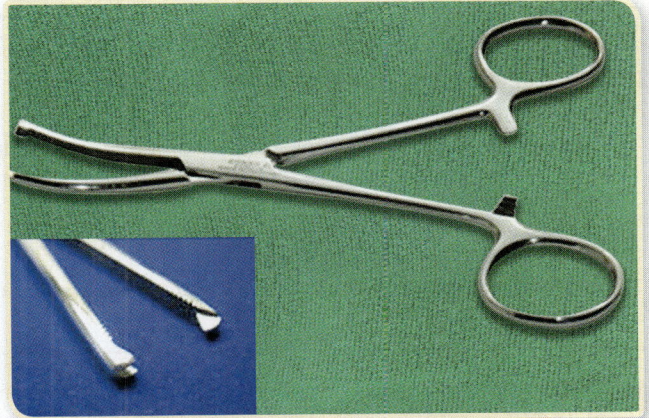

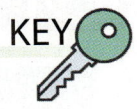

KOCHER'S FORCEPS
- Similar to Spencer Well's forceps except that the tip of blades have tooth on one side and groove on other side and blades are slightly longer than Spencer Well's forceps
- Used during thyroidectomy to be applied around the margins of the gland to be excised to prevent bleeding
- Also used for holding bleeding vessels in tough structures and to hold meniscus during meniscectomy
- In Obstetric practice it is used for artificial rupture of membranes.

SURGERY PLATE 17

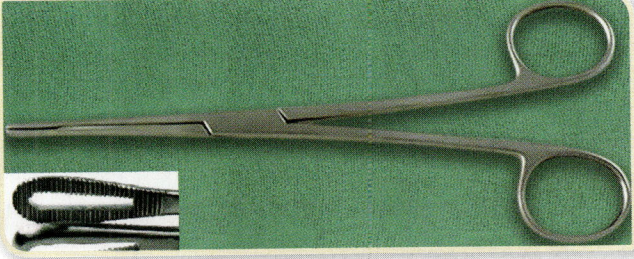

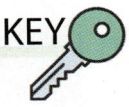

LISTER'S SINUS FORCEPS
- Long slender instrument with pairs of blade having transverse serrations only on tip and their tips are blunt (olive tipped)
- Shaft have no catch to prevent vital structures from crushing
- Used to break loculi and to introduce corrugated rubber tubes or roller pack in abscess cavity and exploring sinus tract.

SURGERY PLATE 18

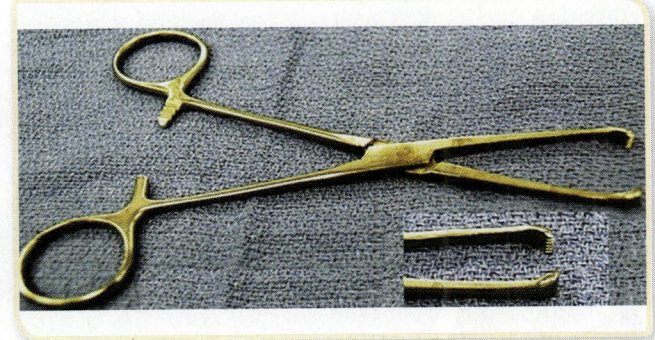

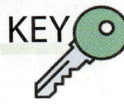

ALLIE'S TISSUE FORCEPS
- **Parts:** Finger bows, shaft with catch, box joint and blades
- Blades are long straight and have gap in between then throughout their length.
- Tip of blades are curved inward with sharp tooth and grooves which interlock to provide grasp.
- It minimally crushes the tissue in between the tip of the blades.
- Used to hold skin flaps and other hard structures.

SURGERY PLATE 19

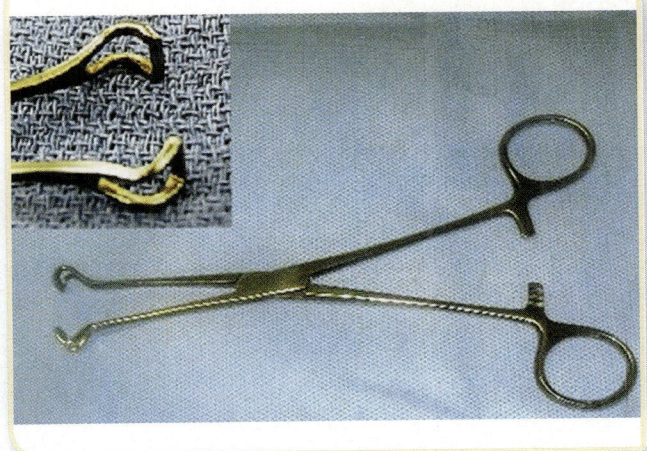

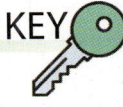

BABCOCK'S TISSUE FORCEPS
- Light and nontraumatic instrument having finger bows, shaft with catch, boxjoint, and blades
- Terminal part of blades are curved with triangular fenestrated to hold delicate structures
- Tip of the blades are nontraumatic with small serrations to provide grip
- Used to hold tubular structures like appendix, bowel, fallopian tubes, ureters, cord, etc.

SURGERY PLATE 20

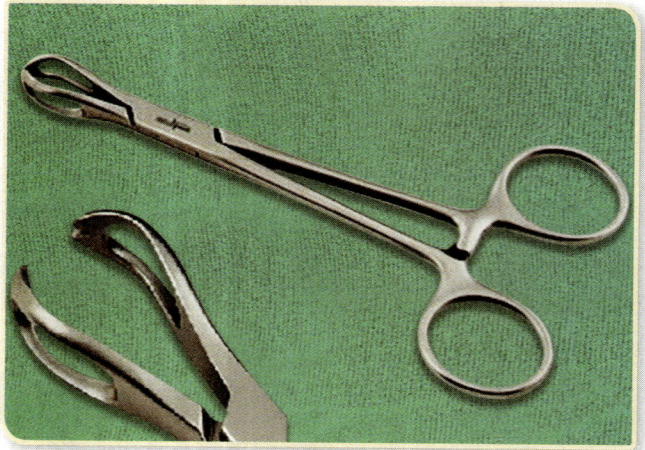

LANE'S TISSUE FORCEPS
- It is short, thick, bulkier and heavy.
- It has finger bows, shaft with catch, box joint and blades.
- Blades are small compared to shaft, and are curved with fenestrations to accommodate bulky tissue.
- The tip of blade have single sharp tooth on one side and groove on other side.
- Used to hold bulky and slippery tissue like fat and breast tissue.
- Can also be used as towel clip.

SURGERY PLATE 21

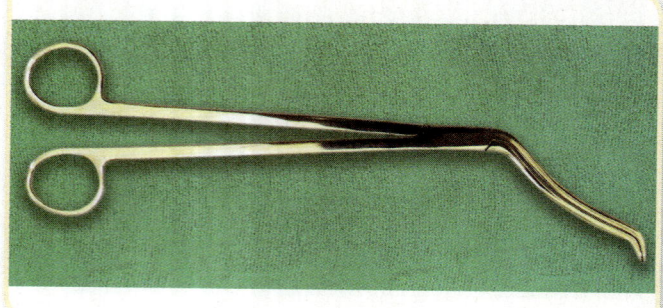

CHEATLE'S FORCEPS
- Parts: Finger bow, shaft, joint and blades but no catch
- Curved dipped blades with large serrations at tip for firm grip
- Always ready to use are it is always dipped in antiseptic solution
- Used to pick the sterilized instruments, linen, etc.

SURGERY PLATE 22

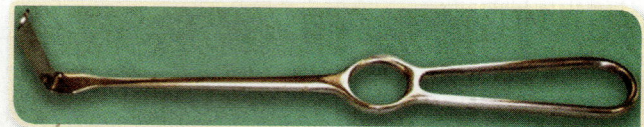

LANGENBECK'S RIGHT ANGLED RETRACTOR
- Comes in different sizes
- Flat solid blade right angled to the shaft for retraction, tip of blade is also curved at right angle to the rest of the blade for better retraction
- Handle is fenestrated for better grip
- Also comes with double blades at both ends
- Used in superficial surgeries like hernia to retract skin, fascia and aponeurosis.

SURGERY PLATE 23

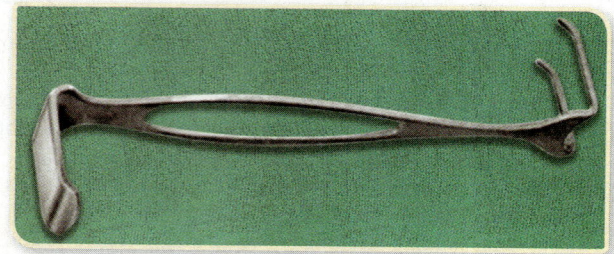

CZERNEY'S RETRACTOR
- Double blades at both ends, one blade is solid while other blade have 2 hooks
- Shaft is fenestrated to reduce weight and better grip
- Flat solid blade is used as Langenback's retractor
- Biflanged blade is used to retract the incision while approximating (suturing) in midline laparotomy as the tissue to be sutured can be seen in between the two flangs.

SURGERY PLATE 24

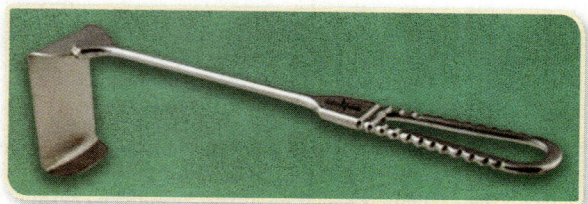

MORRIS RETRACTOR

- Design is same as Langenbeck's retractor except that the blade is wider and slightly concave than Langenbeck's retractor providing more space to work
- Used for retraction of anterior abdominal wall and intra-abdominal viscera.

SURGERY PLATE 25

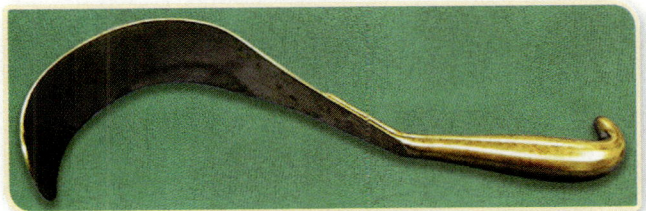

DEAVER'S RETRACTOR[AIIMS PG]

- Large curved retractor like a shape of "S" with solid curved blade at one end to accommodate large structures
- Long handle like a hook for firm grip
- Used to retract abdominal organs in various laparotomies.

SURGERY PLATE 26

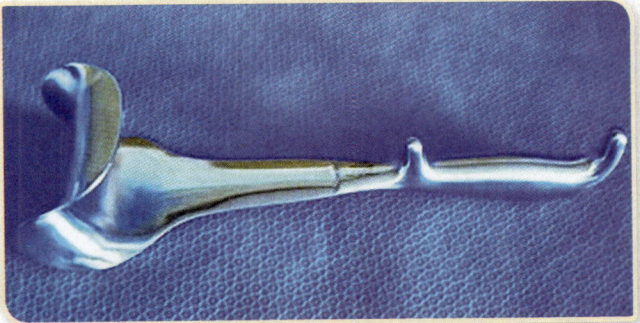

DOYEN'S RETRACTOR[AIIMS PG]

- Solid curved blade and solid non fenestrated handle
- Blade is curved from the shaft, tip of blade is curved from rest of the blade, body of the blade is curved outward laterally and tip of the blade itself is curved (neither pointed nor flat) i.e. every part of blade is curved.
- This quality makes it atraumatic.
- Used in pelvic and gynecological surgeries.
- Used in Cesarean section to retract bladder[AIIMS PG]

SURGERY PLATE 27

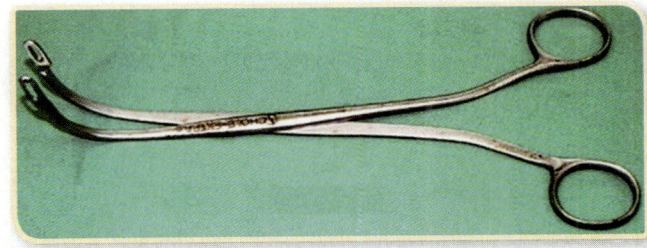

DESJARDIN'S CHOLEDOCHOLITHITOMY FORCEPS

Parts

Long curved blades with no serrations, flat and fenestrated tip with no serrations for stone holding, finger bows, screw type joint, shaft (curved with no catch to avoid crushing of stone while removal)

Uses

- During choledocholithotomy it is inserted in CBD and stones are removed.
- Can also be used in nephrolithotomy, pyelolithotomy and ureterolithotomy.

SURGERY PLATE 28

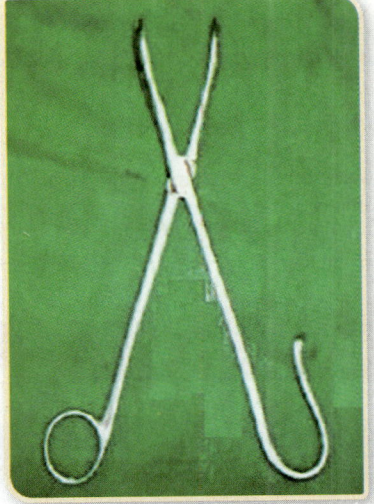

SUPRAPUBIC CYSTOLITHOTOMY FORCEPS

Parts

Shaft (handle) is peculiar with one finger bow for thumb and one incomplete ring like a hook for remaining fingers, for adequate grip without crushing stone. Blades are spoon shaped with concave inside and fine spicules or blunt serrations for stone holding without crushing. No catch.

Uses

To remove bladder stones (vesicle calculus) during suprapubic cystolithotomy.

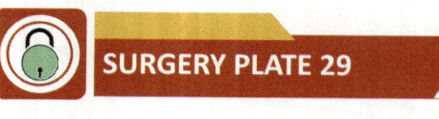
SURGERY PLATE 29

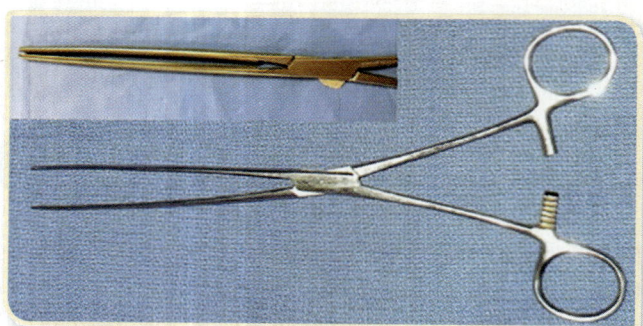

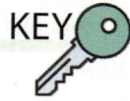

DOYEN GASTROINTESTINAL OCCLUSION (NONCRUSHING) CLAMP

Parts

Finger bows, catch, pair of shaft with long blades

Blades are flat, slightly concave, light weight, thin and springy with vertical serrations throughout the length with minimal depth to avoid crushing. Tips are blunted and rounded. When tip meets on closing the catch, there is small gap between the blades to allow holding intestine without crushing.

Uses

To clamp intestine during resection and anastomosis.

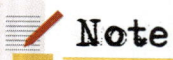**Note**

Kocher's Gastric occlusion clamp is same as Doyen Gastrointestinal occlusion clamp

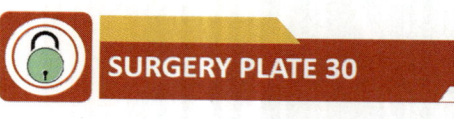
SURGERY PLATE 30

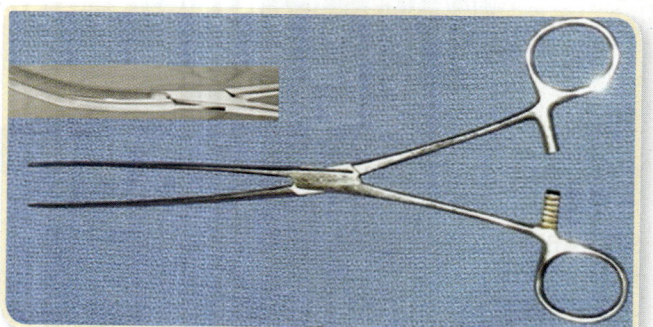

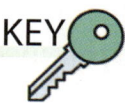

MOYNIHAN'S GASTRIC OCCLUSION (NONCRUSHING) CLAMP

Similar as Doyen's gastric occlusion clamp except that blades can be straight or curve and serrations are transverse

Uses

To hold and occlude stomach in Gastrectomy and Gastrojejunostomy.

SURGERY PLATE 31

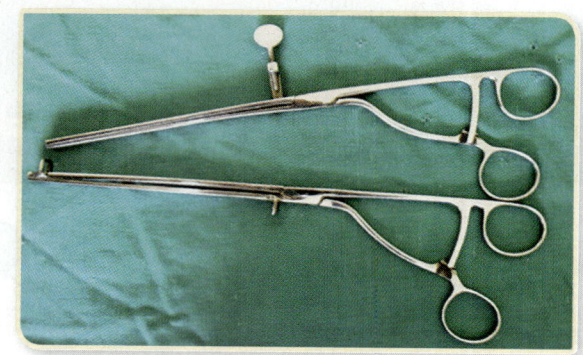

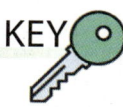

LANE'S TWIN GASTROJEJUNOSTOMY OCCLUSION CLAMP

This is a double or paired non crushing clamps containing two long occlusion clamp joined together by screw and a square ring near the tip. The clamps can be attached to each other with either their handles on same side or opposite side as per convenience. Curved or straight blades with longitudinal serrations

Uses

They are used in gastrojejunostomy. The two instruments are separated and one is applied to each loop of gut. Thereafter the two are fitted together, this allows loops to hold together for anastomosis.

SURGERY PLATE 32

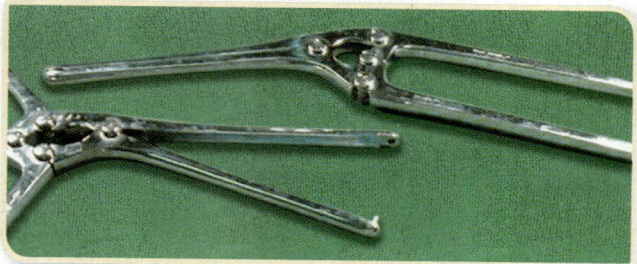

PAYR'S CRUSHING CLAMP

Parts
Heavy instrument with great crushing effect by virtue of double lever action. First lever opposes the blades firmly, second lever multiplies the pressure and crushes the viscus. Vertical serrations (parallel) on the whole length of blades. Blades may be long in gastric clamp and short in duodenal/small intestinal clamp. One tip is having blunt tooth while other tip have a groove for interlocking.

Uses
Gastric resections (Gastrectomy), intestinal resection anastomosis.

SURGERY PLATE 33

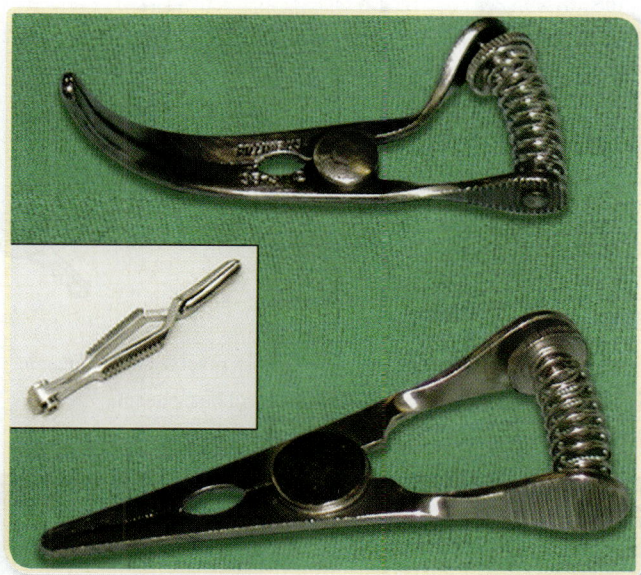

 KEY

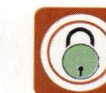 SURGERY PLATE 34

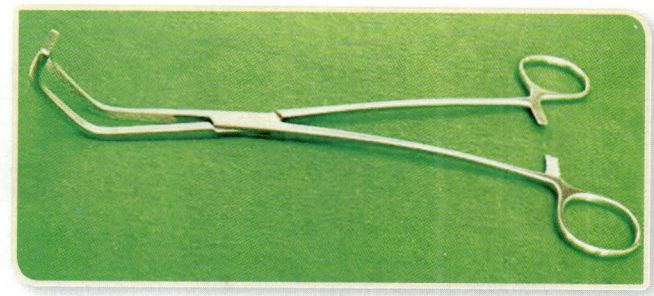

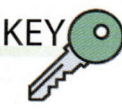 KEY

SATINSKY VASCULAR CLAMP

Parts
Pair of blades and shafts, catch and finger bows. Blades has vertical groove with fine serrations to avoid injury to occluded vessel. Blade is curved with different degrees of angulations at its blades and shaft also to clamp the vessels in depth and also not to obstruct the vision to operating surgeon.

Uses
- To occlude large vessels like IVC, SVC, aorta and large branches
- Aneurysms repair
- Renal, splenic and liver pedicle (porta hepatis) occlusion to stop bleeding from lacerations/blunt trauma.

 SURGERY PLATE 35

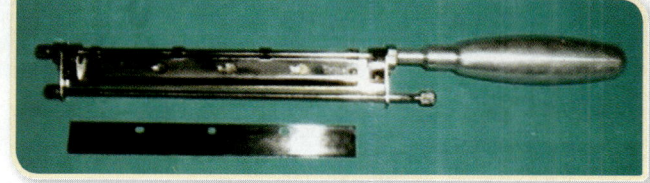

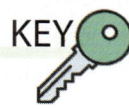 KEY

BULLDOG VASCULAR CLAMP

Parts
Clamp with spring like or pincer like (inset) action. Blades opened on pressing the shaft. Shaft have vertical groove with fine serrations on whole length of blade. Clamp have low closing pressure for noncompressive occlusion.

Uses
To occlude arteries/veins with correct tension to produce minimal trauma to vessels like coronary artery bypass and AV fistula.

 KEY

HUMBY'S KNIFE
- It has a handle, blade and a screw at the tip of the blade to adjust the blade for the thickness of the skin graft to be taken
- Blade is provided with a slot to attach surgical long blade, which is fixed by tightening the screw at the tip
- Used to take partial (split thickness) or full thickness (Wolf) graft from donor site of the patient to be grafted at the recipient site.

SURGERY PLATE 36

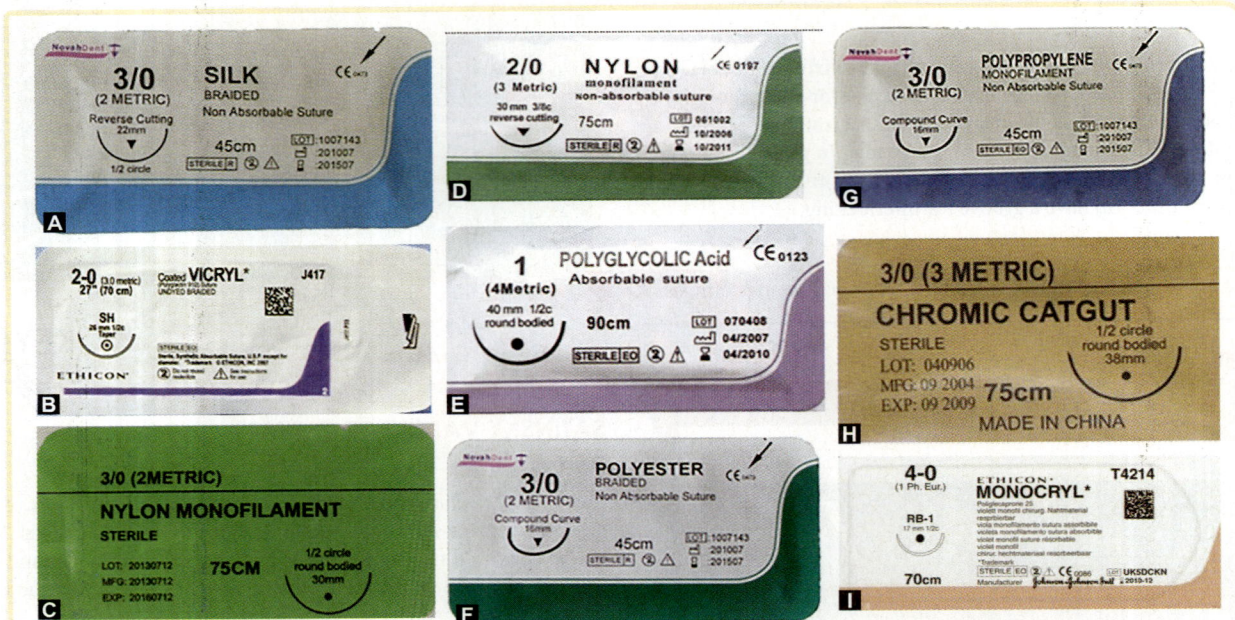

PLATE LEGENDS

A. Mersilk in reverse cutting needle
B. Vicryl in round body needle
C. Nylon in round body needle
D. Nylon in reverse cutting needle
E. Polyglycolic acid in round body needle
F. Polyester in reverse cutting needle
G. Polypropylene (Prolene) in reverse cutting needle
H. Chromic catgut with round body needle
I. Monocryl with round body needle

Characteristics of Absorbable Suture Materials					
Suture (trade name)	Manufacturing process	Effective strength (d)	Complete absorption (d)	Absorption profile		Application
				Tissue reactivity	Handling	
Surgical gut	Collagen from sheep intestine submucosa	4–10	70	High	Poor	Used for quick-healing mucosa
Chromic gut	Catgut treated with chromic acid	10–14	90	Moderate	Poor	Used for quick-healing mucosa
Polyglycolic acid (Dexon)	Synthetic monofilament or braided	14–21	60–120	Minimal	Good	Subcutaneous sutures, mucosa, ligation of vessels
Polyglactin acid (Vicryl)	Synthetic braided, lubricated with polyglactin 370; undyed or purple	20–30	60–90	Minimal	Excellent	Subcuticular and subcutaneous sutures
Monocryl (poliglecaprone 25)	Synthetic, monofilament, made of copolymer of glycolide and epsilon caprolactone.	Best knot strength in absorbable sutures	90 days	Minimal (Less reactive than Vicryl)	Excellent	Indicated for use in general soft tissue approximation, but not for use in CVS, CNS, microsurgery or ophthalmic surgery
Polydioxanone (PDS)	Monofilament polyester	40–60	180	Minimal	Good	Used for extended support
Polyglyconate (Maxon)	Synthetic monofilament	40–60	180–210	Minimal	Excellent	More supple than polydioxanone

Characteristics of Nonabsorbable Suture Materials

Suture (trade name)	Manufacturing process	Tissue reactivity	Handling	Application
Silk	Braided; derived from cocoon of silkworm larva	High	Excellent	Vessel ligation; high capillarity; should be avoided in areas prone to infection
Cotton	Braided	High	Excellent	Same as silk
Polyester	Braided terephthalate (Dacron), polyethylene (Mersilene), coated with Teflon (Tevdek), silicone (Ticron), polybutylate (Ethibond)	Minimal	Good if uncoated; excellent if coated	Commonly used for fascia; uncoated sutures have excellent knot security; coated sutures require five throws for knot security
Nylon	Synthetic polyamide monofilament or braided	Minimal	Good	Used for skin, fascia; requires five throws for knot security
Polypropylene (Prolene, Surgilene)	Plastic monofilament	Minimal	Good	High elasticity; commonly used for skin closure and vascular anastomoses; requires five throws
Polybutester (Novafil)	Plastic monofilament copolymer	Minimal	Good	Very high elasticity; used when tissue swelling is present
Steel	Alloy monofilament	None	Poor	Retention sutures, bone

SURGERY PLATE 37

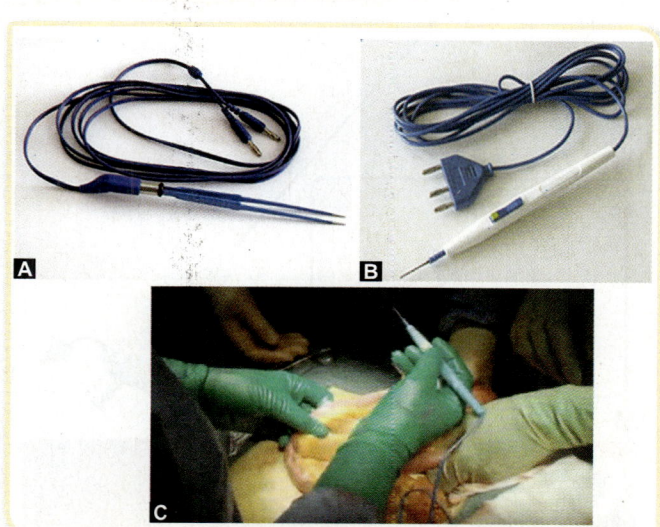

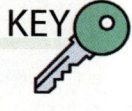 KEY

DIATHERMY
A. Bipolar diathermy
B. Monopolar diathermy
C. Monopolar diathermy intraoperative

PRINCIPLES OF DIATHERMY

The Effects of Electricity on Tissue

At low frequencies, alternating current (a.c.) causes a dangerous shock but with frequencies above 20 kHz, muscular contraction stops, pain stops and the only detectable effect is heat generation within the tissue. The heating is produced because of the **Joule effect**. At high frequencies, the body can be modelled as a resistor, instead of the capacitive + resistive elements as happens in low frequencies. Thus, the heating energy is:

$$E = I^2 R T$$

- Where E is the energy in Joules
- I is the current through the skin in Amperes
- R is the resistance of your body in Ohms
- T is the time in seconds

The Current Density (Current Divided by Area)

- The greater the current through a particular area, the greater is the heating effect.
- The smaller the area through which a particular current flows, the greater the heating effect.

The Size of the Electrode

If the electrodes used are flat plates of equal size, the heating effect produced at both electrodes will be of equal intensity. Maximum heat intensity will be at a depth of approximately **1 cm** from the skin surface. This is the type of effect produced by medical diathermy used in physiotherapy departments. Should one of the electrodes be reduced in size, the current at both electrodes will be almost equal but the current density will increase at the smaller electrode and the heating effect produced by that electrode, will be concentrated. Eventually, if the size is reduced even further, the heat will become intense enough to produce a burn. This is the type of effect produced by surgical diathermy otherwise known as electrosurgery.

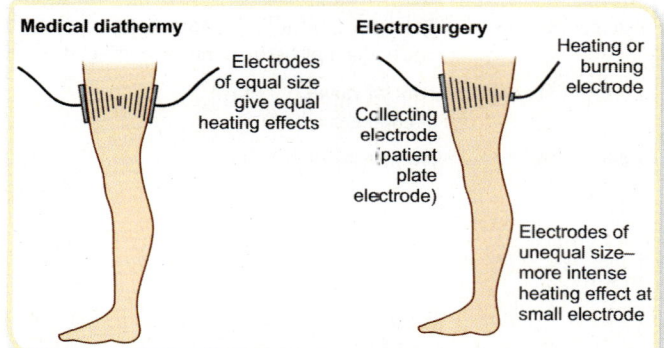

EFFECTS OF DIATHERMY

- **Cutting/Electrotomy:** Continuous output of current between the active electrode and tissue in monopolar diathermy produces temperature up to **100°C**. Cellular water is vaporized causing tissue disruption without much coagulation. This setting is not available in bipolar diathermy. Temperatures of above 100°C in the region around the active electrode lead to the rapid evaporation of the fluid within the cell membrane. As a result, the cell membrane ruptures forming vapor around the electrode which in turn involves other cells lying in the path of the electrode as it moves

- **Coagulation:** Pulsed output from diathermy generator results in sealing of blood vessels with minimum tissue disruption. Temperatures of **60–70°C** in the area around the active electrode lead to a slow boiling of the intra-cellular fluid through the cell membrane. As a result of this effect, the cell shrinks and several cells link up to form chains. A **"welding effect"** is initiated which stops the bleeding.
  - **Desiccation** (otherwise known as **pinpoint coagulation or contact coagulation**) creates rapid localized heat at the end of the blood vessel causing contraction with eventual occlusion of the lumen. This creates precise coagulation of the tissue
  - **Spray coagulation** mode (otherwise known as **fulguration** or non contact coagulation) employs higher voltages. This is because the waveform is off for longer periods of time than any other mode, and because the electrode is not in contact with the tissue (held approximately **2–4 mm** away). This therefore, creates an air gap across which the current must jump. The spray coagulation mode creates a more widespread coagulation than the other coagulation modes and due to the higher voltages employed, should not be used in laparoscopic or endoscopic surgery, where the voltages could break down the insulation of the instruments used.

- **Blended:** Many machines have this setting of monopolar diathermy; a continuous output with pulses to help coagulate as well as cut.

TYPES OF DIATHERMY

There are two main types of diathermy Monopolar and Bipolar. Polarity refers to the number of electrode poles at the site of application

	Types of Diathermy	
	Monopolar	Bipolar
Power	High power generator (400 W)	Low power generator (50 W)
Electrodes	One hand held electrode and one plate electrode (70 cm sq)	2 electrodes in pair of forceps
Uses	Cutting and coagulation	Coagulation only
Adjacent tissue	Should be careful about adjacent tissue	Adjacent tissue is never damaged
Contraindications	Artificial valves, Pacemakers	
Adverse effects	Plate electrode burns	

Contd...

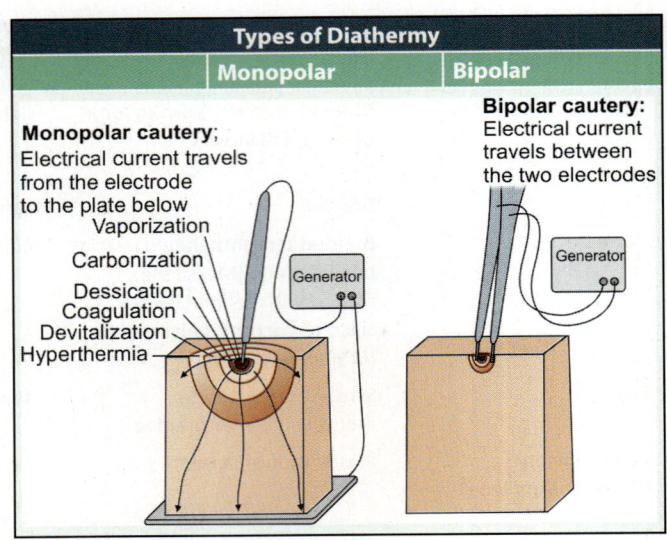

SURGERY PLATE 38

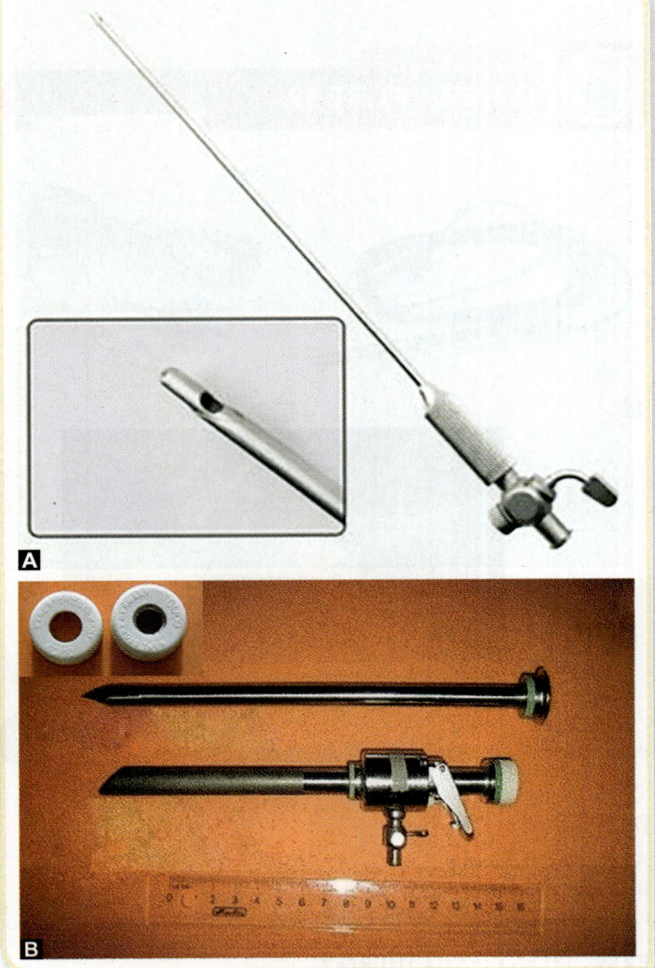

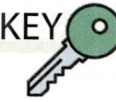

KEY

PLATE LEGENDS

A. A **Veress needle** is a spring-loaded needle used to create pneumoperitoneum for laparoscopic surgery. It was first developed in 1932 by Janos Veress, a Hungarian internist working with tuberculosis patients. Raoul Palmer introduced the use of the Veress needle in laparoscopy to establish a pneumoperitoneum.

Two methods are used for establishing abdominal access during laparoscopic procedures.
- **Hasson technique:** The first, direct puncture laparoscopy, begins with the elevation of the relaxed abdominal wall with two towel clips or a well-placed hand.
- **Veress needle:** A small incision is made in the umbilicus, and a specialized spring-loaded (Veress) needle is placed in the abdominal cavity

Modern needles are **12 to 15 cm long** and external diameter of 2 mm. The outer cannula consists of a beveled needle point for cutting through tissues of the abdominal wall. A spring-loaded, inner stylet is positioned within the outer cannula. This inner stylet has a dull tip to protect any viscera from injury by the sharp, outer cannula. Direct pressure on the tip—as when penetrating through tissue—pushes the dull stylet into the shaft of the outer cannula. When the tip of the needle enters a space such as the peritoneal cavity, the dull, inner stylet springs forward. Carbon dioxide is then passed through the Veress needle to inflate the space, creating a pneumoperitoneum.

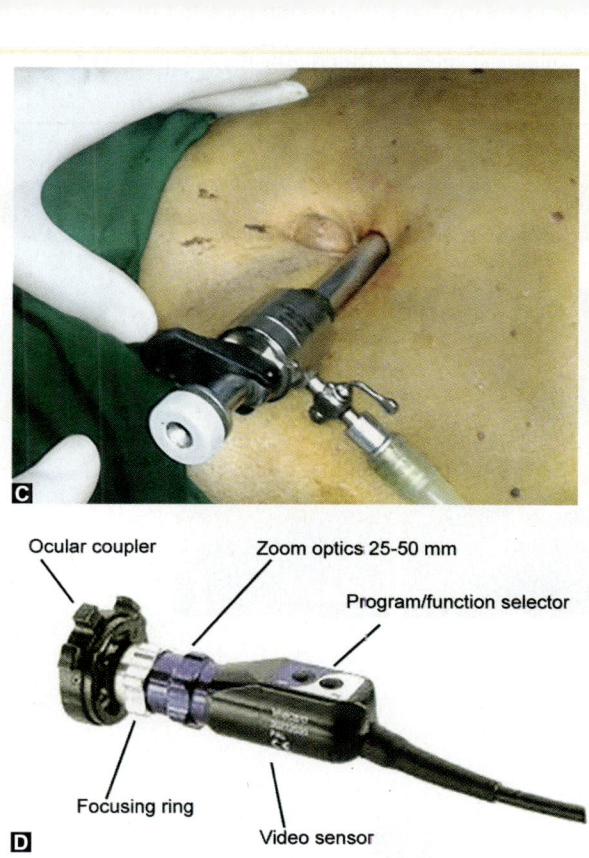

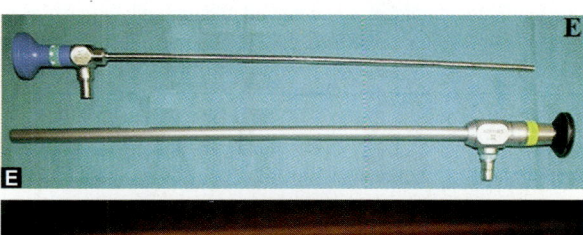

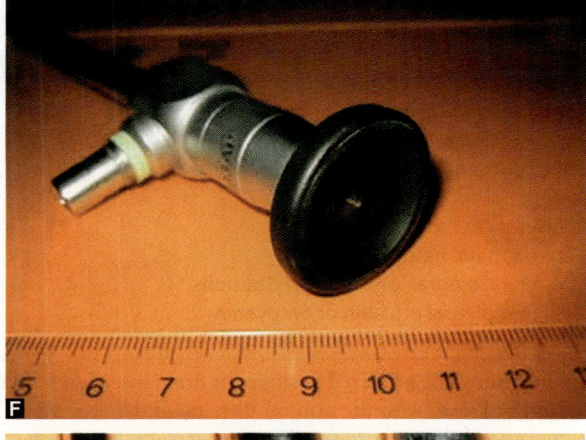

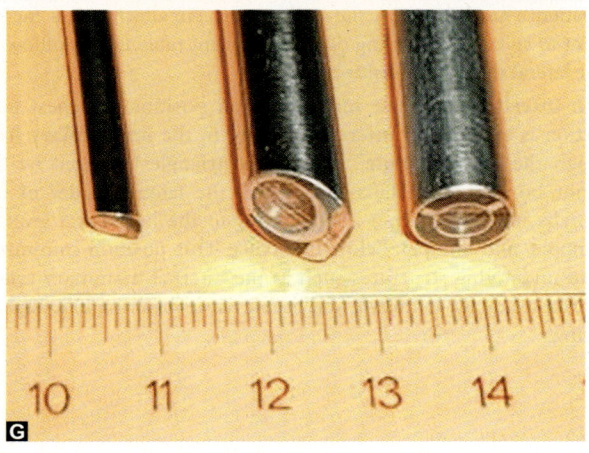

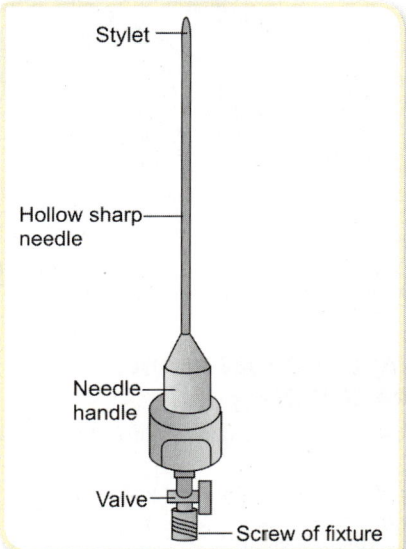

B. Laparoscopy Trocar Assembly: Trocar assembly includes Cannula (below in the picture), Seal (with cannula and insat) and Obturator (Above in the picture).

C. First trocar in place: The given picture shows first trocar in place with obturator removed and pneumoperitoneum CO_2 gas supply in place

D. Laparoscopic Camera (Labelled)

E. Laparoscope 5 mm above and 10 mm below: Laparoscopes vary in their physical dimensions; however, the most practical sizes are the **5 and 10 mm** diameters and 15-30 cm in length. Laparoscope are straight but can be angled.

F. Ocular of Laparoscope: The proximal end is the head or the ocular; this is where the video camera is attached for display on the monitor. This is where one can view the tissue directly with one's own eyes or attach a photographic camera for high-resolution image capture. Below is the input connection for the fiber-optic illumination. The ocular needs to be inspected before attaching the video camera, making sure that it is spotlessly clean.

G. Tip of Laparoscope: Laparoscopic tip can be 0 degrees or 30 degrees (most common- center of picture). Angulations increases the field of vision.

SURGERY PLATE 39

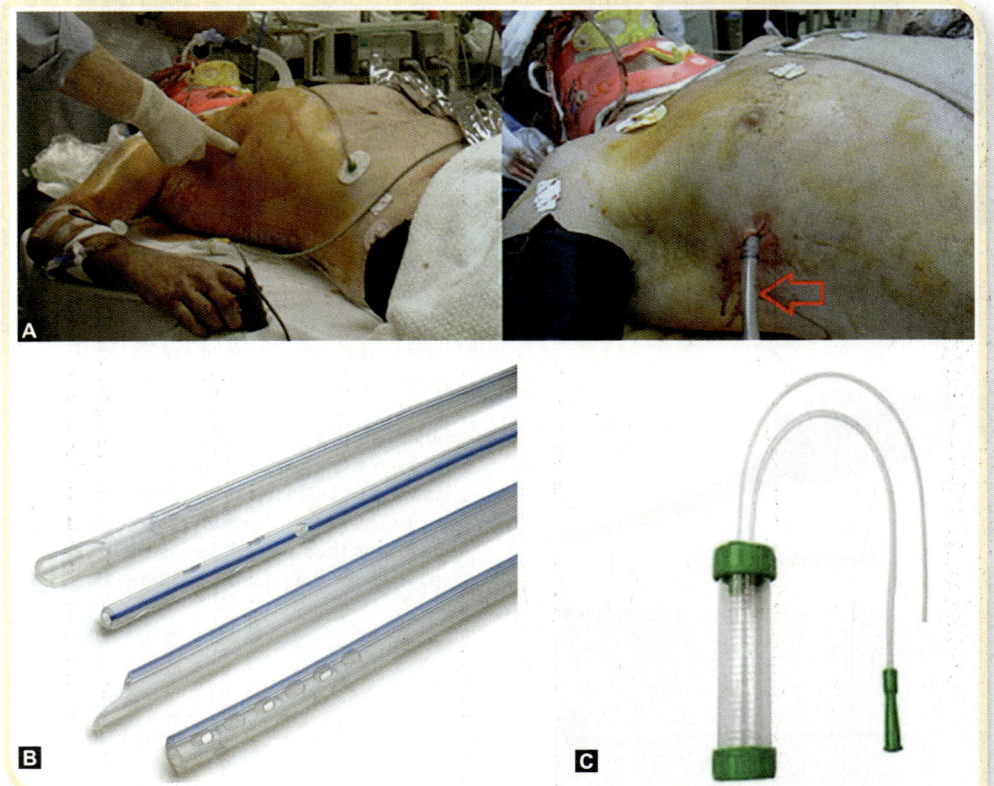

INTERCOSTAL CHEST TUBE DRAIN (TUBE THORACOSTOMY)

A chest tube can be a diagnostic procedure as well as a therapeutic one

A. Chest tube drain in situ in the chest wall of a trauma patient
B. Chest tube drains
C. Mucous trap (Plastic- Single use)

Indications for Chest Tube Drain Insertion
▫ Pneumothorax
▫ Tension pneumothorax after initial needle relief
▫ Malignant and complicated pleural effusion
▫ Hemothorax
▫ Empyema
▫ Chylothorax
▫ Traumatic hemopneumothorax
▫ Postoperative—For example, thoracotomy, esophagectomy, cardiac surgery
▫ To deliver intrapleural local analgesia in Flail chest

Contraindications of Tube Thoracostomy
The need for emergent thoracotomy is an absolute contraindication to tube thoracostomy.
Relative contraindications include the following:
▫ Coagulopathy
▫ Pulmonary bullae
▫ Diaphragmatic hernia
▫ Pulmonary, pleural, or thoracic adhesions
▫ Loculated pleural effusion or empyema
▫ Skin infection over the chest tube insertion site

Patient position: The preferred position for drain insertion is on the bed, slightly rotated, with the arm on the side of the lesion behind the patient's head to expose the axillary area. An alternative is for the patient to sit upright leaning over an adjacent table with a pillow or in the lateral decubitus position.

Drain insertion site: The most common position for chest tube insertion is in the **fifth intercostal space** in the **mid axillary line**, through the "**safe triangle**". This is the triangle bordered by the anterior border of the latissimus dorsi, the lateral border of the pectoralis major muscle, a line superior to the horizontal level of the nipple, and an apex below the axilla. This position minimizes risk to underlying structures such as the internal mammary artery and avoids damage to muscle and breast tissue resulting in unsightly scarring.

- In Open pneumothorax ('sucking chest wound'), a chest tube is inserted as soon as possible in a site remote from the injury site.
- In Tension pneumothorax, a chest tube is inserted through the fifth intercostal space in the anterior axillary line.

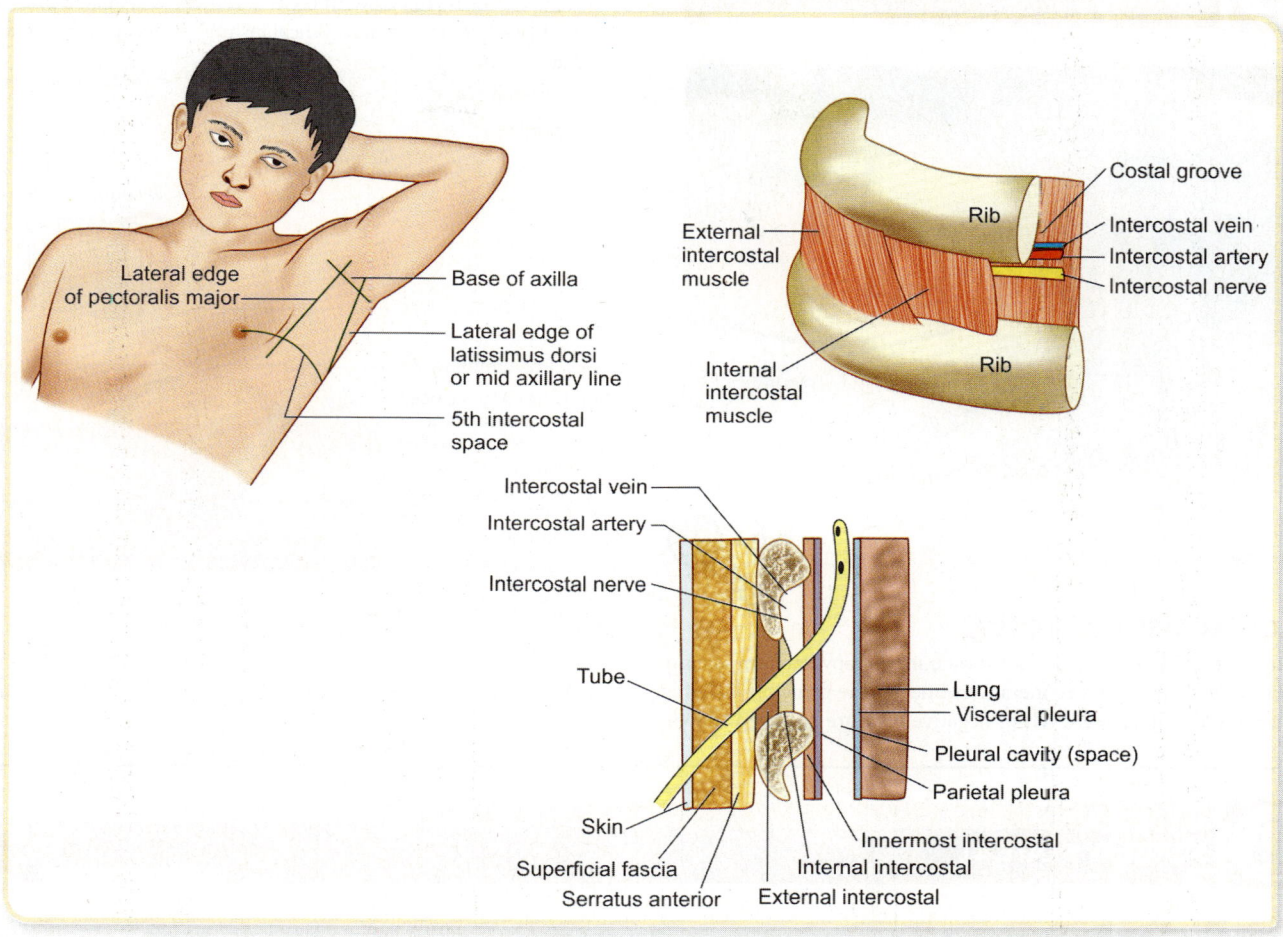

Drain size is selected based on the indication, with No. 20 to 28 French sufficient for pneumothorax, No. 28 to 40 French for hemothorax and empyema, or No. 30 to 36 French in the trauma situation. A large-bore (32-36 French) chest tube should be used in adolescents and adult patients.

Procedure

1. **Local anesthetic** should be infiltrated prior to insertion of the drain.
2. **Skin incision** is made in between the midaxillary and anterior axillary lines over a rib that is below the intercostal level selected for chest tube insertion. The incision for insertion of the chest drain should be similar to the diameter of the tube being inserted. The incision should be made just above and parallel to a rib.
3. **Blunt dissection** of the subcutaneous tissue and muscle into the pleural cavity. A closed and locked **Kelly clamp** is used to enter the chest wall into the pleural cavity to develop the tract and then with finger. The index finger should be inserted into the **pleural space** before tube placement to ensure that the pleural cavity has been entered and is free of adhesions and that any intra-abdominal organs have not herniated through the diaphragm.
4. The tube should be advanced (with or without trocar) posteriorly and superiorly in the pleural cavity. The position of the tip of the chest tube should ideally be aimed apically for a pneumothorax or basally for fluid. However, any tube position can be effective at draining air or fluid and an effectively functioning drain should not be repositioned solely because of its radiographic position.
5. After insertion, the tube should be secured in the skin of the chest wall and connected to a collection system under suction. A chest radiograph is usually obtained after insertion of the chest tube to confirm adequate placement and positioning.
6. All chest tubes should be connected to a single flow drainage system e.g. under water seal bottle or flutter valve. When chest drain suction is required, a high volume/low pressure system should be used.
7. Avoid clamping the ICD, as it may leads to tension pneumothorax, if forget to remove the clamp.

Removal of the chest tube: General criteria for chest tube removal include absence of air leak and **less than 200 mL of fluid drainage over a 24-hour period** (2 consecutive days). The chest tube should be removed either while the patient performs Valsalva's maneuver or during expiration with a brisk firm movement while an assistant ties the previously placed closure suture. In cases of pneumothorax, the chest tube should not be clamped at the time of its removal.

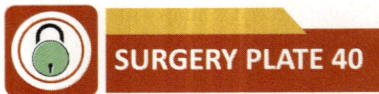

SURGERY PLATE 40

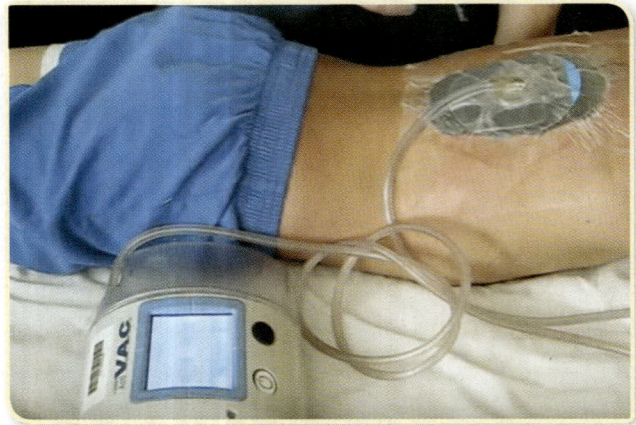

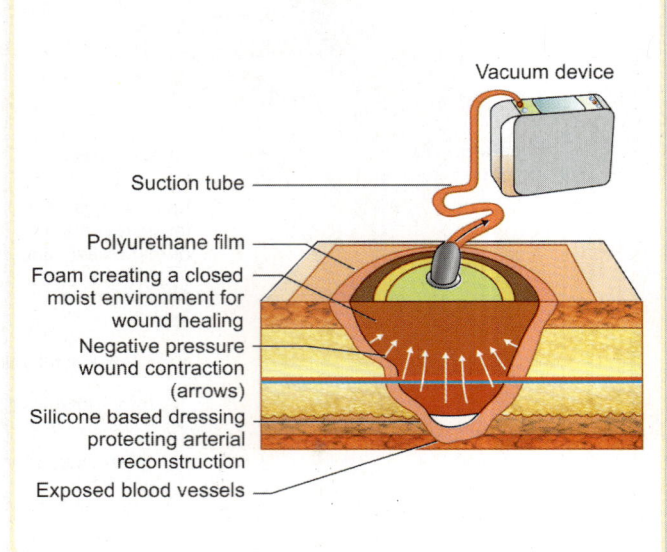

KEY

VACUUM ASSISTED CLOSURE

Vacuum assisted closure (also called vacuum therapy, vacuum sealing or topical negative pressure therapy) works on the principle that the application of controlled levels of negative pressure has been shown to accelerate debridement and promote healing in many different types of wounds. The optimum level of negative pressure appears to be around **125 mm Hg** below ambient and there is evidence that this is most effective if applied in a cyclical fashion of five minutes on and two minutes off.

SURGERY PLATE 41

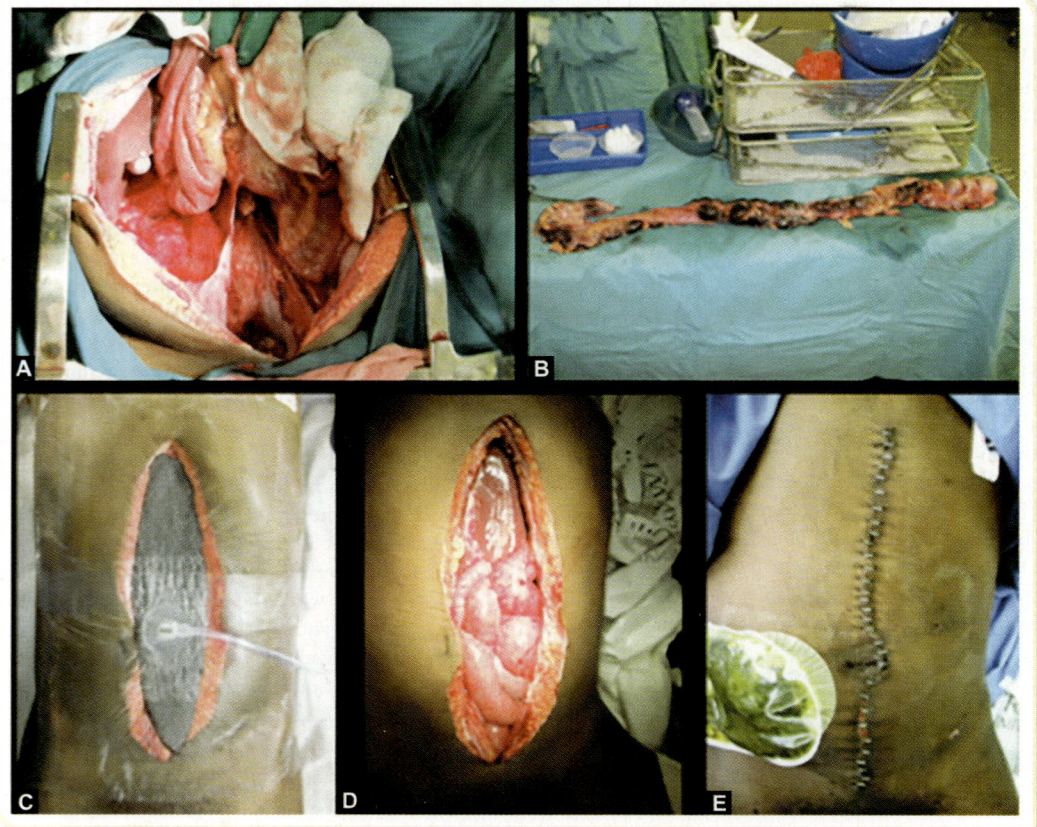

Credit: Navsaria P, Nicol A, Hudson D, Cockwill J, Smith J

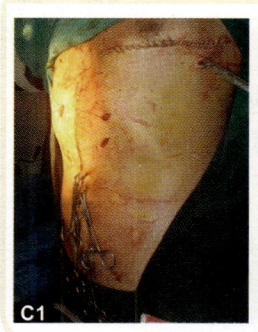 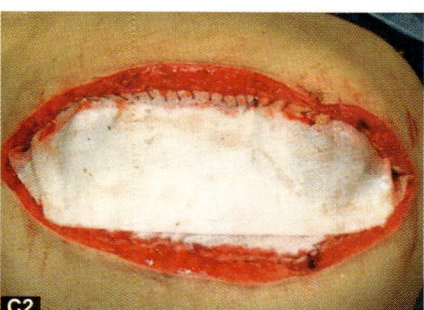 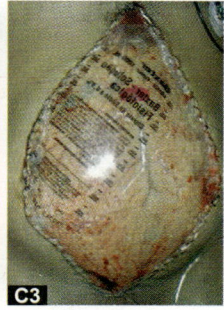 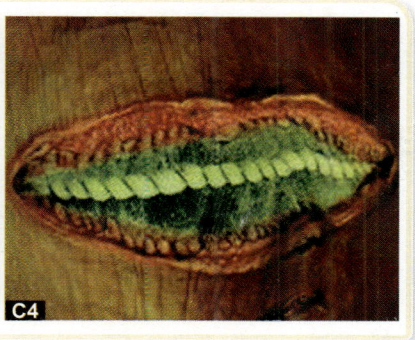

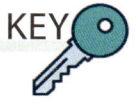 **KEY**

C1 = Towel clip closure
C2 = Witmann patch (overlapping Velcro-like sheets)
C3 = Bogota technique using a presterilized, soft 3-L IV bag
C4 = Polypropylene mess closure

PLATE LEGENDS

A 27-year-old male was admitted with blunt abdominal trauma.
A. A damage control laparotomy was performed
B. 90 cm of necrotic bowel removed
C. Vacuum assisted device closure applied at -80 mm Hg
D. Second look laparotomies were performed at 24 and 48 hours
E. Fascia closed at Day 3 post injury

Steps A, B, D, E are essentially same in all Damage control surgery related to abdominal trauma. Step C depends on the choice of device or dressing used.

TYPES OF TEMPORARY ABDOMINAL CLOSURE (TAC)

- Towel-clipping of skin edges (Simplest and fastest)
- Open packing of abdomen
- Zipper closure
- Whitmann patch (overlapping Velcro-like sheets)
- Synthetic mesh closure
- Silastic (plastic bag) closure (also known as the Bogotá Bag)
- Vacuum assisted device (VAC) closure

 SURGERY PLATE 42

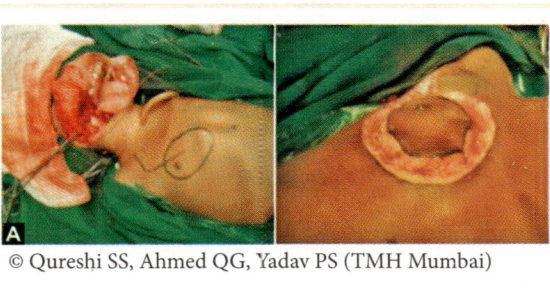

© Qureshi SS, Ahmed QG, Yadav PS (TMH Mumbai)

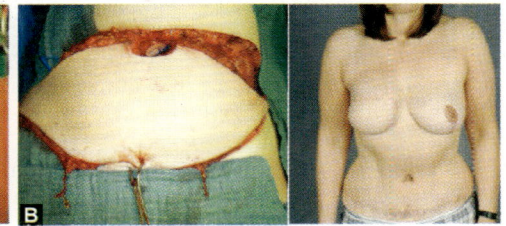

©Daigeler A, Harati K, Kapalschinski N, Goertz O, Hirsch T, Lehnhardt M, Kolbenschlag

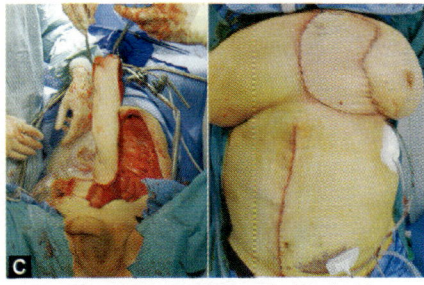 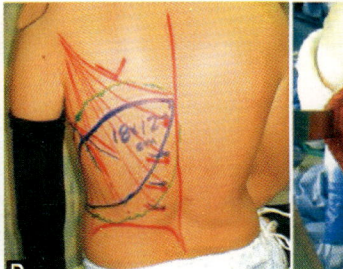 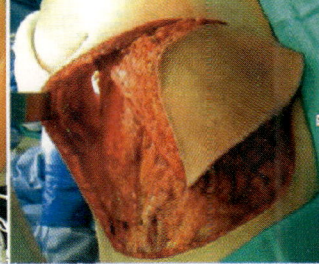

©Daigeler A, Harati K, Kapalschinski N, Goertz O, Hirsch T, Lehnhardt M, Kolbenschlag

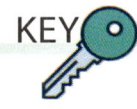 **KEY**

MYOCUTANEOUS FLAPS

A. **Pectoralis Major Myocutaneous Flap (PMMC):** Intraoperative photograph showing the skin paddle of PMMC and its suturing to the surgical defect.

B. **Transverse Abdominis Myocutaneous Flap (TRAM):** Intraoperative and postoperative (used for breast reconstruction)

C. **Vertical Rectus Abdominis Myocutaneous Flap (VRAM):** Intraoperative and immediate postoperative for defect of chest wall

D. **Latissimus dorsi (LD) flap:** Skin markings preoperatively and skin island raised with LD flap intraoperatively.

SURGERY PLATE 43

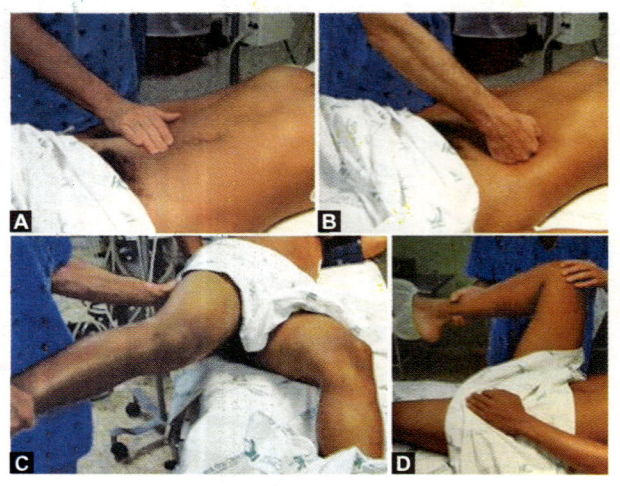

SIGNS OF APPENDICITIS

The sequence of abdominal discomfort and anorexia associated with acute appendicitis is pathognomonic. The pain is described as being located in the periumbilical region initially and then migrating to the right lower quadrant. Rectal and pelvic examinations are most likely to be negative. However, if the appendix is located within the pelvis, tenderness on abdominal examination may be minimal, whereas anterior tenderness may be elicited during rectal examination.

A. **Blumberg sign:** The exact location of the tenderness is directly over the appendix, which is most commonly at McBurney's point (located one third of the distance along a line drawn from the anterior superior iliac spine to the umbilicus).
B. **Rovsing's sign:** Pain in the right lower quadrant during palpation of the left lower quadrant
C. **Psoas sign:** Pain on extension of the right hip (typical of a retrocecal appendix)
D. **Obturator sign:** Pain on internal rotation of the hip (suggesting a pelvic appendix)
   Dunphy's sign: Any movement, including coughing, may cause increased pain (Not shown in picture).

SURGERY PLATE 44

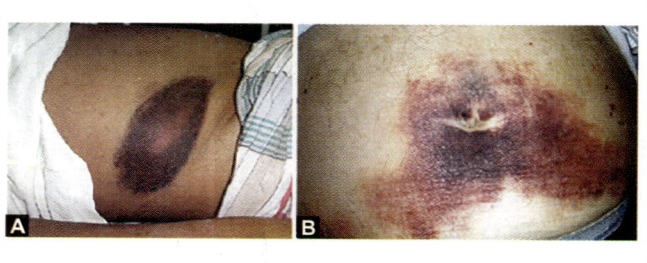

CULLEN'S AND GREY TURNER'S SIGN

On rare occasions, flank ecchymoses; **Grey Turner's sign** (A) or periumbilical ecchymoses; **Cullen's sign** (B) which result from retroperitoneal hemorrhage, can be seen during severe pancreatitis.

Cullen sign	Periumbilical bruising	Hemorrhagic pancreatitis or ectopic pregnancy
Grey turner sign	Bruising of flank	Hemorrhagic pancreatitis

SURGERY PLATE 45

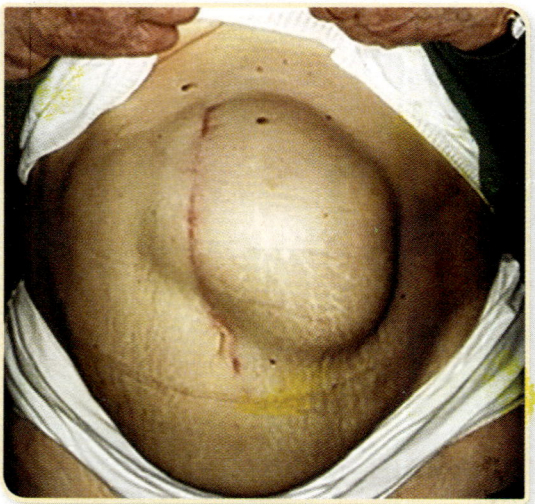

INCISIONAL HERNIA

Swelling/bulge with previous surgery and surgical scar with cough impulse positive almost confirms the clinical diagnosis of incisional hernia.

Acquired hernias may develop through slow architectural deterioration of the muscular aponeuroses or they may develop from failed healing of an anterior abdominal wall incision (*incisional hernia*).

- Cause of incisional hernia in any given case can be difficult to determine, but obesity, primary wound healing defects, multiple prior procedures, prior incisional hernias, and technical errors during repair may all be contributory
- The most common finding is a *mass or bulge on the anterior abdominal wall*, which may increase in size with a Valsalva maneuver. Ventral hernias may be asymptomatic or cause a considerable degree of discomfort, and generally enlarge over time. Physical examination reveals a bulge on the anterior abdominal wall that may reduce spontaneously, with recumbency, or with manual pressure. A hernia that cannot be reduced is described as *incarcerated* and requires emergent surgical correction. Incarceration of an intestinal segment may be accompanied by nausea, vomiting, and significant pain. Should the blood supply to the incarcerated bowel be compromised, the hernia is described as *strangulated*, and the localized ischemia may lead to infarction and perforation.

- *Incisional hernias of the anterior abdominal wall may occur in up to 10–20% of prior abdominal operations of all types.*
- Primary suture repair of abdominal wall incisional hernias is associated with an unacceptably high incidence of hernia recurrence, and has prompted the wide use of prosthetic mesh materials for hernia repair.
- Identified risk factors for recurrence were primary suture repair, postoperative wound infection, prostatism, and surgery for abdominal aortic aneurysm. These investigators concluded that mesh repair was superior to primary repair. **Mesh repair has become the gold standard** in the elective management of most incisional hernias.
- *Laparoscopic incisional hernia repair offers important advantages over open repairs including reduced pain medication use, earlier return to normal function, and possibly superior protection from hernia recurrence*
- In an effort to decrease the suture line tension associated with primary repair, Ramirez first described the **components separation technique**. Components separation entails the creation of large subcutaneous flaps lateral to the fascial defect followed by incision of the external oblique muscles and, if necessary, incision of the posterior rectus sheath bilaterally. These fascial releases allow for primary apposition of the fascia under far less tension than in simple primary repair. Components separation hernia repair is associated with a high wound infection risk (20%) and a recurrence rate of 18.2% at 1 year. Components separation is most applicable for the repair of incisional hernias when there are converging needs to (a) avoid the use of prosthetic materials, and (b) achieve a definitive repair. Most commonly this occurs in the setting of a contaminated or potentially contaminated surgical field.

SURGERY PLATE 46

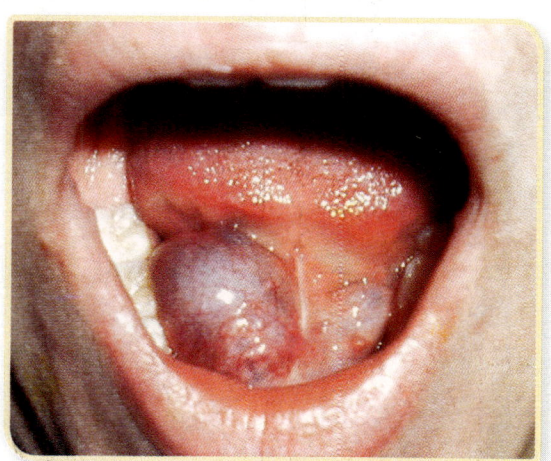

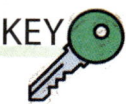

RANULA

Ranula is a retention cyst from the mucous gland of the floor of mouth. It is soft cystic swelling and is brilliantly transilluminant. It may sometimes be communicated into the neck behind the mylohyoid muscle with a characteristic of popping out and in. This is called as **Plunging Ranula.**

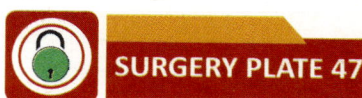

SURGERY PLATE 47

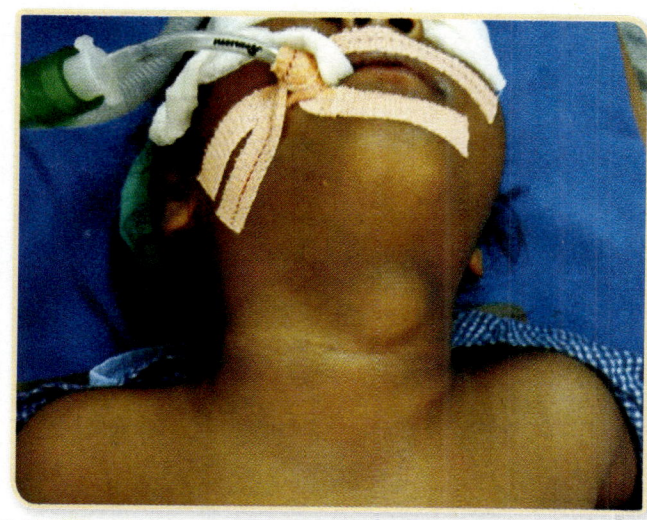

© MedEasy, Dr Prashant Bharadwaj

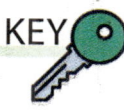

THYROGLOSSUS CYST

Thyroglossus Cyst	
Embryology	The thyroid gland descends early in fetal life from the base of the tongue towards its position in the lower neck with the isthmus lying over the second and third tracheal rings. At the time of its descent, the hyoid bone has not been formed and the track of the descent of the thyroid gland is variable, passing in front, through or behind the eventual position of the hyoid body. Thyroglossal duct cysts represent a persistence of this track and may therefore be found anywhere in or adjacent to the midline from the tongue base to the thyroid isthmus. Rarely, a thyroglossal cyst may contain the only functioning thyroid tissue in the body.

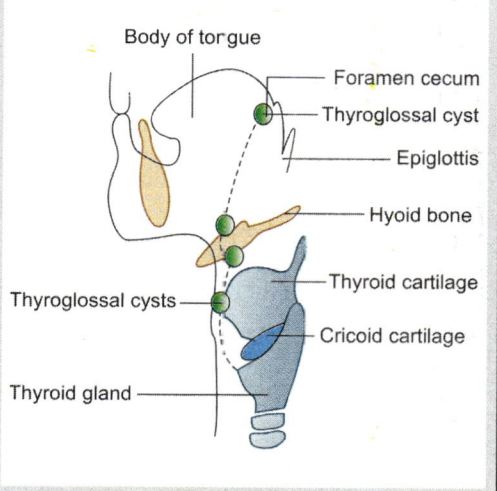

Contd...

Thyroglossus Cyst	
Clinical features	The cysts almost always arise in the midline but, when they are adjacent to the thyroid cartilage, they may lie slightly to one side of the midline. Classically, the cyst moves upwards on swallowing and with tongue protrusion, but this can also occur with other midline cysts such as dermoid cysts, as it merely indicates attachment to the hyoid bone. Thyroglossal cysts may become infected and rupture onto the skin of the neck presenting as a discharging sinus. Although they often occur in children, they may also present in adults, even as late as the sixth or seventh decade of life.
Treatment	Treatment must include excision of the whole thyroglossal tract, which involves removal of the body of the hyoid bone and the suprahyoid tract through the tongue base to the vallecula at the site of the primitive foramen caecum, together with a core of tissue on either side. This operation is known as **Sistrunk's operation** and prevents recurrence, most notably from small side branches of the thyroglossal tract.

In 1901, Hutchinson recognized that there can be multiple causes of Raynaud's observations and coined the term **Raynaud's phenomenon** to indicate the presence of an underlying abnormality causing this disorder. Over the past 100 years, by tradition, we have therefore classified all patients with digital vasospasm into the following two groups based on the presence or absence of associated disease:

- **Raynaud's disease** refers to a primary vasospastic disorder where there is no identifiable underlying cause.
- **Raynaud's phenomenon** refers to individuals where vasospasm is secondary to an underlying condition or disease.

In clinical practice, use of the term Raynaud's disease or Raynaud's phenomenon has not been intuitive. These terms are commonly misunderstood and are often mistakenly interchanged; as a result, they have lost much of their original meaning. For more than 20 years, John Porter and others have advocated replacing the old terms of disease and phenomenon with **Raynaud's syndrome**.

Patients with Raynaud's syndrome can be subdivided into two groups:

1. **Primary Raynaud's syndrome**, indicating those with idiopathic vasospasm
2. **Secondary Raynaud's syndrome**, indicating those who have an underlying disease-causing vasospastic episode.

SURGERY PLATE 48

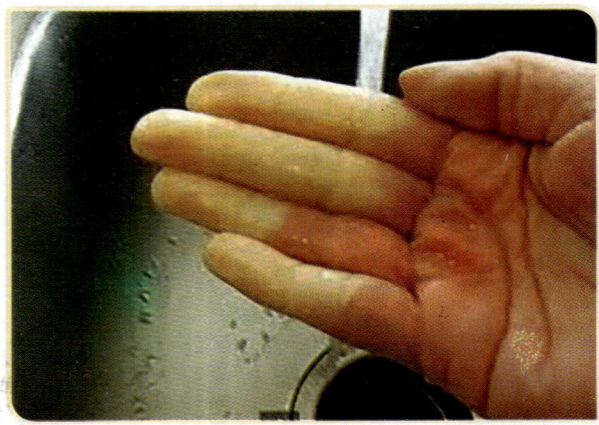

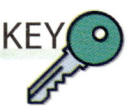

RAYNAUD'S PHENOMENON

In 1882, **Maurice Raynaud,** a French physician, entitled his thesis for the Academy of Medicine "On Local Asphyxia and Symmetrical Gangrene of the Extremities." In this paper he described 25 patients with intermittent digital ischemia and recognized the relationship of local cold and emotional stress in the causation of these episodes. He attributed the attacks of digital ischemia to excessive sympathetic activity producing vasoconstriction of digital arteries. He also described the classic tricolor skin changes of digital pallor, cyanosis, and rubor that are now associated with his name. These patients with intermittent vasospastic episodes of digital ischemia were hence diagnosed as having "Raynaud's disease."

SURGERY PLATE 49

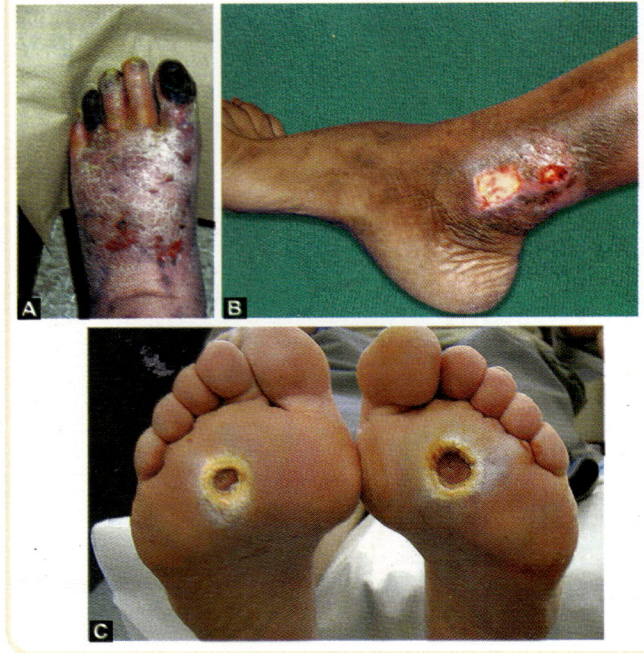

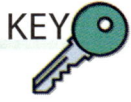

COMMON CAUSES OF LEG ULCERS

A. Arterial ulcer
B. Venous ulcer
C. Neurotrophic ulcer

Differential Diagnosis of Common Leg Ulcers

Type	Usual Location	Pain	Bleeding With Manipulation	Lesion Characteristics	Surrounding Inflammation	Associated Findings
Ischemic (Arterial)	Distal, on dorsum of foot or toes	Severe, particularly at night; relieved by dependency	Little or none	Irregular edge; poor granulation tissue. Punched out when chronic	Absent	Trophic changes of chronic ischemia; absence of pulses
Stasis (Venous)	Lower third of leg (gaiter area)	Mild; relieved by elevation	Venous ooze	Shallow, irregular shape; granulating base; rounded edges	Present	Lipodermatofibrosis, pigmentation
Neurotrophic	Under calluses or pressure points (e.g., plantar aspect of first or fifth metatarsophalangeal joint)	None	May be brisk	Punched-out, with deep sinus	Present	Demonstrable neuropathy

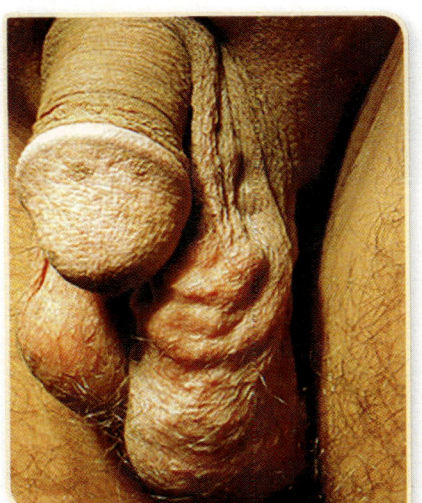

SURGERY PLATE 50

 KEY

VARICOCELE

Idiopathic/Primary varicocele	Secondary varicocele
□ In 95% of cases no cause is found. □ Incompetent or absent valves of **testicular vein and internal spermatic vein** □ **Common on left side** because left testicular vein has longer course and perpendicular entry into the left renal vein	□ A pelvic or abdominal malignancy most commonly **RCC** □ **Post nephrectomy** due to removal of draining renal vein □ **Obstruction of the inferior vena cava.** □ **Retroperitoneal mass**; Sudden onset, older age □ Retroperitoneal fibrosis or adhesions □ One non-malignant cause of a secondary varicocele is the so-called "**Nutcracker syndrome**", a condition in which the superior mesenteric artery compresses the left renal vein, causing increased pressures there to be transmitted retrograde into the left pampiniform plexus.

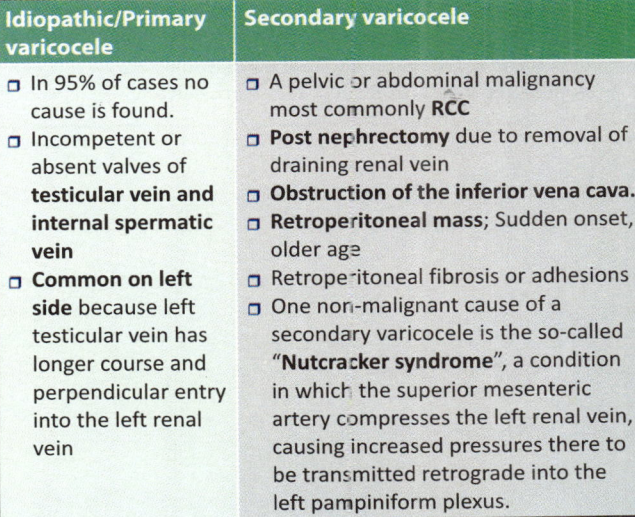

321

- Typically, varicoceles arise secondary to incompetent internal spermatic vein valves. However, the presence of *unilateral right-sided varicocele raises the suspicion of poor drainage at the junction of the right testicular vein and right renal vein, which could be secondary to a large right-sided renal mass.*
- In addition, the sudden onset of varicocele in an older man raises the suspicion of a retroperitoneal mass leading to inadequate drainage of the testicular veins.
- Varicocele is usually symptom less
- Annoying dragging discomfort that is worse if the testis is unsupported.
- Examination of a man with varicocele when he is upright reveals a mass of **dilated, tortuous veins lying posterior to and above the testis**. It may extend up to the external inguinal ring, and the **Coughing/Valsalva maneuver can increase the degree of dilation.**
- Varicocele gives the feeling of **bag of worms**
- Decompress/reduces in supine position
- Characteristically, the varicocele does not decompress in the supine position in RCC.
- **Boe sign:** After holding the varicocele between thumb and fingers, patient is asked to bow. Varicocele reduces in size due to reduced blood flow of testicular vein.
- Sperm concentration and motility is significantly decreased in 65% to 75% of subjects causing **infertility.**
- Varicocele is the most common surgically correctable cause of male infertility.
- Operation is not indicated for asymptomatic varicocele.
- The simplest procedure is **laparoscopic ligation** of the testicular vein above the inguinal ligament where the pampiniform plexus has coalesced into one or two vessels.
- However, when facilities are available, **embolization of the testicular vein** under radiographic control is probably the treatment of choice. Because of the presence of plentiful collateral veins, recurrence is common after all types of varicocele surgery.
- In the **Gat-Goren procedure**, invented by an Israeli Gynecologist, essentially the same thing happens as with an embolization. The difference, however, is that instead of using metal coils or a balloon to stop the blood flow to the site of the varicocele, a liquid which selectively closes off the offending veins is injected.
- **Varicocelectomy**, the surgical correction of a varicocele, is performed on an outpatient basis. The three most common approaches are inguinal (groin), retroperitoneal (abdominal), and infrainguinal/subinguinal (below the groin).
  - **Palomos operation:** Suprainguinal extraperitoneal/retroperitoneal ligation of testicular vein
  - **Ivanissevich approach:** Inguinal approach, easier and safer
  - **Marc Goldstein approach:** Subinguinal approach at superficial inguinal ring outside the external oblique aponeurosis without opening of external oblique aponeurosis
  - **Scrotal approach:** Done in grade 4 varicocele.

SURGERY PLATE 51

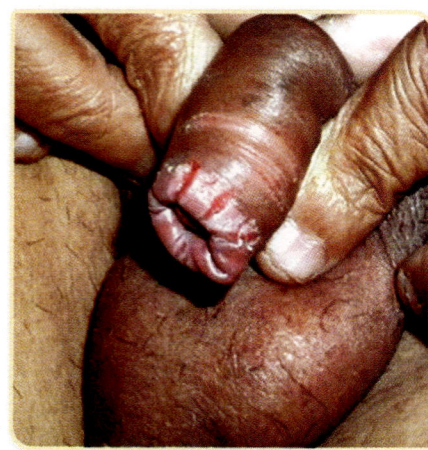

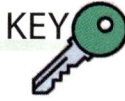

BALANOPOSTHITIS

Defined as the inflammation of the foreskin and glans in uncircumcised males, balanoposthitis occurs over a wide age range and may have any of multiple bacterial or fungal origins or be caused by contact dermatitides. Although not as necessary as in the past, circumcision may be considered for refractory or recurrent balanoposthitis. Balanoposthitis should not be confused with balanitis, which is inflammation of the glans penis or the clitoris. **The preputium skin became edematous, and fissures appear and evolve to ulcers.**

SURGERY PLATE 52

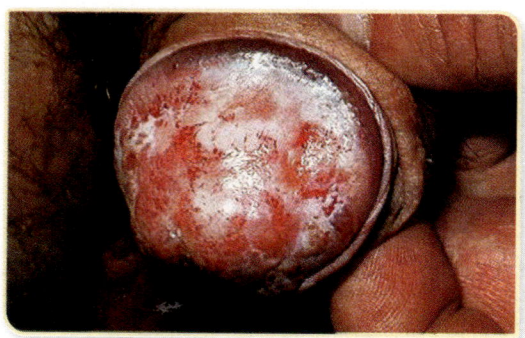

BALANITIS XEROTICA OBLITERANS (BXO)

Lichen sclerosus is a chronic, progressive, sclerosing inflammatory dermatosis of unclear etiology. Most reported lichen sclerosus cases (83%) involve the genitalia. In men, this genital involvement has traditionally been known as balanitis xerotica obliterans (BXO).

Early in its course, penile lichen sclerosus (balanitis xerotica obliterans [BXO]) is relatively asymptomatic with only mild visually observable changes of the penis and glans. Physical changes occur over months or years and may include color or textural changes. Early symptoms are more prevalent in uncircumcised patients. Early penile lichen sclerosus (balanitis xerotica obliterans [BXO]) demonstrates only subtle physical findings (e.g., mild, nonspecific erythema; mild hypopigmentation). **As the condition progresses, single or multiple discrete erythematous papules or macules progress and coalesce into atrophic ivory, white, or purple-white patches or plaques.**

SURGERY PLATE 53

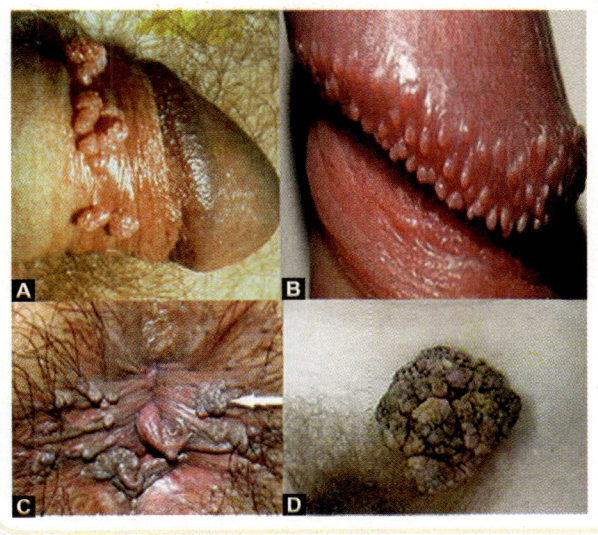

GENITAL WART/CONDYLOMA ACUMINATUM

These lesions are soft, pink, pedunculated papilliferous masses (cauliflower like) with finger-like peduncles and an irregular surface. They are usually seen on moist, partially keratinized epithelium such as the preputial cavity, urinary meatus, labia minora, introitus, vagina, cervix, anus, an anal canal, but may affect intertriginous areas as well (groin, perineum, and anal area). Genital warts are a **sexually transmitted infection** (STI).

A. **Condyloma acuminatum** or genital wart of the foreskin and shaft of penis
B. **Condyloma acuminatum** or genital wart of the glans of penis
C. **Condyloma acuminatum** or genital wart of the anal verge
D. **Buschke-Lowenstein tumor**; Giant condyloma caused by human papillomavirus types 6 or 11 is a very rare variant. First described by Buschke and Löwenstein in 1925. Slow-growing, locally destructive verrucous plaque that typically appears on the penis but may occur elsewhere in the anogenital region.

Etiology: The virus that causes genital warts is called human papilloma virus (HPV). Not all types of HPV cause genital warts. Most cases of infection with HPV cause no visible symptoms. Around 90% of all cases of genital warts are caused by two strains of the virus, **type 6 and type 11**. Genital warts are usually flat, papular, or pedunculated growths on the genital mucosa. Patients with visible warts may be infected simultaneously with oncogenic "high risk" HPVs such as **types 16 and 18**, which mostly give rise to subclinical lesions associated with intraepithelial neoplasia (IN) and anogenital cancer.

Recommended Regimens for External Genital Warts
Patient-Applied:
Podofilox 0.5% solution or gel OR
Imiquimod 5% cream OR
Sinecatechins 15% ointment
Provider–Administered:
Cryotherapy with liquid nitrogen or cryoprobe. Repeat applications every 1–2 weeks. OR
Podophyllin resin 10%–25% in a compound tincture of benzoin OR
Trichloroacetic acid (TCA) or Bichloroacetic acid (BCA) 80%–90% OR
Surgical removal either by tangential scissor excision, tangential shave excision, curettage, or electrosurgery.

SURGERY PLATE 54

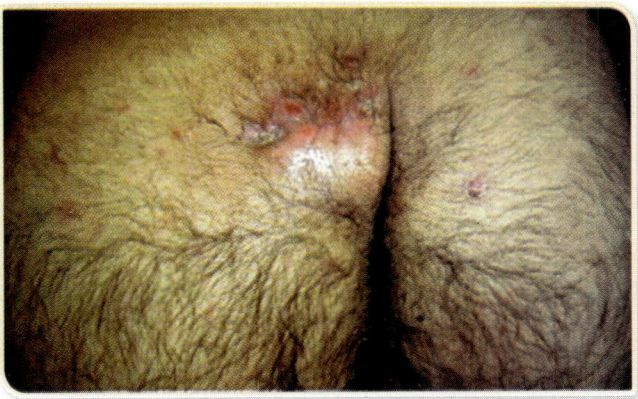

Pilonidal disease (cyst, Sinus, infection) consists of a **hair-containing sinus or abscess** occurring in the intergluteal cleft.

SURGERY PLATE 55

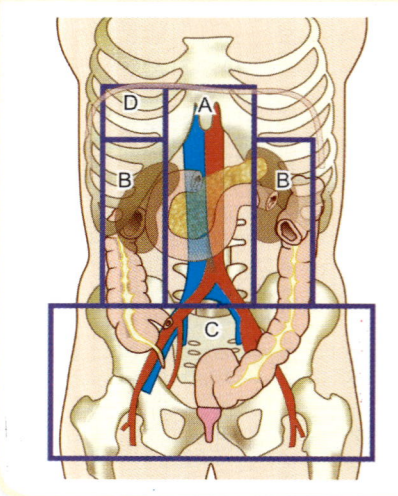

Retroperitoneal Hemorrhage Zones		
D= Zone 4	Portal vein and retro hepatic vena cava	Perihepatic area, which contains the hepatic artery, the portal vein, the retrohepatic IVC, and the hepatic veins

Footnote:
- Nunn et al. proposed first anatomic division of the retroperitoneal space into **three zones** for description and decision making in the treatment of retroperitoneal injury. Zone 4 was added later and hence it is not shown normally in the diagrams
- The major abdominal vasculature is located in the retroperitoneum, and thus injuries may present with contained retroperitoneal hematomas rather than free bleeding
- Zone 3 predominates in blunt trauma (70%), whereas zone 2 is the most commonly seen in penetrating injury (50%). Retroperitoneal hematomas are associated with morbidity of up to 60% and mortality from 13% to 40%

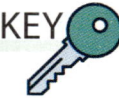

RETROPERITONEAL HEMORRHAGE ZONES

For vascular trauma purposes, the abdomen is conventionally divided into the following four anatomic areas:

Retroperitoneal Hemorrhage Zones		
A= Zone 1 (Central)	Aorta and Vena cava	Midline retroperitoneum extending from the aortic hiatus to the sacral promontory. This zone is subdivided into 1. **Supramesocolic area**: contains the suprarenal aorta and its major branches (celiac axis, superior mesenteric artery [SMA], and renal arteries), the supramesocolic inferior vena cava (IVC) with its major branches, and the superior mesenteric vein (SMV). 2. **Inframesocolic area** contains the infrarenal aorta and IVC.
B= Zone 2 (Lateral)	Renal vessels	(left and right), which includes the kidneys, the paracolic gutter, and the renal vessels
C= Zone 3 (Pelvic)	Iliac vessels	which includes the pelvic retroperitoneum and contains the iliac vessels

Contd...

SURGERY PLATE 56

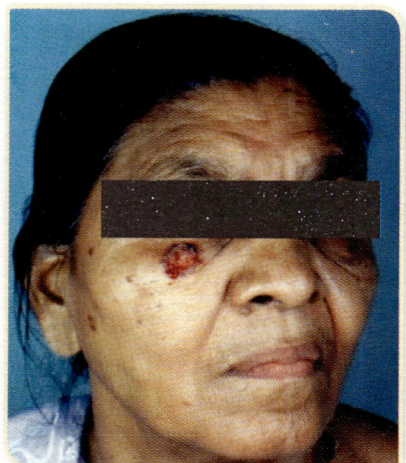

© Patidar S (Baroda Skin Clinic)

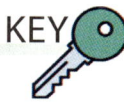

BASAL CELL CARCINOMA

Indurated ulcer with raised margins over right infraorbital region due to Basal cell carcinoma. Basal cell cancer (BCC) or **Rodent Ulcer** often occurs on the face above a *line joining* the *angle* of the *mouth* and the *ear lobe*. There are 5 common clinical subtypes of basal cell carcinoma (BCC).

BCC Clinical Subtype

Subtype	Site	Growth	Lesion	Color	Surface
Solid or Nodular (60-80%)	Face	Slow	Nodule	Skin translucent	Telangiectasia
Rodent ulcer	Face	Faster	Central ulcer, rolled borders	Translucent necrotic, Red	Telangiectasia
Pigmented	Face	Slow	Nodule	Brown	Telangiectasia
Adenocystic	Face	Slow	Lobulated cyst + rolled edges	Erythematous/ + squamous	Telangiectasia
Superficial	Trunk, Limbs	Slow	Plaque, pearly border	Red scaly	Well defined
Morphoeic (2-6% of BCC)	Face	Slow	Scar like plaque	Yellowish	Undefined
Metatypical or Basosquamous	Face	Rapid	Plaque + Metastasis	Yellowish	Undefined Telangiectasia

Risk Categories of BCC

	Low risk BCC	High risk BCC
Site		Mid face, Ear region
Size	<2 cm	>2 cm
Histology	Non Basosquamous	Basosquamous/Metatypical
Course	Primary	Recurrent
Immunity	Normal	Compromised

SURGERY PLATE 57

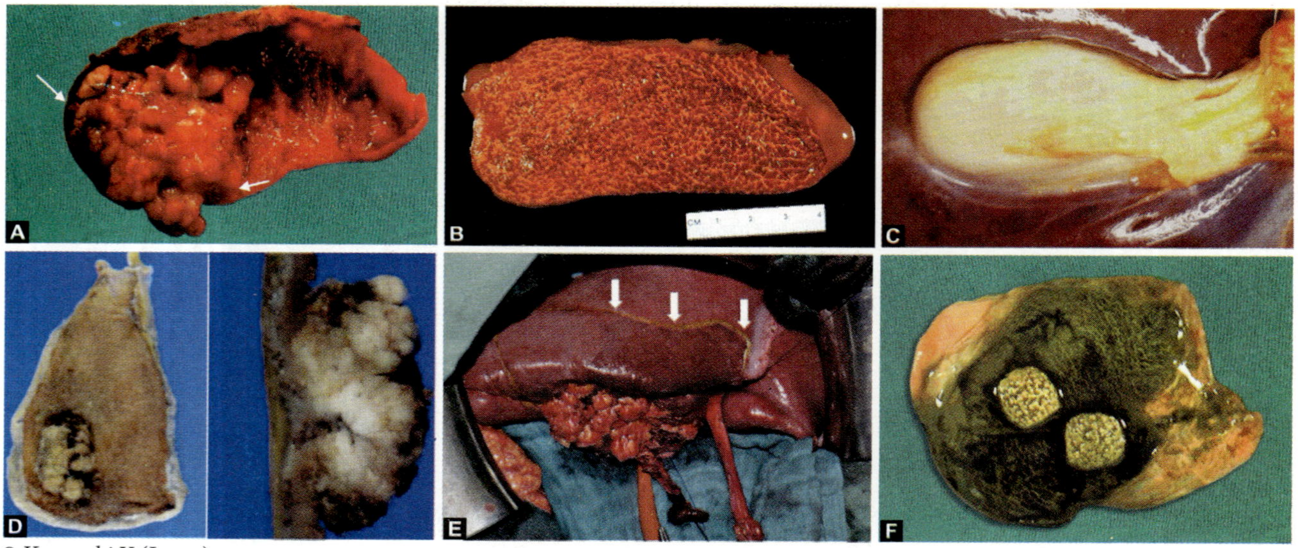

© Kawasaki Y (Japan)   © Scheingraber S (Germany)

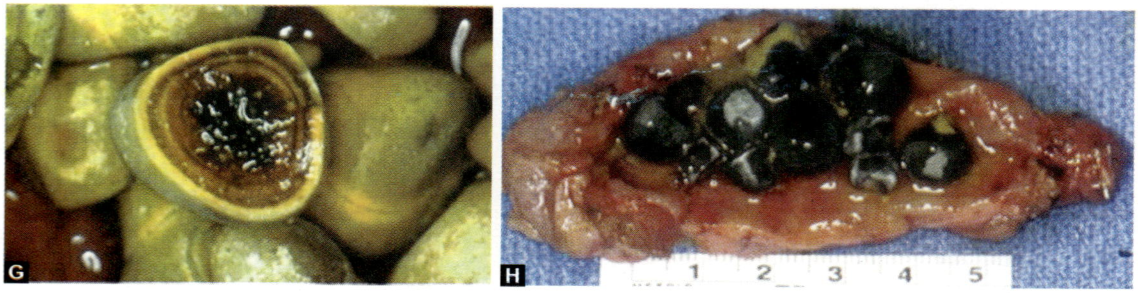

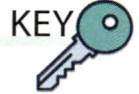 KEY

GALLBLADDER PATHOLOGY SPECIMENS

 Note

Gallbladder pathologies are often seen mixed rather isolated. Example stone with cholesterolosis, stone with polyp, Polyp with carcinoma etc.

A. Gallbladder polyps: Gross photo showing a sessile polypoid mass (yellow arrows) located at the fundic region of the opened gallbladder

B. Gallbladder cholesterolosis/Strawberry Gallbladder: The appearance of the gallbladder mucosa seen here is consistent with cholesterolosis (containing cholesterol crystal deposits). Microscopically, the mucosa in cholesterolosis of the gallbladder contains many foamy macrophages which produce the grossly visible strawberry-like appearance.

C. Porcelain gallbladder: This is a gross appearance of the gallbladder termed "porcelain gallbladder" because the wall and surfaces of the gallbladder are hard and tan-white like a porcelain vase. This is one end result of chronic cholecystitis.

D. Gallbladder cancer: Macroscopic appearance of the gall bladder mass located in the fundus. Tumor infiltration to the muscularis layer is evident macroscopically in the cut section side view. Adenocarcinomas are divided into infiltrative (65%), papillary (15%), and colloid (10%) subtypes. Nearly 60% of carcinomas originate in the fundus, 30% in the body, and 10% in the neck.

E. Gallbladder cancer infiltrating the liver: En bloc resection of the tumor mass with liver segments IVb and V. Arrows demonstrate demarcation of segment IVb after round ligament approach.

F. Gallbladder Cholesterol stones: Two composite cholesterol gallstones are seen here with a yellowish green appearance.

G. **Gallbladder Mixed stones:** Yellow tan faceted mixed gallstones are present. These Gallstones consist of a mixture of cholesterol, bilirubin, and calcium. These stones are squared off (faceted) because they sat together. Hint: if you find one faceted stone, there is probably at least one more somewhere else.

H. **Gallbladder Pigment stones:** These are black or dark brown pigmented hard stones.

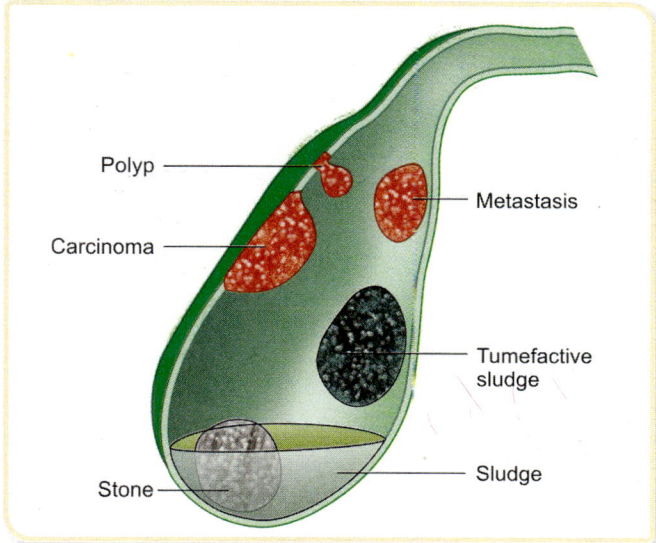

TRICHOBEZOARS

Trichobezoars (hair balls) are unusual and are almost exclusively found in female psychiatric patients, often young. They are caused by the *pathological ingestion of hair*, which remains undigested in the stomach. Trichobezoars tend to form a *cast of the stomach*, with strands of hair having been observed as far distally as the transverse colon.

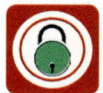

SURGERY PLATE 59

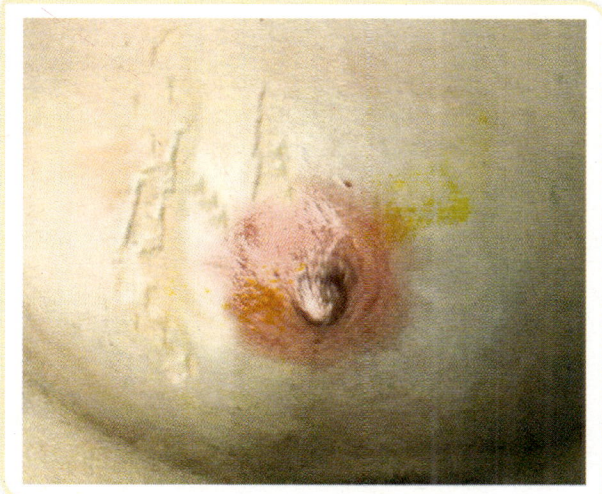

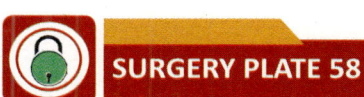

SURGERY PLATE 58

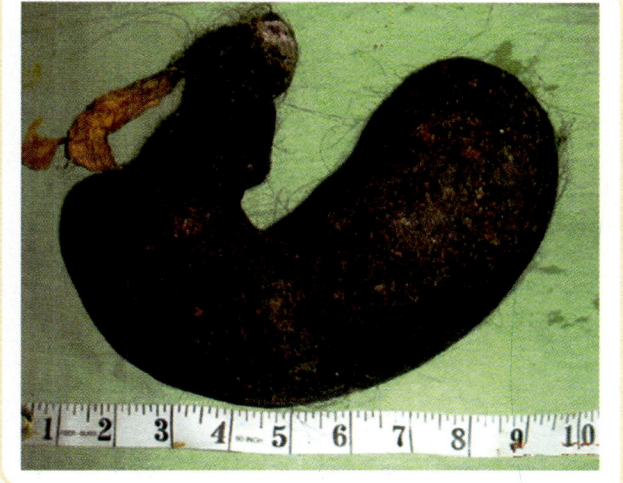

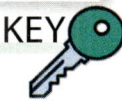

MONDOR'S DISEASE

Mondor's disease[AIIMSPG] is a rare self-limiting benign condition which involves thrombophlebitis of the subcutaneous veins of the breast and anterior chest wall. It can also occur in the arm and penis. It is usually unilateral and bilaterality is uncommon.

NOTES

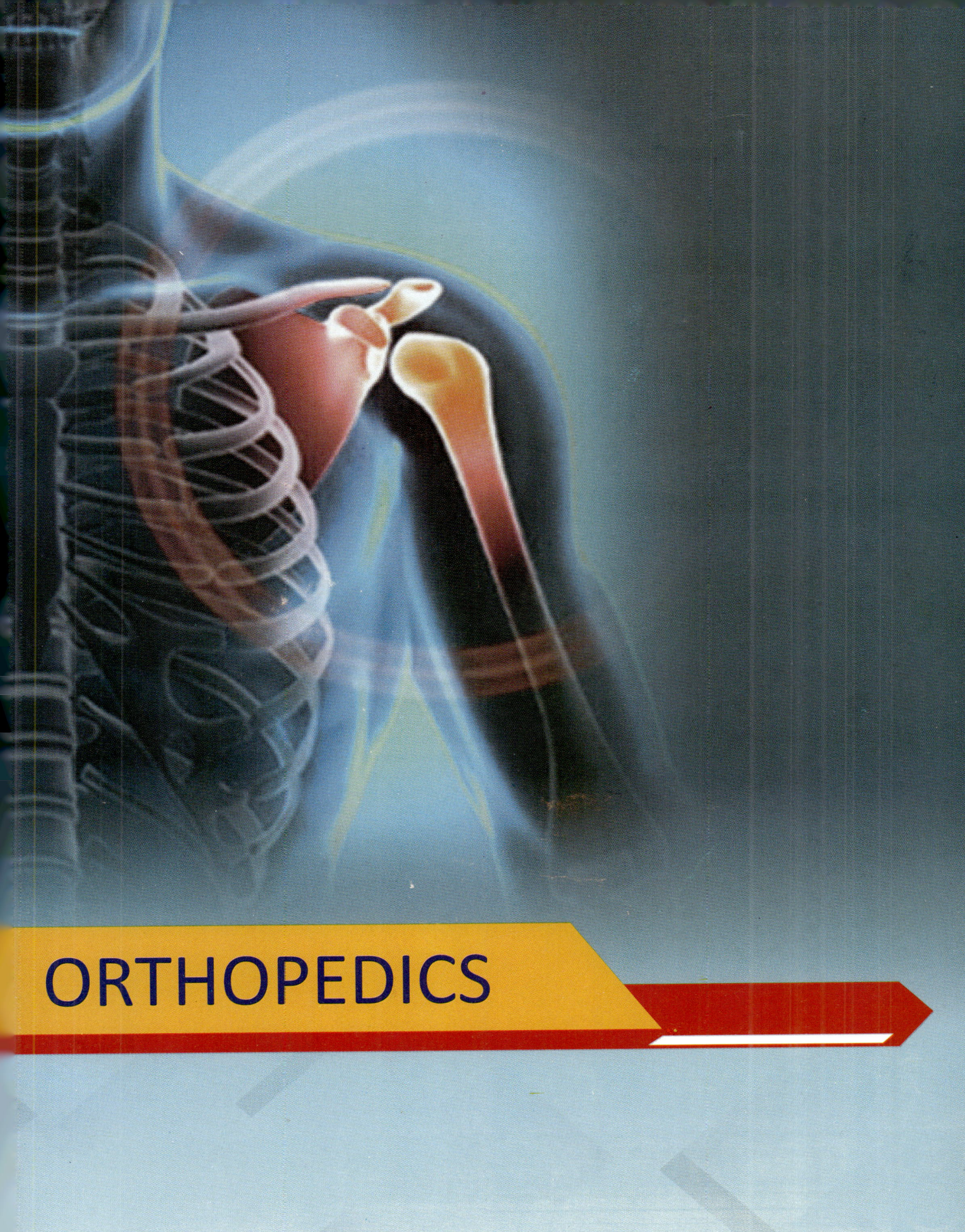

ORTHO PLATE 1

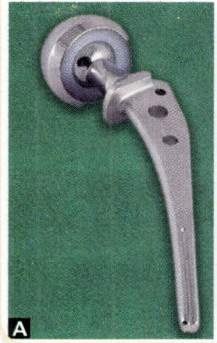
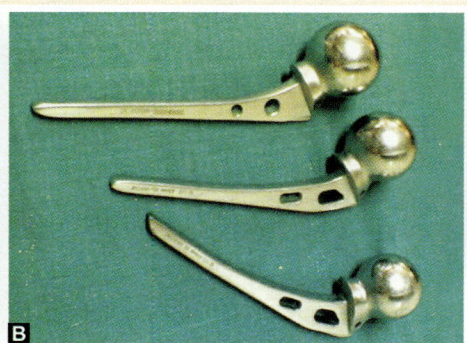
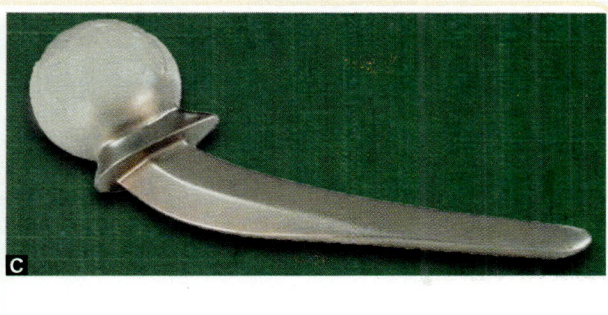
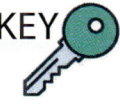

HIP PROSTHESIS

A. **Bipolar hip prosthesis:** Bipolar prosthesis is used for total hip replacement (THR). Motion is present between metal head and polyethylene socket (inner bearing). Range of motion is greater than Unipolar prosthesis.

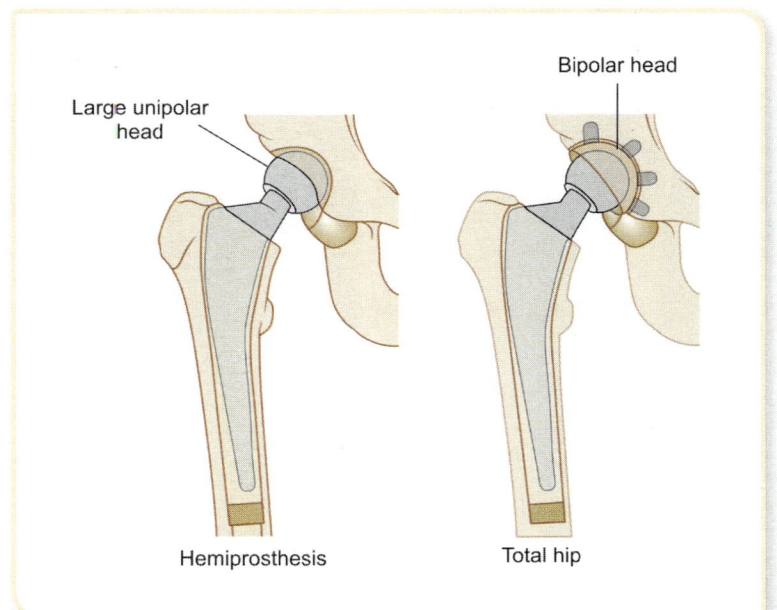

B. **Austin moore prosthesis:** Fenestrated unipolar hip prosthesis used in hemiarthroplasty (acetabulum is retained).
C. **Thompson prosthesis:** Non fenestrated unipolar hip prosthesis used in hemiarthroplasty (acetabulum is retained). Designed for non union of fracture neck of femur, when there is no neck available.

	Unipolar Hip Prosthesis	
	Austin Moore	**Thompson**
Parts	Head, neck, collar, shoulder, stem	Head, neck, collar, stem (no shoulder)
Fixing	Without bone cement	With bone cement
Extraction	Easier	Very difficult
Stem fenestrations	Two in number	Nil
Collar hole	Present (to check position)	Absent
Self-locking	Present	Absent
Weight	Light weight	Heavier
Used when	Calcar femorale >1.25 cm	Calcar femorale <1.25 cm

Contd...

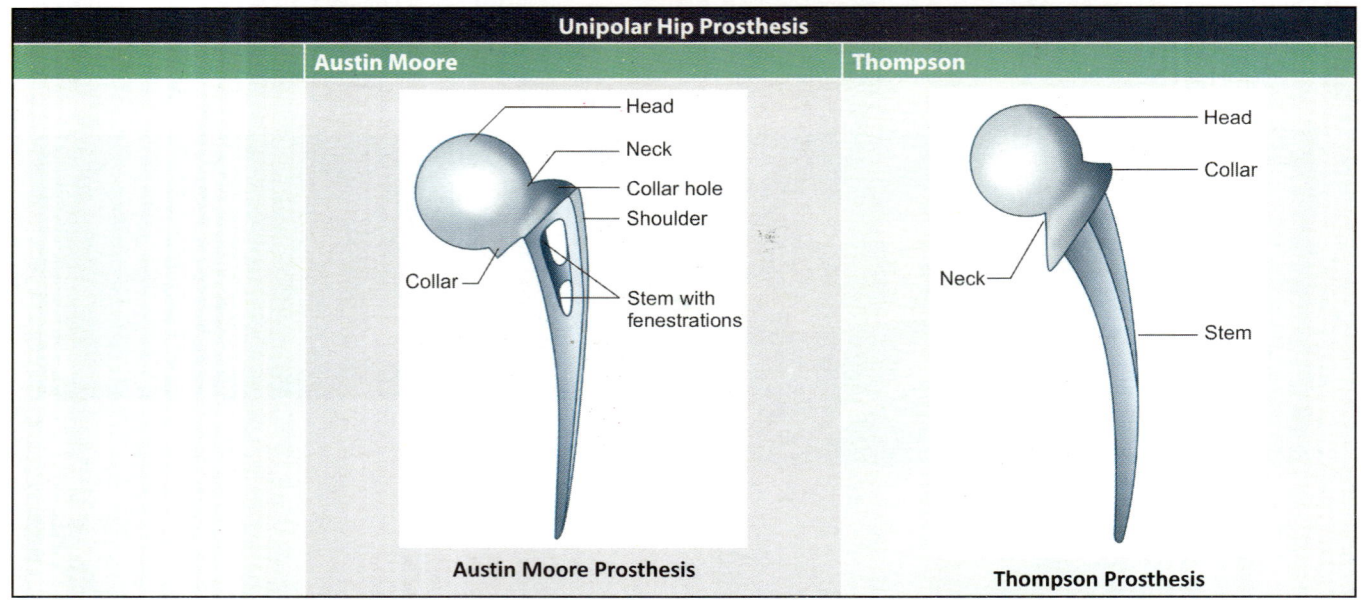

ORTHO PLATE 2

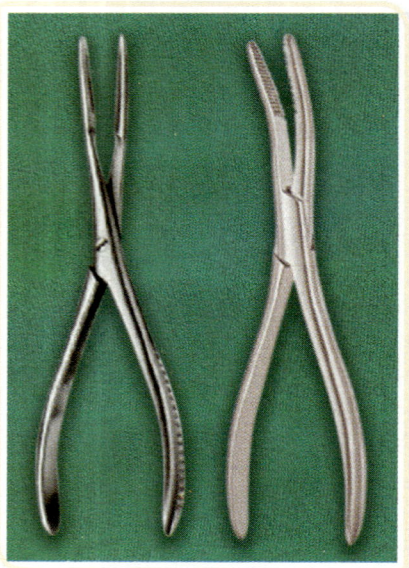

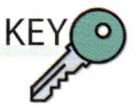 KEY

SEQUESTRUM HOLDING FORCEPS

A forceps with small, powerful teeth used for extracting necrotic or sharp fragments of bone from surrounding tissue. It has a stout blade with thick transverse serrations with a groove in the middle without a ratchet. Sequestrum should be formed before removal, hence X-ray is mandatory.
Uses: Used to remove sequestrum in osteomyelitis.
Two types; Straight (left) and curved (right)

> **Note**
> The instrument appears like the crocodile bone holding forceps, but does not have a catch to prevent crushing of the sequestrum

ORTHO PLATE 3

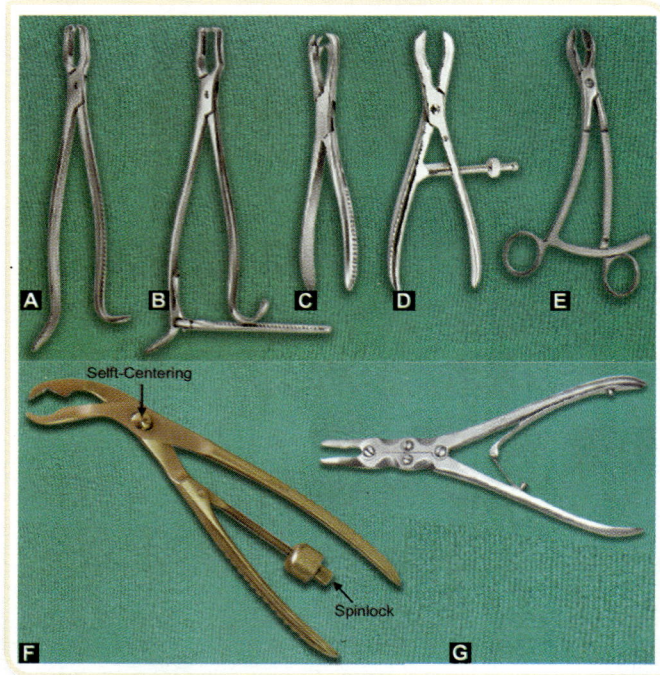

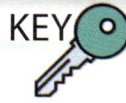 KEY

BONE HOLDING FORCEPS[AIIMS PG]

There are different types of Bone holding forceps, Each with curved and straight models.
A. **Lane's Bone holding forceps without Ratchet:** For holding femur and tibia. Like all other instruments designed by lane, this instrument is also long. Kern bone holding forceps is similar to Lane except that it is shorter than Lane.
B. **Lane's Bone holding forceps without Ratchet:**
C. **Fergusson's Bone holding forceps:** AKA Lion tooth bone holding forceps.
D. **AO Type forceps:** For radius and ulna, self-retaining

E. **Burn's bone holding forceps:** Used for radius, ulna and fibula. Blades are triangular, curved and serrated with pointed tip. Catch lock mechanism for locking.
F. **Verbrugge Bone Holding Forceps**[AIIMS PG]**:** with pincer-like jaws and a ratchet mechanism .
G. **Rongeur bone nibbler**[AIIMS PG]**:** Hand piece with spring action. Double action hinge. Used for removing excess bone and smoothening its surface i.e. Nibbling.

ORTHO PLATE 4

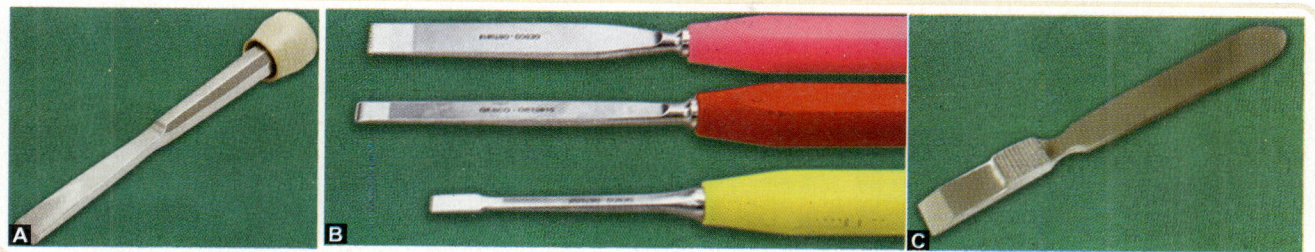

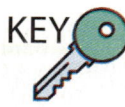
KEY

PLATE LEGENDS
A. **Bone Chisel** is used to chip the bone. Only one edge is beveled.
B. **Osteotome** is used to cut and divide the bone. These are long handled instruments with both edges are beveled.
C. **Periosteal elevators** are instruments designed to strip (or elevate) periosteum from bone. The look of a periosteal elevator can have the tip being rounded or squared, narrow, or wide.

ORTHO PLATE 5

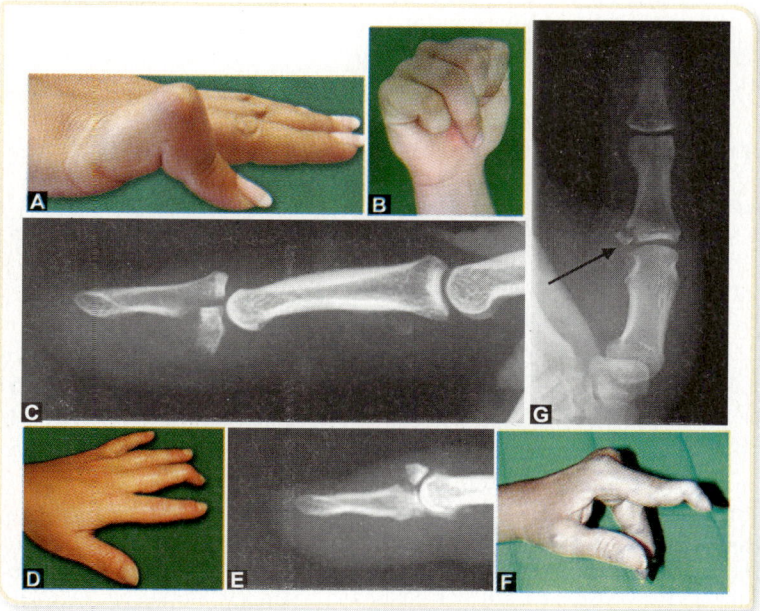

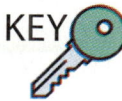
KEY

LIGAMENT INJURIES OF FINGERS
A. **Boutonnière deformity** of the little finger
B. **Jersey finger** of the ring finger (most common)
C. **Jersey finger X-ray:** Avulsion fracture arising from the FDP insertion site on the volar/palmar aspect of the base of the distal phalanx leading to Jersey finger

333

D. **Mallet finger:** Mallet finger is a traumatic zone I lesion of the extensor tendon with either tendon rupture or bony avulsion at the base of the distal phalanx.
E. **Mallet Finger X-ray:** Avulsion fracture of the base of distal phalanx on dorsal aspect in type IV mallet finger.
F. **Swan neck deformity**[NEETPG] characterized by hyperextension of PIP and flexion of DIP
G. **Gamekeeper's fracture:** Avulsion fractures of the ulnar base of the proximal phalanx of the thumb

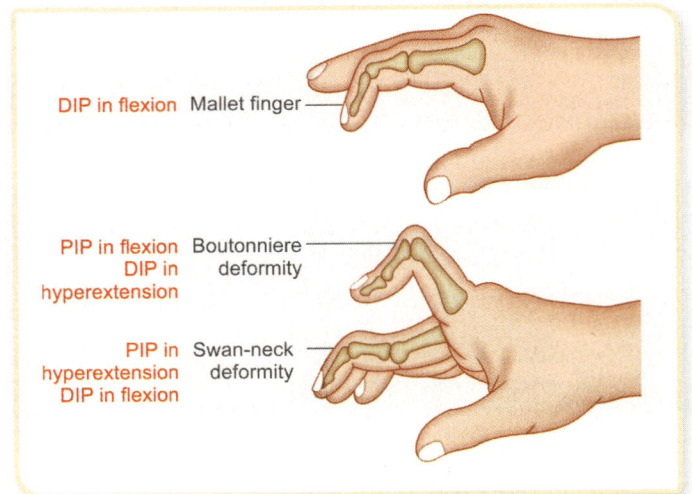

	Ligament Injuries of Finger			
	Description	**History/Physical Exam**	**Work-Up/ Findings**	**Treatment**
Boutonniere Deformity	□ **Extensor tendon** (central slip injury) at PIP ruptures. DIP is hyperextended and PIP is hyperflexed □ Associated with RA	Hx: Hand trauma PE: PIP flexed, no active extension, DIP extended	XR: Hand series: normal	□ Splint PIP in extension, DIP free □ Reconstruct central slip and bands □ Severe: fusion or arthroplasty
Jersey Finger	**Flexor digitorum profundus (FDP)** tendon injury by forceful extension on a flexed digit, typically in an athlete grabbing opponent's jersey. (also called a Zone 1 Flexor tendon injury). Occur mostly in rugby/football. Occurs most commonly in the ring finger (75%).	Hx: Extension injury, 1/2 pain. PE: FDS: 1 sublimis test FDP: 1 profundus test	XR: Rule out fracture (1/2 avulsion fracture)	□ Primary repair □ Older patient: DIP fusion
Mallet Finger	AKA: **baseball, dropped, dolphin finger** - Hyperflexion **Extensor digitorum tendon injury** of the fingers at DIP (zone I) □ FDP unopposed so DIP flexes	H/O: **Hyperflexion** injury of Extensor digitorum, usually occurs when a ball, while being caught, hits an outstretched finger Exm: Cannot extend DIP, minimal pain & swelling, hyperextended PIP Jt	X-Ray: 1/2 avulsion fracture	□ **Constant splint** (DIP only) for 8 weeks followed by 4 weeks night only splint □ Operative treatment is considered only if there is a large fragment (>50%) & subluxation of DIP.
Swanneck Deformity	□ FDS rupture/volar plate injury □ Lateral bands subluxes dorsally, PIP hyperextends & DIP flexes	Hx: Caused by rheumatoid arthritis[NEET PG] or Trauma, spastic PE: PIP hyperextended, DIP flexed	XR: Hand series	□ Early: splint □ Late: surgical repair (individualize each case)
Gamekeeper's Thumb	- AKA; **SKIER'S THUMB** - **Ulnar collateral ligament** tear of the thumb metacarpophalangeal joint □ Mechanism: forceful radial deviation or fall on extended thumb causing **hyperabduction**	H/O: Trauma. Pain & swelling. Exm: **partial rupture:** only the ligament proper is torn and the thumb is unstable in flexion but stable in full extension because the palmar plate is intact. **Complete rupture**, both ligament proper & palmar plate are torn & thumb is unstable in all positions	XR: 1/2 avulsion fracture. Stress view shows injury	□ **Incomplete:** splint 2-4 weeks, avoid pinch for 6-8 weeks □ **Complete:** surgical repair (treat **Stener lesion;** proximal end of torn ligament gets trapped in front of the adductor pollicis aponeurosis)

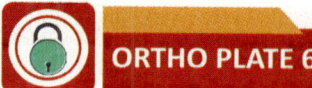

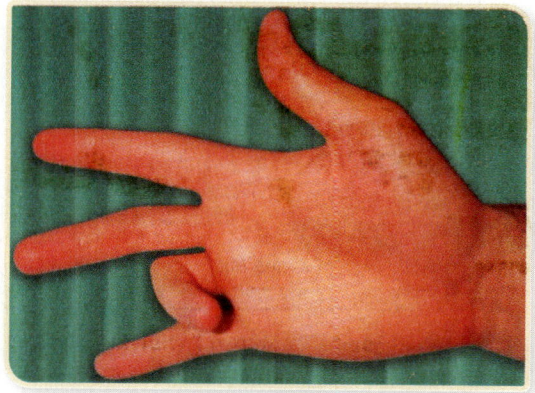

- In more advanced cases, the finger may be locked in flexion and very painful to reduce. The patients may complain of the occurrence more in the morning hours than later in the day.
- On physical examination, actual triggering may not be elicited but tenderness directly over the A1 pulley usually is present.
- The condition is more frequently seen in patients with rheumatoid arthritis, gout, diabetes, and degenerative arthritis. Patients usually present in the fifth to seventh decade of life.
- Initial treatment is non operative. Simple splinting with the use of NSAIDs has been shown to be effective in some patients. Injection of corticosteroid into the flexor tendon sheath has been shown to be effective in 70% of patients.
- Flexor tendon sheath release or trigger finger release is indicated when non operative management fails. This is done at the opening of the flexor tendon sheath, or at the level of the A1 pulley.

STENOSING TENOSYNOVITIS (TRIGGER FINGER)

- Stenosing tenosynovitis condition is a mechanical problem of a mismatch in size of the flexor tendons within their flexor tendon sheath.
- The result is a bunching or catching of the tendons as they pass through the orifice of the A1 pulley.
- This mismatch in size results in the mechanical problem of triggering that is the clinical hallmark of the condition.
- **A fibrocartilagnous dysplasia develops at the A1 pulley, leading to a similar lesion on the corresponding surface of the flexor tendon. This results in degenerative tendinopathy over time.**
- The process can occur at any digit but more commonly affects the **ring finger**.
- Patients usually present with a complaint of a painful catching of the finger with gripping.

ORTHO PLATE 7

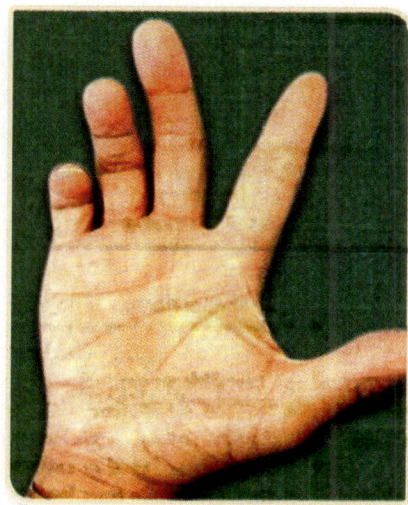

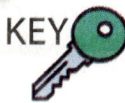

ULNAR CLAW HAND

Brachial Plexus Nerve Lesions		
Nerve (segment)	**Motor deficit(s)**	**Sensory deficits**
Long Thoracic (C 5,6,7)	**Winged Scapula-** *Serratus Anterior*	None
Suprascapular (C 5,6)	Hard to start shoulder abduction - *Supraspinatus*	None
Axillary (C 5,6)	Difficult abducting arm to horizontal - *Deltoid*	Lateral side of arm below point of shoulder
	Loss of shoulder roundness - Deltoid	
Musculocutaneous C 5,6,(7)	Very weak flexion of elbow joint- *Biceps & Brachialis*	Lateral forearm
	Weak supination of radioulnar joint -*Biceps*	
Radial (C 5 - T1)	Low lesions are usually due to fractures or dislocations at the elbow, or to a local wound. Wrist extension is preserved	Posterior lateral & arm; dorsum of hand
	High lesions occur with fractures of the humerus or after prolonged tourniquet pressure. There is an obvious **wrist drop**, due to weakness of the radial extensors of the wrist, as well as inability to extend the metacarpophalangeal joints or elevate the thumb.	Sensory loss is limited to a small patch on the dorsum around the **anatomical snuffbox.**

Contd...

Brachial Plexus Nerve Lesions

Nerve (segment)	Motor deficit(s)	Sensory deficits
	Very high lesions may be caused by trauma or operations around the shoulder. More often, though, they are due to chronic compression in the axilla; this is seen in drink and drug addicts who fall into a stupor with the arm dangling over the back of a chair ('**Saturday night palsy**') or in thin elderly patients using crutches ('**crutch palsy**'). In addition to weakness of the wrist and hand, the triceps is paralyzed and the triceps reflex is absent.	Posterior lateral & arm; dorsum of hand
Median C 5 - T1) at Elbow	Pronation of radioulnar joints-Pronator teres & quadratus	Radial portion of palm; palmar surface & tips of radial 3½ digits
	Bishop/Benediction Hand/Pope's Blessings Hand (When the patient tries to make a fist, they are *unable to flex the index and middle fingers* while the ring & index fingers flex due to loss of lateral lumbrical action	
	Weak wrist flexion - *Fl. carpi radialis*	
	Weakened opposition of thumb - *thenar muscles*	
	Ape hand- Thumb hyper extended and adducted - *thenar muscles*	
	"Papal Hand" Loss of flexion of I.P. joints of thumb & fingers 1 & 2 - *Fl. pollices longus ; Fl. digit. superficialis, Fl. digit profundus*	
Median (C 5 - T1) at Wrist	**Ape/Simian hand deformity (MC):** Thumb hyper extended and adducted (unopposable thumb like an ape), Weakened opposition of thumb due to week thenar. Seen at rest	Palmar surface & tips of radial 3½ digits including thumb
Ulnar (C 8, T1) at Elbow	**"Ulnar Claw hand"** (AKA 'intrinsic minus' hand)- Loss of flexion/hyperextension of 4th & 5th MCP joints and loss of extension (i.e. Flexion) of IP joints. Due to paralysis of palmar and dorsal interossei and medial 2 lumbricals. Typical presentation at rest. Wasted hypothenar eminence and loss of adduction of thumb. Similar to the hand of benediction except that Ulnar claw is seen at rest while Benediction hand is seen while trying to make fist	Ulnar and dorsal aspect of palm and of ulnar 1½ digits
	Ulnar Paradox: In lesion of the ulnar nerve at the elbow, in addition to the muscles of the hand Medial half of Flexor Digitorum Profundus (FDP) & Flexor Carpi Ulnaris are also paralysed. The ulnar claw will develop as before, but with one key difference. There will not be any flexion of the ring and little fingers. Now the ulnar claw only consists of hyperextension at the MCP joints, giving a less evident claw hand. This is known as the 'ulnar paradox. The worse injury, lesion at elbow, looks less serious than a lesion at the wrist. Ulnar nerve injury of Elbow is more prominent when patient is asked to make a fist.	

Contd...

Brachial Plexus Nerve Lesions

Nerve (segment)	Motor deficit(s)	Sensory deficits
Ulnar (C 8, T1) at Wrist	**"Ulnar Claw hand" (AKA 'intrinsic minus' hand)**- Loss of flexion/ hyperextension of 4th & 5th MCP joints and loss of extension (i.e. Flexion) of IP joints. Due to paralysis of palmar and dorsal interossei and medial 2 lumbricals. Typical presentation at rest. Wasted hypothenar eminence and loss of adduction of thumb. Unlike Ulnar nerve injury at elbow, the FDP is spared and hence Clawing is more prominent	
	Note: Dupuytren's contracture: This typically involves the little and ring fingers and can mimic a claw hand, but the metacarpophalangeal joint is flexed and the contracted fingers cannot passively be extended. Palpation of the Dupuytren's tissue in the palm confirms the diagnosis.	
Combined median & ulnar nerve palsy at wrist	**Full claw hand** with thenar and hypothenar flattening, and thumb adduction and flexion. **[AKA- Simian hand or Ape Hand (true)]**	Palm and digits

ORTHO PLATE 8

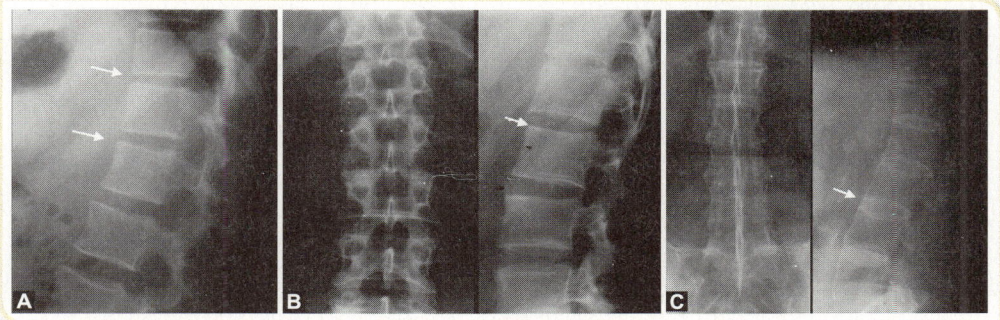

KEY

ANKYLOSING SPONDYLITIS

A. Lateral view of the thoracolumbar region showing slight abnormalities in the form of slight vertebral squaring (arrows)
B. Frontal and lateral view of the lumbar spine showing bridging syndesmophytes (arrows)
C. Frontal and lateral view of the lumbar spine showing fusion of several vertebral bodies (arrow)

Ankylosing Spondylitis	
Ankylosing spondylitis (AS) is an inflammatory disorder of unknown cause that primarily affects the axial skeleton; peripheral joints and extra articular structures are also frequently involved.	
Ankylosing spondylitis, Reiter's disease and psoriatic arthritis characteristically test negative for rheumatoid factor; they have been grouped together as the 'seronegative spondarthritides'. The term *axial spondyloarthritis*, coming into common use, includes early or mild forms that do not meet classical criteria for AS	
Age of onset	15 and 25 years
Genetic marker	HLA B 27 in 95% cases HLA-B27 is associated with AS and Aortic Root Dilatation with AR
Clinical features	**Sacroiliitis** is often the earliest manifestations of AS. The initial symptom is usually dull pain, insidious in onset, felt deep in the lower lumbar or gluteal region, accompanied **by low-back morning stiffness of up to a few hours'** duration that improves with activity and returns following inactivity. The most specific findings involve **loss of spinal mobility, with limitation of anterior and lateral flexion and extension of the lumbar spine and of chest expansion.**

Contd...

	Ankylosing Spondylitis
Posture	In established cases the posture is typical: **loss of the normal lumbar lordosis, increased thoracic kyphosis** and a forward thrust of the neck; upright posture and balance are maintained by standing with the hips and knees slightly flexed, and in late cases these may become fixed deformities. Spinal movements are diminished in all directions, but loss of extension is always the earliest and the most severe disability. It is revealed dramatically by the **'wall test'**: the patient is asked to stand with his back to the wall; heels, buttocks, scapulae and occiput should all be able to touch the wall simultaneously.
Extra skeletal manifestations	General fatigue and loss of weight are common. **Acute anterior uveitis** (most common extra skeletal manifestation 25-40%); it usually responds well to treatment but, if neglected, may lead to permanent damage including **glaucoma**. Other extra skeletal disorders, such as **aortic valve disease**, carditis and **pulmonary fibrosis** (apical), are rare and occur very late in the disease. **Chest expansion**, which should be at least 7 cm in young men, is often markedly decreased. About 10% of patients meeting criteria for AS have **psoriasis.**
X-ray (See **ORTHO PLATE 6**)	The cardinal sign – and often the earliest – **is erosion and fuzziness of the sacroiliac joints.** The earliest vertebral change is flattening of the normal anterior concavity of the vertebral body ('squaring'). Later, ossification of the ligaments around the intervertebral discs produces delicate bridges **(syndesmophytes)** between adjacent vertebrae. Bridging at several levels gives the appearance of a **'bamboo spine'.**
	SASSS = Stoke Ankylosing Spondylitis Spine Score: Anterior and posterior changes in the lumbar spine Grade 0: Normal findings Grade 1: Erosion, sclerosis and/or squaring Grade 2: Syndesmophytes Grade 3: Total ankylosis
Special investigations	The ESR and CRP are usually elevated during active phases of the disease. **HLA-B27** is present in 95% of cases. Serological tests for rheumatoid factor are usually negative.
Management	All management of AS should include an exercise program designed to maintain posture and range of motion. Nonsteroidal anti-inflammatory drugs (NSAIDs) are the first line of pharmacologic therapy for AS. Anti TNF alpha drugs are being tried.

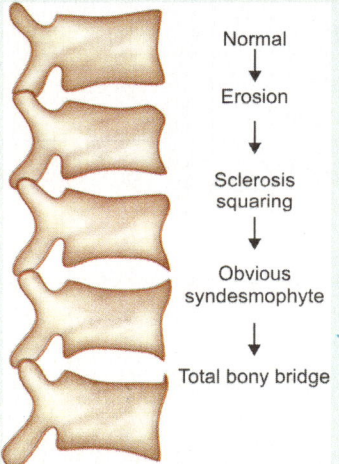

ORTHO PLATE 9

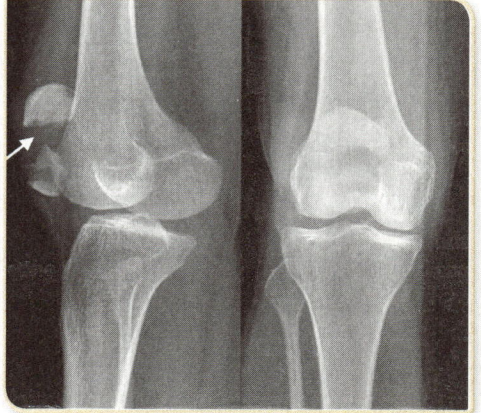

FRACTURE OF PATELLA

The lateral and AP radiograph of knee shows a displaced transverse fracture of patella, the treatment of which should be Tension band wiring

Patella Fracture			
Description	**Evaluation**	**Classification**	**Treatment**
Mechanism: direct & indirect: (e.g. fall, dashboard or kicking injury) ☐ Pull of quadriceps and patella tendons displace most fractures ☐ If intact, retinaculum resists displacement ☐ Do not confuse with bipartite patella	**H/O**: Trauma, Pain, cannot extend knee, swelling. **EXM**: Dome effusion. Tenderness, +/- palpable defect. Inability to extend knee. **X-Ray**: Knee trauma series **CT**: Not usually needed	☐ Descriptive & location: ☐ Nondisplaced ☐ Transverse ☐ Vertical ☐ Stellate ☐ Inferior/superior pole ☐ Comminuted	☐ **Nondisplaced or comminuted**: cylinder cast for 6 wks ☐ **Displaced (>3 mm)**: ORIF (e.g. tension band wiring) to restore articular surface ☐ **Severely comminuted**: May require patellectomy

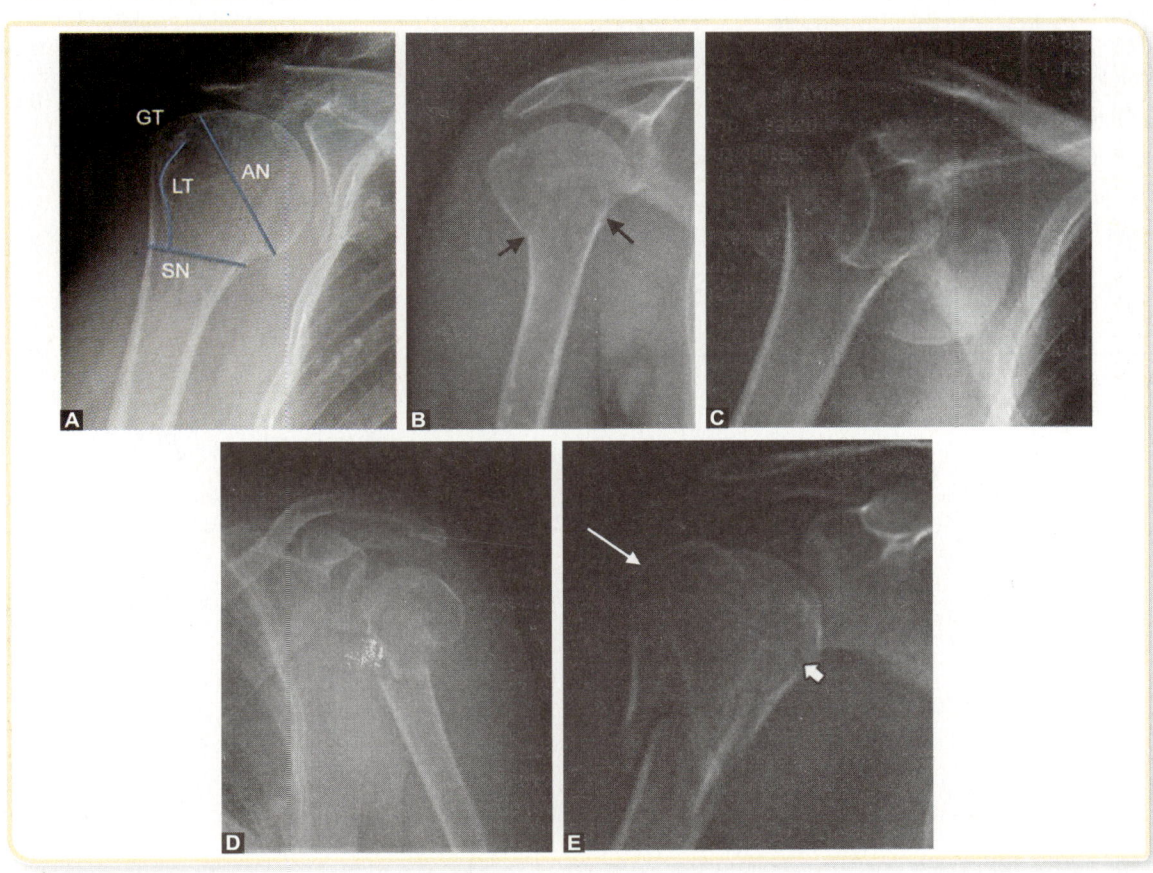

ORTHO PLATE 10

NEER CLASSIFICATION OF PROXIMAL HUMERUS FRACTURE

A. **Normal Proximal Humerus X-ray**: AN = Anatomical neck, GT = Greater tuberosity, LT = Lesser tuberosity, SN = Surgical neck
B. **Type I- Minimal displacement:** Fracture of greater tuberosity and surgical neck but no displacement and no angulation.
C. **Type II- Anatomical neck 2 part NEER fracture:**
D. **Type III- Surgical neck 2 part NEER fracture;** Surgical neck is displaced more than 1 cm from the humeral head.
E. **Type IV- 2 Greater Tuberosity part NEER fracture;** Greater tuberosity (long arrow) is displaced more than 1 cm from the humeral head (short arrow) which remains at anatomic position.

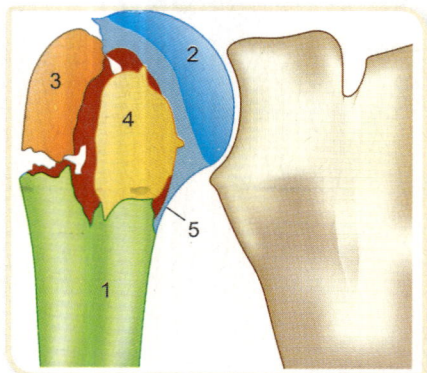

Fractures of the proximal humerus Diagram of a fractured proximal humerus, showing the four main fragments, two or more of which are seen in almost all proximal humeral fractures. 1 = shaft of humerus; 2 = head of humerus; 3 = greater tuberosity; 4 = lesser tuberosity.

	Neer Classification of Proximal Humerus Fracture	
	Type	Subtype
I	Minimal displacement	1-part
II	Anatomical neck	2-part
III	Surgical neck	2-part
IV	Greater tuberosity	2, 3, or 4-part
V	Lesser tuberosity	2, 3, or 4-part
VI	Fracture dislocation	Anterior - 2, 3, 4-part, or articular surface involvement Posterior - 2, 3, 4-part, or articular surface involvement

ORTHO PLATE 11

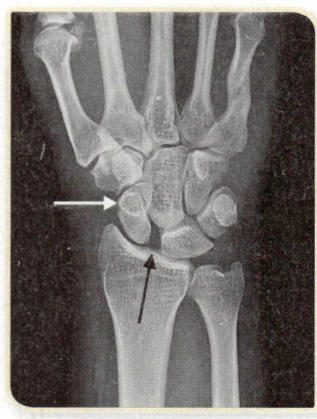

SCAPHOID FRACTURE

The scaphoid is potentially the most unstable of all the carpal bones. As the wrist flexes and extends, so does the scaphoid bone; the lunate and triquetrum follow passively. Tenderness in the anatomical snuffbox is typical of a scaphoid injury

Pain X-ray shows a gap between the scaphoid and lunate, the **Terry-Thomas sign** (Black arrow); Named after British comedian Terry Thomas' midline diastema. The actor Terry Thomas with the trademark gap between his front teeth) and rotation of the scaphoid. If the scaphoid is flexed, it will look foreshortened and the tubercle may appear as a dense 'ring' in the bone (**Scaphoid Signet ring sign-** white arrow)

A true lateral view is examined to assess the relative alignment of the distal radius, the lunate, capitate and scaphoid. In a normal wrist, the articular surfaces of the radius, lunate and capitate are parallel. Following a fracture of the scaphoid or rupture of the scapholunate ligament (scapholunate dissociation), the lunate no longer passively follows the scaphoid. The scaphoid tends to flex and the lunate assumes its default position of extension (dorsal tilt). (**Ref Apley 9th ed page 395**)

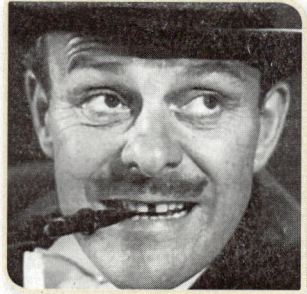

Fig: British comedian Terry Thomas' with midline diastema

ORTHO PLATE 12

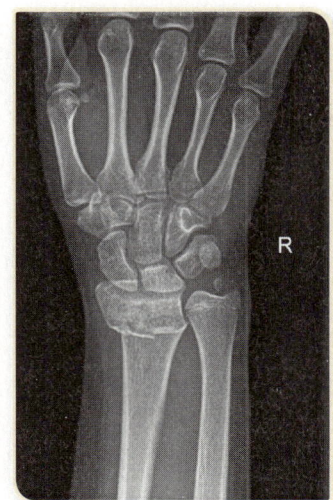

COLLE'S FRACTURE

Colles' fracture is distal radius fracture with dorsal angulation, impaction and radial drift due to fall on outstretched hand

Colles' Fracture	
Described by **Abraham Colles** in 1814. Fracture of distal radius at corticocancellous junction which is typically dorsally displaced and angulated	
Mechanism	▫ Fracture is also caused by a forced dorsiflexion of the wrist ▫ Occurs in pts >50 years of age(**Post-menopausal elderly women**) ▫ Fall on out stretched hand ▫ Dorsal surface undergoes compression while volar surface undergoes tension
Displacements	**Mnemonic**: SLIP (L and P comes twice, so total 6 displacements) ▫ Supination (External rotation) ▫ Lateral displacement ▫ Lateral tilt/angulation ▫ Impaction ▫ Posterior/Dorsal displacement ▫ Posterior/Dorsal tilt
Deformity	**Dinner fork/Silver fork/Spoon shaped deformity**
Complications	▫ Finger and joints stiffness is **most common complication** ▫ Malunion is **2nd most common** ▫ Sudeck's osteo dystrophy (colles # is MC cause of Sudeck of upper limb) ▫ Shoulder hand syndrome ▫ Rupture of extensor pollicis tendon ▫ Carpal tunnel syndrome ▫ Carpal instability ▫ Triangular fibro cartilage complex (TFCC) injury ▫ Delayed and nonunion are rare

ORTHO PLATE 13

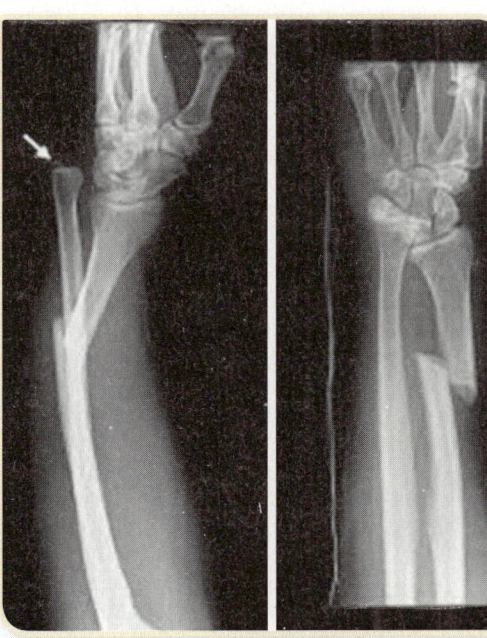

GALEAZZI FRACTURE

The X-ray shows a fracture of the distal radius and distal radio-ulnar joint dislocation typically seen in **Galeazzi fracture**[AIIMS PG]

Galeazzi Fracture	
Mechanism of injury	This injury was first described in 1934 by Galeazzi. The usual cause is a **fall on the hand; probably with a superimposed rotation force.** The radius fractures in its **lower third and the inferior radio-ulnar joint** subluxates or dislocates.
Site and components	Fracture of distal radius (between middle 1/3rd and distal 1/3rd) with disruption and dislocation of distal radioulnar joint. It is associated with tearing of interosseus membrane and the triangular fibrocartilage complex. It has been proposed that major cause of dislocation and poor response to conservative management in Galeazzi fracture is because of Injury to TFCC and intraosseus membrane.
Clinical features	More common than Monteggia. **Prominence or tenderness over the lower end of the ulna is the striking feature.** It may be possible to demonstrate the instability of the radio-ulnar joint by 'balloting' the distal end of the ulna (**the 'piano-key sign'**) or by rotating the wrist. It is important also to test for an ulnar nerve lesion, which may occur.
X-ray	A transverse or short oblique fracture is seen in the lower third of the radius, with angulation or overlap. The distal radioulnar joint is subluxated or dislocated (**better demonstrated in lateral view**)

Contd...

Galeazzi Fracture	
Treatment	The important step is to restore the length of the fractured bone. In children, closed reduction is often successful; in adults, reduction is best achieved by open operation and compression plating of the radius. An X-ray is taken to ensure that the distal radio-ulnar joint is reduced. *If the distal radioulnar joint is reduced and stable:* No further action is needed. The arm is rested for a few days, then gentle active movements are encouraged. The radioulnar joint should be checked, both clinically and radiologically, during the next 6 weeks. □ *If the distal radioulnar joint is reduced but unstable*: The forearm should be immobilized in the position of stability (usually supination), supplemented if required by a transverse K-wire. The forearm is splinted in an above-elbow cast for 6 weeks. If there is a large ulnar styloid fragment, it should be reduced and fixed. □ *If the distal radioulnar joint is irreducible.* This is unusual. Open reduction is needed to remove the interposed soft tissues. The triangular fibrocartilage complex (TFCC) and dorsal capsule are then carefully repaired and the forearm immobilized in the position of stability (again, usually supination, supported by a wire if needed) for 6 weeks.

Monteggia Fracture Dislocation	
	Bado classification: (based on radial head location): I. **Anterior (Most common)** II. Posterior III: Lateral IV: Anterior with associated both bone fracture.
X-ray	Fracture of upper third of ulna with forward bowing Forward dislocation of radial head
Treatment	Ulna: ORIF (plates/screws) Radial head: closed reduction (open if irreducible or unstable). Peds: closed reduction & cast.

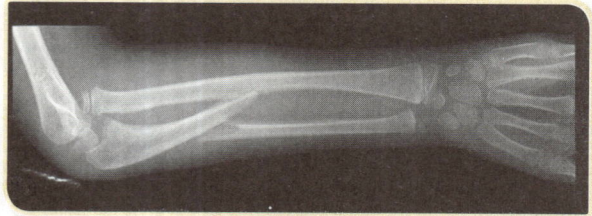

Monteggia   Galeazzi

ORTHO PLATE 14

ORTHO PLATE 15

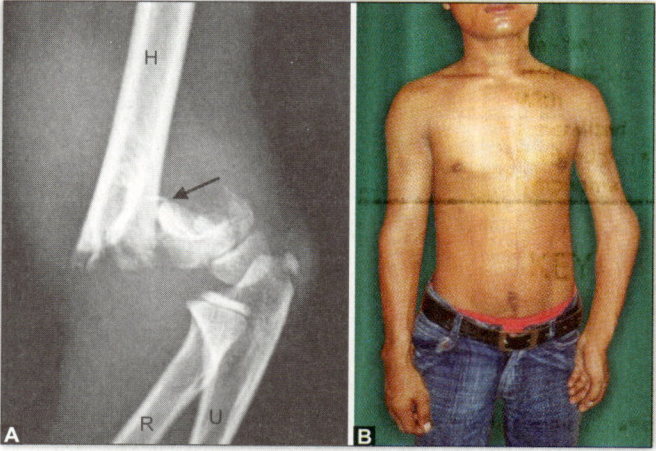

By James Heilman, MD (Own work) [CC BY-SA 3.0 (http://creativecommons.org/licenses/by-sa/3.0)]

MONTEGGIA FRACTURE

Fracture of shaft of ulna with dislocation of proximal radio ulnar joint

Monteggia Fracture Dislocation	
Definition	Fracture of proximal/ shaft of ulna with anterior angulation of ulna and anterior dislocation of radial dead. In less common type the angulation and dislocation is posteriorly
Mechanism of injury	Direct blow or fall on outstretched hand.
Clinical features	Pain and tenderness on lateral side of elbow. Dislocated head of radius is masked by swelling. Ulnar deformity is visible

Contd...

SUPRACONDYLAR FRACTURE OF HUMERUS

A. **Supracondylar Fracture** radiograph showing extension type injury with posterior displacement of the distal segment
B. **Cubitus Varus ('Gun-Stock' Deformity):** The deformity is *most obvious when the elbow is extended and the arms are elevated*. The most common cause is malunion of a **supracondylar fracture.** The deformity can be corrected by a wedge osteotomy of the lower humerus but this is best left until skeletal maturity.

	Supracondylar Fracture of Humerus
Age group	Most common in children and elderly patients, but it may occur at any age
Mechanism	Flexion type or an extension type, depending upon the **displacement of the distal fragment** of bone ▫ **Posterior angulation or displacement or Extension type (95%)** suggests a hyperextension injury, usually due to a fall on the outstretched hand and is stable only in significant flexion. ▫ **Anterior angulation or displacement or flexion type** is produced by a fall on the flexed elbow and is relatively stable in extension
Classification	**Gartland classification** is useful for determining appropriate treatment for supracondylar fractures: ▫ **Type I:** undisplaced ▫ **Type II:** displaced with intact posterior cortex ▫ **Type III:** is a completely displaced fracture (although the posterior periosteum is usually still preserved, which will assist surgical reduction).
Clinical features	Pain, swelling, S shaped deformity, Loss of anatomical landmark, signs of neurovascular injury can accompany and should be checked.
Adequacy of reduction	**Baumann angle** usually is considered the angle formed by the intersection of a line perpendicular to the long axis of the humeral shaft and the physeal line of the lateral condyle; reported **normal values range from 9° to 26°**. A common rule of thumb is that a Baumann angle of at least 10° is acceptable
Treatment	▫ Side-arm skin traction for Type 1 injury **(Dunlop traction)** ▫ Overhead skeletal traction for Type 1 injury ▫ **CRPP** (closed reduction percutaneous pinning) for type 2 injury ▫ **ORIF** (open reduction and internal fixation) for type 3 injury. performed emergently (<8 hours) or urgently (≤24 hours) or after the swelling has decreased, but not later than 5 days after injury because the possibility of myositis ossificans apparently increases after that time
Early complications	▫ **Brachial artery injury** (earlier 5%, nowadays < 1%) - perform angiography, or Doppler ▫ Compartment syndrome (uncommon) ▫ **Nerve injury:** Most commonly *median nerve (particularly the anterior interosseous branch)*. Most nerve injuries are associated with type III displaced supracondylar fractures. The radial nerve lies posterolateral to the supracondylar fractures thus less commonly involved. Ulnar nerve which is posteriorly located is uncommonly injured. Conclusion: **MEDIAN > ULNAR > RADIAL** ▫ **Neuropraxia**—is reported to occur in 3% to 22% and is transitory
Late complications	▫ **Malunion** ▫ **Cubitus varus** (carrying angle < 5°) and Cubitus valgus (carrying angle >15°) (**Cubitus varus AKA Gun stock deformity is far more common**). Cubitus varus is the most common angular deformity that results from supracondylar fractures in children. The most common cause is malunion of a supracondylar fracture. ▫ **Cubitus valgus**, although mentioned in the literature as causing tardy ulnar nerve palsy, rarely occurs and is more often caused by nonunion of lateral condylar fractures. ▫ **Tardy ulnar nerve palsy** (Not due to supracondylar fracture per se but its complication as valgus) ▫ Elbow stiffness and myositis ossificans
Management of cubitus varus	Three basic types of osteotomies have been described: a medial opening wedge osteotomy with a bone graft, an oblique osteotomy with derotation, and a lateral closing wedge osteotomy (easiest, safest and most stable osteotomy)

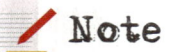

Note

Baumann angle is different from Carrying angle. **Carrying angle** is a small degree of cubitus valgus, formed between the axis of a radially deviated forearm and the axis of the humerus. The normal carrying angle of the elbow is 5–15 degrees of valgus; anything more than this is regarded as a valgus deformity.

Carrying angle (normal 5-15°)	Negative (<5°)	**Cubitus varus:** Physeal damage (e.g. malunion supracondylar fracture)
	Positive (>15°)	**Cubitus Valgus:** Physeal damage (e.g. lateral epicondyle fracture)

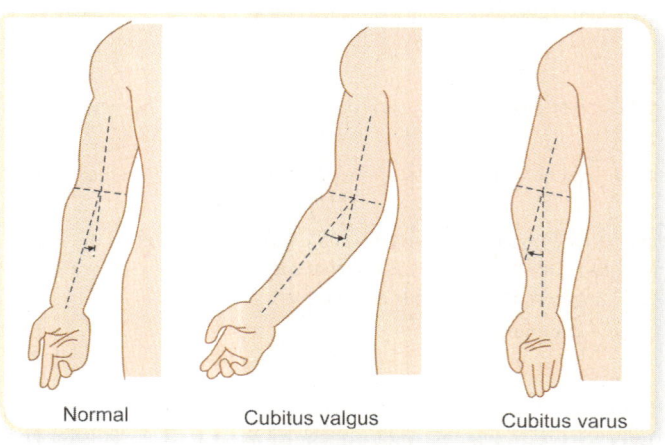

Normal — Cubitus valgus — Cubitus varus

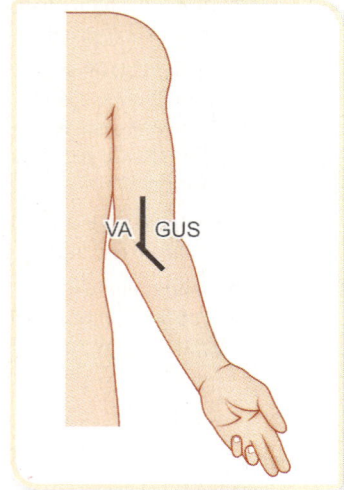

 ORTHO PLATE 16

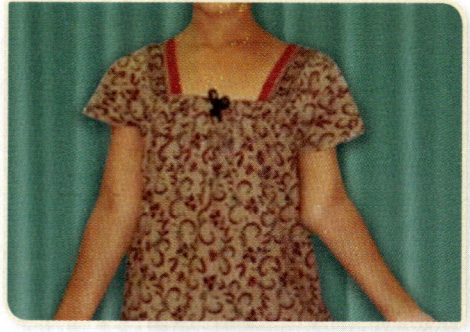

 KEY

 **ORTHO PLATE 17**

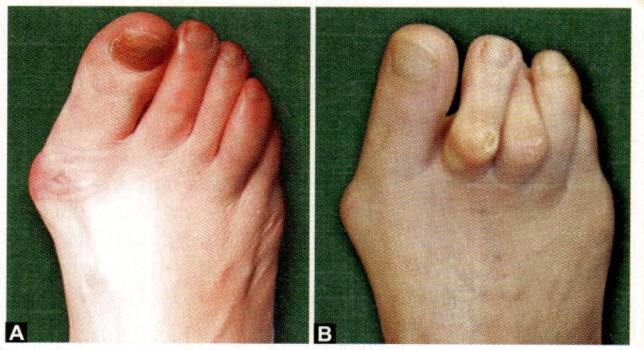

 KEY

CUBITUS VALGUS

The normal carrying angle of the elbow is 5–15 degrees of valgus; anything more than this is regarded as a valgus deformity, which is usually quite obvious when the patient stands with arms to the sides and palms facing forwards. The commonest cause is longstanding **non-union of a fractured lateral condyle**; the deformity may be associated with marked prominence of the medial condylar outline. The importance of cubitus valgus is the liability to delayed ulnar palsy; years after the causal injury the patient notices weakness of the hand, with numbness and tingling of the ulnar fingers. The deformity itself needs no treatment, but for delayed ulnar palsy the nerve should be transposed to the front of the elbow. Great care is needed in performing the operation. Excessive dissection of the nerve or rough handling can impair nerve function.

Varus and valgus deformities (cubitus varus and cubitus valgus) are usually the result of trauma around the elbow. By far the best way to demonstrate a varus deformity is to ask the patient to lift his or her arms sideways to shoulder height; in this position the deformity becomes much more obvious, the arm taking on the appearance of a rifle butt (gunstock deformity

HALLUX VALGUS (BUNION)

A. Hallux Valgus deformity
B. Hallux Valgus with Hammertoe deformity of 2nd and 3rd toe

Hallux valgus (lateral deviation of the great toe) is not a single disorder, as the name implies, but a complex deformity of the first ray that frequently is accompanied by deformity and symptoms in the lesser toes.

Hallux abductus (or hallux valgus) angle – The angle created by the bisection of the longitudinal axis of the hallux and the longitudinal axis of the first metatarsal. Historically, a hallux abductus (HA) angle of greater than 15 degrees was considered abnormal, but such deformities are not always symptomatic, and some cases of an HA angle greater than 15 degrees occur naturally due to the shape of the articular surfaces involved. Contemporary research suggests an *HA angle of 20 degrees or greater is abnormal.* If the **valgus angle of the first metatarsophalangeal joint exceeds 30 to 35 degrees,** pronation of the great toe usually results.

Intermetatarsal (IM) angle – The angle determined by the bisection of the longitudinal axes of the first and second metatarsals. An IM angle less than 9 degrees is considered normal.

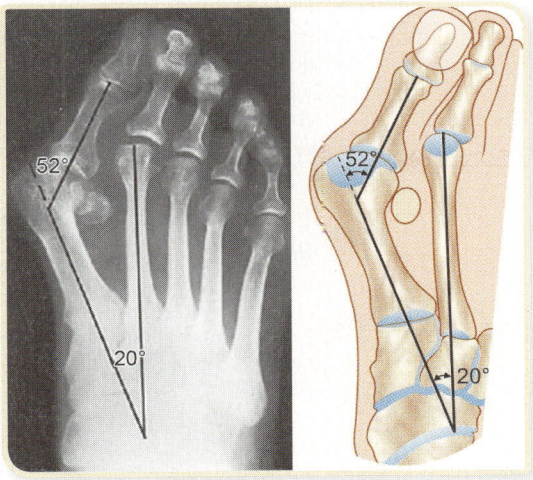

The valgus posture of the great toe frequently causes a **hammer toe–like deformity of the second toe**. In addition, the splaying of the forefoot makes the wearing of shoes more difficult; with shoes that have a narrow toe box, corns often develop, as does bursal hypertrophy over the medial eminence of the first metatarsal head **(bunion)**. Amputation of the second toe frequently is followed by severe hallux valgus because the great toe tends to drift toward the third to fill the gap left by amputation.

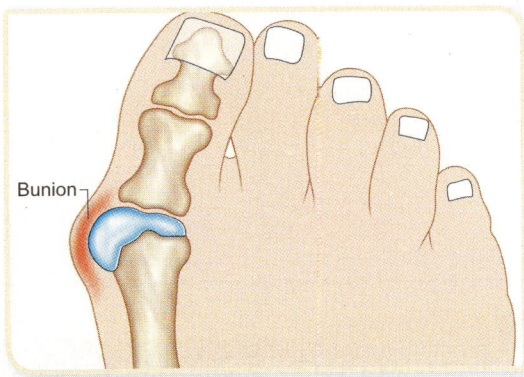

Hallux valgus complex. Note increase in intermetatarsal angle, lateral dislocation of sesamoids, subluxation of first metatarsophalangeal joint (leaving metatarsal head uncovered), and pronation of great toe associated with marked hallux valgus.

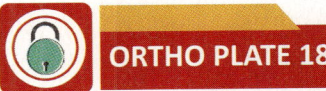

ORTHO PLATE 18

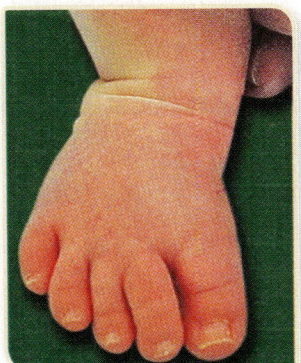

KEY

FOREFOOT ADDUCTION DEFORMITY

It is also known as Metatarsus Adductus affects Lisfranc Joint and causes Adduction of Metatarsal Bones with foot inversion causing in toeing. It can occur in patients with cerebral palsy as an isolated deformity or in association with other deformities, such as in an incompletely corrected or recurrent clubfoot.

ORTHO PLATE 19

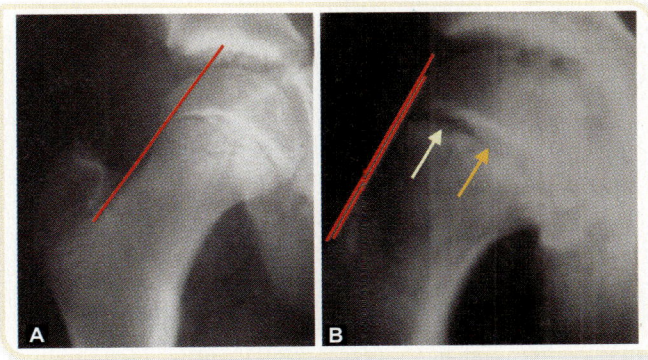

KEY

SLIPPED CAPITAL FEMORAL EPIPHYSIS (SCFE)

A. **Normal hip joint with Klein line** (red line) along the anterior or superior aspect of the femoral neck that normally is intersected by the capital femoral epiphysis is flush with or below this line.
B. In a Slipped capital femoral epiphysis the epiphysis may be flush with or even below Klein line (Trethowan's sign).

Slipped Capital Femoral Epiphysis (SCFE)	
Definition: Displacement of the proximal femoral epiphysis – also known as femoral capital epiphysiolysis or slipped capital femoral epiphysis (SCFE)	
Age group: 10-15 years	
Epidemiology	Approximately **3 in 100,000**; Boys > Girls (2:1). **Left hip > Right Hip (2:1)** Bilateral involvement occurs in between 20% and 60% of cases. SCFE is associated with **obesity**. Patients with an underlying **hormonal or endocrine disorder** have an associated increased risk for development of SCFE. When bilateral slips occur, the second slip usually occurs within 12 to 18 months of the initial slip.
Classification	**Temporal:** Acute <3 weeks, chronic >3 weeks, and acute-on-chronic is a sudden exacerbation of subclinical symptoms of long-standing duration
	This classification system has gained greater popularity because it appears to be clinically more useful. ☐ **Stable SCFE** is able to walk without assistance, with mild pain, or a slight limp ☐ **Unstable SCFE** are unable to walk or to bear weight. Unstable SCFEs are associated with a higher rate of complications.

Contd...

Slipped Capital Femoral Epiphysis (SCFE)

Clinical features	Pain in the groin, medial thigh, or knee and limitation of hip motion, especially internal rotation. Limp also occurs early and is more constant. On examination the leg is externally rotated and is 1–2 cm short. Characteristically there is limitation of flexion, abduction and medial rotation
Complications	Primary complications associated with SCFE are ❏ **Avascular necrosis:** Avascular necrosis is uncommon with stable SCFE treated with pinning in situ. There is a greater incidence of avascular necrosis associated with unstable SCFE. A vigorous attempt at reduction of an unstable SCFE should NOT be performed ❏ **Chondrolysis:** Chondrolysis is a gradual loss of the joint space following stabilization of the SCFE. It has been associated with treatment with one or more pins as well as with a spica cast in which no internal fixation was used
Diagnosis	❏ **Radiograph:** The diagnosis of SCFE usually is apparent from anteroposterior radiographs, but special views may be helpful. A cross-table, or true, lateral view can help determine the extent of posterior displacement of the epiphysis, and a "frog-leg" lateral view best shows subtle slipping. The **Klein line** is a line along the anterior or superior aspect of the femoral neck that normally is intersected by the epiphysis is flush with or below this line. In an early slip the epiphysis may be flush with or even below this line *(Trethowan's sign).* Often a double density is seen at the metaphysis when a femoral head is even mildly slipped posteriorly on the regular radiograph as compared with the contralateral hip; this has been called a *"blanch" sign of steel.* In the anteroposterior view the epiphyseal plate seems to be too wide and too 'woolly'. *Capener's sign* describes loss of the intracapsular area at the medial aspect of the femoral neck, which normally overlaps the posterior wall of the acetabulum creating a dense triangular shadow. Decreased epiphyseal height, physeal ❏ **CT scan** may help confirm the diagnosis in patients with early, mild slipping that is not apparent on radiographs. ❏ **Magnetic resonance imaging MRI** has been used to detect and stage avascular necrosis (AVN) of the femoral head) ❏ **Ultrasonography** may detect a hip effusion associated with an acute event, and may also show metaphyseal remodelling in a chronic slip.
Treatment	The most widely recommended form of treatment is surgical stabilization with **percutaneous pinning in situ.** For a stable SCFE, this can usually be accomplished with a single, cannulated screw inserted under fluoroscopic control.

Contd...

Slipped Capital Femoral Epiphysis (SCFE)

The aim of the procedure is to insert the screw perpendicular to the femoral head in both the AP and lateral planes with close attention to avoid penetrating the femoral head and entering the hip joint. In cases of an unstable SCFE, a second screw may be inserted to further stabilize the femoral head

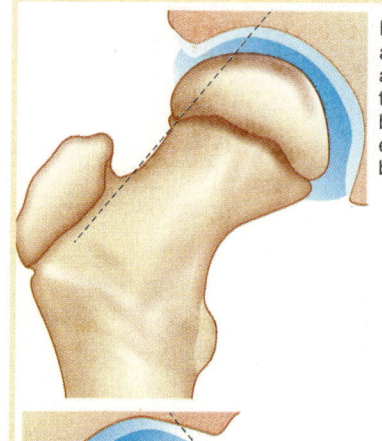

Normal hip joint with klein line along the anterior or superior aspect of the femoral neck that normally is intersected by the capital femoral epiphysis is flush with or below this line.

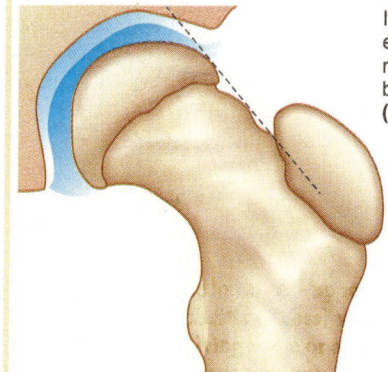

In a slipped capital femoral epiphysis, the epiphysis may be flush with or even below klein line **(Trethowan's sign).**

 ORTHO PLATE 20

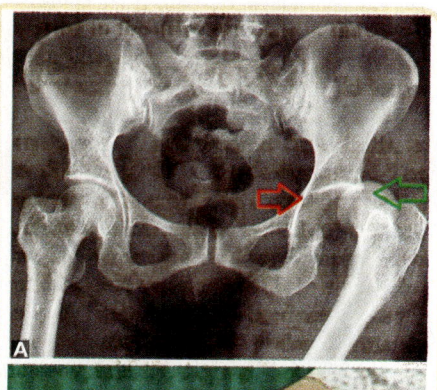

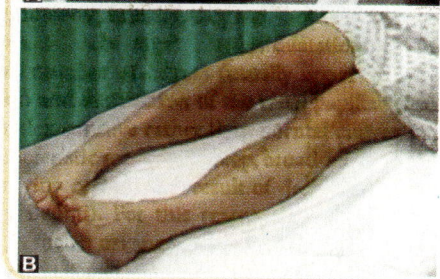

POSTERIOR DISLOCATION OF HIP

A. In the AP film the femoral head is seen out of its socket and above the acetabulum. The Right femoral head (green arrow) lies superior (and posterior) to the acetabulum (Red arrow). No Pelvic fracture is seen.
B. Position of limb in Posterior dislocation of hip: Typical attitude of the limb is **Flexion, Adduction, Internal rotation (FADIR)**

HIP Dislocation

Description	Evaluation	Treatment
☐ High energy trauma (esp. Motor Vehicle Accident-dashboard injury or significant fall.) ☐ Orthopedic emergency ☐ Multiple associated injuries +/- fractures, (e.g. femoral head & neck)	☐ H/O: Trauma. Severe pain, Cannot move thigh/hip. ☐ Pain (esp. with motion), good neurovascular exam ☐ X-ray: AP pelvis, frog lateral (Femoral head is different size) Also femur & knee series CT: Rule out fracture or bony fragments	Early reduction essential, then repeat X-ray & neurologic exam **Posterior I:** Closed reduction & abduction pillow **Posterior II-V:** ☐ Closed Reduction (open if irreducible) ☐ ORIF fracture or excise fragment **Anterior:** closed reduction, ORIF if necessary.

Classification

Anterior	Posterior	Central
Epstein classification	**Thompson classification**	**Not a true dislocation**
10% hip dislocation	Most common (85-90%), 10% associated with sciatic nerve injury	Although this is called 'central dislocation', it is really a fracture of the acetabulum.
I. Superior (A, B, C) II. Inferior (A, B, C) A: No associated fracture B: Femoral head fracture C: Acetabular fracture	I. Simple, no posterior fragment II. Simple, large posterior fragment III. Comminuted posterior fragment IV. Acetabular fracture V. Femoral head fracture	Head of femur is felt in Per rectal examinations
No shortening, may be true lengthening of limb	Shortening of limb	Shortening of limb
Abducted, flexed, Externally rotated leg	Adducted, flexed, Internally rotated leg	Adducted or abducted, Externally or internally rotated depending on the extent of penetration into the pelvis

Complications: Osteonecrosis (AVN) reduced risk with early reduction; Sciatic nerve injury (posterior dislocations); Femoral artery & nerve injury (anterior dislocations); Instability & recurrence; Osteoarthritis; Heterotopic ossification
Vascular sign of narath is positive in posterior dislocation of hip joint. Due to posterior dislocation, the hip joint falls on the femoral artery, and this causes feeble or absent femoral pulse.

ORTHO PLATE 21

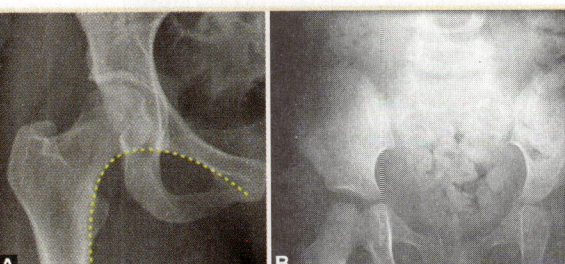
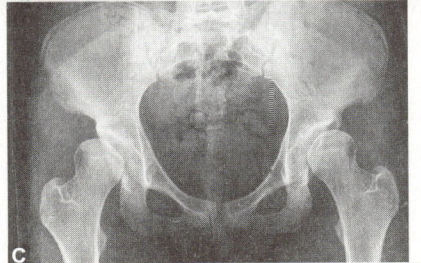

DEVELOPMENTAL DYSPLASIA OF THE HIP

A. Figure shows the normal shenton line: **Shenton line** is an imaginary line drawn along the inferior border of the superior pubic ramus (superior border of the obturator foramen) and along the inferomedial border of the neck of femur. This line should be continuous and smooth. Interruption of the Shenton line can indicates:
   • Developmental dysplasia of the hip (DDH)
   • Fractured neck of femur
B. Unilateral DDH
C. Bilateral DDH

DDH – X-rays: Numerous radiographic measurements have been used to assist in the evaluation of DDH (a typical radiographic evaluation is described in the image below). From an anteroposterior radiograph of the hips, a horizontal line (**Hilgenreiner line**) is drawn between the triradiate epiphyses. Next, lines are drawn perpendicular to the Hilgenreiner line through the superolateral edge of the acetabulum (**Perkin line**), dividing the hip into four quadrants. The proximal medial femur should be in the lower medial quadrant, or

347

the ossific nucleus of the femoral head, if present (usually observed in patients aged 4 to 7 months), should be in the lower medial quadrant.

- **The acetabular index** is the angle between the Hilgenreiner line and a line drawn from the triradiate epiphysis to the lateral edge of the acetabulum. Typically, this angle decreases with age and should measure less than 20 degrees by the time the child is 2 years old. The angle should not exceed 30°
- **The acetabular roof Shenton line** is an imaginary line drawn along the inferior border of the superior pubic ramus (superior border of the obturator foramen) and along the inferomedial border of the neck of femur. This line should be continuous and smooth.
- **Von Rosen's lines:** With the hips abducted 45° the femoral shafts should point into the acetabula. In each case the left side is shown to be abnormal.

Graf Classification			
Class	Alfa angle	Beta angle	Description
I	>60 degree	<55 degree	Normal
II	43-60 degree	55-77 degree	Delayed ossification
III	<43 degree	>77 degree	Lateralization
IV	Not measurable		Dislocation

ORTHO PLATE 22

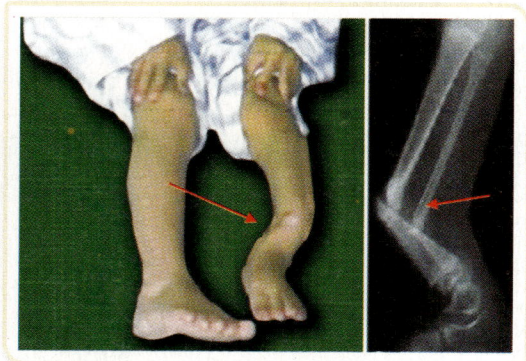

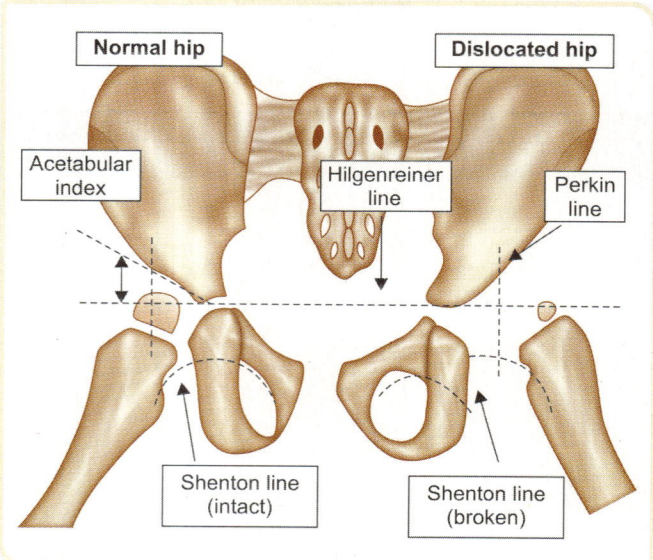

Ultrasound scanning has replaced radiography for imaging hips in the newborn. **Ultrasound is the test of choice in the infant (<6 months)** as the proximal femoral epiphysis has not yet significantly ossified. The radiographically 'invisible' acetabulum and femoral head can, with practice, be displayed with static and dynamic ultrasound

Alpha angle: Angle formed by the acetabular roof to the vertical cortex of the ilium. This is a similar measurement as that of the acetabular angle. The normal value is greater than or equal to 60 degrees.

Beta angle: Angle formed between the vertical cortex of the ilium and the triangular labral fibrocartilage (echogenic triangle). The normal value is less than 77 degrees, but is only useful in assessing immature hips when combined with the alpha angle.

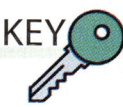

CONGENITAL TIBIAL PSEUDOARTHROSIS

Congenital tibial pseudoarthrosis of the tibia describes abnormal bowing that can progress to a segment of bone loss simulating the appearance of a false joint. Overall, 10% of patients with NF1 are diagnosed with tibial pseudoarthrosis.

ORTHO PLATE 23

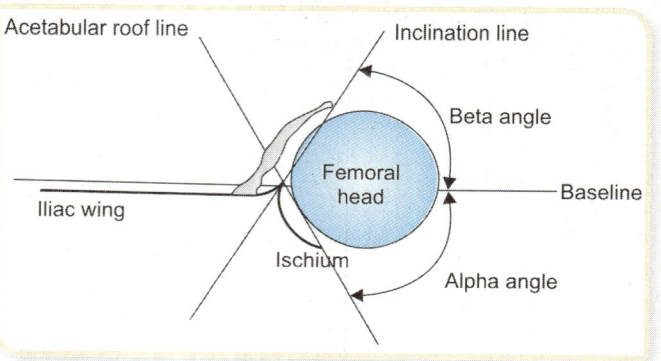

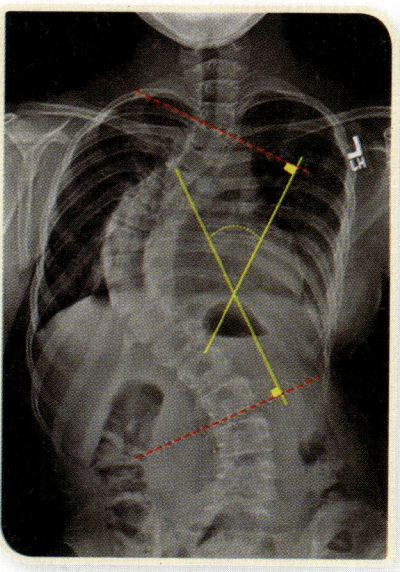

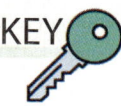

COBB'S ANGLE IN SCOLIOSIS

Scoliosis is defined as a lateral deviation of the normal vertical line of the spine. Scoliosis also can be classified based on the etiology. Idiopathic scoliosis is the most common type, but the exact etiology is unknown. Congenital scoliosis is caused by a failure in vertebral formation or segmentation of the involved vertebrae

The most common quantification of scoliosis is the Cobb angle. The Cobb angle was first described in 1948 by American orthopedic surgeon John R Cobb (1903-1967). Measurement consists of three steps: (1) locating the superior end vertebra, (2) locating the inferior end vertebra, and (3) drawing intersecting perpendicular lines from the superior surface of the superior end vertebra and from the inferior. The angle of deviation of these perpendicular lines from a straight line is the angle of the curve. If the endplates are obscured, the pedicles can be used instead.

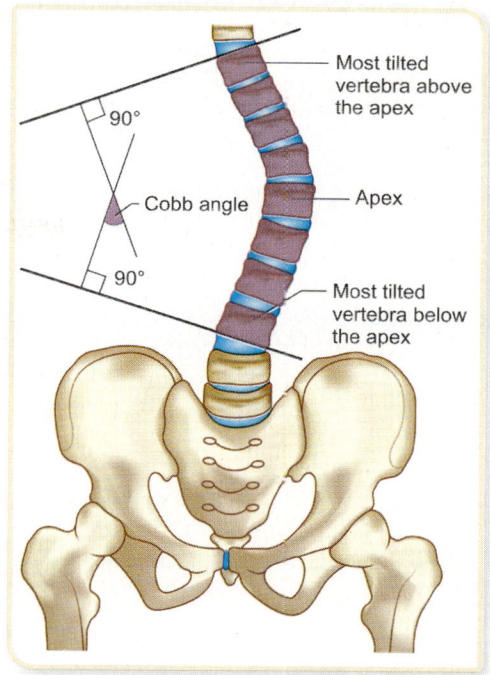

Cobb angle	Definition
0°–10°	Spinal curve
10°–20°	Mild scoliosis
20°–40°	Moderate scoliosis
>40°	Severe scoliosis

ORTHO PLATE 24

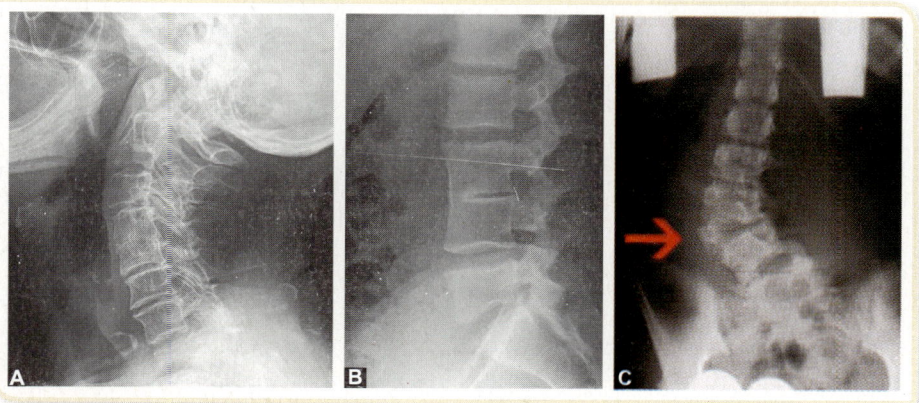

VERTEBRAL ANOMALIES

A. Block vertebra of C4 C5 cervical vertebrae
B. Partial block vertebra of L3- L4 lumbar vertebrae
C. Hemivertebrae are wedge-shaped vertebrae and therefore can cause an angle in the spine (kyphosis, scoliosis, and lordosis). Among the congenital vertebral anomalies, hemivertebrae are the most likely to cause neurologic problems. The most common location is the midthoracic vertebrae, especially T8

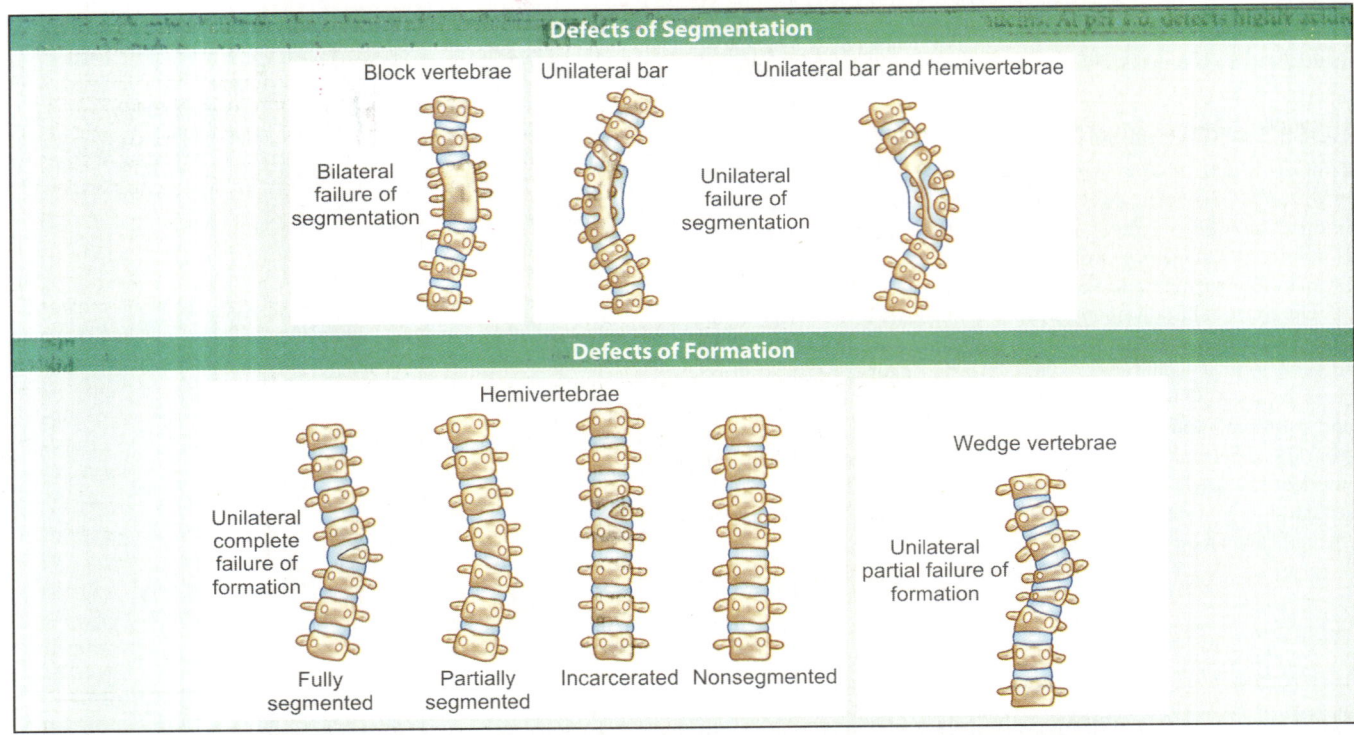

ORTHO PLATE 25

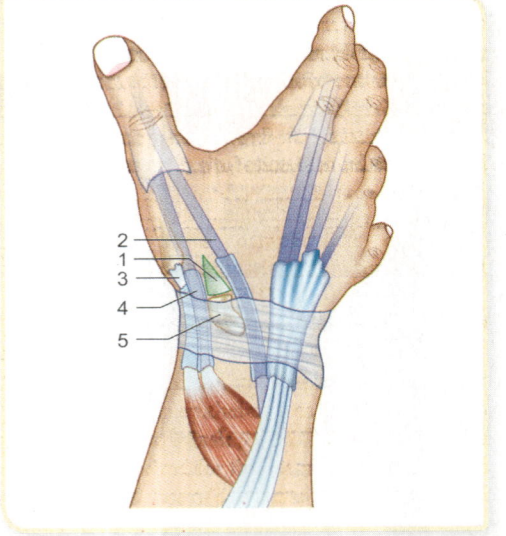

ANATOMICAL SNUFF BOX
1. Anatomical snuff box
2. Extensor pollicis brevis[NEET PG]
3. Abductor pollicis longus[NEET PG]
4. Extensor pollicis brevis
5. Scaphoid

De Quervain's Tenosynovitis

When the extensor pollicis brevis and the abductor pollicis longus tendons in the first dorsal compartment are affected, the condition is named after the Swiss physician Fritz de Quervain, who described his experience in 1895. The cause is almost always related to overuse, either in the home or at work, or is associated with rheumatoid arthritis. The presenting symptoms usually are pain and tenderness at the radial styloid. Sometimes a thickening of the fibrous sheath is palpable. **Finkelstein test** (most pathognomonic objective but not diagnostic) is usually positive. Technique: Ulnar deviation to the wrist while grasping the thumb. Interpretation: Pain over radial styloid = de Quervain's tenosynovitis.

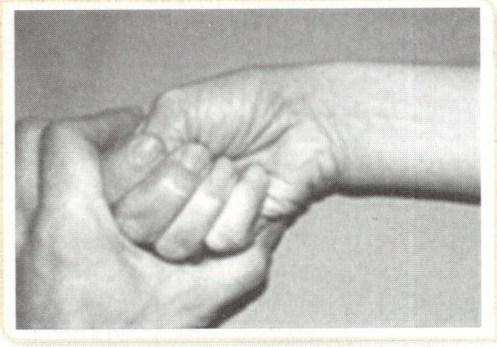

Fig: Finkelstein test

ORTHO PLATE 26

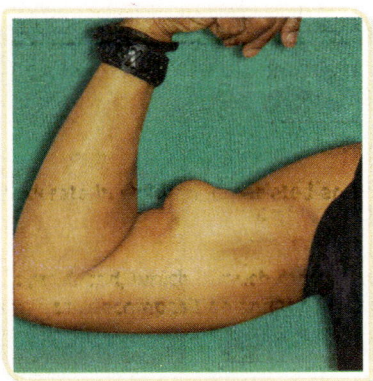

POPEYE DEFORMITY

Acute proximal long head of biceps tendon rupture is classically associated with the bulbous palpable mass near the elbow or in the mid-upper arm which becomes prominent on elbow flexion, this is known as "Popeye deformity".

The deformity is named after the famous cartoon character Popeye

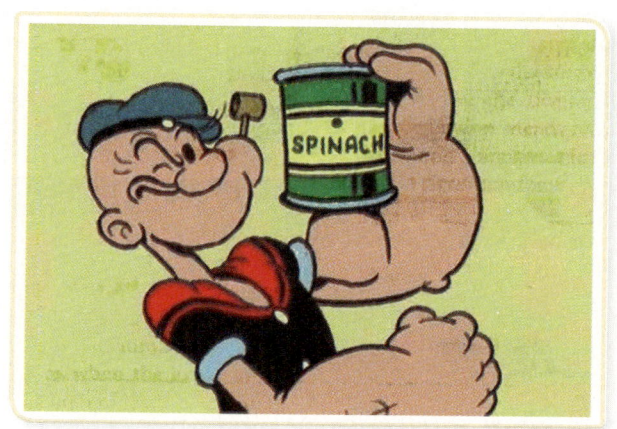

ORTHO PLATE 27

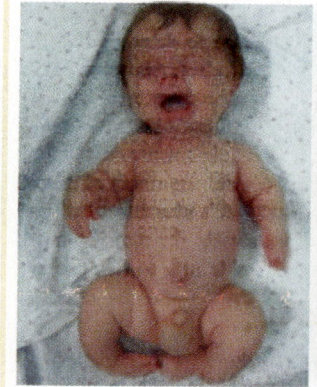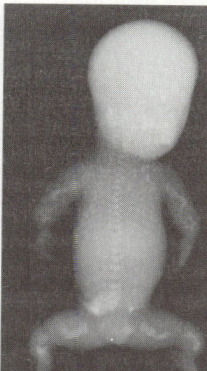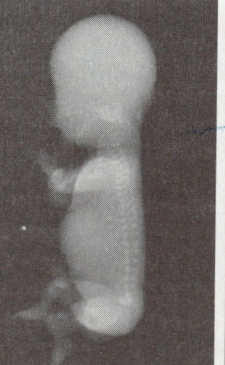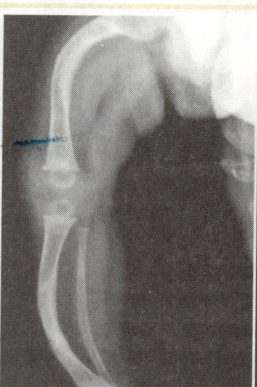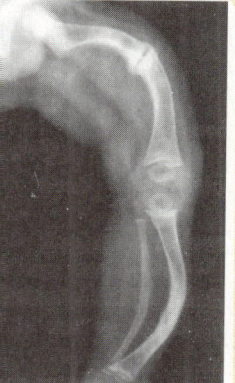

© Georgescu I et al

OSTEOGENESIS IMPERFECTA

Osteogenesis imperfecta refers to a heterogeneous group of congenital, non-sex-linked, genetic disorders. It is characterized by bone fragility resulting from abnormal quality and/or quantity of type I collagen. Generalized osteoporosis, Kyphoscoliosis, bowing of long bones, multiple fractures, Wormian bones, slender and twisted long bones with sclerosis of the metaphyseal ends, bowing of long bones, periosteal thickening and bilateral dislocation of the radial heads.

ORTHO PLATE 28

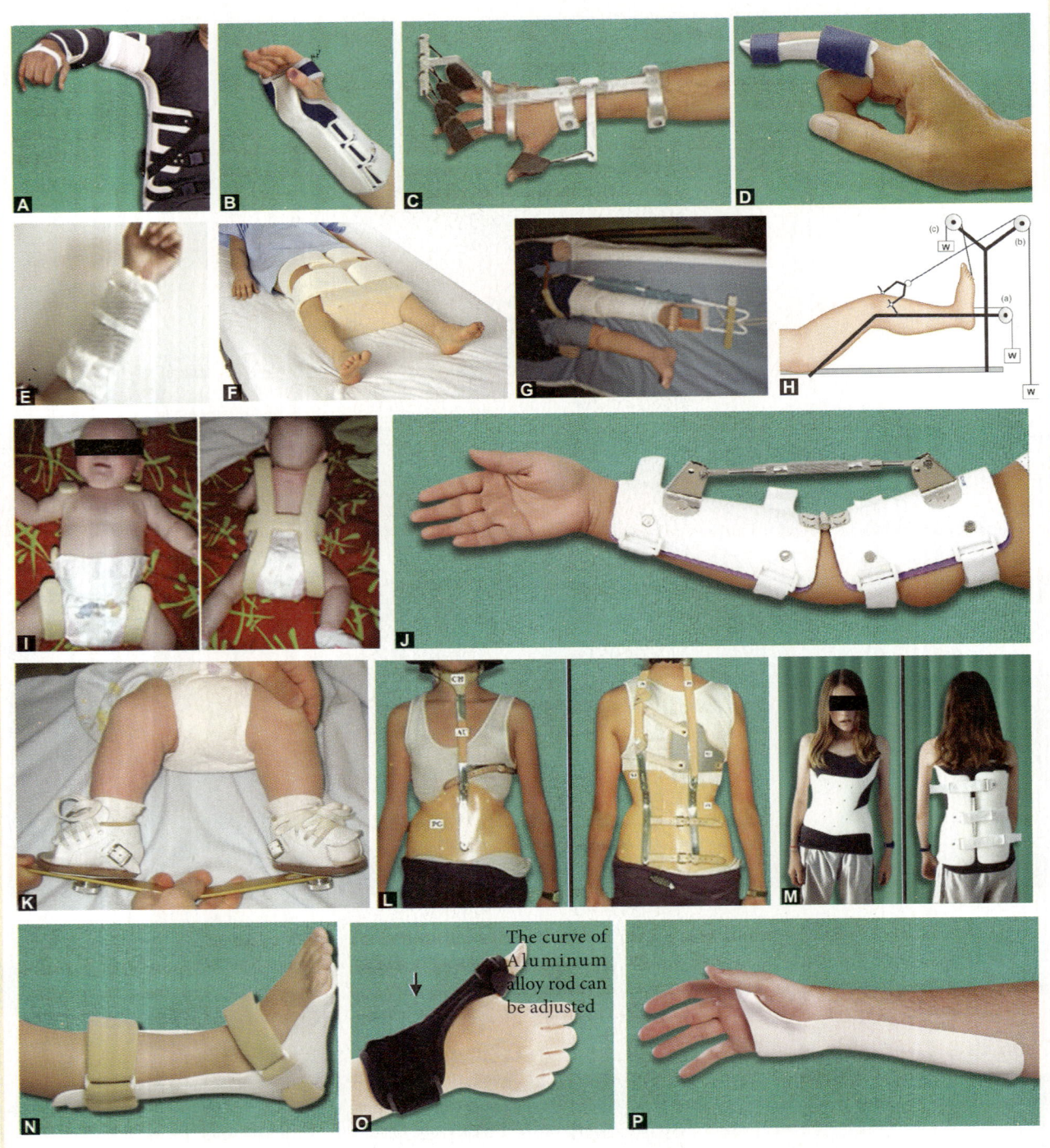

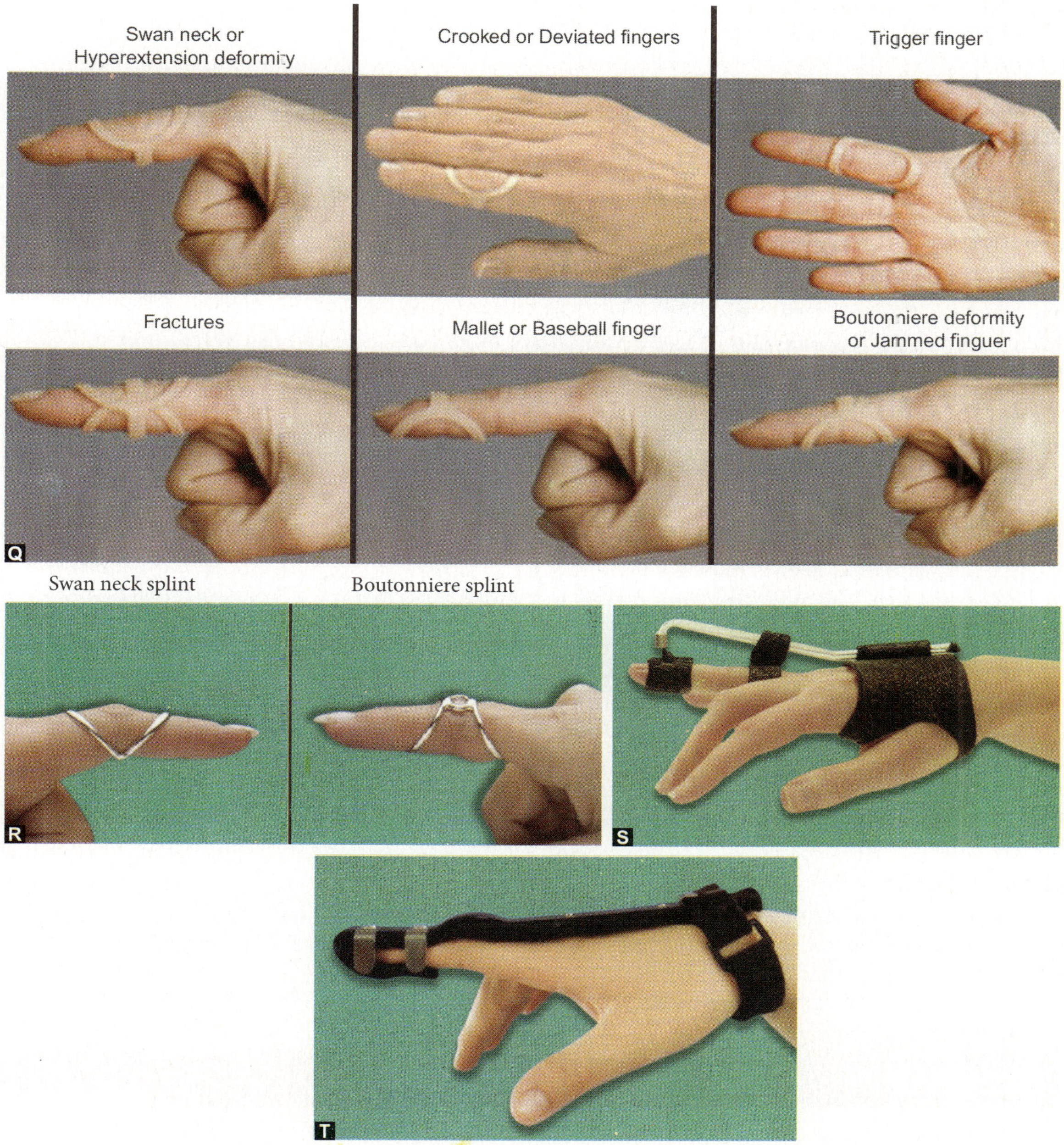

SPLINTS IN ORTHOPEDICS

A. **Aeroplane splint:** Also known as arm abduction splint. Keeps arm in 90-degree abduction, Used in Brachial plexus injury
B. **Cock up splint** used in wrist drop i.e. radial nerve injury
C. **Dynamic cock up splint** used in wrist drop i.e. radial nerve injury
D. **Aluminum splint:** Used for Finger immobilization
E. **Cramer wire splint:** Used in Emergency immobilization
F. **Triangular pillow splint:** Used to keep hip abducted and neutrally rotated
G. **Thomas knee splint:** Used for knee immobilization, femur fracture
H. **Bohler brown splint:** (3 pulley- Proximal pulley to prevent foot drop, 2nd pulley for traction in line with femur, 3rd Pulley for traction in line with the leg). Used in Femur fracture (proximal)
I. **Von Rosen splint:** Used in Developmental dysplasia of Hip
J. **Volkman's turn buckle splint:** Used in Volkmann's ischemic contracture
K. **Dennis brown splint:** Used in CTEV
L. **Milwaukee brace:** It was developed in 1940. It is made of plastic and metal to span the entire length of the spine from neck to pelvis. Most commonly used scoliosis brace post-surgical treatment.
M. **Boston brace:** Developed in 1972, it lacks the metal components of the Milwaukee brace. This brace is most commonly used with adolescents undergoing a non-surgical treatment of Scoliosis

N. **Toe raising/ foot drop splint:** Used in Common peroneal / Sciatic nerve palsy
O. **Radial gutter splint or Dr Quervain's splint:** used for Quervain's Tenosynovitis
P. **Ulnar gutter splint:** Used for Boxer (5th Metacarpal) fracture
Q. **Oval 8 finger splint:** Ready-made splint available in different sizes and made of molded plastic. Applies 3 point of control for support, correct and protect the finger joint. Applied in different locations to treat multiple finger conditions like arthritis, mallet finger, trigger finger, boutonniere deformity, crooked fingers or fractures, all with the same splint.
R. **Silver Ring Splints** are custom made splints of silver with double-loop design that fit comfortably on the finger. Applied in different locations to treat Swan neck splint (prevent PIP hyperextension), Boutonniere splint (immobilize IP in extension) and Realignment splint.
S. **Bunnell Finger extension splint:** Used for reducing swan neck deformity
T. **Dynamic finger splint:** with positive pressure. Used for reducing swan neck deformity

 ORTHO PLATE 29

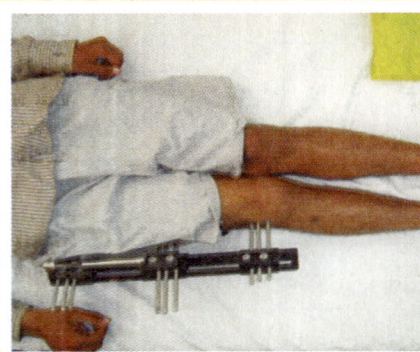 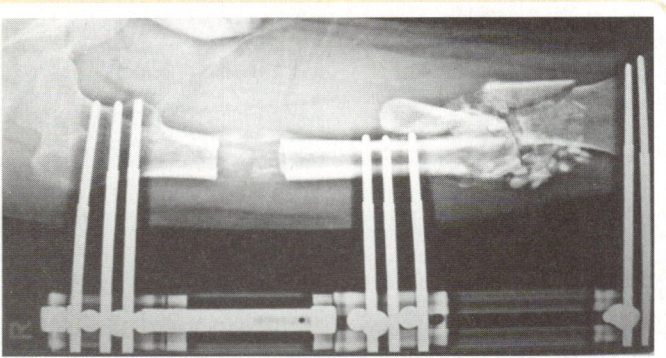

RAIL EXTERNAL FIXATOR AIIMS PG

This is monolateral external fixator available in the form of a rail or a telescoping multi joint assembly. This is used for bone lengthening and tension is supplied through the external fixator gradually distracting the bone ends, normally at a rate of 1mm per day. It can also be used for deformity correction.

 ORTHO PLATE 30

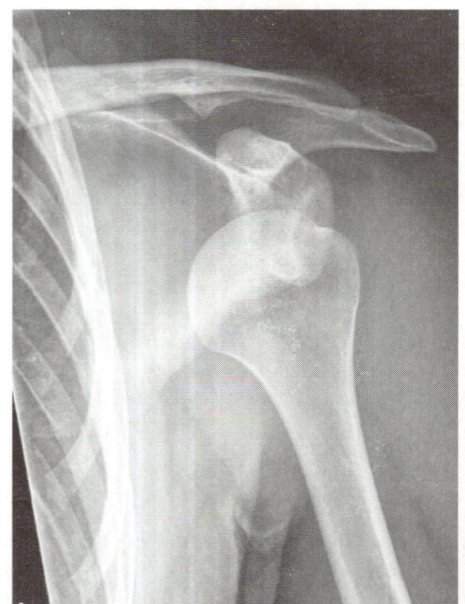 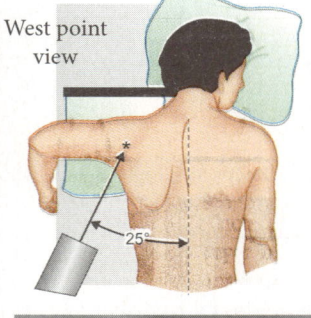 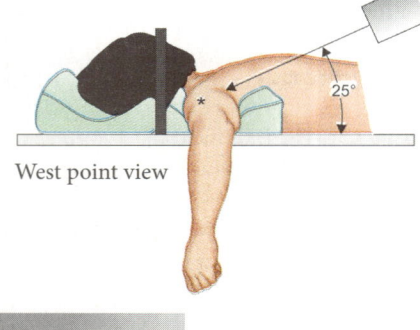

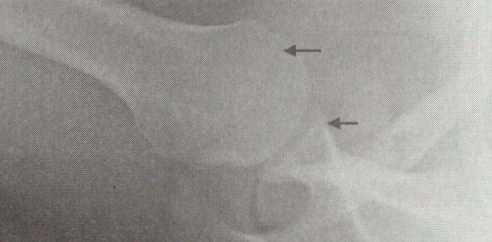

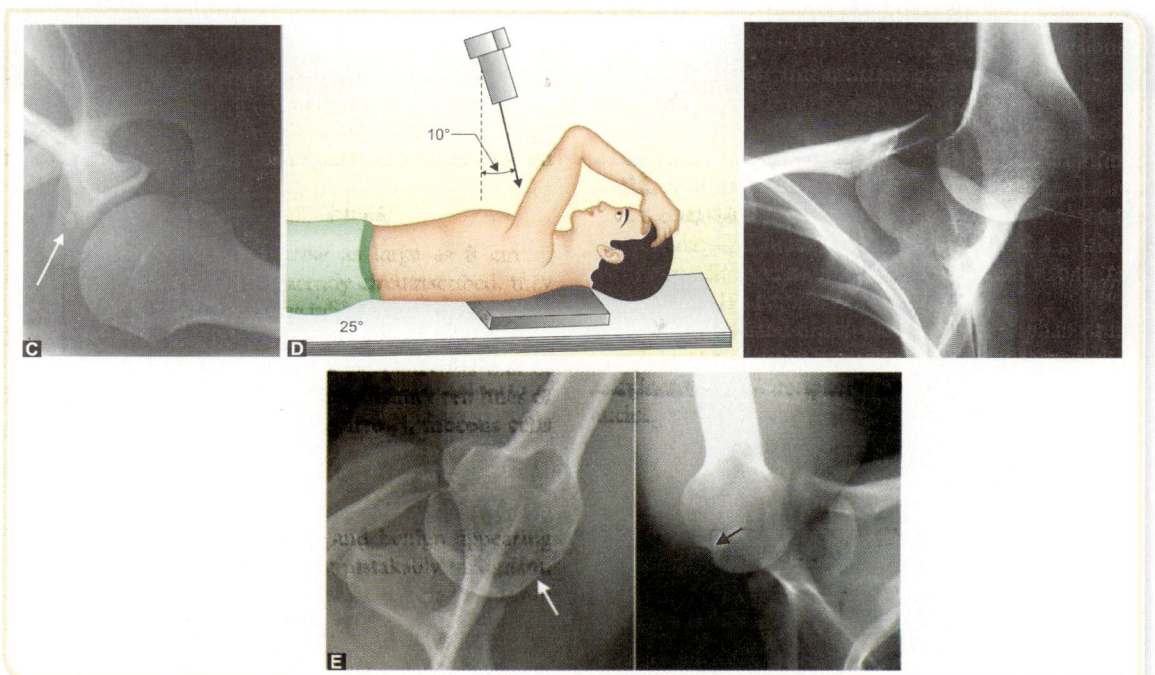

ANTERIOR DISLOCATION OF SHOULDER JOINT

A. **Anterior dislocation of shoulder joint** [AIIMSPG]: Complications may include a Bankart lesion, Hill-Sachs lesion, rotator cuff tear, or injury to the axillary nerve.
B. **West point view x ray of shoulder joint:** Normal anatomy
C. **West Point axillary view is used to evaluate bony Bankart lesions**: It is used to evaluate the glenoid. This radiograph reveals an avulsion of the anteroinferior corner of the glenoid (bony Bankart lesion; arrow)
D. **Stryker notch view:** Normal anatomy. X-Ray Beam is directed from anterior to posterior, centered at the coracoid and angled 10-degrees cephalad.
E. **Stryker notch view demonstrates Hill-Sachs lesion:** defect in posterolateral humeral head as minimal flattening (first image) and defect (2nd image) of the posterolateral contour of the humeral head (arrow).

ORTHO PLATE 31

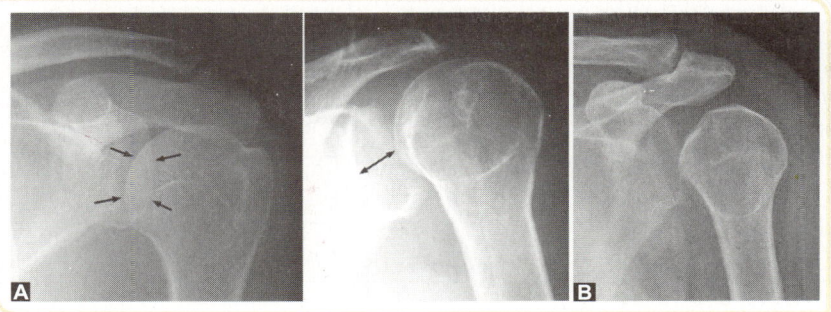

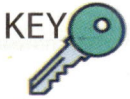

POSTERIOR DISLOCATION OF SHOULDER JOINT

A. **Half moon sign:** Normally the medial part of the head of the humerus overlaps the glenoid fossa to form a shadow shaped like a half-moon which reaches down to the inferior border of the fossa. This disappears in posterior dislocation.
B. **Lightbulb sign** is seen in AP radiograph appearance of the humeral head in posterior shoulder dislocation. The humerus head internally rotates such that the head contour projects like a light bulb when viewed from the front.

Notes

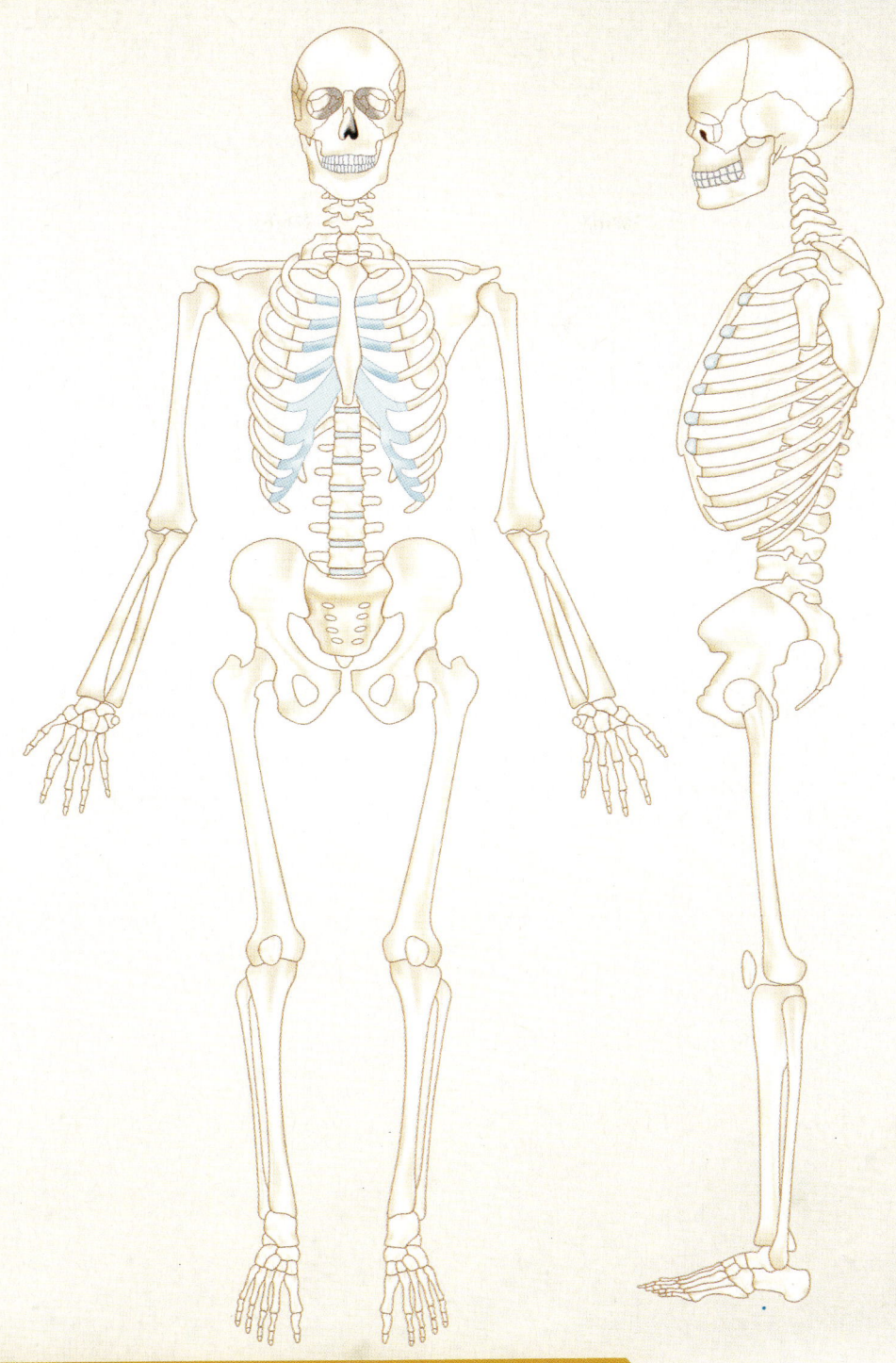

OSTEOLOGY

OSTEO PLATE 1

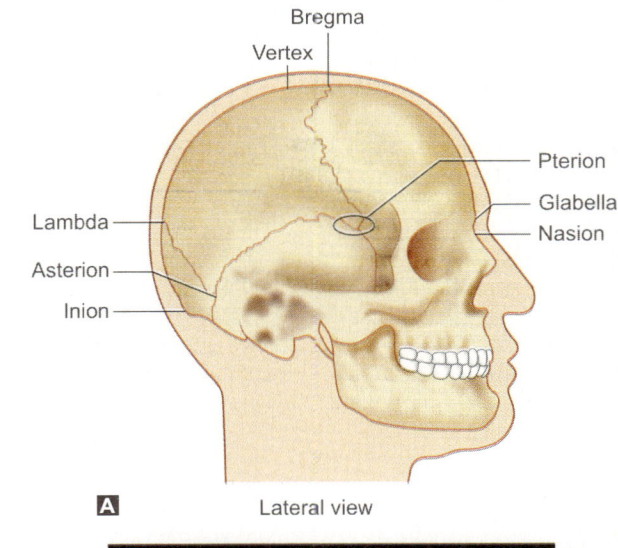

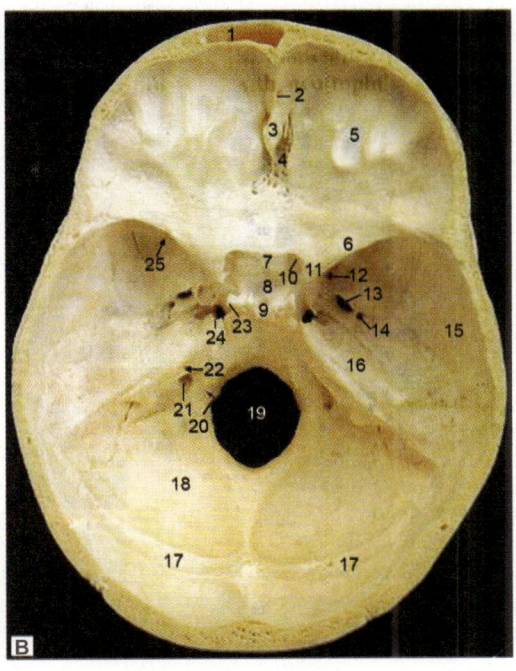

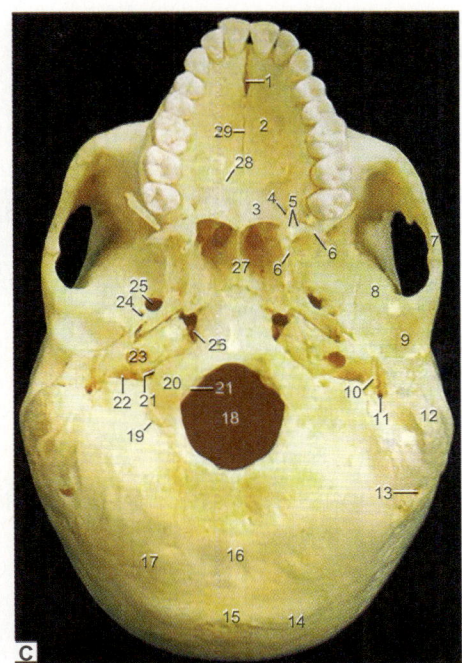

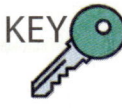

PLATE LEGENDS

A. Craniometric points on Lateral view of the skull

Pterion[NEETPG]- Junction of greater wing of sphenoid, squamous temporal parietal and frontal bone. Overlies the course of middle meningeal artery[NEETPG]

Lambda- Junction of lambdoid and sagittal sutures

Bregma- Junction of coronal and sagittal suture

Glabella- Smooth prominence in frontal bone superior to the root of nose. Most anterior projecting part of forehead.

Nasion- Junction of frontonasal and internasal sutures.

Asterion- Star shaped. Located at the junction of 3 sutures namely; Parietomastoid, Occipitomastoid and lambdoid suture.

B. Legends	C. Legends
1. Frontal sinus 2. Foramen cecum 3. Crista galli 4. Cribriform plate 5. Anterior Cranial Fossa 6. Lesser Wing of Sphenoid 7. Chiasmatic Groove 8. Sella Turcica 9. Dorsum Sella 10. Optic Canal 11. Anterior Clinoid Process 12. Foramen Rotundum 13. Foramen Ovale 14. Foramen Spinosum 15. Squamous Part of Temporal Bone 16. Petrous Part of Temporal bone 17. Groove for Transverse Sinus 18. Posterior Cranial Fossa 19. Foramen Magnum 20. Hypoglossal Canal 21. Jugular Foramen 22. Internal Acoustic Meatus 23. Posterior Clinoid Process 24. Foramen Lacerum 25. Superior Orbital Fissure	1. Anterior Palatine Foramen 2. Palatine Process of Maxilla 3. Palatine 4. Greater Palatine Foramen 5. Lesser Palatine Foramen 6. Pterygoid Processes of Sphenoid 7. Zygomatic Process 8. Squamous Part of Temporal Bone 9. Mandibular Fossa 10. Styloid Process 11. Stylomastoid Foramen 12. Mastoid Process 13. Mastoid Foramen 14. Superior Nuchal Line 15. External Occipital Protuberance 16. Median Nuchal Line 17. Inferior Nuchal Line 18. Foramen Magnum 19. Condyloid Canal 20. Occipital Condyle 21. Hypoglossal Canal 22. Jugular Foramen 23. Carotid Canal 24. Foramen Spinosum 25. Foramen Ovale 26. Foramen Lacerum 27. Vomer 28. Transverse Palatine Suture 29. Median Palatine Suture

Foramina of the Skull

Bone	Foramina	Vessels	Nerves
Foramina in the anterior cranial fossa			
Ethmoid	Cribriform Plate		Olfactory Nerve
Frontal	Foramen Cecum	Emissary Veins to Superior Sagittal Sinus	-
Ethmoid	Anterior Ethmoidal Foramen	Anterior Ethmoidal Vessels	Anterior Ethmoidal Nerve
Ethmoid	Posterior Ethmoidal Foramen	Posterior Ethmoidal Vessels	Posterior Ethmoidal Nerve
Foramina in the middle cranial fossa			
Sphenoid	Optic Canal	Ophthalmic Artery Central retinal artery & vein	Optic Nerve (II)
Sphenoid	Superior Orbital Fissure	Superior Ophthalmic Vein	Oculomotor Nerve (III), Trochlear Nerve (IV), Lacrimal, Frontal & nasociliary branches of ophthalmic nerve (V_1), Abducent Nerve (VI)
Sphenoid and maxilla	Inferior Orbital Fissure	Inferior ophthalmic veins, Infraorbital vessels	Zygomatic Nerve, Infraorbital branch of maxillary Nerve (V_2), Orbital Branches of pterygopalatine Ganglion
Sphenoid	Foramen Rotundum	-	Maxillary division of trigeminal nerve (CN V_2)
Sphenoid	Foramen Ovale (Mnemonic: OVALE)	**A**ccessory Meningeal Artery, **E**missary veins	**O**tic ganglion, Mandibular division of trigeminal nerve (V_3) **L**esser Petrosal Nerve (Occasionally)
Sphenoid	Foramen Spinosum	Middle Meningeal Artery	Meningeal Branch of The Mandibular Nerve (V_3)
Sphenoid	Foramen Lacerum	Internal Carotid Artery, Artery of Pterygoid Canal	Nerve Of Pterygoid Canal, Greater and deep petrosal nerve
	Carotid canal	Internal carotid artery	Sympathetic carotid plexus
	Hiatus of facial canal		Greater petrosal nerve

Contd...

		Foramina in the Posterior cranial fossa	
Temporal	**Internal Acoustic Meatus/canal:** [Vertical crest (AKA- **Bill's bar**) divides the superior compartment of IAC into anterior & posterior compartment. The transverse crest (AKA- **crista falciformis**) divides upper 2 quadrants from lower 2 quadrants	Labyrinthine artery, occasionally by branches of the anterior inferior cerebellar artery (AICA) or a loop of the AICA itself	Five nerves pass through the internal auditory canal (IAC): **Anteriosuperior quadrant:** Facial (motor root), nervus intermedius (sensory component of Facial nerve) **Anteroinferior quadrant:** Cochlear nerve **Posterosuperior quadrant:** Superior vestibular nerve **Posteroinferior quadrant:** Inferior vestibular nerve (**Mnemonic:** 7up- 7th cranial nerve is Up/superior, Coke - Cochlear nerve is down/inferior)
Temporal	Jugular Foramen (**Mnemonic:** Juggles with three cranial nerves; 9, 10, 11)	Anterior part: Inferior Petrosal Sinus Middle part: Meningeal branch of Ascending Pharyngeal Artery Posterior part: Internal Jugular vein, Inferior Petrosal Sinus, Sigmoid Sinus	Middle part: Glossopharyngeal Nerve (IX), Vagus nerve (X), Spinal accessory Nerve (XI)
Occipital	Hypoglossal Canal	Meningeal artery	Hypoglossal Nerve (XII)
Occipital	Foramen Magnum	Anterior and Posterior Spinal arteries, Vertebral arteries, venous plexus of vertebral canal.	Medulla Oblongata, Ascending Spinal Fibers of Accessory Nerve (XI)
	Condyloid foramen	condyloid emissary vein	
	Mastoid foramen	Branch of occipital artery to dura mater, Mastoid emissary vein	
		Foramina in the front of the skull	
Frontal	Supraorbital Foramen	Supraorbital vessels	Supraorbital Nerve
Maxilla	Infraorbital Foramen	Infraorbital vessels	Infraorbital Nerve
	Mental foramen	Mental vessels	Mental nerve
	Zygomatico facial foramen		Zygomaticofacial nerve

Contd...

Foramina in the base of the skull

Bone	Foramen	Vessels	Nerve
Temporal	Stylomastoid Foramen	Stylomastoid Artery	Facial Nerve
Temporal	Petrotympanic fissure	Anterior tympanic artery (often)	Chorda tympani
Maxilla	Incisive Foramen/ Incisive Canal	Terminal part of sphenopalatine or greater palatine vessels	Nasopalatine nerve(V_2)
Palatine	Greater Palatine Foramen	Greater Palatine vessels	Greater Palatine nerve
Palatine and maxilla	Lesser Palatine Foramina	Lesser Palatine vessels	Lesser Palatine nerve
	Palatine canal	Descending palatine vessels	Greater and lesser palatine nerves
	Pterygoid canal		Nerve of the pterygoid canal (Vidian nerve)
	Sphenopalatine foramen	Sphenopalatine vessels	Nasopalatine nerve

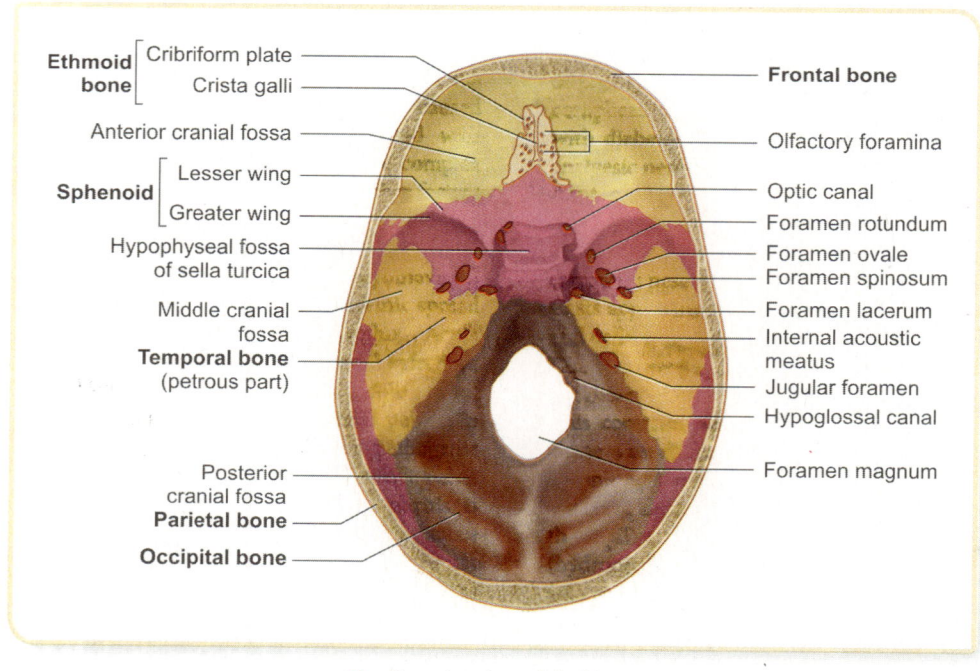

Fig: Superior view of skull base

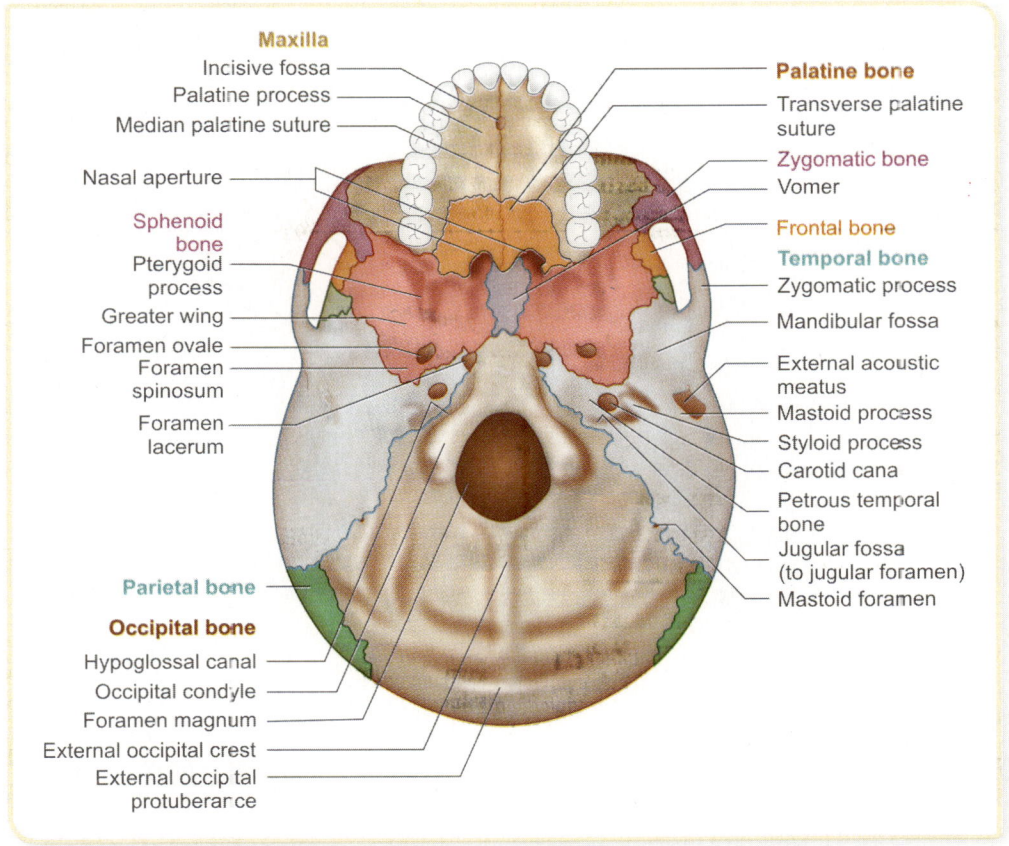

Fig: Inferior surface of skull

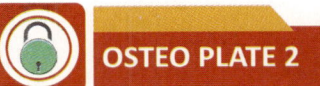

OSTEO PLATE 2

4. Ramus
5. Angle
6. Oblique Line
7. Body
8. Alveolar Process
9. Mental Foramen
10. Mylohyoid Line/Grove
11. Mandibular Foramen[NEETPG]

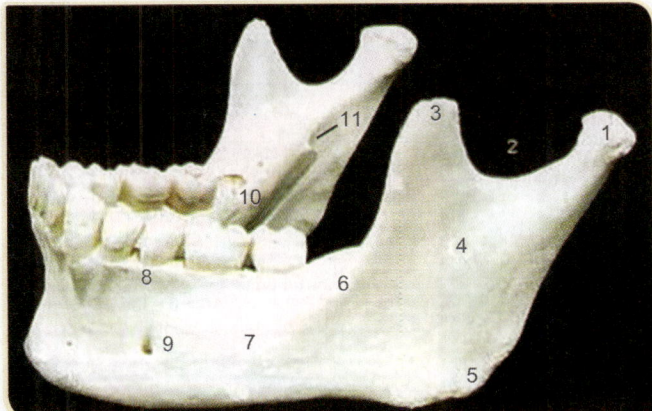

MANDIBLE SUPERIOR ANTERIOLATERAL VIEW
1. Mandibular Condyle
2. Mandibular Notch
3. Coronoid Process

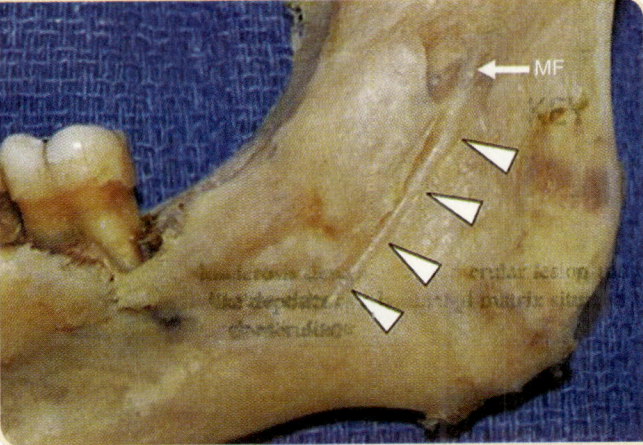

Fig: Medial view of the right mandible and mylohyoid groove (arrow heads). MF= mandibular foramen

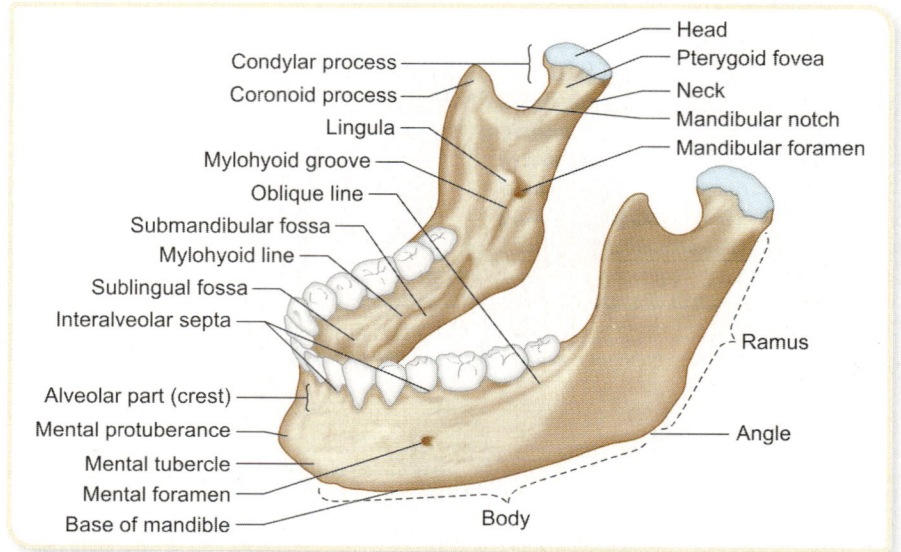

Fig: Mandible superioanterior lateral view (Labelled)

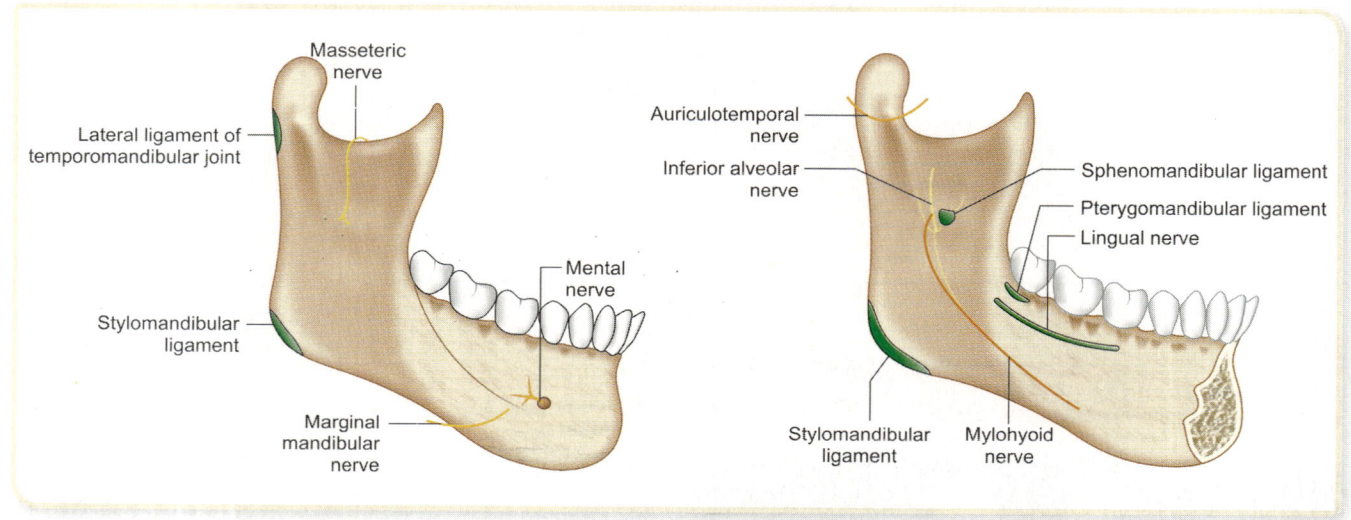

OSTEO PLATE 3

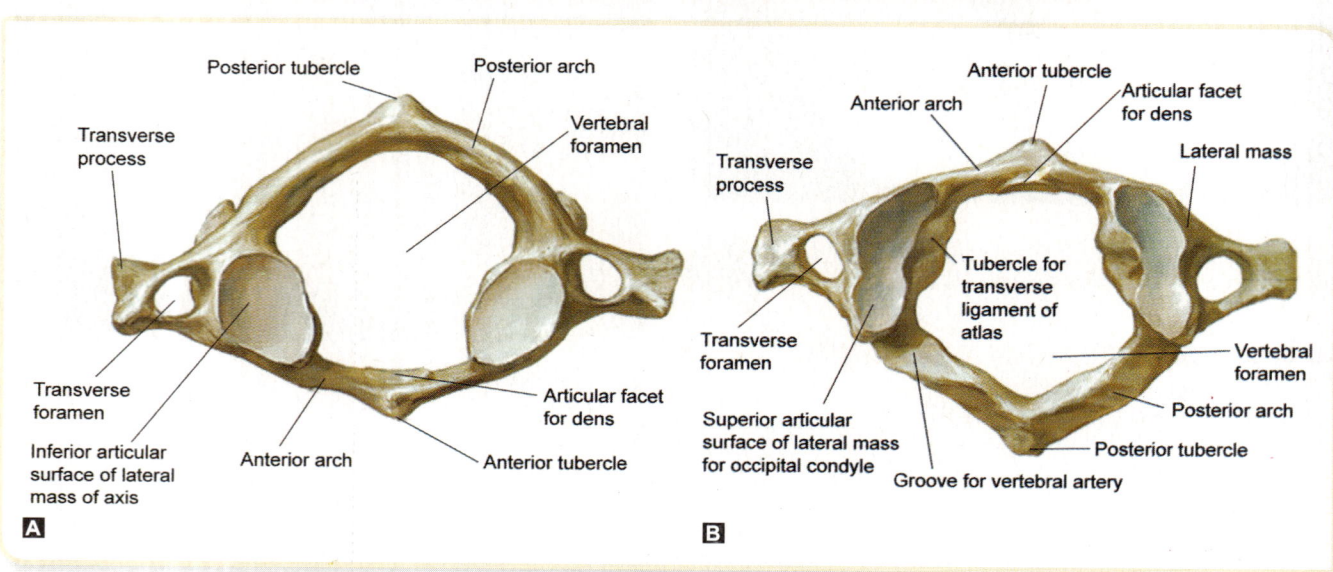

ATLAS (C1) INFERIOR AND SUPERIOR VIEW

A. Atlas (C1) inferior view (Labeled)
B. Atlas (C1) superior view (Labeled) - with groove for vertebral artery[AIIMSPG]

OSTEO PLATE 4

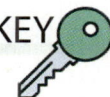

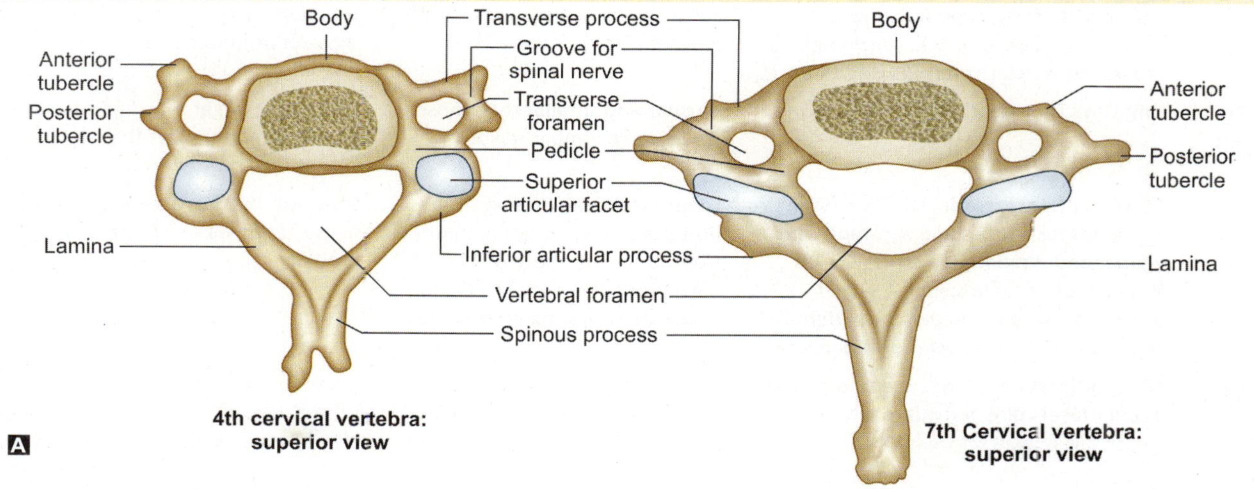

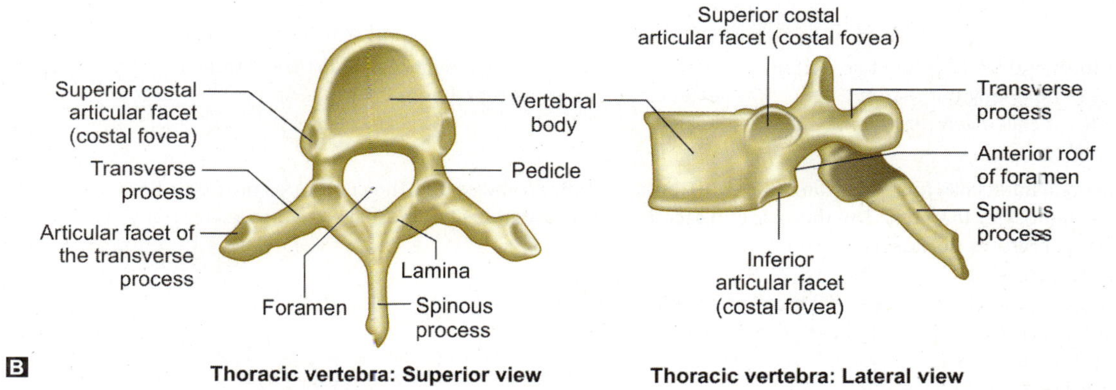

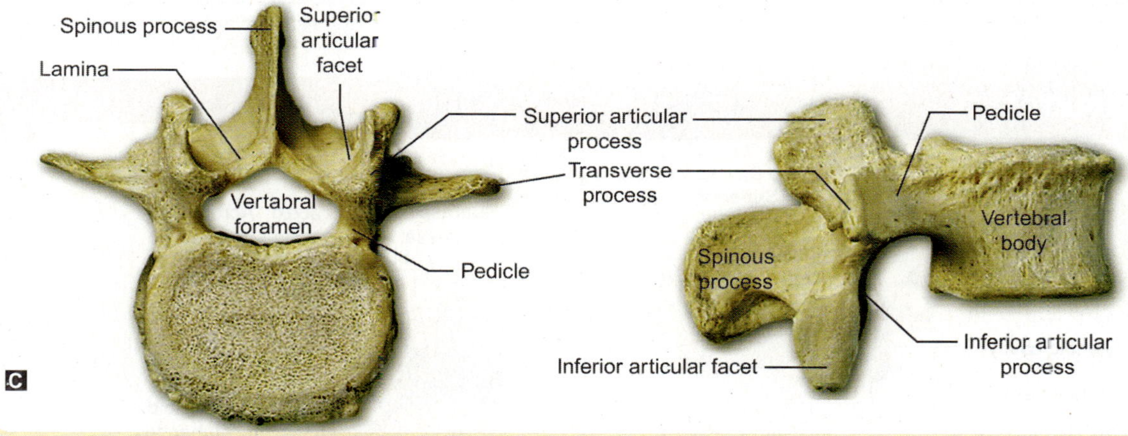

CERVICAL, THORACIC AND LUMBAR VERTEBRA

A. Cervical vertebra labelled
B. Thoracic vertebra labelled
C. Lumbar vertebra labelled

Vertebral Column			
The adult vertebral column typically consists of 33 vertebrae arranged in five regions: 7 cervical, 12 thoracic, 5 lumbar, 5 sacral, and 4 coccygeal			
	Cervical vertebrae (C1 -C7)	**Thoracic vertebrae (T1 -T12)**	**Lumbar vertebrae**
Body	Small and wider from side to side than anteroposteriorly; superior surface is concave between adjacent (uncinate) processes; inferior surface is convex	**Heart-shaped**; bears one or two costal facets for articulation with head of rib (H)	Massive; **kidney-shaped** when viewed superiorly; larger and heavier than those of other regions
Vertebral foramen	Large and triangular	**Circular and smaller** than those in cervical and lumbar regions	**Triangular**; larger than in thoracic vertebrae and smaller than in cervical vertebrae
Transverse processes	**Foramina transversaria**; small or absent in C7; vertebral arteries and accompanying venous and sympathetic plexuses pass through foramina (except C7, which transmits only small accessory vertebral veins); anterior and posterior tubercles	Long and strong; extends posterolaterally; length diminishes from T1 to T12; those of T1-T10 have transverse costal facets for articulation with tubercle of rib	Long and slender; accessory process on posterior surface of base of each process
Articular processes	Superior facets directed superoposteriorly; inferior facets directed inferoanteriorly	Superior articular facets directed posteriorly and slightly laterally; inferior articular facets directed anteriorly and slightly medially	Superior articular facets directed posteromedially (or medially); inferior articular facets directed anterolaterally (or laterally); mammillary process on posterior surface of each superior articular process
Spinous process	C3-C5 short and bifid (split in two parts); process of C6 is long but that of C7 is longer (C7 is called *vertebra prominens*)	Long; slopes posteroinferiorly; tip extends to level of vertebral body below	Short and sturdy; hatchet-shaped

Footnote:
- The vertebral column in adults has four curvatures: cervical, thoracic, lumbar, and sacral. The curvatures provide a flexible support (shockabsorbing resilience) for the body. The **thoracic** and **sacral** (pelvic) **curvatures** (**kyphoses**) are concave anteriorly, whereas the **cervical** and **lumbar curvatures** (**lordoses**) are concave posteriorly
- C2 is strongest cervical vertebra
- Process of C6 is long but that of C7 is longer (C7 is called **vertebra prominens**)
- Most visible spinous process C7 (C7 is called **vertebra prominens**)
- Most prominent spinous process T1
- C1 has no spinous process

OSTEO PLATE 5

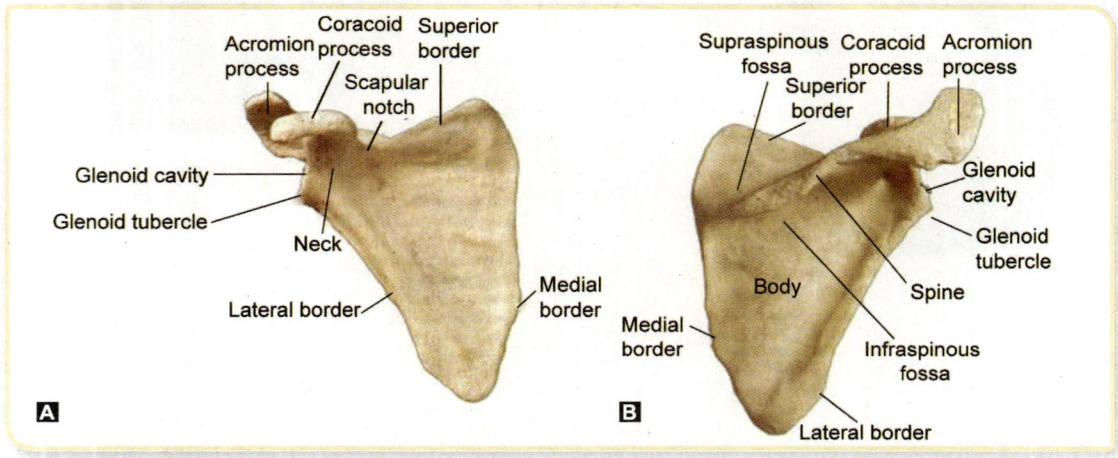

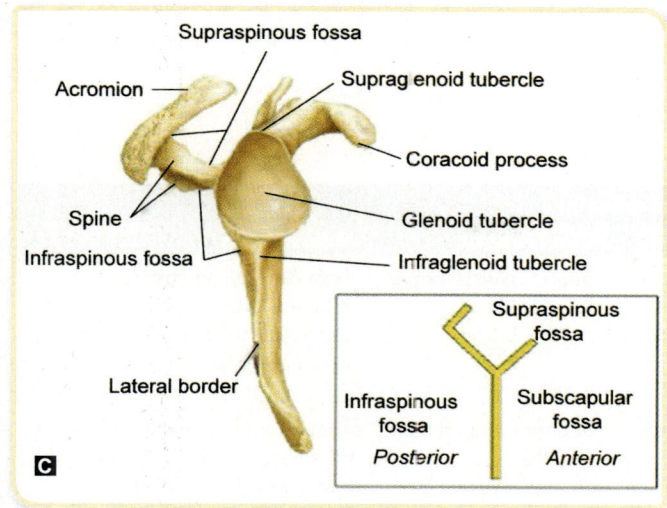

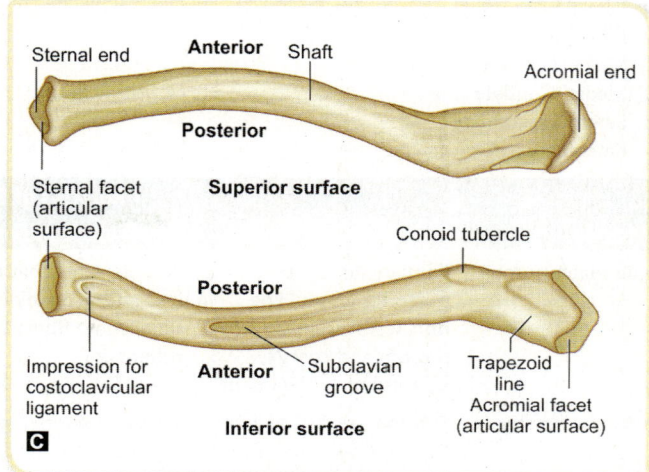

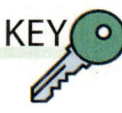

SCAPULA BONE

The scapula is a large, flat, triangular bone which lies on the posterolateral aspect of the chest wall, covering parts of the 2nd to 7th ribs. It has **2 surfaces**; costal and dorsal, **3 borders**; superior, lateral and medial, and **3 angles**; inferior, superior and lateral angles, and **3 processes**, the spine, its continuation, the acromion and the coracoid process.

A. Costal surface of scapula (labelled): costal surface can easily be distinguished from the dorsal surface, which is interrupted by the shelf-like projection of the spine.
B. Dorsal surface of scapula (labelled)
C. Lateral border of scapula showing Glenoid cavity (labelled)

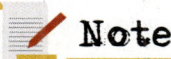

Coracoid process can be palpated subcutaneously[AIIMSPG]

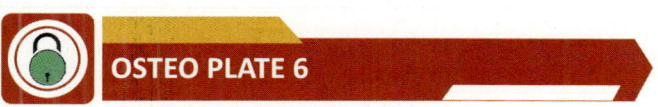

CLAVICLE

A. Right clavicle superior surface
B. Right clavicle inferior surface
C. Right clavicle superior and inferior surface (labelled).

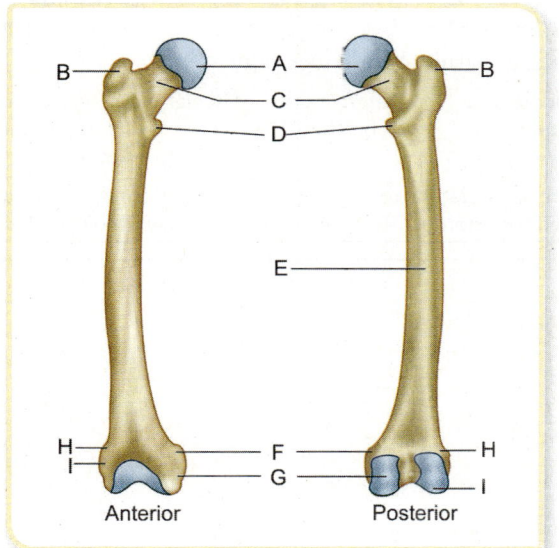

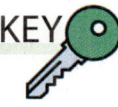

FEMUR

A. Head
B. Greater trochanter [AIIMSPG] (Muscles attached to greater trochanter are gluteus medius and minimus both of which abducts and medially rotates thigh)
C. Neck

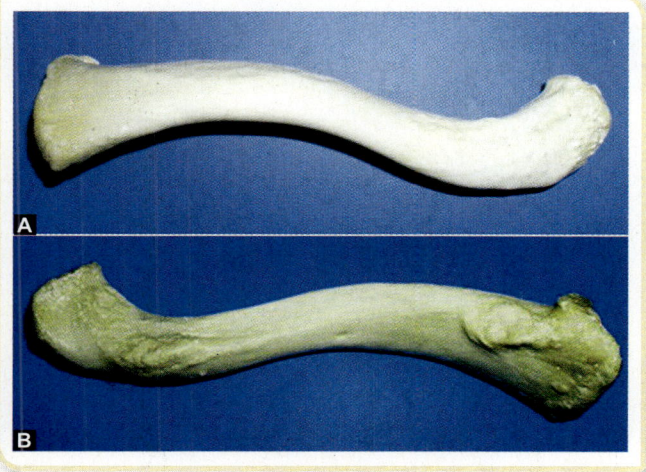

367

D. Lesser trochanter
E. Linea Aspera
F. Medical epicondyle
G. Medial Condyle
H. Lateral epicondyle
I. Lateral condyle

| Muscles of Gluteal Region |||||
Muscle	Proximal attachment	Distal attachment	Innervation	Main actions
Gluteus maximus	Ilium posterior to posterior gluteal line, dorsal surface of sacrum and coccyx, sacrotuberous ligament	Iliotibial tract that inserts into lateral condyle of tibia; some fibers to gluteal tuberosity	Inferior gluteal nerve (L5, **S1, S2**)	Extends thigh and assists in lateral rotation; steadies thigh and assists in raising trunk from flexed position
Gluteus medius	External surface of ilium between anterior and posterior gluteal lines; gluteal fascia	Lateral surface of greater trochanter of femur	Superior gluteal nerve (L5, S1)	Abducts and medially rotates thigh; keeps pelvis level when opposite leg is off ground and advances pelvis during swing phase of gait; TFL also contributes to stability of extended knee
Gluteus minimus	External surface of ilium between anterior and inferior gluteal lines	Anterior surface of greater trochanter of femur		
Tensor fasciae latae (TFL)	Anterior superior iliac spine and iliac crest	Iliotibial tract that attaches to lateral condyle (Gerdy tubercle) of tibia		
Piriformis	Anterior surface of sacrum and sacrotuberous ligament	Superior border of greater trochanter of femur	Anterior rami of S1 and S2	
Obturator internus	Pelvic surface of obturator membrane and surrounding bones	Medial surface of greater trochanter of femur by common tendons	Nerve to obturator internus (L5, S1) Nerve to quadratus femoris (L5, S1)	Laterally rotate extended thigh and abduct flexed thigh; steady femoral head in acetabulum
Superior gemellus	Ischial spine			
Inferior gemellus	Ischial tuberosity			
Quadratus femoris	Lateral border of ischial tuberosity	Quadrate tubercle on intertrochanteric crest of femur		Laterally rotates thigh,c steadies femoral head in acetabulum
There are six lateral rotators of the thigh: piriformis, obturator internus, gemelli (superior and inferior), quadratus femoris, and obturator externus. These muscles also stabilize the hip joint.				

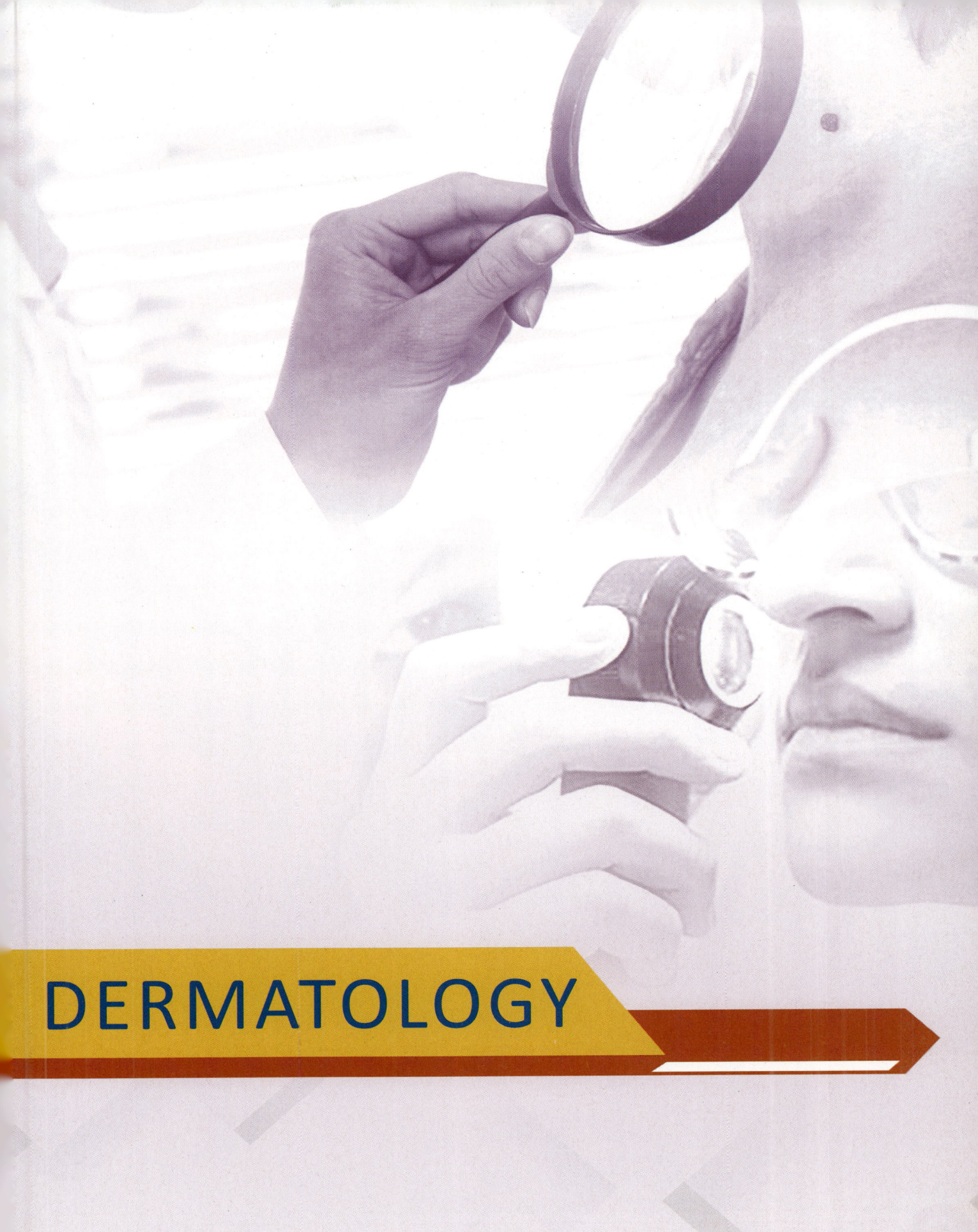

DERMATOLOGY

DERMATOLOGY PLATE 1

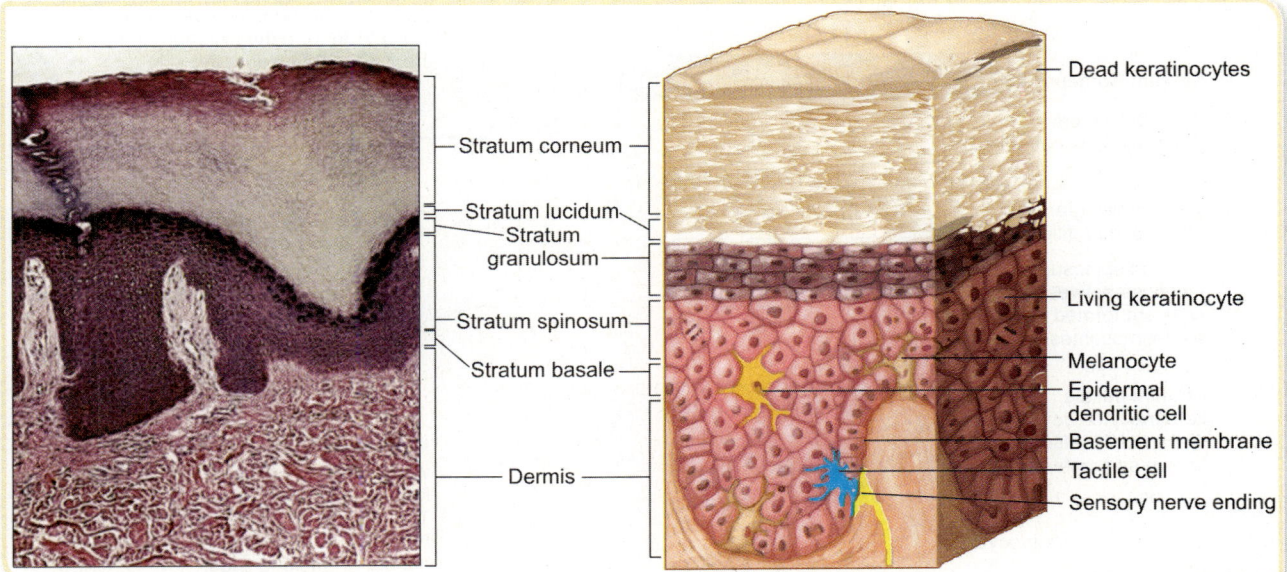

HISTOLOGY OF SKIN

	Histology of Skin		
	Layer	**Cells**	**Comments**
EPIDERMIS	Stratum corneum	☐ Many flattened, **dead "cells"**, called squames, packed with keratin filaments	☐ Most superficial layer of epidermis ☐ Dead cells containing **Keratin** with hard protein envelop. Intracellular lipid
	Stratum lucidum	☐ Dead cells ☐ Indistinct homogeneous layer of keratinocytes, present only in thick skin	☐ Dead cells containing dispersed **Keratohyalin** ☐ Cells *lack nuclei* and organelles ☐ Cytoplasm is packed with keratin filaments and eleidin
	Stratum granulosum	☐ Flattened nucleated keratinocytes arranged in 3 to 5 layers ☐ Keratinocytes contained Keratin and **Profilaggrin**	☐ Cells contain many coarse **keratohyalin** granules associated with tonofilaments ☐ Membrane-coating (**waterproofing**) granules occasionally present
	Stratum spinosum	☐ Several layers of keratinocytes (called **"prickle cells"**). Keratinization begins at Stratum Spinosum ☐ **Langerhans cells** also are present in this layer	☐ Keratinocytes are mitotically active, especially in the deeper layers. ☐ Keratinocytes contain membrane-coating (**waterproofing**) granules
	Stratum basale (germinativum)	☐ **Keratinocytes** are mitotically active ☐ **Melanocytes** and **Merkel cells** also present	Deepest layer of epidermis, composed of a single layer of tall cuboidal keratinocytes
DERMIS	**Papillary layer**	☐ Superficial thin layer of connective tissue that interdigitates with epidermal ridges of the epidermis. ☐ Forms dermal papillae where **Meissner corpuscles** and **capillary loops** may be found. ☐ Contains delicate collagen (**type I and type III**) fibers. ☐ Contains anchoring fibrils (**type VII collagen**), microfibrils (fibrillin) and elastic fibers.	
	Reticular layer	☐ Extensive part of the dermis, lying deep to the papillary layer ☐ Contains thick bundles of collagen (**type I**) fibers and elastic fibers ☐ **Arteries**, **veins**, and **lymphatics** are present ☐ Location of **sweat glands** and their ducts, Pacinian corpuscles, and nerves. ☐ In thin skin, contains **hair follicles, sebaceous glands, and arrector pili muscles**	

Contd...

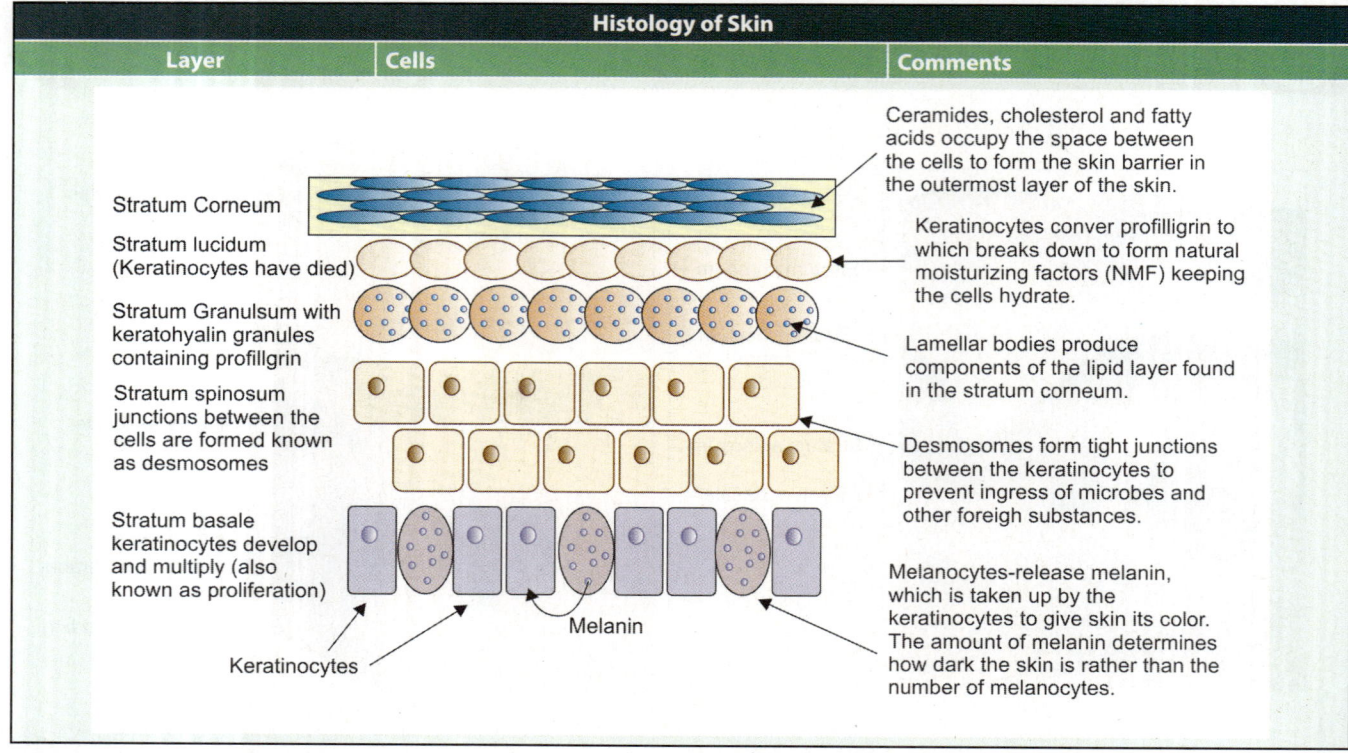

DERMATOLOGY PLATE 2

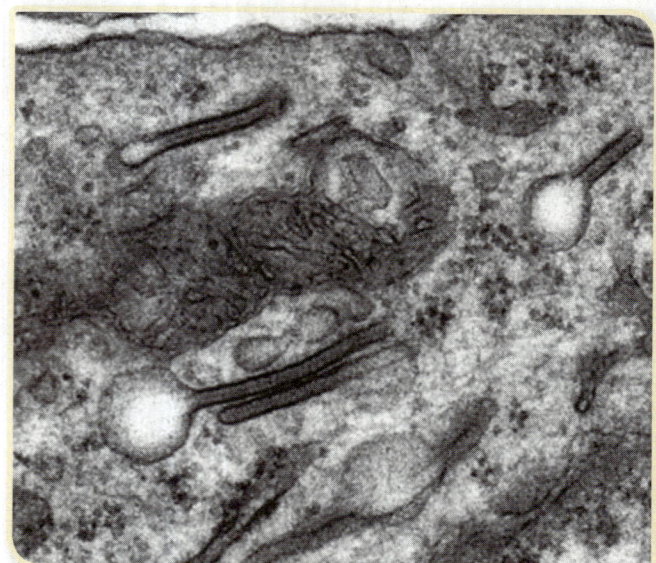

 KEY

BIRBECK GRANULES

The image shows Birbeck granules. Birbeck granules or Birbeck bodies, are "tennis-racket" cytoplasmic organelles found in Langerhans cells. The most reliable means for identification of Langerhans cells on electron microscopy is Birbeck granules. Langerhans' cells, named for Paul Langerhans who, while a medical student in Berlin in 1868, was the first to describe them.

Langerhans cells are antigen presenting cells similar to macrophages and, like them, possess cell surface HLA-DR, which is necessary for presentation of antigen to lymphocytes, and membrane receptors for both the C3b component of complement and the Fc portion of IgG and IgE. Langerhans cell has distinct morphology and plays a crucial role in various immune processes, among them are: allergic contact dermatitis, allograft rejection, immune tolerance, and surveillance for incipient neoplasia. Langerhans cells express CD1a and S100 antigens that permit them to be recognized by immunohistochemical techniques.

DERMATOLOGY PLATE 3

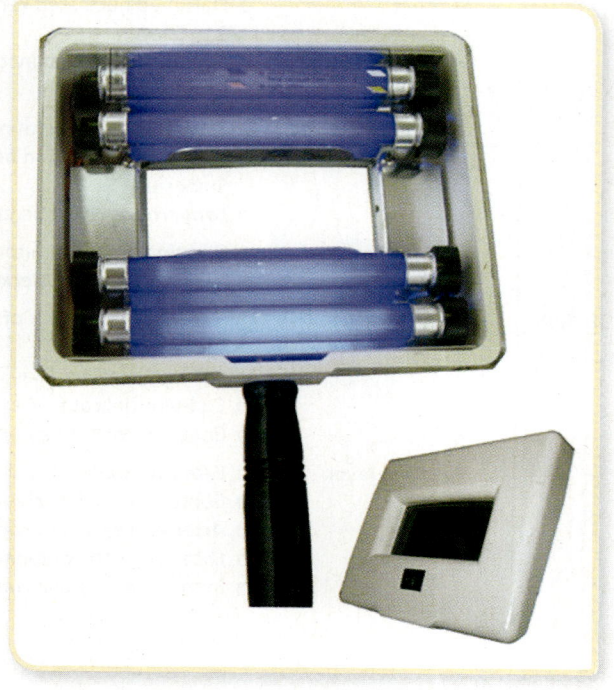

WOOD'S LAMP

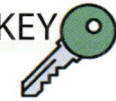

Wood's Lamp in Dermatology

Wood's lamp was invented in 1903 by a Baltimore physicist, **Robert W. Wood**

Principle: Wood's *lamp emits long-wave UV radiation (UVR), also called black light, generated by a high-pressure mercury arc fitted with a compound filter made of barium silicate with 9% nickel oxide, the* **"Wood's filter."** *This filter is opaque to all light rays except a band between 320 and 400 nm with a peak at 365 nm. Fluorescence of tissues occurs when Wood's (UV) light is absorbed and radiation of a longer wavelength, usually visible light, is emitted. The output of Wood's lamp is generally low (< 1 mw/cm2). The fluorescence of normal skin is very faint or absent and is mainly due to constituents of elastin, aromatic amino acids and precursors or products of melanin.*

Condition	Description of Findings
Superficial fungal infections	
Tinea capitis	**Blue-green fluorescence.** Wood's lamp is helpful in the diagnosis and treatment of an individual patient as well as for mass screening and control of epidemics in schools. It can also help to assess the length and response to treatment; the end point being emergence of non-fluorescent hair
P. versicolor	*Malassezia furfur* emits a **yellowish-white or copper-orange fluorescence.** Wood's lamp can detect sub-clinical infection and the extent of infection. It can also help distinguish Pityrosporum folliculitis from other causes of folliculitis
Bacterial infections	
Pseudomonas	Pathogenic *Pseudomonas* species produce a pigment 'pyoverdine' or 'fluorescein' which **shows green fluorescence** under Wood's light. Fluorescence is detected when the bacterial count exceeds $105/cm^2$, the number required for infections.
Erythrasma	*Corynebacterium minutissimum* **shows coral red fluorescence** under Wood's light due to water soluble coproporphyrin III produced by the organisms. Hence, washing the area will remove the fluorescence
Acne vulgaris	Coproporphyrin is the major porphyrin produced by *P. acnes* that imparts **orange-red fluorescence** to the comedones inhabited by *P. acnes*. Facial follicular fluorescence correlates well with the *P. acnes* population.
Pigmentary disorders	
Hypopigmented lesions	In hypopigmented or depigmented lesions, there is less or no epidermal melanin. Consequently, there is a window through which the light induced autofluorescence of dermal collagen can be seen. The lesions **appear bright blue-white due to autofluorescence.** Wood's lamp is therefore helpful in making a diagnosis of vitiligo, chemical leukoderma, ash leaf macules. Wood's lamp can also help to differentiate nevus depigmentosus from nevus anemicus; the latter does not show accentuation with Wood's light.
Hyperpigmented lesions	Wood's lamp can be used to determine the depth of melanin in the skin in skin conditions like **melasma.**
Porphyria	**Red pink fluorescence** in teeth, hair, nails, urine and feces
Photodynamic diagnosis of premalignant and malignant conditions after application of ALA. This photodynamic diagnosis has proved very useful in the diagnosis **of basal cell epithelioma, squamous cell epithelioma, Bowen's disease, solar keratosis and extramammary Paget's disease.**	
Demonstration of a burrow in scabies	

DERMATOLOGY PLATE 4

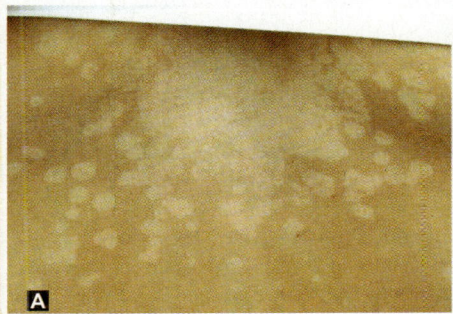
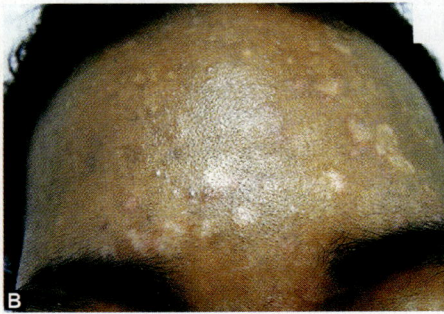

By Sarahrosenau on Flickr.com © Grook Da Oger © Warfieldian on wikimedia

TINEA VERSICOLOR

A. It presents with multiple hypo or hyperpigmented macules with fine granny scales predominantly over chest, neck and back. The macules tend to coalesce with each other.
B. *Pityriasis versicolor* commonly causes hypopigmentation in people with dark skin tones.
C. *Tinea versicolor* fluorescence under Wood's lamp: *Malassezia furfur* emits a **yellowish-white or copper-orange fluorescence**. Wood's lamp can detect sub-clinical infection and the extent of infection. It can also help distinguish *Pityrosporum folliculitis* from other causes of folliculitis.
- Caused by **Malassezia furfur** (*Pityrosporum ovale*)
- Presents multiple, small, hypo pigmented macules over chest and back of young adults
- Perifollicular macules to begin with and then merge together.
- **Diagnosis:** 10% KOH mount – short and round hyphae (spaghetti and meat ball appearance). Green fluorescence on wood's lamp
- **Treatment:**
  - Ketoconazole/Itraconazole/for systemic treatment and Miconazole/clotrimazole for local application.
  - Griesofulvin is not effective.

ERYTHRASMA

A. Clinical picture of a patient with erythrasma.
B. Wood's lamp image of a patient with erythrasma. Note the coral red color.
- *Erythrasma* is a cutaneous infection producing reddish-brown, macular, scaly, pruritic intertriginous patches.
- The dermatologic presentation under the Wood's lamp is of **coral-red fluorescence**. *C. minutissimum* appears to be a common cause of erythrasma, although there is evidence for a polymicrobial etiology in certain settings. In addition, this fluorescent microbe has been associated with bacteremia in patients with hematologic malignancy.
- Erythrasma responds to topical erythromycin, clarithromycin, clindamycin, or fusidic acid, although more severe infections may require oral macrolide therapy.

DERMATOLOGY PLATE 5

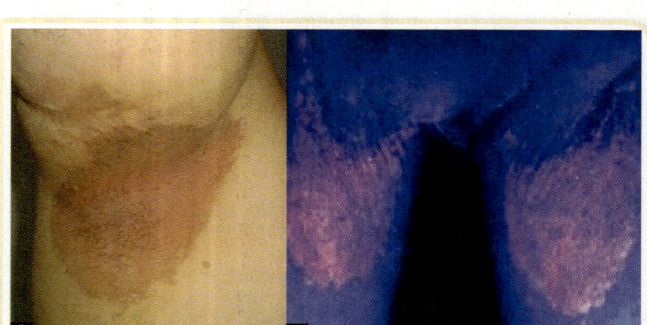

DERMATOLOGY PLATE 6

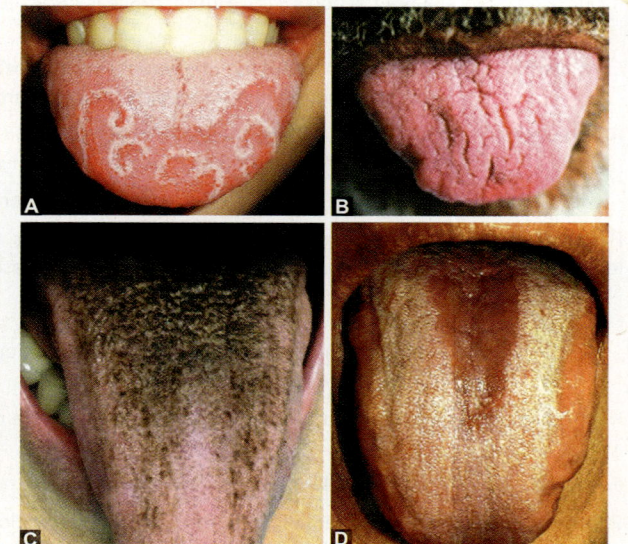

SOME IMPORTANT CONDITIONS OF THE TONGUE

A. Geographical Tongue
B. Fissured tongue
C. Hairy tongue or Black hairy
D. Median rhomboid glossitis or central papillary atrophy

Some Important Conditions of the Tongue	
Condition	Remarks
Geographic tongue or benign migratory glossitis/stomatitis or Psorasiform mucositis	Geographic tongue typically presents itself on the dorsum of the tongue as multiple well-delineated areas of erythema surrounded by a yellowish-white serpiginous border the erythema is a result of atrophy of the filiform papillae. Geographic tongue is usually asymptomatic, although some patients may experience a burning sensation or sensitivity to hot or spicy foods. Seen in normal individuals, Psoriasis, Atopic dermatitis, Fissured tongue. Geographic tongue generally requires no treatment other than assuring the patient that it represents a benign condition. If symptoms such as burning, sensitivity, pain or tenderness are present to a severe extent and interfere with the patient's lifestyle, application of a potent topical corticosteroid gel may provide some relief

Contd...

Some Important Conditions of the Tongue	
Condition	**Remarks**
Fissured tongue or Scrotal tongue or Plicated tongue or Furrowed tongue or Lingua plicata	Common, benign clinical condition of unknown etiology. Few to numerous furrows or grooves are seen on the dorsum of the tongue. Grooves are usually 2-3 mm in depth. Seen in Melkersson–Rosenthal syndrome, Down's syndrome, Cowden's syndrome, Pachyonychia congenital, Acromegaly. Fissured tongue is a benign condition requiring no treatment.
Hairy tongue or Black hairy tongue or Lingua villosa nigra	Hairy tongue is a common, benign clinical condition that basically represents accumulation of varying amounts of keratin on the dorsum of the tongue. It s not a sign of underlying systemic disease in an otherwise healthy and non-debilitated patient, as was historically believed. Hairy tongue presents as diffuse hair-like projections on the dorsum of the tongue, especially in the middle region. The elongated papillae are usually yellow to brown–black, although a wide range of color presentations may occur due to differential exogenous staining from food, tobacco or chromogenic bacteria. **Overgrowth of the latter may occur in the setting of oral or systemic antibiotic therap**y. Some patients complain of bad breath, bad taste, or a gagging sensation when the tongue contacts the palate. Microscopic examination reveals pronounced accumulation of parakeratosis at the tips of otherwise normal filiform papillae. Often, bacteria can be seen colonizing the surface. Hairy tongue is a benign condition requiring no treatment. Some patients desire treatment due to the unaesthetic nature of the process, or because of the altered taste, bad breath, or gagging sensation. In such cases, patients should be encouraged to scrape the tongue with a tongue scraper or brush it during tooth brushing.
Median rhomboid glossitis or central papillary atrophy	Median rhomboid glossitis was formerly thought to be a developmental defect resulting from failure of the embryonic tuberculum impar to be covered by the lateral processes of the tongue. Median rhomboid glossitis appears as a well-demarcated diamond- or oval-shaped area of erythema and atrophy on the dorsum of the tongue anterior to the circumvallate papillae. Median rhomboid glossitis accompanied by palatal inflammation in the area of contact with the tongue lesion may represent a sign of HIV infection or other immunodeficient states. When biopsied, median rhomboid glossitis demonstrates loss of the filiform papillae and tubular hyphae of *Candida albicans* embedded in the parakeratin layer. However, the diagnosis is usually made clinically and confirmed by potassium hydroxide preparation showing budding yeast and pseudohyphae. The mucosal alteration seen in median rhomboid glossitis resolves completely or partially after a course of appropriate anticandidal therapy such as clotrimazole troches or oral fluconazole.

DERMATOLOGY PLATE 7

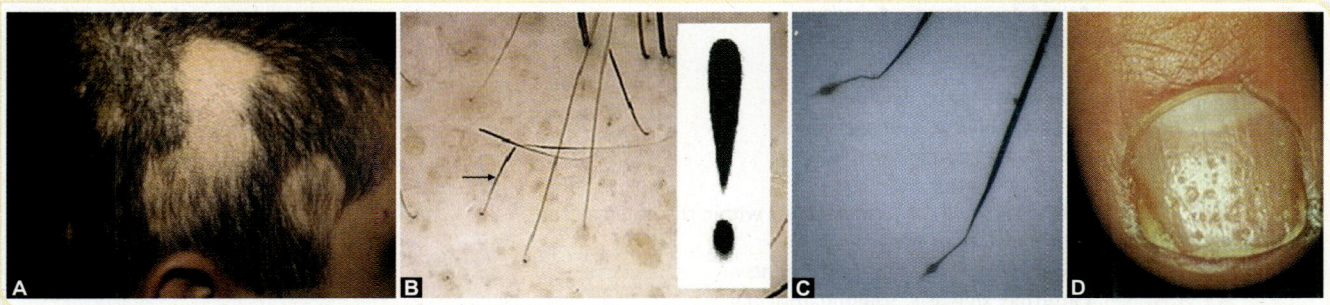

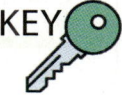

KEY

ALOPECIA AREATA

A. Alopecia areata
B. Exclamation mark sign of scalp hairs
C. Removed scalp hair with exclamation mark sign
D. Nail changes in Alopecia areata

Alopecia Areata

Alopecia areata (AA) is a non-scarring alopecia characterized by a patchy loss of hair without atrophy. It may affect any hairy area of the body and is usually reversible

Synonym	Davey Kirts syndrome, Spot baldness
Etiology	Autoimmunity, Heredity, Emotional stress, Atopy, Psychology, Down's Syndrome
Autoimmune conditions associated with Alopecia areata	Hashimoto's thyroiditis, Addison's disease, pernicious anemia, vitiligo, lichen planus, morphea, lichen sclerosus et atrophicus, pemphigus foliaceus, systemic lupus erythematosus, Sjögren's syndrome, ulcerative colitis, myasthenia gravis, autoimmune hemolytic anemia, diabetes mellitus, autoimmune testicular and ovarian disease, and chronic mucocutaneous candidiasis with endocrinopathy
Pathogenesis	CD 8+ cell mediated immunity against follicular melanocytes
Types	Ikeda types: atopic, pre hypertensive, autoimmune Scalp: patchy, sisaipho, ophiasis, reticulate, diffuse, subtotal, alopecia totalis ☐ Ophiasis (ophidion means serpent) is a form of AA that begins at the occiput and slowly progresses anteriorly, as well as bilaterally along the scalp margins in a band-like fashion. ☐ An inverse ophiasis pattern (called sisaipho) spares the occipital fringe and affects the rest of the scalp. ☐ Small patches closely arranged in a reticulate pattern Generalized alopecia universalis Severe forms of Alpecia areata: Confluence of patches of Alopecia areata may lead to Diffuse AA AA totalis: complete loss of hair from scalp and eyebrows AA universalis: Complete loss of hair from all parts of the body
Clinical features	The scalp is the commonest site of affection, although any hairy area may be affected M>F : 2:1 A pathognomonic sign for alopecia areata is the **"Exclamation mark hair"**, which is wide distally and narrower at the base. These hairs are often found at the periphery of a patch of hair loss. Hair that regrows in the area of alopecia areata is in many cases white. Nail pitting may be also present. The treatment consists of injection of intralesional steroids and topical steroids. Most experience complete regrowth of hair. **"Coudability" sign** in AA, a normal looking hair kinks when forced inwards or bent, the kink being situated 5–10 mm above the surface. At the margins of a new or expanding patch, the characteristic **exclamation mark hair** can be found. These are seen as 2–4 mm long broken hair, the shafts of which reduce progressively in thickness and pigmentation toward the bulb end. A hand lens shows that their free ends are splayed giving a **"frayed rope" appearance.** **The frequency of nail involvement (10%–20%):** The commonest change is superficial, uniform, minute pits arranged regularly along and across the nail giving a "scotch plaid" effect or coalescing into "ripples". Red or mottled lunulae, nail thinning and ridging, discoloration (including longitudinally arranged punctate leukonychia), splitting, dystrophy, onycholysis, and even onychomadesis have been described. **Nail changes:** In about 10% of cases of alopecia areata, especially in long-standing cases with extensive involvement, the nails develop uniform pits that may form transverse or longitudinal lines. Trachyonychia, onychomadesis, and red or spotted lunulae occur, but less commonly. Dermoscopic examination typically demonstrates diffuse, round, or polycyclic perifollicular yellow dots.
Poor prognostic factors	**Early age of onset** **Nail changes:** Pits, onychodystrophy, onycholysis, anonychia **Extensive scalp involvement** (>50% scalp) , Alopecia universalis , Alopecia totalis **Associated systemic disorders** **Atopy** **Hypertension** **Connective tissue disorders** **Loss of eyebrows and eyelashes** **Associated genetic disorder** **Down syndrome** **Patchy regrowth of terminal hairs within the patch** **Family history of AA** **Recurrent episode MIF-173*C gene** **Patterns—ophiasis, sisaipho, reticular**
Treatment	1. Self-limiting disorder, hence reassurance 2. Topical or intralesional therapy with corticosteroids remains the most common mode and first line therapy 3. Irritants anthralin, phenol, salicylic acid, sulfur, oil of cade, cantharidin, croton oil, tretinoin 4. Photochemotherapy Topical PUVA, turban-PUVA 5. Systemic therapy with ciclosporin, corticosteroids, biologics like alefacept 6. Contact sensitizers SADBE= squaric acid dibutyl ester, DNCB= dinitrochlorobenzene, and diphencyprone can be useful in refractory cases. 7. Topical minoxidil

DERMATOLOGY PLATE 8

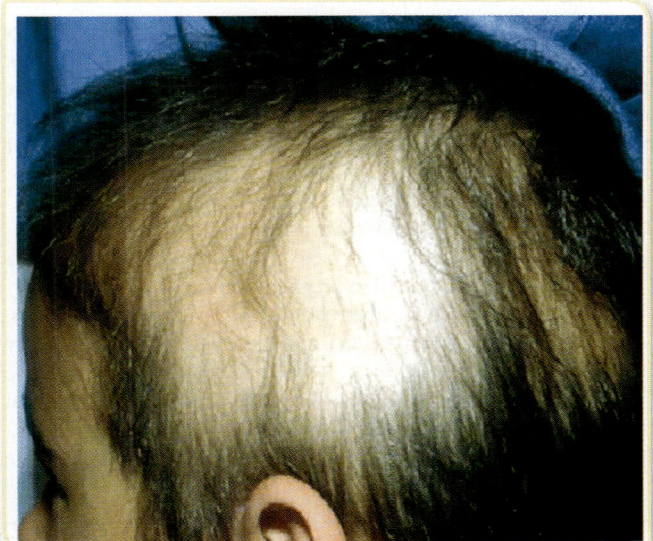

Alopecia areata	Trichotileomania
On HPE you can see a *swarm of bees appearance* due to dense peri bulbar (around hair bulb) lymphocytic infiltrate	On HPE you can see deformed hair, empty follicles with keratin, excess catagen hair and aggregation of melanin.
Dermoscopic clues: preponderance of yellow dots. Exclamation mark hair, coudability	Dermoscopic clues: coiled hair with fraying and split ends

TRICHOTILEOMANIA

The term trichotileomania (TM) literally means a morbid craving/impulsivity to pull out hairs. It is one of the types of traumatic alopecia. Hair plucking is most common from the scalp and rarely from eyebrows, eyelashes, pubic hair, etc. Hair loss may be minimal to extensive. Hairs are short, broken, irregular in length and distorted. Plucked hairs may be stroked, licked, and sometimes swallowed (trichophagia), leading to trichobezoar.

Main differential diagnosis of Trichotilomania (Dermatological point of view) is Alopecia areata

Alopecia areata	Trichotileomania
It presents with a patch of non-scarring alopecia. The skin of the patch is normal or slightly reddened/inflamed. Length of hair are uniform. The hair in margin are easily extractable and show exclamation mark morphology and coudability (kinking of hair when bent inwards)	It also presents as a patch of non-scarring alopecia. The skin of the patch is generally normal. The commonly affected areas are frontotemporal zones. **Friar Tuck sign:** This common presentation of TT includes areas of hair loss arranged in a circular pattern with **hair of different lengths** because of mechanical pulling. Thus, unaffected hairs surround an area of hair loss. Absence of skin abnormalities or inflammation
Associated features of atopy, nail pitting, autoimmune disorders	History of **Psychiatric illness.** Associated features may be bleeding from some areas, trichobezoar, onychophagia, onytotillomania

Contd...

DERMATOLOGY PLATE 9

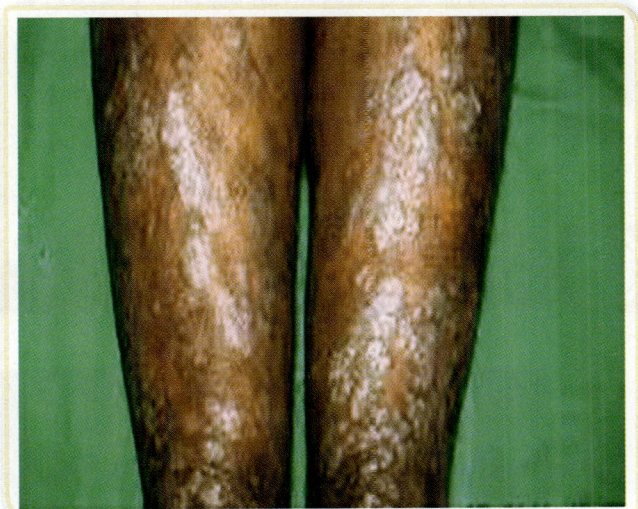

PSORIASIS VULGARIS

Typical lesion of **Psoriasis vulgaris.** Note the red scaly plaques. Scales are silvery white. It manifests as coin-sized to large palm-sized well defined erythematosquamous plaques distributed bilaterally. The extensor surfaces of the body (particularly the elbows and knees), lumbosacral area and back are commonly involved.

- The **Auspitz sign** refers to the appearance of small bleeding points after successive layers of scale have been removed from the surface of psoriatic papules or plaques.
- The **Koebner phenomenon** or Köbner phenomenon, also called the Koebner response or the isomorphic response, attributed to Heinrich Köbner, is the appearance of skin lesions on lines of trauma.

Use of corticosteroids in psoriasis: Although dramatic in short-term effectiveness, they are not recommended for psoriasis because of their toxicity and the propensity of the disease to recur in a more severe form on cessation of therapy. However, it is used in:

- Erythrodermic psoriasis
- Severe generalized plaque psoriasis
- Acute exacerbation while changing to other agents or waiting for them to take effect
- Both corticosteroids and ciclosporin can be used in pustular psoriasis in pregnancy.

DERMATOLOGY PLATE 10

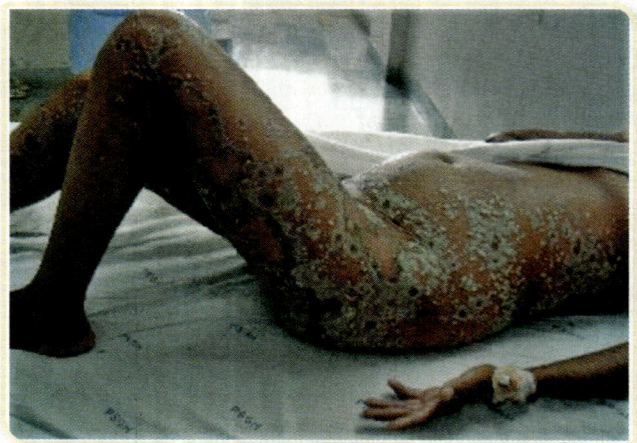

© Lakshmi C, Srinivas CR, Paul S, Chitra TV, Kanchanamalai K, Somasundaram LS

IMPETIGO HERPETIFORMIS

Erythematous, scaly, figurative lesions, with pustules on the periphery on the trunk in pregnancy is consistent with Impetigo herpetiformis. It is a rare dermatosis of pregnancy with typical onset during the last trimester of pregnancy and rapid resolution in the postpartum period. Clinically and histologically, it is consistent with pustular psoriasis. This similarity has led some authors to name the disease "the pustular psoriasis of pregnancy.

Treatment modalities for pustular psoriasis

- **Oral retinoids:** Drug of choice. It is teratogenic and hence absolutely contraindicated in pregnant women
- **Cyclosporine:** Second line treatment for pustular psoriasis. Cyclosporine is not teratogenic, and it is classified as a pregnancy prescribing category C drug. Use during pregnancy should be considered only in exceptional patients for whom the potential benefits of cyclosporine therapy dramatically outweigh the risks.
- **Oral corticosteroids:** Used in pustular psoriasis. They are pregnancy category C drugs.

DERMATOLOGY PLATE 11

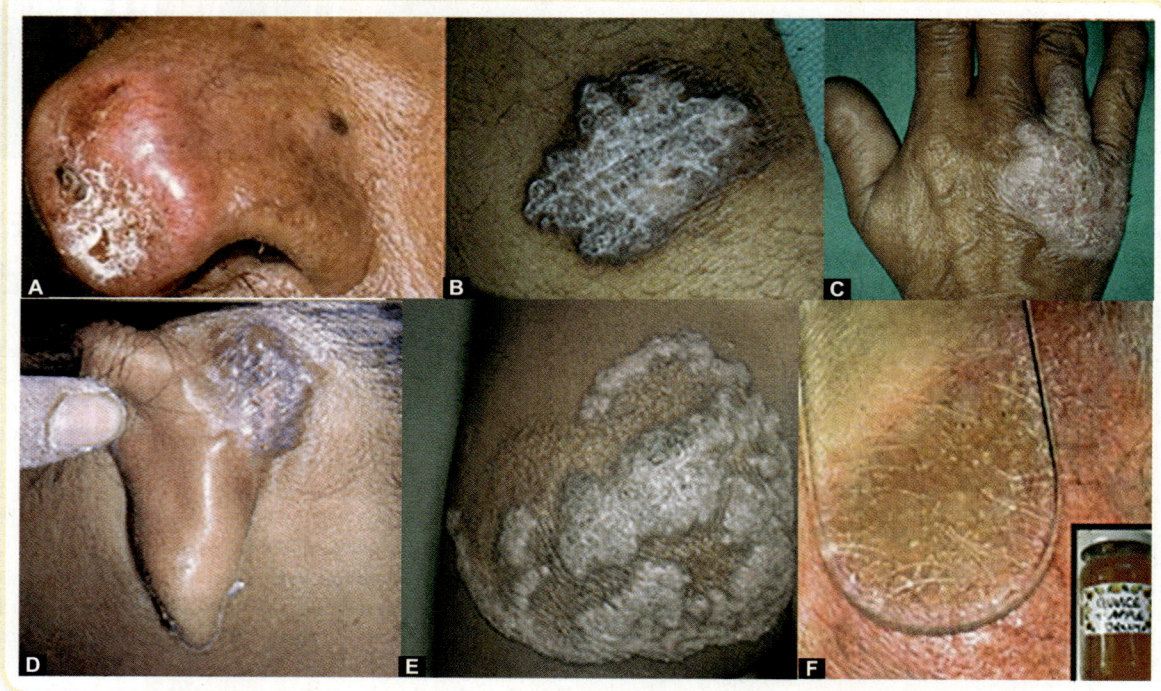

Credit: Pic A; Dwari BC, Ghosh A, Paudel R, Kishore P, Nepal, Pic B-E; Dr Mary Thomas, Dr Meryl Antony

LUPUS VULGARIS

A. Erythematous plaque type of lupus vulgaris on the dorsum of the nose
B. Psoriasiform lupus vulgaris: Solitary plaque with silvery scaling
C. Erythematous plaque type of lupus vulgaris on the dorsum of the hand
D. Nodular lupus vulgaris on the retroauricular area
E. Giant plaque of lupus vulgaris on the gluteal region

F. **Diascopy:** Pressing a glass slide on the lesion compresses the blood out of the small vessels. Diascopy is of particular value in detecting granulomatous nodule which have a translucent brownish colour known as Apple jelly nodules (e.g. Lupus vulgaris, Sarcoidosis of skin).
Note: It is not the Nodule shape of consistency which but the colour on blanching which name it as Apple Jelly Nodule. Apple jelly colour can be seen in inset for the reference.

Cutaneous TB Classification		
Host immunity	Method of inoculation	Disease
Naive host	Direct inoculation	Tuberculous chancre (primary inoculation)
Multibacillary: Low host immunity		
	Contiguous spread	Scrofuloderma
	Autoinoculation	Orificial TB
	Hematogenous spread	Acute miliary TB, TB gumma
Paucibacillary or high host immunity		
	Direct inoculation	Tuberculosis verrucosa cutis, lupus vulgaris
	Hematogenous	Lupus vulgaris
Tuberculids		Lichen scrofulosorum, papulonecrotic tuberculid, erythema induratum of bazin

Lupus vulgaris:
- Most common form of cutaneous TB in India
- Most common site: In India it is **Buttock > Thigh > Legs**, worldwide it is **face** (particularly around nose)
- **Clinical forms**: Psoriasiform, plaque, Nodular, ulcerative, vegetative, popular and tumor-like
- Lupus vulgaris in advanced stages may show similarity with scarring lesions of DLE. Whereas fresh lesions of lupus vulgaris are characterized by reddish brown macule and papule of soft friable consistency and soft erythematous Nodule. A few surrounding nodules may appear and later coalesce to form a soft plaque
- Extension of the plaque is a slow process; gradually it becomes infiltrated and may show scaling. In the classical descriptions of lupus vulgaris, the presence of yellowish-brown **apple-jelly nodules** at the edge of a plaque is often seen on diascopic examination
- The edges of the lesion gradually extend in some areas and heal with **atrophic central scarring.** Sometimes causing considerable tissue destruction over many years. The plaque is characterised by evidence of healing and atrophic scarring in some areas interspersed between areas of activity giving a **wolf bitten appearance** (Hence the name Lupus, Latin for wolf)
- Lupus vulgaris has a tendency to ulcerate, which is very uncommon in DLE
- Pigmentation is absent in Lupus vulgaris which is common in DLE
- Mutilation of acral sites like nose and earlobes is a common feature of both Lupus vulgaris and DLE
- Lupus Vulgaris of ear lobule is called **Turkey Ear** (Named after Istanbul, Turkey)

Scrofuloderma:
- Scrofuloderma results from the involvement and breakdown of the skin overlying a contiguous tuberculosis focus. This is usually a lymph gland, an infected bone or joint, or a lacrimal gland or duct.
- A bluish-red nodule overlying the infected gland or joint breaks down to form undermined ulceration with granulating tissue at the base. Numerous fistulae may intercommunicate beneath ridges of a bluish skin. Progression and scarring produce irregular adherent masses, densely fibrous in places and fluctuant or discharging in others. Excessive granulation tissue may give rise to fungating tumors. After healing, characteristic puckered scarring marks the site of the infection.

DERMATOLOGY PLATE 12

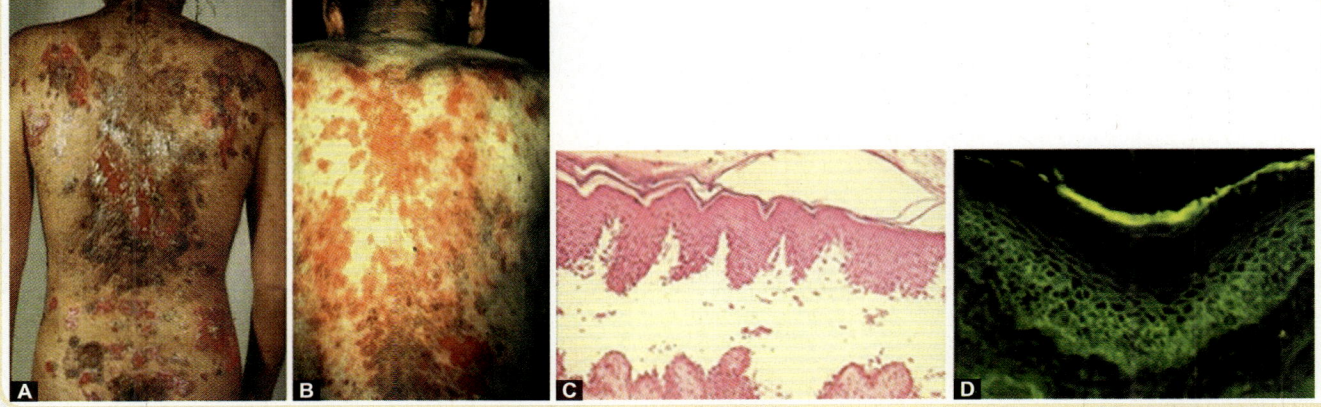

© Otten JV, Hashimoto T, Hertl M, Payne AS, Sitaru C

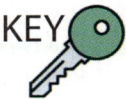

PEMPHIGUS VULGARIS (AND VARIANTS)

A. **Pemphigus vulgaris (PV):** Patients suffering from muco-cutaneous pemphigus vulgaris (PV) usually have flaccid blisters and erosions on the trunk with crusts and hyperpigmentation accompanied by mucosal ulcerations in the mouth

B. **Pemphigus foliaceus (PF):** Patients are characterized by crusted epidermal erosions whereas involvement of mucous membranes is absent

C. **Pemphigus vulgaris Histopathology:** Suprabasal acantholysis (cleft); **C1**; In PV, the epidermal cleavage plane is located in the deep epidermis, usually right above the basal layer (Suprabasal cleft). A single layer of basal keratinocytes remains attached to the basement membrane as a "**Row of tombstones**" appearance. In PF, epidermal splitting occurs between granular layers (subcorneal blisters within the epidermis)

D. **Pemphigus Vulgaris Immunohistochemistry:** Direct immunofluorescence showing granular deposits of immunoglobulin IgG3 and C3 in intracellular space (**fish net pattern**)

Classification of Bullae	
Intraepidermal	
Sub cornea	Subcorneal pustular dermatosis
Granular cell layer	Pemphigus foliaceous and erythematosus Bullous ichthyosiform erythroderma Subcorneal pustular dermatosis Staphylococcal scalded skin syndrome Bullous impetigo
Spinous layer	Familial benign pemphigus
Suprabasal	Pemphigus vulgaris Acantholytic disorders like Hailey Hailey disease, Darier's disease and Grover's disease (transient acantholytic dermatosis)
Basal layer	Epidermolysis bullosa simplex Toxic epidermal necrolysis Erythema multiforme Lupus erythematosus Lichen planus
Sub epidermal bullae (Dermoepidermal junction)	
Lamina lucida	Bullous and cicatricial pemphigoid, pemphigoid (herpes) gestatiois, dermatitis herpetiformis, thermal burns
Lamina densa	Bullous SLE, Epidermolysis bullosa dystrophica, epidermolysis bullosa acquisita, porphyria cutanea tarda

Granular cell layer
- Pemphigus foliacous
- Pemphigus erythematous

Spinous layer (upper and mid epidermis)
- Eczematous blisters
- Frictional blisters
- Viral blisters

Spinous layer (suprabasal area)
- Pemphigus vulgaris

Basal cell area
- Epidermolysis bullosa simplex
- Lichen planus
- Toxic epidermolysis
- Necrosis (TEN)

Laminal lucida
- Bullous pemphigoid
- Cicatrical pemphigoid
- Epidermolysis bullosa acquisita
- Dermatitis herpatiformis

Sublaminar connective tissue
- Epidermolysis bullosa dystrophica
- Erythema multiforme (dermal type)

Pemphigus foliaceus — Subcorneal
Pemphigus vulgaris — Suprabasal
Bullous pemphigoid — Subepithelial

Blistering Diseases of the Skin

	Pemphigus Vulgaris	Pemphigoid	Linear IgA Dermatosis	Herpes gestationis	CBDC*	Dermatitis Herpetiformis
Age of onset	30-50 years	50-80 years	Middle age	Pregnant women	1st decade of life	3rd decade of life (20-30yrs)
HLA association	HLA DR4, HLA A-10, A26	NIL	NIL	NIL	HLA-BM8	HLA-B8, DRW-3
Clinical Features	Discrete, flaccid, bullae arising over normal skin, scalp, chest, back intertriginous areas, **Nikolsky and bulla spread +ve**	Tense bullae over urticarial plaques. Flexures Nikolsky and Bulla spread sign -ve	Blister smaller than pemphigoid> DH, Flexural areas	Large Bulla, Erythematous, papulovesicles and plaque abdomen, palms, soles, chest	Grouped tense vesicles and bullae **'cluster of jewels' pattern** flexure and pelvic region	Vesicles and papulo vesicles 3-6 mm in size, Symmetrical over extensor surface Elbow, knees
Mucosal involvement	Involved in almost all cases	Oral lesions 20%	Infrequent	Mucosa spared	Spared	Spared
Variants	Pemphigus foliaceus, vegetans, erythematous	Classical bullous vesicular, nodular	NIL	NIL	NIL	NIL
Associated features	Myasthenia Gravis, Thymoma	NIL	NIL	NI	NIL	Gluten sensitive Enteropathy
Precipitating features	Drugs #	NIL	NIL	Pregnancy	NIL	Ingestion of Gluten
Location of Blister	Intra Epidermal Supra basal cleft in epidermis (Pemphigus vulgaris), Subcorneal (Pemphigus foliaceous), Row of tombstones (keratinocytes attached to BM but not with each other)	Complete Sub Epidermal Breaks Lamina ducida BM	Sub Epidermal	Sub Epidermal	Sub Epidermal	Papillary tip microabscess
Immuno florescence	Deposition of IgG3 and C3 in intracellular space **(fish net pattern)**	Linear deposition of IgG and C3 at the Lamina Lucida of BM	Linear deposition of IgA at BMZ	Linear deposition of C3 at BMZ IgG also	Linear deposition of IgA BMZ	Granular deposits of IgA at tips of papilla uninvolved skin
Treatment	High Doses Cortico Steroids, Immuno suppressive, IVIG	Mod.- High doses of steroids, Immuno suppressive	Dapsone alone or with steroids	Corticosteroids	Dapsone	Dapsone

CBDC* - Chronic bullous dermatosis of childhood
BM= Basement membrane
Drugs #- **Drug induced pemphigus** is seen with (Mnemonic PCR); Penicillin, Penicillamine, Captopril and Rifampicin

DERMATOLOGY PLATE 13

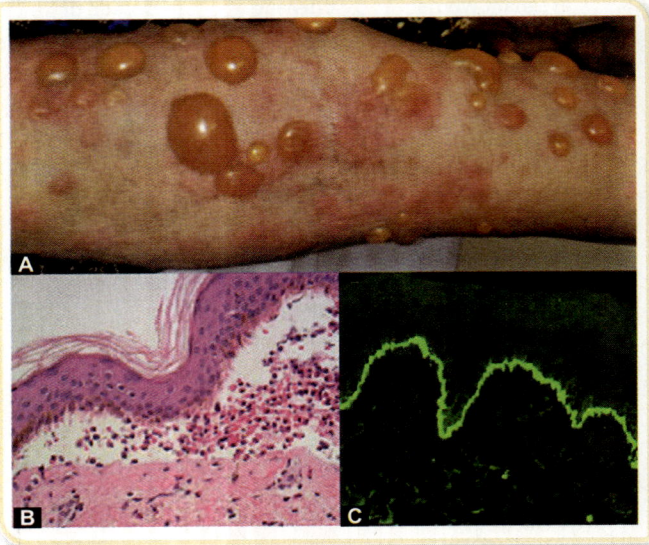

DERMATOLOGY PLATE 14

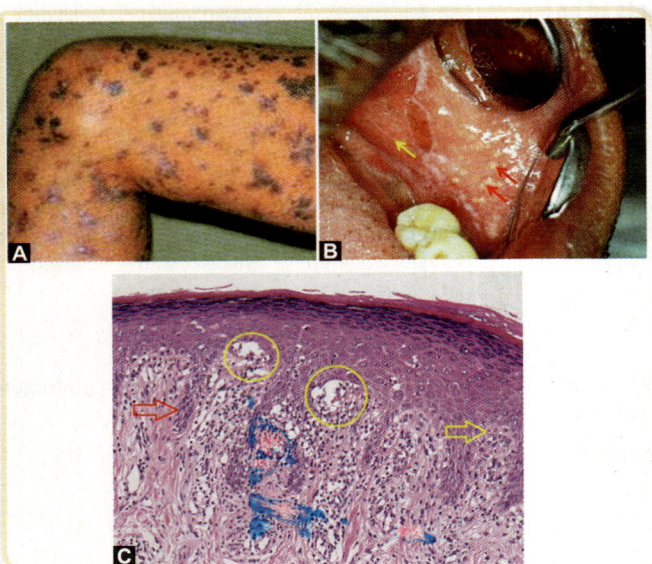

BULLOUS PEMPHIGOID

A. **Bullous pemphigoid clinical picture:** intensely pruritic eruption with widespread blister formation. Erythematous plaques covered with large, **tense blisters** with clear fluid, located symmetrically on the flexural site of the upper limbs, the trunk, the cervical region and the lower limbs, an erosion of 2-3cm diameter on the anterior thorax covered by hematic crust, erythematous plaques with clearly defined edges, covered with pearly white scales, located in the sacral region; hypochromic plates located on the posterior sites of the upper limbs and the lower limbs, atrophic skin covered by fine scales on the lower limbs

B. **Bullous pemphigoid histopathology:** There is a subepidermal blister and a superficial, perivascular infiltrate predominantly of eosinophils and neutrophils. There are numerous eosinophils within the blister cavity. The adjacent epidermis is irregularly hyperplastic with prominent hypergranulosis and compact orthokeratosis

C. **Bullous pemphigoid: Direct immunofluorescence:** Homogenous, linear deposition of IgG in the basement membrane at desmoepithelial junction.

LICHEN PLANUS

A. **Typical plaques of lichen planus:** Pruritic, Polygonal, Purple (Violaceous), Plain (flat) topped papule and Plaque (**Mnemonic 5P**)

B. **Wickham Striae in Lichen Planus of left buccal mucosa:** Note the while lacy pattern AKA- Wickham striae posteriorly (yellow line) and the Fordyce granules anteriorly (red arrow), which appears as a small yellow nodule.

C. **Histopathology**
1. The primary features are hyperkeratosis without parakeratosis, focal increases in the granular cell layer, irregular acanthosis with a **"sawtooth" appearance of Rete Ridges** (Red arrow), **Basal epidermal liquefactive degeneration** and a band-like lymphocytic infiltrate at the dermal– epidermal junction.
2. Apoptotic or dyskeratotic keratinocytes (also referred to as **Civatte, hyaline or cytoid bodies**) are usually present in the basal layer (Yellow arrow tip)
3. Subepidermal Lichenoid Band due to deposition of lymphocytes and histiocytes
4. Vacuolar changes within the basal cell layer may become confluent and result in small separations between the epidermis and the dermis (called **"Max-Joseph spaces"** - yellow circles). There is often incontinence of pigment with multiple dermal melanophages.

Lichen Planus	
Lichen planus (LP), is **self-limiting, papulosquamous prototype of lichenoid dermatoses**, is an idiopathic inflammatory disease of the skin and mucous membranes. **Classic LP** Pruritic, Polygonal, Purple (Violaceous), Plain (flat) topped papule and Plaque (**Mnemonic 5P**) that favor the extremities.	
Pathogenesis	LP represents **T-cell-mediated autoimmune** damage to basal keratinocytes that express altered self-antigens on their surface. CD8 cell is the major effector cell
Etioogy	☐ Unknown but associated with 1. **HCV:** In several case–control studies, the prevalence of HCV (3.4– 38%) was 2- to 13.5-fold higher in patients with LP than in control. Of the various types of LP, it is the oral form that is most commonly viewed as a manifestation of HCV infection 2. Vaccines 3. *H. pylori* bacteria

Contd...

	Lichen Planus
	4. Contact allergens : Dental amalgams, heavy metals 5. Drugs 6. Autoantigens
Cutaneous	**Typical plaques of lichen planus:** Pruritic, Polygonal, Purple (Violaceous), Plain (flat) topped papule and Plaque (**Mnemonic 5P**). Although the **Koebner phenomenon** (i.e. isomorphic response) is commonly seen in LP, excoriations and impetiginization are unusual. Face is generally spared.
Oral Mucosal	▫ Oral LP can appear in at least seven forms, which occur separately or simultaneously: atrophic, bullous, erosive, papular, pigmented, plaque like and reticular. ▫ The most common and characteristic form of oral LP is the **reticular**. It is characterized by slightly raised whitish linear lines in a lace-like pattern **"Wickham's striae"** or in rings with short radiating spines. This form is usually asymptomatic and the most common site of involvement is the **buccal mucosa**; lesions are often bilateral and symmetric. ▫ Gingival involvement is common, and oral LP affecting the gingivae exclusively is seen in approximately 10% of cases. It typically presents as chronic desquamative gingivitis
Types	Hypertrophic, Atrophic, Guttate (eruptive), Annular, Linear, Vesiculobullous, Follicular or Lichen planopilaris, Ulcerative (erosive), Lichen planus pigmentosus, Actinic or Lichen planus subtropicus, Lichen planus pemphigoides
Nail	**Pterygium (diagnostic), Onychorrhexia,** Thinning
Genital	**Annular** shaped genital mucosal lesion
Scalp	Scarring alopecia
Treatment	**Steroid** is the mainstay of treatment

DERMATOLOGY PLATE 15

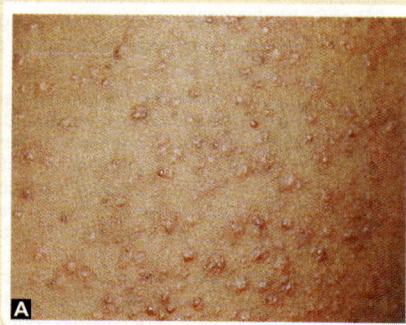
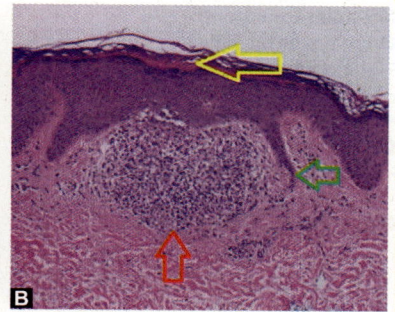

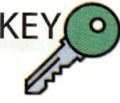
KEY

LICHEN NITIDUS

A. Shiny discrete pin head sized papules seen in **lichen nitidus**
B. **Histology of lichen nitidus** showing **parakeratosis** (yellow arrow), **well-defined granuloma** (red arrow) infiltrate composed of lymphocytes, epithelioid cells and occasional Langhans giant cells, enclosed by hyperplastic **rete ridges** (Green arrow) giving the appearance of **"claw clutching a ball"** on scanning magnification (H and E, × 40). Similar resemblance can be seen in histology of early lesions of juvenile xanthogranuloma (JXG) and lichenoid eruptive histiocytoma. Occasionally, micropapular lichen planus and tuberculoid leprosy may show such appearance, although with shorter "claws."

Lichen Nitidus (LN)	
Lichen nitidus (LN) is an idiopathic lichenoid dermatosis clinically characterized by a monomorphic eruption of asymptomatic, minute, skin-colored papules	
Children and young adults are the usual sufferers	
Usual sites: Common sites of involvement are the forearm, penis (glans and shaft), buttocks, lower abdomen and chest. Some cases may have a generalized distribution.	**Description of lesions** Individual lesions of LN are flesh-colored, pinpoint to pinhead-sized, flat to dome-shaped, shiny, discrete papules
Other features **Koebnerization** may be present. The lesions are usually asymptomatic, but rarely mild to intense pruritus may be associated. Healing occurs without scarring or pigmentary changes.	
Types: Linear, spinous, vesicular, follicular, perforating, hemorrhagic and actinic	
Mucous membrane is spared i.e. Wickham Striae is not seen. (Note; Mucous membrane is involved in Lichen planus)	

DERMATOLOGY PLATE 16

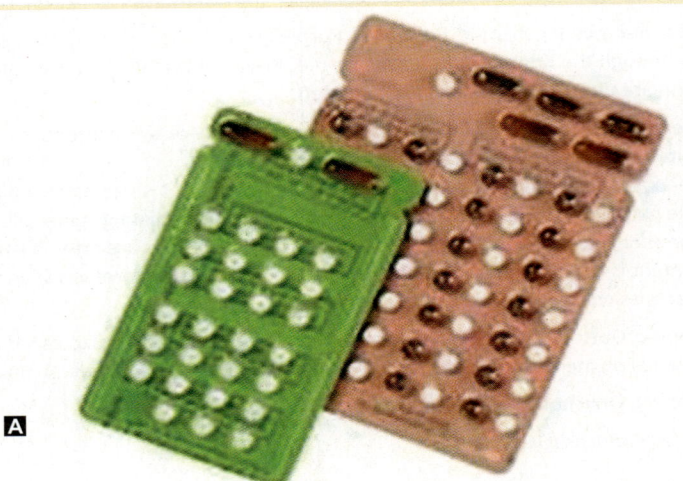

A

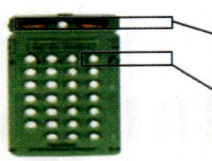

PB adult blister pack

PB adult treatment:
Once a month: Day 1
-2 capsules of rifampicin (300 mg X 2)
-1 tablet of dapsone (100 mg)
Once a day: Days 2-28
-1 tablet of dapsone (100 mg)
Full course: 6 blister packs

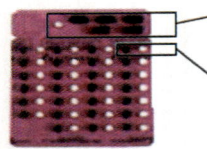

MB adult blister pack

B

MB adult treatment:
Once a month: Day 1
- 2 capsules of rifampicin (300 mg x 2)
- 3 capsules of clofazimine (100 mg x 3)
- 1 tablet of dapsone (100 mg)
Once a day: 2-28
-1 capsule of clofazimine (50 mg)
-1 tablet of dapsone (100 mg)
Full course: 12 blister packs

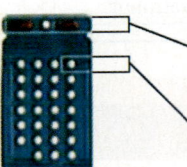

PB child blister pack

PB child treatment (10-14 years):
Once a month: Day 1
-2 capsules of rifampicin
(300 mg + 150 mg)
-1 tablet of dapsone (50 mg)
Once a day: 2-28
-1 tablet of dapsone (50 mg)
Full course: 6 blister packs
For children younger than 10 the dose must be adjusted according to body weight

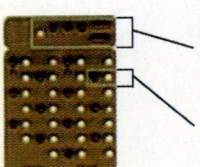

MB child blister pack

MB child treatment (10-14 years):
Once a month: Day 1
-2 capsules of rifampicin (300 mg + 150 mg
-3 capsules of clofazimine (50 mg X 3)
-1 tablet of dapsone (50 mg)
Once a day: Days 2-28
-1 capsule of clofazimine every other day (50 mg)
-1 tablet of dopasone (50 mg)
Full course: 12 blister packs
For children younger than 10, the dose must be adjusted according to body weight

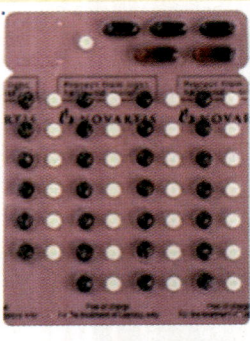

Top 2 lines break off: (detachable):
Clofazimine 300 mg (three capsules of 100 mg), Rifampicin 600 mg (two capsules of 300 mg) and Dapsone 100 mg (one tablet of 100 mg)

Unsupervised Daily Treatment (DAY S2-28): Clofazimine 50 mg (one capsule of 50 mg) EVERY DAY and Dapsone 100 mg (one tablet of 100 mg) EVERY DAY **Duration of Treatment:** 12 blister packs to be taken within 12-18 months

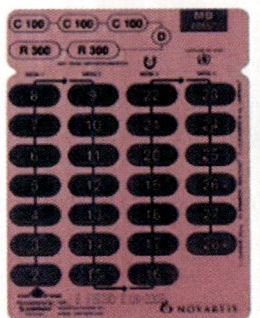

C

Back view of the MB Adult MDT blister pack
R = Rifampicin: Monthly supervised dose is 600 mg (2 capsule, each of 300 mg)
C = Clofazimine 100 mg: monthly supervised dose is 300 mg (3 capsules)
D = Dapsone: Monthly supervised dose is 100 mg (1 tablet).
The figures 2-28 represent 4 weeks of unsupervised Clofazimine (50 mg) every day and Dapsone (100 mg) daily.
Actual size of blister pack: 106 mm × 140 mm

BLISTER PACKS OF MDT OF LEPROSY

The treatment of leprosy is in the form of Multi Drug Therapy (MDT), which is the combination of two or three of the following drugs:
1. Cap. Rifampicin
2. Tab. Dapsone
3. Cap. Clofazimine

Four types of standard regimens are available in blister packs for treatment of leprosy; MDT is provided in convenient-to-use blister calendar packs (BCPs) with medicine for four weeks or 28 days, which is loosely referred to as one month. BCPs for PB leprosy contain two medicines and that for MB leprosy contain three medicines. BCPs for children contain the same medicines as the BCPs for adults but in smaller doses.

Leprosy Regimen			
Adult MB leprosy	▫ Rifampicin: 600 mg once a month supervised ▫ Clofazimine 300 mg once monthly supervised and 100 mg on alternate days or 50 mg daily self-administered ▫ Dapsone 100 mg once monthly supervised with 100 mg daily self-administered	Duration: 12 months (12 blister packs)	Follow up: Once a year for 5 years
Child (ages 10–14) MB leprosy	▫ Rifampicin: 450 mg once a month supervised ▫ Clofazimine 150 mg once monthly supervised and 50 mg on alternate days ▫ Dapsone 50 mg once monthly supervised with 50 mg daily self-administered	Duration: 12 months (12 blister packs)	Follow up: Once a year for 5 years
Child (ages 6–9) MB leprosy	▫ Rifampicin 300 mg once monthly + ▫ Clofazimine 100 mg once monthly supervised and 50 mg twice weekly + ▫ Dapsone 25 mg once monthly supervised with 50 mg daily self-administered	Duration: 12 months (12 blister packs)	Follow up: Once a year for 5 years
Adult PB leprosy	▫ Rifampicin: 600 mg once a month supervised ▫ Dapsone: 100 mg daily self administered ▫ (For adults with body weight below 45 kg the dose of rifampicin should be 450 mg once monthly and dapsone 50 mg daily)	Duration: Six months (six blister packs)	Follow up: Once a year for 2 years
Child PB leprosy	▫ Rifampicin 300 mg (0–5 years) or 450 mg (6–14 years) once monthly supervised ▫ Dapsone 25 mg (0–5 years) or 50 mg (6–14 years) daily	Duration: Six months (six blister packs)	Follow up: Once a year for 5 years

1. The appropriate dose for children under 10 years of age can be decided on the basis of body weight. [Rifampicin: 10 mg per kilogram body weight, clofazimine: 1 mg per kilogram per body weight daily and 6 mg per kilogram monthly, dapsone: 2 mg per kilogram body weight daily. The standard child blister pack may be broken up so that the appropriate dose is given to children under 10 years of age. Clofazimine can be spaced out as required.
2. Rarely, it may be considered advisable to treat a patient with a high bacillary index (BI) for more than 12 months. This decision may only be taken by specialists at referral units after careful consideration of the clinical and bacteriological evidence.

DERMATOLOGY PLATE 17

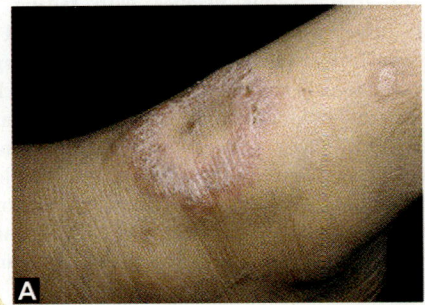
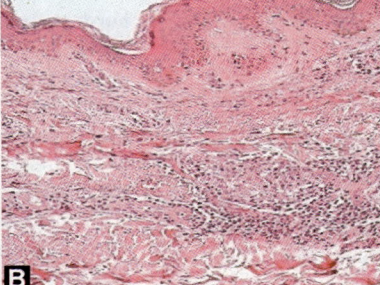
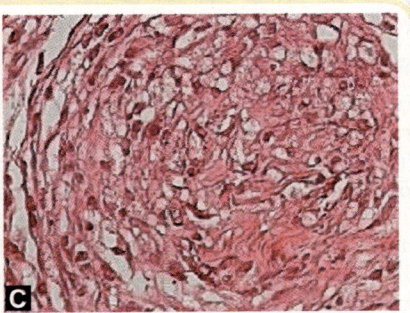

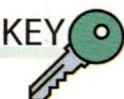

TUBERCULOID LEPROSY (TT)/ PAUCIBACILLARY

A. **Morphology:** Tuberculoid leprosy begins with **localized flat, red skin lesions** that enlarge and develop **Saucer right up (side up) lesion:** Annular lesion with indurated elevated hyperpigmented margins and depressed pale centers (central healing). Sharp outer edge and vague inner edge that slopes towards the center of the lesion. Neuronal involvement dominates tuberculoid leprosy. Nerves become enclosed within granulomatous inflammatory reactions and, if small (e.g., the peripheral twigs), are destroyed. Microscopy: All sites of involvement have granulomatous lesions closely resembling those found in tuberculosis, and bacilli are almost never found, hence the name "paucibacillary" leprosy. *The presence of granulomas and absence of bacteria reflect strong T-cell immunity.*

B. Granulomatous inflammation in the dermis is composed of epithelioid cells surrounded by T cells.

C. Granuloma in tuberculoid leprosy, showing **foamy histiocytes** arranged in a concentric pattern.

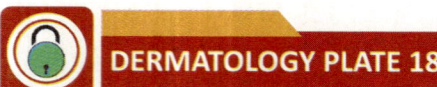

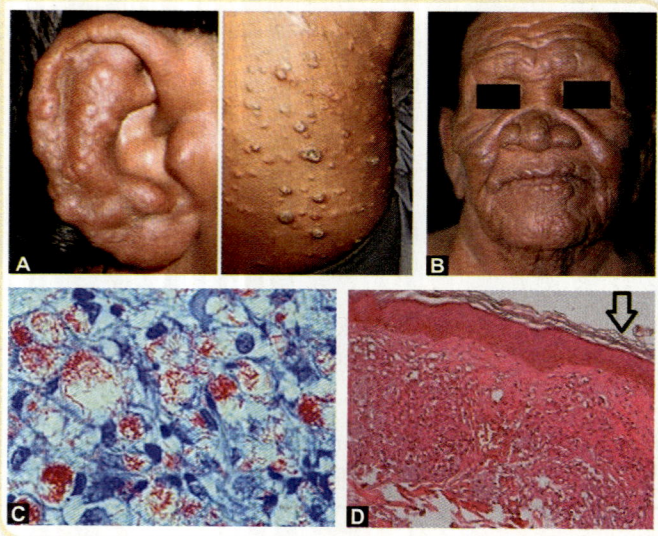

LEPROMATOUS LEPROSY (LL)/ MULTIBACILLARY
Morphology

A. Macular, papular, or **nodular lesions** form on the face, ears, wrists, elbows, back and knees.
B. With progression, the nodular lesions coalesce to yield distinctive **leonine facies**. Most skin lesions are hypoesthetic or anesthetic.
C. Acid-fast bacilli ("**red snappers**") are densely clustered within the cytoplasmic vacuoles of foamy histiocytes. This unique structure called "**globi**" is demonstrated by the Fite's method of **Ziehl-Neelsen stain**
D. On E and H staining: Lepromatous lesions contain large aggregates of *lipid-laden foamy macrophages (lepra cells)*. Because of the abundant bacteria, lepromatous leprosy is referred to as "**multibacillary**". Epidermal atrophy with a **Grenz zone** (down arrow).

Involves the skin, peripheral nerves, anterior chamber of the eye, upper airways (down to the larynx), testes, hands, and feet. The vital organs and CNS are rarely affected, presumably because the core temperature is too high for growth of M. leprae. The peripheral nerves, particularly the ulnar and peroneal nerves where they approach the skin surface, are symmetrically invaded with mycobacteria, with minimal inflammation. The testes are usually extensively involved, leading to destruction of the seminiferous tubules and consequent sterility.

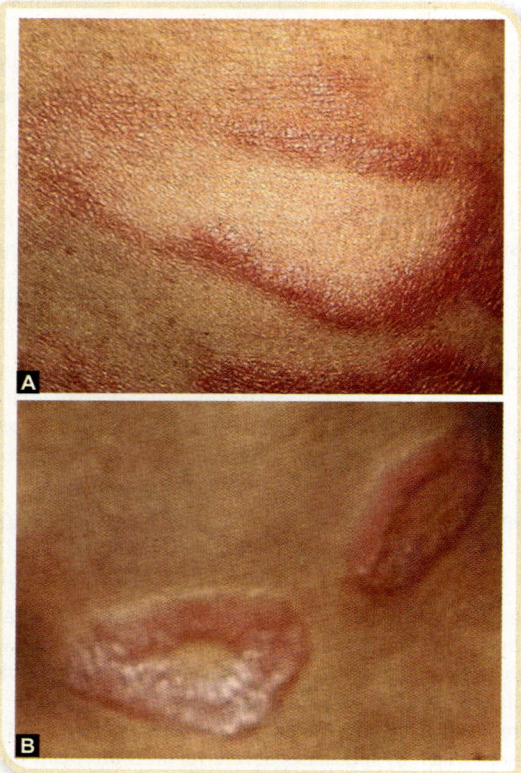

BORDERLINE BORDERLINE LEPROSY

A. The presence of erythematous plaques with **fading outer borders, clear inner borders, and hypopigmented oval center (foveal spot) is suggestive of the BB subgroup**. BB leprosy is the immunologic midpoint in the fascinating clinical spectrum of the granulomatous disease. It is the most unstable and uncommon form. These patients upgrade or downgrade to a more stable clinical form at the earliest. Cutaneous lesions are characteristically annular plaques with sharp interior and exterior borders. Large plaques with islands of clinically normal skin within the plaques give rise to a **"Swiss cheese" appearance**. Lesions are numerous but are asymmetrical.

B. **Total Annular lesion:** With both inner and outer edges being sharp and clear cut consistent with BB Leprosy

Types of lesion	Top view	Side view	Seen in
Saucer right up (side up) lesion: Annular lesion with a sharp outer edge and vague inner edge that slopes towards the center of the lesion			TT, BT Leprosy (DERM PLATE 12 A)
Punched out lesion/ Swiss cheese: Annular lesion with sharp central punch with clear inner but vague and sloping outer edges			BB Leprosy (DERM PLATE 14)
Total Annular lesion: with both inner and outer edges being sharp and clear cut			BB Leprosy
Inverted saucer lesion: A dome shaped lesion with central infiltration and gradual peripheral sloping			BL Leprosy

- ---------- ⇨ Ill-defined/sloping edges
- ────── ⬇ Well-Defined Edges

Ridley Jopling Classification of Leprosy

The Ridley-Jopling classification is based on **clinical** (Skin and nerve involvement), **histopathological, bacteriological** (bacteriological/morphological index in skin and nasal smear), **and immunological** (lepromin test) parameters. It is mainly based on histopathology, reflecting the immunological status of an individual patient and consists of a 5-group system

	Tuberculoid leprosy (TT)	Borderline tuberculoid (BT)	Borderline borderline (BB)	Bborderline lepromatous (BL)	Lepromatous leprosy (LL)
Hypopigmentation	+	+	+	+	+
No. Of lesions	<3	3–10	Numerous but countable	Numerous and uncountable	Numerous and uncountable
Symmetry	Unilateral Assymetrical	Unilateral Assymetrical	Bilateral but Assymetrical	Bilateral and Symetrical	Bilateral and Symetrical
Anhydrosis, sensory loss and hair loss	Complete loss	Impaired	Decreased	Slightly Decreased	Normal
Types of lesion	Macules or plaques (0.5 cm- 30 cm).	Plaques	Plaques	Macular, annular plaques or nodule	Early Macules and late Nodules

Contd...

Ridley Jopling Classification of Leprosy

Lesion	Mostly single (or 2-3) Asymmetrical and usually unilateral. Erythermatous, raised edges central flattening. Loss of sensation hair and sweeting, the surface is dry, rough, and irregular, and the lesions feel firm on palpation. Thickened nerves may be palpable	Commonest presenting form of leprosy. **Welldefined infiltrated plaques.** Margins raised or flat well defined or vague in parts. The surface is dry and anhidrotic. Lesions may also be hypopigmented, slightly erythematous macules	Features of both TT and LL. widespread bilateral but asymmetrical erythematous infiltrated plaques with a punched out or annular appearance. Plaque is **depressed in the centre and has a sharp inner edge and sloping outer border.** Lesions are of varied sizes, bizarre shapes with irregular borders and may have **geographic appearance.**	Lesions tend to be more widespread than BB but are not as symmetrical as in lepromatous leprosy. The nodular or Punched out plaques lesions. Diffuse infiltration of pinna and eyebrows seen in LL start making their appearance in BL leprosy.	**Early Macules**: numerous, small (<2 cm), bilaterally symmetrical, smooth, shiny, ill-defined macules, hypopigmented, erythematous or coppery. **Late Nodules**: macules enlarge and coalesce. The lesions are bilaterally symmetrical and smooth surfaced with sloping edges. If a patient is not treated at this stage, the skin becomes more infiltrated and assumes a **waxy appearance.**
Satellite lesion	Absent	Present	Absent	Absent	Absent
Site	Any site but preferable sites are face, lateral or dorsal aspects of the extremities, and the buttock	Any site	Any site.	More at the sites of LL	Face including Nose, Ear. Nose: **saddle nose**, epistaxis, Anosmia, discharge, **Larynx**: hoarseness, stridor, Asphyxia, Tongue and Palate, Neuritis, iritis, orchitis. Deformity and ulceration of hands, feet
Sensations	Anesthetic macule	Anesthesia is less severe than TT	Anesthesia is less than BT	Anesthesia is often absent	Sensations of touch and pain (pin-prick) are usually unimpaired
Nerve thickening	Thick or tender nerve trunks and nerve to lesion	Thickened or tender or both	Thickened or tender or both	Thickened or tender or both	Multiple thickened nerves
Lepromin test	+++	++ or +	Variable + or -	-	-
Cutaneous nerve	Destroyed/ swollen	Cellular infiltrate	Cellular infiltrate	Infiltrate	Cutaneous Nerve preserved
Granuloma	Compact/ tuberculoid granuloma eroding epidermis	Tuberculoid granuloma but less well defined	Diffuse epithelioid granuloma	Granuloma composed of lymphocytes and macrophage	Thin epidermis, flat rete ridges, diffuse leproma of foamy macrophages, plasma cells and lymphocytes
Acid fast bacilli	AFB are not found except in areas of caseation.	AFB may still be found in the nerve	AFB are easily detectable and numerous	AFB = as numerous as in LL	AFB are seen in large numbers in macrophages, nerves and skin appendages.
Grenz zone (clear zone b/n epidermis and dermis)	Absent	Present	Present	Present	Present
Slit smear (AFB)	NO AFB	Nil to scanty	Moderate	Many	Numerous + globi

Contd...

Ridley Jopling Classification of Leprosy					
Lepra reactions	LEPRA I	LEPRA I	LEPRA I	LEPRA I and II	LEPRA II
Enl				ENL+	ENL +
Comments		Satellite lesion	Punched out lesion, Inverted saucer lesion, Swiss cheese pattern lesion	Onion peel appearance of nerves	Leonine facies, Oil paint appearance on face, Onion peel appearance of nerves, Most infectious stage

Indian classification
1. Tuberculoid
2. Borderline tuberculoid
3. Mid borderline
4. Borderline lepromatous
5. Lepromatous
6. Pure neuritic type

WHO classification
- For treatment purposes, in 1982, the WHO Study Group on Chemotherapy of Leprosy for Control Programs classified leprosy into two types: paucibacillary (PB) (including the tuberculoid, indeterminate, and borderline tuberculoid forms), and multibacillary (MB) (including lepromatous, borderline lepromatous, and midborderline forms)
- Pure neuritic has not been classified
- A simple classification based on the number of lesions has been recommended for use by field workers: 1–5 lesions as paucibacillary, and 6 or more as multibacillary leprosy
- All slit skin smear positive cases are MB

DERMATOLOGY PLATE 20

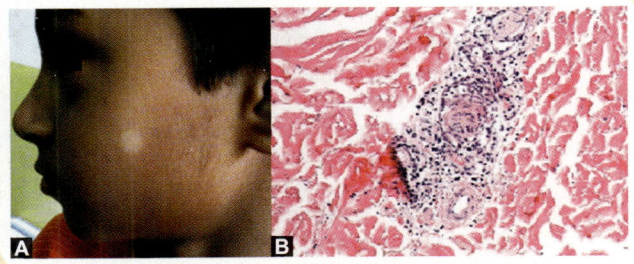

INTERMEDIATE LEPROSY

A. Morphology: It appears as poorly defined areas of slight hypopigmentation or erythema, without systemic or neural changes. The condition is only likely to be recognized readily in endemic areas where there is a high awareness of leprosy.

B. Microscopy: Scanty superficial and deep lymphohistiocytic infiltrate in the dermis, with some tendency to localization around appendages. **Bacilli are infrequent,** but scantily present in nerves. Perineural and peri appendageal inflammatory infiltrate consisting of lymphocytes and histiocytes

INTERMEDIATE LEPROSY
(refers to a very early form of leprosy)
- Classically seen in Resident of endemic area and children
- Not classified under Ridley Jopling classification
- The first lesion to appear is a medium to large sized hypopigmented patch often on the external aspect of thigh, face, extensor surface of the limbs

Contd...

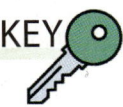

INTERMEDIATE LEPROSY
(refers to a very early form of leprosy)
- The edges are vague and there is some loss of tactile and thermal sensations
- Shiny due to epidermal atrophy
- Hair growth and nerve functions are usually unaffected
- Nerves not enlarged
- Variable lepromin test
- No neurological sequel
- The diagnosis of indeterminate leprosy can only be confirmed on a biopsy which shows presence of bacilli or typical perineural infiltration.
- AFB are mostly not demonstrable.
- Three out of four cases of indeterminate leprosy undergo self healing
- The prognosis with treatment is excellent.

DERMATOLOGY PLATE 21

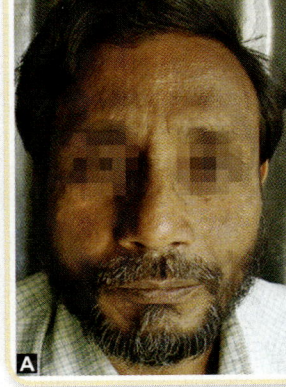
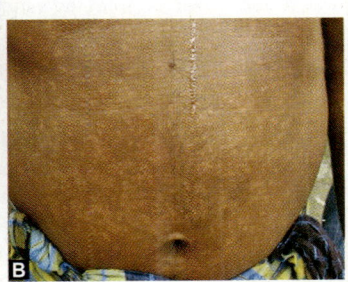

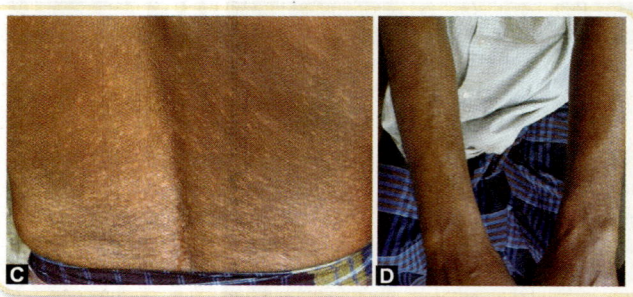

© Islam S, Ashraful Alam Bhuiyan M, Bern C

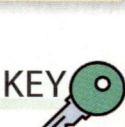

KEY

POST KALA AZAR DERMAL LEISHMANIASIS

This is a case of Post Kala Azar Dermal Leishmaniasis:

A. The patient has hypopigmented papules and plaques over the face, most concentrated on forehead, peri-orally and on the cheeks, common areas of involvement for post-kala-azar dermal leishmaniasis (PKDL).

B. Hypopigmented papules on the abdomen

C. Hypopigmented papules are seen on the back. The lesions are **roughly symmetrical**, a common characteristic of post-kala-azar dermal leishmaniasis (PKDL), and are painless and non-pruritic

D. The patient has hypopigmented papules and plaques on both forearms. The **absence of sensorineural changes** helps to distinguish post-kala-azar dermal leishmaniasis (PKDL) from leprosy, which commonly presents with hypopigmented macules or patches associated with hypoesthesia or anesthesia, and neural thickening.

Case: A 50-year-old man from Mymensingh district, Bangladesh, presented with a 3-month history of non-pruritic, painless hypopigmented papules, and plaques, beginning on the face and subsequently spreading to the forearms, torso, and legs. Fifteen months before the onset of skin lesions, the patient had visceral leishmaniasis (kala-azar), successfully treated with 30 intramuscular injections of sodium stibogluconate (SSG). Polymerase chain reaction showed **Leishmania donovani** DNA in a buffy coat specimen.

Cutaneous Leishmaniasis	
Types	▫ Old world cutaneous leishmaniasis (syn. oriental sore, Biskra button, Delhi boil, Baghdad boil) ▫ Disseminated cutaneous leishmaniasis (syn. leishmaniasis cutis diffusa leproid, cheloid leishmaniasis, leishmaniasis cutanea pseudolepromatosa) ▫ American cutaneous and mucocutaneous leishmaniasis ▫ Visceral leishmaniasis (syn. kala-azar) and post-kala-azar dermal leishmaniasis (syn. dermal leishmanoid)
Infectious agent and vector	L. major, L. tropica, L. aethiopica, and L. infantum. Vector: Infected sandfly P. papatasii and P. sergenti
Reservoir	Humans, canines of the dog family, rodents. In India, the zoonotic reservoir is the desert gerbil.
Clinical features	**Cutaneous leishmaniasis:** The skin is the usual site of entry for the promastigotes. Nodules which may ulcerate with crateriform or cribriform scar. Satellite lesions present. Sporotrichoid spread present. Distribution of lesions on exposed sites.

Contd...

	Visceral leishmaniasis, also known as kala-azar, is characterized by irregular bouts of fever, substantial weight loss, swelling of the spleen and liver, and anaemia (which may be serious). If the disease is not treated, the fatality rate in developing countries can be as high as 100% within 2 years
Diagnosis and Treatment	Demonstration of parasite on smear Lieshmanin test Histopathology showing amastigotes Culture on NNN Medium

Post Kala Azar Dermal Leishmaniasis	
Infectious agent	L. infantum (Mediterranean area, Middle East, Northern Africa, and China), L. chagasi (South America), and L. donovani (India, East Africa, and parts of China).
Reservoir	For L. infantum and L. chagasi, the reservoir is usually dogs and other canines, whereas in L. donovani the reservoir is man.
Vector	P. argentipes
Clinical features	Post-kala-azar dermal leishmaniasis (PKDL) is a complication of visceral leishmaniasis (VL) in areas where Leishmania donovani is endemic; it is characterized by a hypopigmented macular, maculopapular, and nodular rash usually in patients who have recovered from VL. **Two types of morphological lesions are usually seen, the early hypopigmented macules and the later nodular lesions.** It usually appears 6 months to 1 or more years after apparent cure of the disease but may occur earlier or even concurrently with visceral leishmaniasis especially in the Sudan. PKDL heals spontaneously in the majority of cases in Africa but rarely in patients in India. It is considered to have an important role in maintaining and contributing to transmission of the disease particularly in interepidemic periods of VL, acting as a reservoir for parasites. **Systemic features may be seen. Generalized lymphadenopathy may be seen.**
Diagnosis	Histopathology of skin may show the amastigote and clinch the diagnosis or may help to differentiate it from the other conditions such as leprosy, fungal infections, leucoderma, syphilis, yaws, and keloid.

DERMATOLOGY PLATE 22

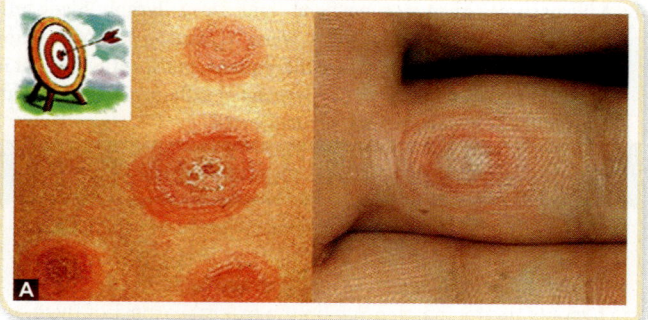

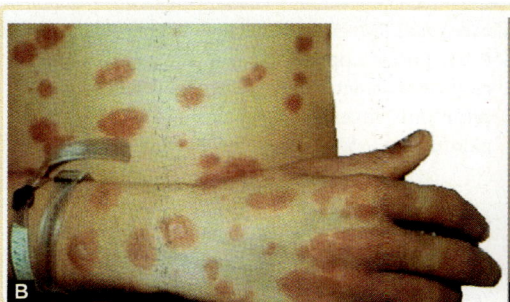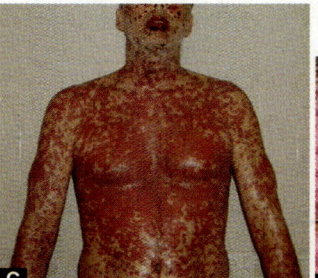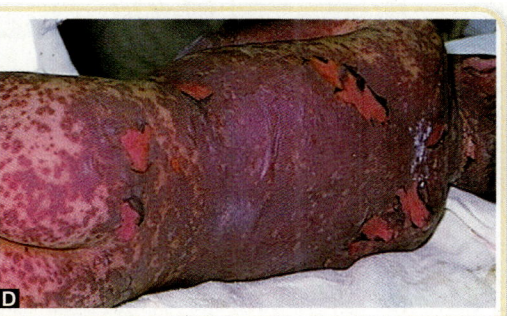

KEY

A. **Erythema multiforme** showing target lesion consisting of three zones: a central dusky discoloration or bulla surrounded by a pale colored edematous ring encircled by erythema
B. **Erythema multiforme** rash with discrete target lesions of the trunk and extremity, with confluence distally; dorsal wrist lesions have central bullae. Note the symmetric distribution of the target macules.
C. **Stevens-Johnson Syndrome** Note there is no exploitation of epidermis. Targetoid lesions on the trunk of patient, as well as the mucosal involvement on the lips.
D. **4 Toxic Epidermal Necrolysis** The initial bullae have coalesced, leading to extensive exfoliation of the epidermis. Scattered apoptotic keratinocytes in the basal and suprabasal layers of the epidermis immediately. In later stages: sub-epidermal cleavage covered with confluent necrosis of the whole epidermis. There is a thrifty/mild perivascular inflammatory infiltrate, especially consisting of lymphocytes. Immunopathology: Variable numbers of lymphocytes (CD 8+) and epidermal macrophages, lymphocytes (CD4 +) in the papillary dermis.

			EM- SJS- Ten Complex		
Clinical criteria allow the distinction of both forms of EM from SJS/ TEN in the vast majority of patients. These clinical criteria are as follows: (1) the type of elementary skin lesion; (2) the distribution of skin lesions (topography); (3) the presence or absence of overt mucosal lesions; and (4) the presence or absence of systemic symptoms					
	EM minor	**EM major**	**Stevens-Johnson syndrome (SJS)**	**SJS/TEN overlap syndrome**	**Toxic epidermal necrolysis (TEN), or Lyell's syndrome**
Common cause	Infection	Infection	Medication	Medication	Medication
Type of skin lesions	Typical targets ▫ ± Papular atypical targets	Typical targets ▫ ± Papular atypical targets ▫ Occasionally bullous lesions	Dusky red lesions, Flat atypical targets (Targetoid lesion with 2 zones)	Dusky red lesions, Flat atypical targets (Targetoid lesion with 2 zones)	Poorly delineated erythematous plaques, Epidermal detachment, Dusky red lesions, Flat atypical targets (Targetoid lesion with 2 zones)
Distribution	Extremities (especially elbows, knees, wrists, hands), face	Extremities, face	Trunk and face; Isolated lesion **Confluence (+)** on face and trunk	Trunk and face; Isolated lesions. **Confluence (++)** on face and trunk	Trunk and face; Isolated lesions are rare. **Confluence (+++)** on face, trunk, and elsewhere
%BSA involved in detachment	< 10 %	< 10 %	<10 %. The skin lesions progress to epidermal necrosis and sloughing.	10- 30 %	> 30%. The skin lesions progress to **full-thickness epidermal necrosis.**
Mucosal involvement	Absent or mild	Severe	**Mucosal membranes are affected in 92 to 100 percent of patients, usually at two or more distinct sites (ocular, oral, and genital)**	Mucosal involvement seen	Severe: **Mucous membranes are involved in nearly all cases**
Systemic symptoms	Absent	Present	Present	Present	Present

Contd...

EM- SJS- Ten Complex

Prodrome	Nil	Mild if any	It is characterized by a **prodrome of malaise and fever**, followed by the rapid onset of erythematous or purpuric macules and plaques.	Prodrome of upper respiratory tract symptoms, fever and painful skin	TEN also begins with a prodrome of fever and malaise, although temperatures are typically higher than those seen with SJS, often **exceeding 39 degrees Celsius**.
Progression to TEN	No	No	Yes	Yes	--
Precipitating factors	Herpes simplex virus Other infectious agent	Herpes simplex virus, Mycoplasma pneumoniae, Other infectious agents Rarely drugs	Drugs, Occasionally Mycoplasma pneumoniae, Rarely immunizations	Drugs, Occasionally Mycoplasma pneumoniae, Rarely immunizations	Drugs, Occasionally Mycoplasma pneumoniae, Rarely immunizations
Mortality	Rare	Rare	1–5%	Between SJS and TEN	25–35 %

Footnote:
- Currently, TEN and SJS are considered to be two ends of a spectrum of severe epidermolytic adverse cutaneous drug reactions, differing only by their extent of skin detachment.
- Drugs are assumed or identified as the main cause of SJS/TEN in most cases, but **Mycoplasma pneumoniae and Herpes simplex virus** infections are well documented causes alongside rare cases in which the etiology remains unknown.
- TEN and SJS usually occur **7–21 days** after initiation of the responsible drug
- The medications most frequently incriminated are allopurinol, nonsteroidal anti-inflammatory drugs, antibiotics and anticonvulsants.
- Historically, these three presentations were considered to form a spectrum from mild to fulminatingly severe cases. *More recently, there has been a re-evaluation of this concept and a tendency to consider erythema multiforme minor and major as part of one spectrum*, often related to infections (especially herpesvirus) and perhaps on occasion to drug reactions.
- On this basis SJS and TEN are separable from erythema multiforme and are more closely linked to drug sensitivities, and may be regarded as severe variants of a single disease.
- Exfoliation is due to extensive death of **keratinocytes via apoptosis;** the latter is mediated via the cytotoxic secretory protein granulysin and interaction of the death receptor–ligand pair Fas–FasL
- Optimal medical management of SJS and TEN requires early diagnosis, immediate discontinuation of the causative drug(s), and rapid initiation of supportive care and specific therapy
- Specific therapies that have the potential to selectively block keratinocyte apoptosis, such as high- dose **IVIg,** may provide added benefit over supportive care alone.

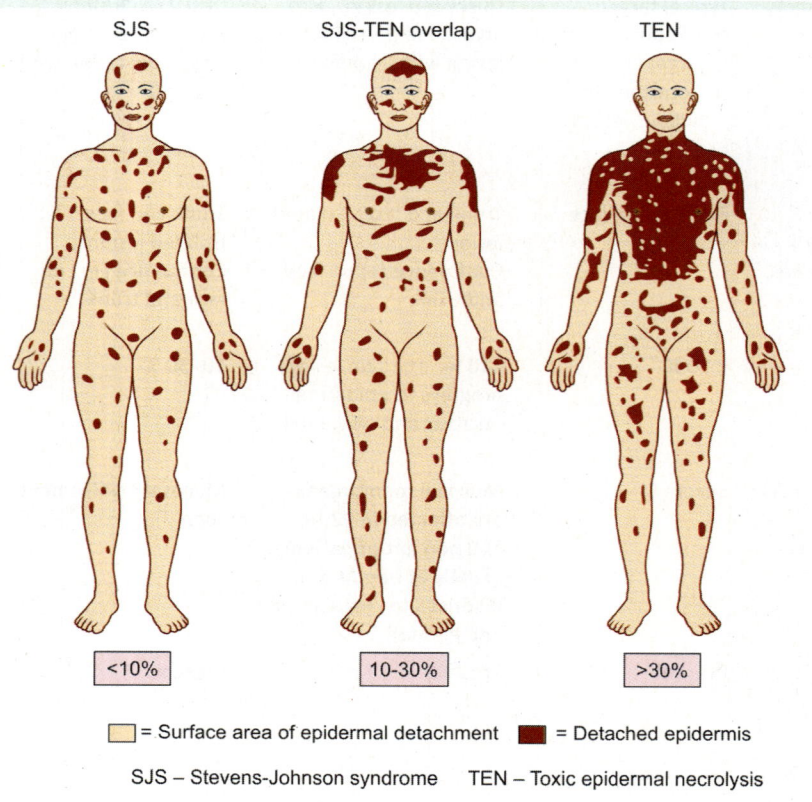

SJS – Stevens-Johnson syndrome   TEN – Toxic epidermal necrolysis

DERMATOLOGY PLATE 23

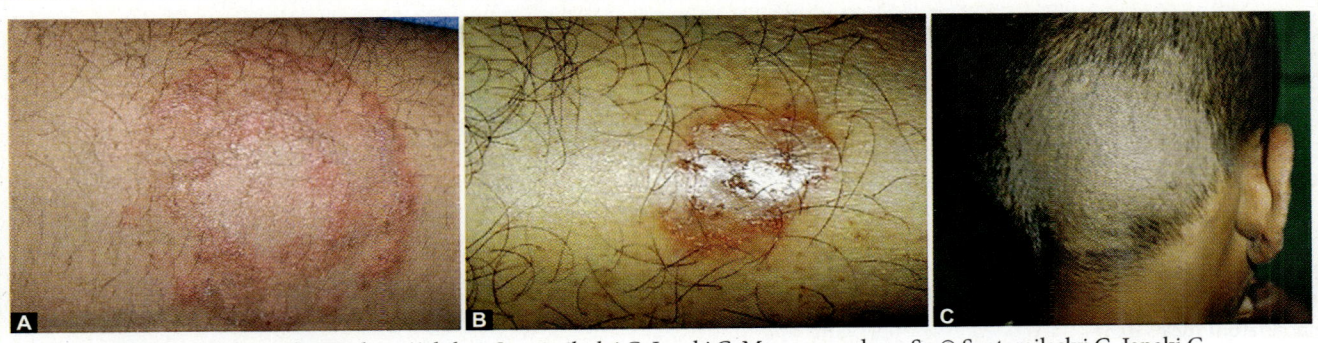
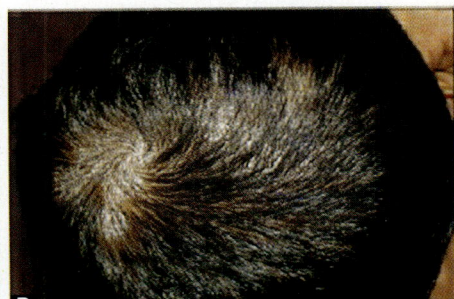
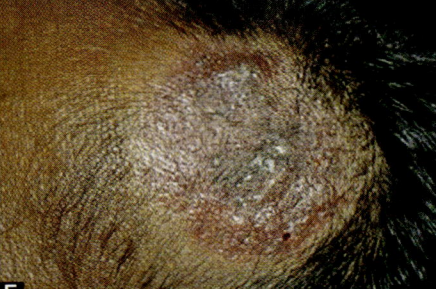
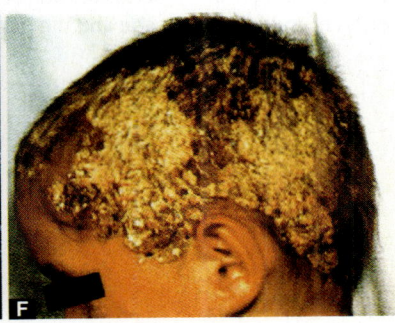

Public Health Image Library (PHIL, http://phil.cdc.gov/phil/home.asp)   © Sentamilselvi G, Janaki C, Murugusundram S   © Sentamilselvi G, Janaki C, Murugusundram S

© Sentamilselvi G, Janaki C, Murugusundram   © Sentamilselvi G, Janaki C, Murugusundram

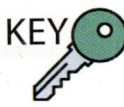
KEY

DERMATOPHYTE

Tineas are dermatophyte infections of the skin. From top to bottom, left to right: fungal infections of a) hair (Tinea capitis); b) face (Tinea capitis /ringworm); c) arm (Tinea corporis); d) close-up of ringworm; e) torso with concentric rings (Tinea imbricata/tinea corporis); f) groin (Tinea cruris); g) toe webbing (Tinea pedis); h) foot (Tinea pedis/"moccasin" type); and i) nails (onychomycosis).

A. **Tines cruris**[NEETPG]: The itchy lesion in picture is a typical dermatophyte infection, and its known **Jock's itch** or **Tinea cruris**. It is also known as **Dhobi's itch**. Although prevalent worldwide, tinea cruris is more common in tropical regions. It is more common in young (18–25 years) males. It may be more common in men than in women probably because tinea pedis (with which tinea cruris is frequently associated) is more prevalent in men, males perspire more than females, anatomical differences (greater areas of occlusive skin where the scrotum is in contact with the thigh), and clothing differences. Tinea cruris is frequently recurrent; factors favoring recurrence are high environmental temperature and sweating, and the wearing of athletic supporters or shorts that produce chafing in the groins. In obese persons, there is constant mechanical irritation of apposed surfaces, decreased aeration, increased sweating, and difficulty in maintaining hygiene and inspecting the area involved.

B. **Tinea corporis** with intra lesional papules suggestive of hair invasion
C. **Tinea capitis black dot type** with Tinea facei involving the pinna
D. **Tinea capitis grey patch type**[AIIMS PG] (Drug of choice Griseofulvin)[AIIMS PG]
E. **Tinea capitis kerion**
F. **Tinea capitis favus**

Dermatophyte
▫ Group of filamentous fungi which affect only the superficial keratinised layers of the skin
▫ Classified into three genera: Trichophyton, Microsporum, Epidermophyton
▫ In cultures on **Sabouraud's agar** they form characteristic hyphae and two types of sexual spores, microconidia and macroconidia
▫ Differentiation of species is dependent upon macroconidia
▫ Trichophyton species infect skin, nails and hair. **T. rubrum is the most common species affecting human beings**
▫ Epidermophyton species affect skin and nails but not the hair. Only one specie is known: *E. floccosum*
▫ Laboratory investigation: Scrapings are taken from the edge of the lesion mixed with 10% KOH on a slide, after placing a cover slip and the preparation heated to bring about a clearing. They are seen under microscope for septate hyphae.
▫ Wood's lamp may also be useful.

Contd...

	Dermatophyte		
Skin Disease	**Location of Lesions**	**Clinical Features**	**Fungi Most Frequently Responsible**
Tinea corporis (ringworm)	Nonhairy, smooth skin.	Circular patches with advancing red, vesiculated border and central scaling. Pruritic.	All dermatophytes can cause. **Mc= T. rubrum**
Tinea imbricata	Subtype of tinea corporis	Concentric rings are seen	T. circinata
Tinea pedis[1] (**Athlete's foot**)	Interdigital spaces on feet of persons wearing shoes.	Acute: itching, red vesicular. Chronic: Itching, scaling, fissures.	T rubrum, T mentagrophytes, E floccosum
Tinea cruris (Ringworm of the groin /**Dhobie itch** /Eczema marginatum **Jock's itch**)	Groin	Erythematous scaling lesion in intertriginous area. Pruritic.	T rubrum (m.c), T mentagrophytes, E floccosum
Tinea capitis (Mainly seen in children, MC mycosis of children)	Scalp hair. Classification according to the size and the location of the spore 1. **Endothrix:** fungus inside hair shaft. 2. **Ectothrix:** fungus on surface of hair.	**Inflammatory variety:** 1. **Kerion:** Is rare and presents with boggy swelling on scalp of a child which is indurated and studded with broken hair and pustules. Lymphadenopathy is commonly seen. It heals with scarring.	T. verrucosum and T. mentagrophytes
		2. **Favus:** Presents with a yellow cup shaped crust composed of dense mat of mycelia and epithelial debris. Called scutulum due to its shield-like shape.	The commonest cause of favus is *T. schoenleinii*. At times, *T. violaceum* and *M. gypseum*
		Non-inflammatory variety: 1. **Gray patch tinea:** Presents as papules which spreads to involve all hair in its path, multiple such partial hairless patches showing numerous broken hair and dandruff like scaling. This type of Tinea capitis is usually observed in epidemics in schools.	*Microsporum audouinii.*
		2. **Black dot Tinea capitis** is an endothrix type of infection. Hair shaft breaks at the level of scalp and remnant of hair appears as black dot.	
Tinea barbae (**Barber's itch**)	Moustache and beard area of face	Edematous, erythematous lesion.	T mentagrophytes
Tinea Faciei	Non hair bearing areas of face		T. mentagrophytes and T. rubrum
Tinea unguium (onychomycosis)	Nail. (Toe nail more common than finger nail)	Nails thickened or crumbling distally; discolored; lusterless. Usually associated with Tinea pedis.	All dermatophytes. But Most commonly T rubrum, T mentagrophytes, E floccosum
Dermatophytid (**id reaction**)	Usually sides and flexor aspects of fingers and Palm. Any site	Pruritic vesicular to bullous lesions. Most commonly associated with Tinea pedis.	No fungi present in lesion. May become secondarily infected with bacteria.

[1]May be associated with lesions of hands and nails (onychomycosis)

	Dermatophyte Involvement		
	Skin	**Hair**	**Nails**
Trichophyton	✓	✓	✓
Microsporum	✓	✓	
Epidermophyton	✓		✓

Tinea unguium (Onychomycosis)	
Distal and Lateral Subungual Onychomycosis	**Most common type.** The most common etiologic agent is *T. rubrum*. Toenails> fingernails. It starts by invasion of the stratum corneum of the hyponychium of the distal nail bed or the lateral nail fold. Subsequently, the infection moves proximally in the nail bed and invades the ventral surface of the nail plate. Subungual hyperkeratosis and splinter hemorrhages are seen

Contd...

	Dermatophyte
White Superficial Onychomycosis	**Second most common type:** Primarily invasion of the dorsal surface of the nail plate. It is usually caused by Trichophyton mentagrophytes and is characterized by well circumscribed powdery white patches away from the free edge of the nail
Proximal Subungual Onychomycosis	**Least common** variant of onychomycosis. It is most commonly caused by T. rubrum; other causes are T. mentagrophytes and T. tonsurans. The first clinical sign is a whitish to brownish area on the proximal part of the nail plate. This rare type is an early indicator of **HIV infection** and is also associated with peripheral vascular compromise
Total dystrophic	End point of all the types

DERMATOLOGY PLATE 24

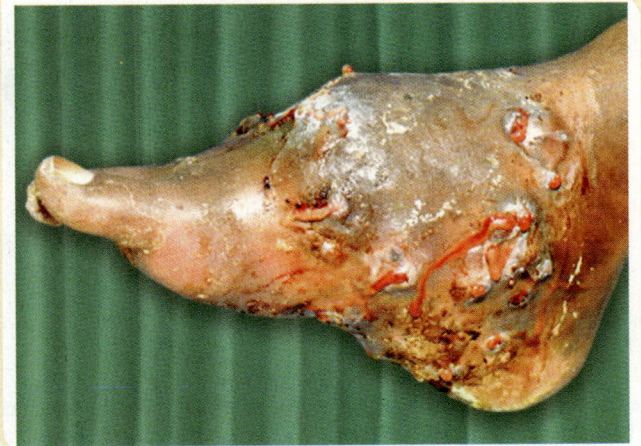

© Fahal A, Mahgoub el S (Sudan)

MYCETOMA

Mycetoma is a chronic, suppurative, granulomatous disease of subcutaneous tissue and bones, characterized by localized swellings with multiple sinuses discharging **granules** that are micro colonies of the causative agents.
Etiology: Bacterial (Actinomycetoma) or Fungal (Eumycetoma), In India actinomycetoma is more common.
Clinical features: Mycetoma begins as soft, small, painless subcutaneous nodules, which ulcerate and drain through sinus tracts. The discharge may be serosanguinous, seropurulent or purulent and often contains characterstic granules. The granules colonies of the organisms. Mycetoma may remain localized or may extend slowly along fascial planes invading subcutaneous tissues, fat, ligaments, muscles, bones but sparing tendons. In eumycetoma, the lesions form single or multiple punched out lytic lesions without little bone reaction. In actinomycetoma, both osteolytic and osteosclerotic changes are seen.
Granules: The granules can be of many colors but Actinomycetoma is mostly yellow and Eumycetoma granules are mostly black. Actinomycetoma visible granules (clumps of organism) are called "sulfur granules", which are gritty and yellow. (Although sulfur is not found in the granule)

Grain	Eumycetoma species	Actinomycetoma species
White		Nocardia asteroides, N. brasiliensis, Actinomadura madurae

Grain	Eumycetoma species	Actinomycetoma species
White to yellow	Pseudoallescheria. Boydii, acremonium species	Streptomyces. somaliensis
Red		Actinomadura. pelleteri
Black	Madurella. Mycetomatis, M.grisea	
Brown	P. jeanselmei	

Treatment: The main mode of therapy is surgical and anti-fungals such as itraconazole, Amphotericin B, Posaconazole have been used, but itraconazole has been most extensively used.

DERMATOLOGY PLATE 25

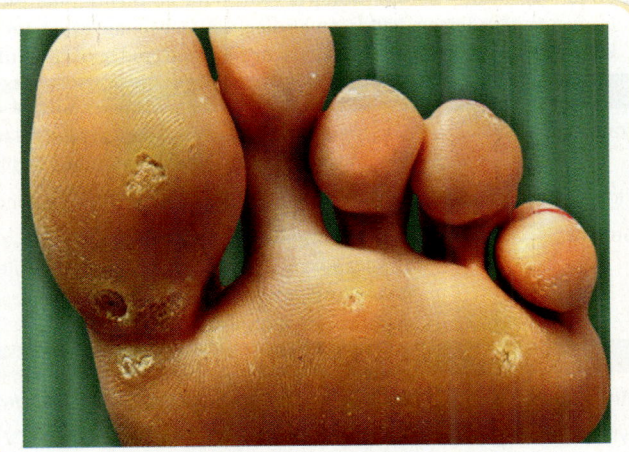

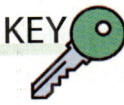

PLANTAR WARTS

- Seen mainly on pressure points like heads of metatarsals
- Caused commonly by HPV 1, 2, 4, 57
- Mosaic plantar warts are caused by HPV-2

Plantar wart and callosity are clinically differentiated by following points
- Lateral pressure causes pain in warts
- Breakage of dermatoglyphics occurs on warts
- Appearance of bleeding points occur on pairing in warts

Contd...

DERMATOLOGY PLATE 26

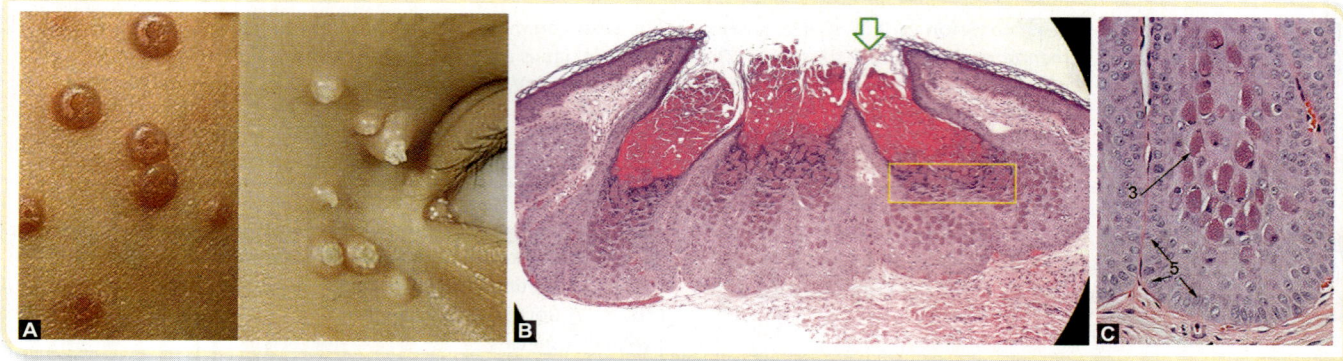

Images courtesy of Ed Uthman from Houston, TX, USA

KEY

MOLLUSCUM CONTAGIOSUM

A. Lesions of *Molluscum contagiosum*: Dome shaped, grouped pink/skincoloured or pearly, with central umblication/pore of papules which are asymptomatic. Enlarging slowly, it may reach a diameter of 5–10 mm in 6–12 weeks. (and by history of presence in immediate family members, indicate contagious nature)

B. Histopathology of *Molluscum contagiosum*:
- Pear shaped nodules of epidermis growing into the dermis as a closed packed lobule which on the surface appears as volcanic micro craters (green downwards arrow) separated by the epidermal lips of the crater.
- *Epidermal acanthosis*; increased thickness of surrounding epidermis (yellow rectangle)

C. High resolution Histopathology: Within the epithelium there are large intracytoplasmic eosinophilic inclusion bodies called Molluscum bodies or Henderson-Patterson bodies, which become more and more basophilic as it rises to the surface. These bodies appear about 1-2 layers above the basal cell layer (arrow 5) of the epidermis as pink to red inclusions (arrow 3).

	Pox Virus
Transmission	Spread is mainly by **direct-contact inoculation**, with droplet spread in some, for example variola, which produce respiratory tract lesions. Some grow readily in eggs and tissue culture, others not at all.
Viral inclusion bodies	Within the cytoplasm, they produce eosinophilic inclusion bodies (**Guarnieri bodies**).
Genera	☐ Orthopoxviruses—variola (smallpox), vaccinia, monkeypox and cowpox, which are ovoid, 300 Å~ 250 nm ☐ Parapoxviruses—orf and milker's nodule viruses, which are cylindrical, 260 Å~ 160 nm ☐ Molluscipox—molluscum contagiosum, intermediate in structure and 275 Å~ 200 nm ☐ Yatapox—tanapox virus.
	Molluscum Contagiosum
Etiology	Molluscum contagiosum virus (MCV), a complex **Double stranded DNA poxvirus,** most common genotype is MCV-1
Types	Two molecular subtypes of the virus, **MCV I and MCV II,** result in indistinguishable skin lesions. The virus occurs throughout the world, most commonly causing disease in childhood. Type 1 MCV is found in the majority of infections (76–97%)
Transmission	Transmission is via skin-to-skin contact and less commonly fomites.
Clinical picture	MC is a common, self-limited condition in children. It also occurs in adults, usually as a sexually transmitted disease, and has been observed with increasing frequency in immunocompromised hosts, most notably HIV-infected individuals. The age of peak incidence is reported as between 2 and 5 years.
Incubation period	14 days to 6 months
Lesion	**Dome-shaped**, grouped pink/skin coloured or pearly, with **central umblication/pore** of papules which are asymptomatic. Enlarging slowly it may reach a diameter of 5–10 mm in 6–12 weeks.
Site	Axilla, popliteal fossa, Genitals and Groin (in sexually active adults, not involved in children). Face is most commonly involved in children
Histopathology	**Molluscum bodies** on Geimsa stain. **Cup-shaped epidermal thickening** with degenerative changes in granular layer. Hypertrophied, Hyperplastic epidermis with intact basal layer
Treatment	Topical and oral **CIDOFOVIR** Curettage, Cautery, Imiquimod and Salicylic acid Topical cantharidin

DERMATOLOGY PLATE 27

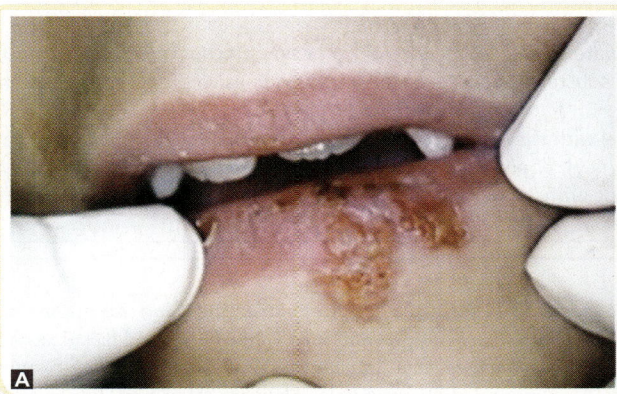
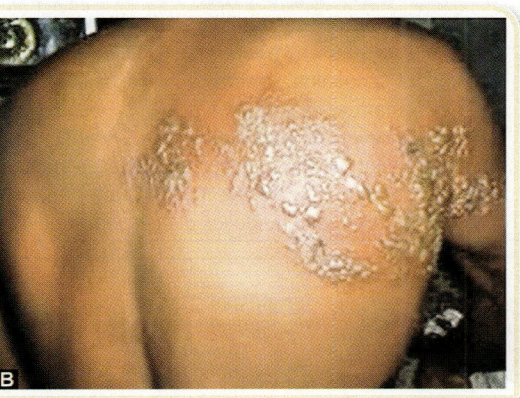

HERPES ZOSTER (SHINGLES)

A. **Herpes labialis**[NEETPG] **of the lower lip** blisters in a group. Burning pain followed by small blisters or sores, which are painful and recurrent. Caused by herpes simplex virus type 1 (direct contact).

B. Note the painful, grouped vesicles in unilateral dermatomal distribution, which is typical of **Herpes zoster.**

	Herpes Zoster (Shingles)
	Herpes zoster (shingles) is a sporadic disease that results from **reactivation of latent Varicella zoster virus (VZV) from dorsal root ganglia.** Most patients with shingles have no history of recent exposure to other individuals with VZV infection. Herpes zoster (HZ) is a localized disease characterized by unilateral radicular pain and grouped vesicular eruption limited to the dermatome innervated by a single spinal or cranial sensory ganglion.
	HZ is seen in adults who previously have had chicken pox. It is more common among patients with leukemia, lymphoma, oatcell carcinoma of lung, bone marrow transplant recipients, renal transplant recipients and HIV infection. More common in **patients > 60 years**
Pathogenesis	During the course of varicella, VZV passes from lesions in the skin and mucosal surfaces into the endings of sensory nerves and is transported centripetally up the sensory fibers to sensory ganglia. In the sensory ganglia, it remains latent. The latent period may seem to last for many years after the primary infection. Clinical manifestations result when the virus is reactivated. The newly synthesized VZV virions are transported along the sensory nerves and released into the skin. Then a unilateral vesicular eruption involving one or two dermatomes forms along the distribution of the sensory nerves. The total duration of disease is generally **7–10 days**; however, it may take as long as **2–4 weeks** for the skin to return to normal. Patients with herpes zoster can transmit infection to seronegative individuals, with consequent chickenpox.
Clinical features	1. There may be a prodrome of symptoms such as fever, malaise, paresthesia or dysesthesia before the lesions erupt. 2. Herpes zoster is characterized by a **unilateral vesicular dermatomal eruption**, and does not cross the midline, often associated with severe pain. The dermatomes from **T3 to L3 are most frequently involved thoracic (53%), cervical (usually C2 and C3; 4%–20%), trigeminal, including ophthalmic (15%), and lumbosacral (11%)** 3. When branches of the trigeminal nerve are involved, lesions may appear on the face, in the mouth, in the eye, or on the tongue. If the ophthalmic branch of the trigeminal nerve is involved, *zoster ophthalmicus* results. 4. In children, reactivation is usually benign; in adults, it can be debilitating because of pain. The onset of disease is heralded by **pain within the dermatome**, which may precede lesions by **48–72 h**; an **erythematous maculopapular rash** evolves rapidly into vesicular lesions 5. In a few patients, characteristic localization of pain to a dermatome with serologic evidence of herpes zoster has been reported in the absence of skin lesions, an entity known as *zoster sine herpetica* 6. In the **Ramsay Hunt syndrome**, pain and vesicles appear in the external auditory canal or tympanic membrane with or without tinnitus, vertigo and deafness, and patients lose their sense of taste in the anterior two-thirds of the tongue while developing **ipsilateral facial palsy**. The geniculate ganglion of the sensory branch of the facial nerve is involved.
Complications	**Cutaneous complications:** Bacterial infection, scarring, zoster gangrenosum and cutaneous dissemination. **Visceral complications:** Pneumonitis, hepatitis, esophagitis, pericarditis, gastritis, cystitis and arthritis. **Neurological complications:** *Postherpetic neuralgia (most common complication)*, meningo-encephalitis, transverse myelitis, peripheral and cranial nerve palsies, sensory loss, deafness and ocular complication

Contd...

Herpes Zoster (Shingles)	
Treatment	Ideally the drug should be administered within 48 to 72 h after the appearance of the rash. □ **Uncomplicated cases:** Acyclovir (800 mg five times daily for 5 days), valacyclovir (1 g t.i.d. for 5 days) and famciclovir (0.5 g t.i.d. for 7 days). □ **Immunocompromised patients:** Acyclovir 10 mg/kg for longer duration □ **Post herpetic neuralgia:** Application of cold water or ice cubes. Topical lignocaine patches or local infiltration of lignocaine. Topical capsaicin, a depletor of substance-P stores in the nerve endings. Oral analgesics and anti inflammatory drugs □ **In severe or persistent pain:** Systemic therapy with tricyclic antidepressants like amitriptyline (25–75 mg/day), anti-epileptics like carbamazepine (600–1000 mg/day), or phenytoin (300–400 mg per day) or lamotrigine (200–400 mg per day) may be effective. Gabapentin, starting with 300 mg per day and gradually increased up to 3600 mg per day in three divided doses over a period of 4 weeks.

DERMATOLOGY PLATE 28

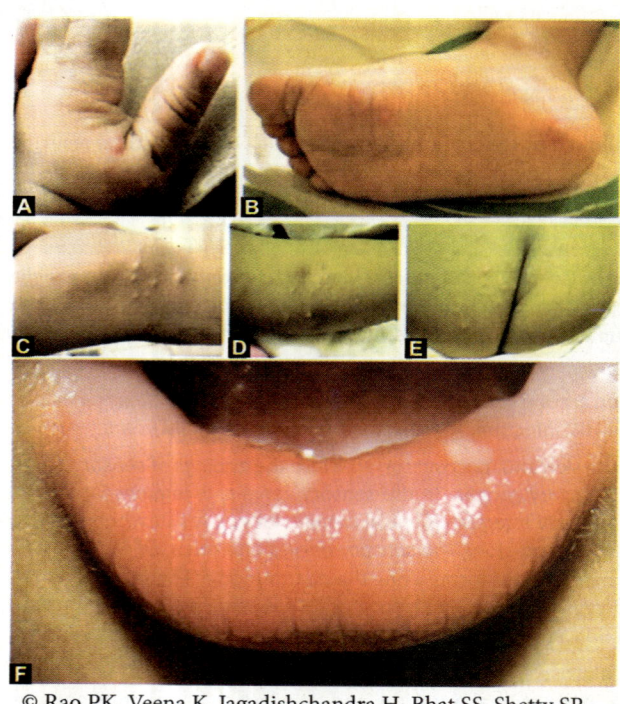

© Rao PK, Veena K, Jagadishchandra H, Bhat SS, Shetty SR

A. to E. Multiple eruptions over the hand, feet, knee, elbow and buttocks: Multiple eruptions on the hands and feet are asymptomatic red papules that quickly become small, grey, 3–7 mm vesicles surrounded by a red halo. They are often oval, linear, or crescentic, and run parallel to the skin lines on the fingers and toes. Especially in children who wear diapers, vesicles and erythematous, edematous papules may occur on the buttocks. Treatment is supportive, with the use of oral topical anesthetics.

F. Oral ulcers on the labial mucosa of lower lip: In 90% of cases oral lesions develop; these consist of small (4–8 mm), irregular shape, rapidly ulcerating vesicles surrounded by a red areola on the **lower lip, buccal mucosa, tongue, soft palate, and gingiva.** The lower lip was edematous. Lesions are self-limiting and heals without scarring

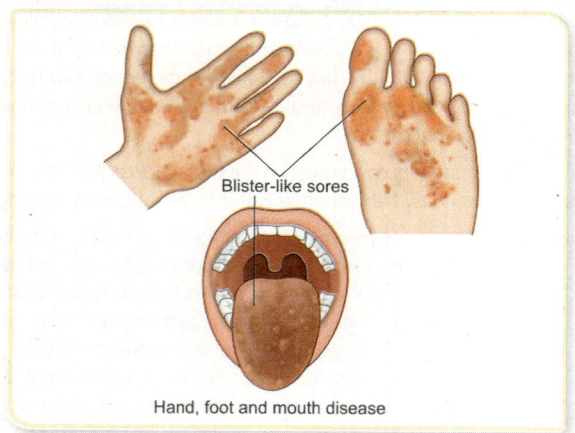

HAND, FOOT AND MOUTH DISEASE (HFMD)

Hand, foot and mouth disease (HFMD) was first described in Canada in 1957 by Robinson and Alsop et al coined the term hand, foot and mouth disease 1959.

Etiology

Hand foot and mouth disease is most frequently caused by Coxsackie virus A—16 and less commonly by other Coxsackie viruses (A5, A7, A 9, A10, B1, B3, and B5). Transmission is mainly via fecal oral contact and less commonly by respiratory droplets. During epidemics, transmission can occur via mother to fetus. Children from 2-10 years are commonly affected. Incubation period ranges from 2-5 days and virus shedding lasts up to 5 weeks.

An abrupt onset of scattered papules that progress to oval or linear vesicles in an acral distribution should suggest hand-foot-and-mouth disease.

DERMATOLOGY PLATE 29

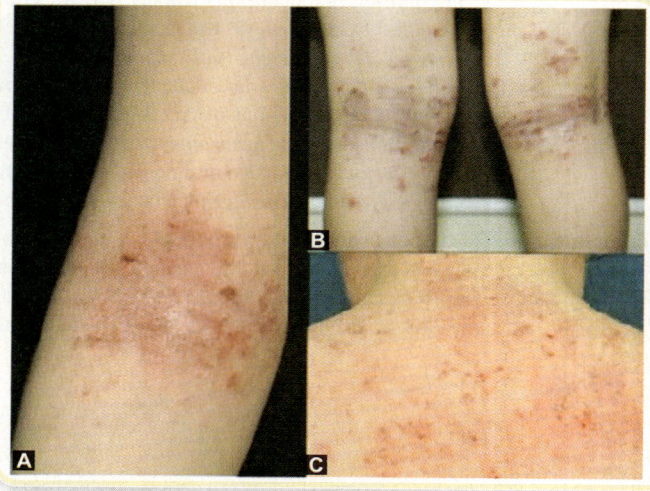

ATOPIC DERMATITIS

Atopic dermatitis (which is synonymous with atopic eczema) is an itchy, chronic, or chronically relapsing, inflammatory skin condition. The rash is characterized by itchy papules (occasionally vesicles in infants) which become excoriated and lichenified, and typically have a flexural distribution. The eruption is frequently associated with other atopic conditions in the individual or other family members.

Hanifin and Rajka Criteria of Atopic Dermatitis 3 major and 3 minor criteria need to be fulfilled
Major criteria
▫ Pruritus
▫ Typical morphology and distribution (flexural lichenification or linearity in adults and facial and extensor involvement in infants and children)
▫ Chronic or chronically relapsing dermatitis
▫ Personal or family history of atopy (asthma, allergic rhinitis, or atopic dermatitis)
Minor or less characteristic features:
▫ Xerosis
▫ Ichthyosis, palmar hyperlinearity or keratosis pilaris
▫ Immediate (type 1) skin test reactivity
▫ Elevated serum IgE
▫ Early age of onset
▫ Tendency toward cutaneous infections (esp. Staph. Aureus and HSV infection)/impaired cell mediated immunity
▫ Tendency toward nonspecific hand or foot dermatitis
▫ Nipple eczema
▫ Cheilitis
▫ Recurrent conjunctivitis
▫ Dennie–Morgan infraorbital folds (bilateral symmetrical folds formed by two additional creases beneath the eyelids)
▫ Keratoconus (conical cornea resulting from degenerative changes, leading to the cornea being pushed outwards due to intraocular pressure)
▫ Posterior and anterior subcapsular cataracts (small opacities and translucent globules seen in the lens at the pole in front of the posterior or anterior capsule)
▫ Orbital darkening (bluish to greyish periorbital pigmentation, possibly following chronic rubbing)
▫ White dermographism/delayed blanch (development of a delayed white line on firm stroking of the skin, instead of the usual red line seen normally)
▫ Facial pallor/facial erythema
▫ Pityriasis alba
▫ Anterior neck folds
▫ Itch when sweating
▫ Intolerance to wool or lipid solvents
▫ Perifollicular accentuation
▫ Food intolerance
▫ Course influenced by environmental/emotional factors

Modified Hanifin Rajka criteria of Atopic dermatitis
In order to qualify as a case of atopic dermatitis with the UK diagnostic criteria, the child must have: ▫ An itchy skin condition (or parental report of scratching or rubbing in a child) Plus three or more of the following: 1. Onset below age 2 years (not used if child is under 4 years) 2. History of skin crease involvement (including cheeks in children under 10 years) 3. History of a generally dry skin 4. Personal history of other atopic disease (or history of any atopic disease in a first degree relative in children under 4 years) 5. Visible flexural dermatitis (or dermatitis of cheeks/forehead and outer limbs in children under 4 years)

DERMATOLOGY PLATE 30

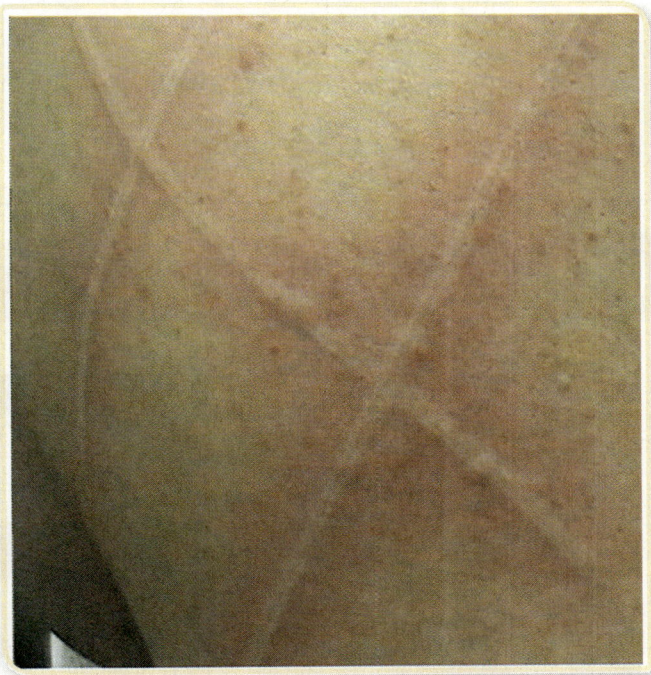

DERMOGRAPHIC URTICARIA

Note the linear shape of Wheal, one can literally draw/see spider web and chemistry molecules on the skin. Variety of google images can be searched.

Dermographic Urticaria (Factitious urticaria)	
The term Dermographism literally means **Writing on the skin**	
Etiology	Unknown, Idiopathic
Epidemiology	Most common physical Urticaria More common in young adults with peak incidence at 2nd and 3rd decade of life
Mechanism	Firm stroke on skin produces initial red line (due to capillary dilatation) → **Axon reflex flare** with erythema (ateriolar dilatation) → formation of linear wheal (Transudation of fluid/edema). Collectively these 3 steps are called as **TRIPLE RESPONSE OF LEWIS**. This reaction is normal, but in 2-5% of normal people this physiological response is sufficiently exaggerated to warrant the term **dermographism**.

Contd...

Dermographic Urticaria (Factitious urticaria)	
Clinical features	□ Patients complain of whealing within **5- 10 min** of stroking which persists for **15-30 min** this is known as Simple dermatographism
□ If itching is present along with wheal, it is symptomatic dermatogaphism. Which gets aggravated by and trauma, heat, pressure, stress, emotions, friction with clothing or scratching the skin. The itching is often disproportionately severe compared with whealing and is often most **severe at night.**
□ The eliciting stimulus determines the shape of the wheals, but they are often linear from scratching or stroking.
Types	□ **Simple dermatogaphism:** Whealing but no itching

Dermographic Urticaria (Factitious urticaria)	
	□ **Symptomatic dermatographism:** Whealing with Itching
□ **White dermographism** (due to capillary vasoconstriction following light stroking of the skin) occurs normally and is particularly pronounced in atopic subjects.
□ **Black dermographism** is discolouration of the skin after pressure from a metallic object.
□ **Red dermographism**, where repeated rubbing is necessary to induce small, punctate wheals.
Treatment	Avoid physical stimuli, reduce stress and anxiety
H1 Antihistaminics are drug of choice
Omalizumab (monoclonal antibodies against IgE) has been successfully used.

Contd...

DERMATOLOGY PLATE 31

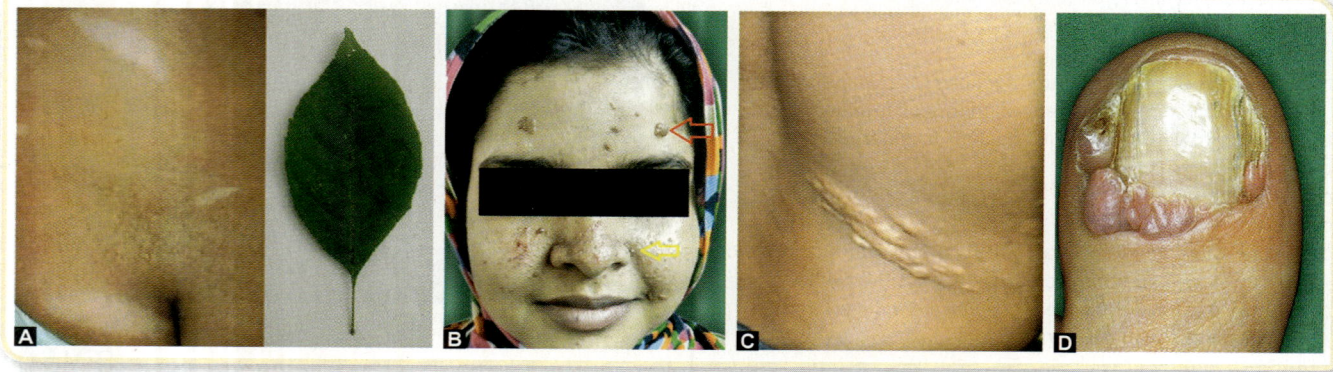

© MedEasy © Dr Ishad Aggarwal IPGIMER Kolkata

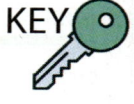

KEY

TUBEROUS SCLEROSIS (BOURNEVILLE'S DISEASE)

A. Ash Leaf spots
B. **Adenoma sebaceum** (yellow arrow), **Forehead Plaque** (red arrow)
C. Shagreen patches
D. **Periungual fibromas:** Also known as **Koenen's tumors**

Tuberous Sclerosis (Bourneville's Disease)	
Genetics	Autosomal dominant inheritance due to mutation of:
1. TSC1 gene on chromosome 9q34 encoding **hamartin** or
2. TSC2 on chromosome 16p13 encoding **tuberin**
Cutaneous	□ **Ash Leaf spots:**
1. **Earliest cutaneous and non-cutaneous sign of TS**
2. Hypomelanic 1-3 cm macules, polygonal and lance-ovate, usually multiple, that may appear anywhere on the body. Hypomelanotic but not amelanotic
3. These are usually the only visible sign of TSC at birth.
4. In fair-skinned individuals a Wood's lamp (ultraviolet light) may be required to see them.
□ **Adenoma sebaceum:** Multiple angiofibromas of the face. A rash of reddish spots or bumps, which appear on the nose and cheeks in a butterfly distribution. They consist of blood vessels and fibrous tissue. Can be removed using dermabrasion or laser treatment. A recent publication indicates that topical rapamycin is helpful for treatment of facial angiofibromas.

Contd...

Tuberous Sclerosis (Bourneville's Disease)	
	□ **Forehead plaques:** Raised, discolored areas on the forehead. □ **Shagreen patches:** Areas of thick leathery skin that are dimpled like an orange peel, usually found on the lower back or nape of the neck. □ Other skin features are not unique to individuals with TSC, including **molluscum fibrosum** or skin tags, which typically occur across the back of the neck and shoulders, **café au lait spots** or flat brown marks, and poliosis, a tuft or patch of white hair on the scalp or eyelids.
Nail	**Periungual fibromas:** Also known as **Koenen's tumours,** these are small fleshy tumours that grow around and under the toenails or fingernails and may need to be surgically removed if they enlarge or cause bleeding. These are very rare in childhood but common by middle age.
Systemic	**Kidneys** (renal angiomyolipomas > renal cysts > RCC) are affected in 80% of patients. CNS: **seizures, mental retardation,** Subependymal giant cell astrocytoma, ependymomas, glioma, ganglioneuroma, hamartoma **Retinal hamartomas**, pulmonary lymphangioleiomyomatosis (women), and cardiac rhabdomyomas.
Carcinoma	Renal cell carcinoma, Astrocytoma, CNS Hamartomas

DERMATOLOGY PLATE 32

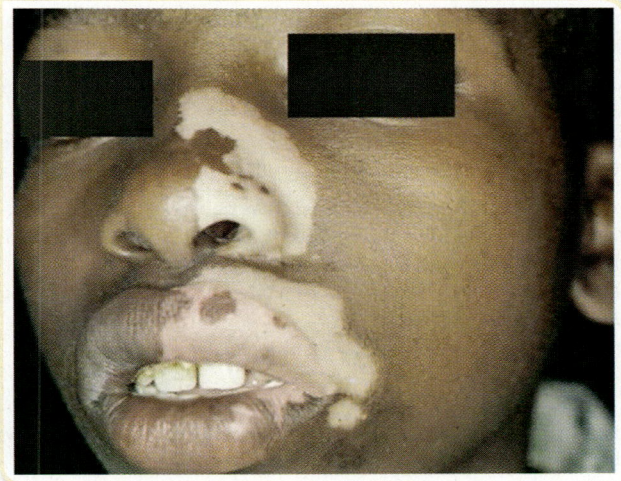

UNILATERAL (SEGMENTAL) VITILIGO
Unilateral (segmental) vitiligo affecting one side of the face of a young boy. Note that the depigmentation does not correspond to a dermatome.

Vitiligo	
Vitiligo is an acquired disorder characterized by circumscribed depigmented macules and patches that result from a progressive loss of functional melanocytes.	
Prevalance	□ 0.5–2% of the general population worldwide □ 3%–4% in India
Clinical features	□ The most common presentation of vitiligo is totally **amelanotic** (i.e. milk- or chalk-white) macules or patches surrounded by normal skin. The lesions characteristically have discrete margins, and they can be round, oval, irregular or linear in shape. □ The borders are usually convex, as if the depigmenting process were "**invading**" the surrounding normally pigmented skin. □ Lesions enlarge centrifugally over time, and the rate may be slow or rapid. Vitiligo macules and patches range from millimeters to centimeters in diameter and often vary in size within areas of involvement. □ The incidence of body leukotrichia varies from 10% to >60%, as follicular melanocytes are often spared in vitiligo. □ One of the manifestations of vitiligo is the **isomorphic Koebner phenomenon** (IKP), characterized by the development of vitiligo in sites of trauma (e.g. a laceration, burn or abrasion).

Contd...

Vitiligo

Classification	Two major forms are generally recognized:
	□ Segmental
	□ **Non-segmental form**, also called **vitiligo vulgaris**
	a. **Localized:**
	  1. **Focal:** one or more macules in one area, but not clearly in a segmental distribution
	  2. **Unilateral/segmental:** One or more macules involving a unilateral segment of the body; lesions usually stop abruptly at the midline
	  3. **Mucosal:** mucous membranes alone
	b. **Generalized:**
	  1. **Vulgaris:** Scattered patches that are widely distributed
	  2. **Acrofacial:** Distal extremities and face
	  3. **Mixed:** Various combinations of segmental, acrofacial and/or vulgaris
	c. **Universal:** Complete or nearly complete depigmentation	

Clinical variants and other features	□ **Vitiligo ponctué:** Multiple small (confetti-like), discrete amelanotic macules, sometimes superimposed upon a hyperpigmented macule. □ **Inflammatory vitiligo:** Vitiligo with raised inflammatory borders □ **Blue vitiligo:** Vitiligo develops in areas already affected by post inflammatory hyperpigmentation. □ **Trichrome vitiligo:** Hypopigmented zone between normal and totally depigmented skin. The intermediate zone (with intermediate melanocytes) does not have a gradation of color from white to normal, but rather a fairly uniform hue. □ In **quadrichrome vitiligo**, a fourth darker color is present at sites of perifollicular repigmentation. □ **Pentachrome vitiligo** with five shades of color (black, dark brown, medium brown [unaffected skin], tan and white) has also been described.	
Associated disorders	**Autoimmune disorders:** Pernicious anemia, Addison's disease, Graves' disease, hyperthyroidism, hypothyroidism, thyroiditis, hyperparathyroidism, DM. Internal malignancy, Antibodies against adrenal, thyroglobulin, and gastric parietal cell antigens have been detected. Gastritis, gastric carcinoma, and IgA deficiency are other associations occasionally reported	
Poor prognostic factors	□ Lesions on the so-called resistant sites, such as bony prominences, non-fleshy areas, non-hairy areas and mucosal areas. They comprise the sides of the ankles, front of the wrists, back of the elbows, dorsum of feet and hands, palms, soles, nipples and areola □ The greater the percentage of associated white hair, the worse the prognosis □ Extensive long-standing disease □ Associated ailments, especially systemic ones □ Heredo-familial background □ Old age □ Iatrogenic factors, including injudicious administration of topical and systemic medicines, particularly photochemotherapeutic agents	
Psoralen and PUVA	Psoralen	Photosensitising agent which is a fluorocoumarin derivative. Natural: 8 methoxy psoralen and 5 methoxy psoralen. Synthetic: 4,5,8 trimethylpsoralen
	Photochemotherapy	Topically, treatment using a combination of psoralen derivatives or other photosensitizing agent, followed by irradiation with long wave ultraviolet light
	PUVA therapy	Topical psoralen + UVA (320-400 nm)
	PUVASOL	Topical psoralen + sun exposure as source of UVA
	ORAL PUVA	Oral psoralen (0.6 mg/kg/body TMP , 0.3 mg/kg/ body weight 8-MOP) + UVA
	Narrow band UVB	311 nm
	Excimer laser	308 nm Xenon chloride laser
	Calcipotriol + PUVA	
	Khellin + UVA	
	Phenylalanine + UVA	
Topical therapy	Topical Corticosteroids	First line of treatment for patients with a few localized lesions
	Calcineurin inhibitors	Tacrolimus (0.03%, 0.1%)
	Basic fibroblast factor	
	Placental extracts	
Oral therapy	Corticosteroids	Oral mini pulse, ACTH + Corticosteroids
	Immunosuppresants	Azathioprine, cyclophosphamide , levamisole
Surgical treatment	Used mainly for stable vitiligo. Punch excision and grafting, Mini punch grafting, Split skin grafting , Theirsch grafting, non-melanocyte cultured suspension , cultured melanocyte transplant	
Others	Cosmetic camouflaging, Bleaching	

Vitiligo Vs Leprosy		
	Vitiligo	**Leprosy**
Lesion	Depigmented, no change in texture, non-scaly	Hypopigmented, infiltrated and raised, scaly
Hair in the patch	Depigmentated	Number may be decreased
Sensation	No loss	May be impaired
Nerve	No thickening	May be thickened

DERMATOLOGY PLATE 33

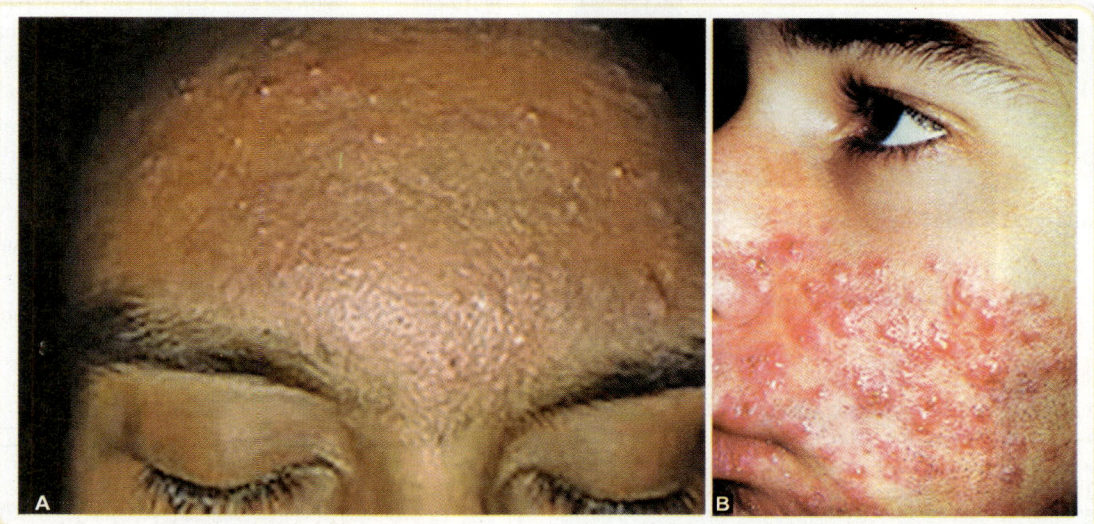

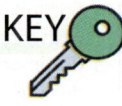

KEY

TYPES OF ACNE

A. **Acne vulgaris:** Acne vulgaris is a disorder in which hair follicles characterised by Comedones. Blackheads or comedones are formed by follicular plugs (follicular debris and compacted sebum). The skin becomes greasy. Blackheads or comedones often occur over the sides of the nose and the forehead, but can occur anywhere.

B. **Nodulocystic acne:** In severe cases of acne the nodules liquefy centrally to form fluctuant cysts which are actually pseudocysts, as they have no epithelial lining. This type of severe acne is known as cystic or nodulocystic acne

Classification and Treatment of Acne					
	Mild acne (No comedones, no inflammatory lesions, some papules and/or pustules)		**Moderate acne (Many inflammatory papules, pustules, 1-2 nodules and/or scarring)**		**Severe acne(> 2 nodules, cysts, abscesses, bridging scars)**
	Comedonal	Papular pustular	Papular/pustular	Nodular	Nodular/conglobate
1st Choice	Topical retinoid	Topical retinoid +topical antimicrobial	Oral antibiotic + topical retinoid ± BPO	Oral antibiotic + topical retincid ± BPO	Oral isotretinoin
2nd Choice	Alternate topical retinoid or azelaic acid or salicylic acid	Alternate topical antimicrobial + alternate topical retinoid Or azelaic acid	Alternate oral antibiotic + alternate topical retinoid ± BPO	Oral isotretinoin or Alternate oral antibiotic + alternate topical retinoid ± BPO/ azelaic acid	High-dose oral antibiotic + topical retinoid + BPO

DERMATOLOGY PLATE 34

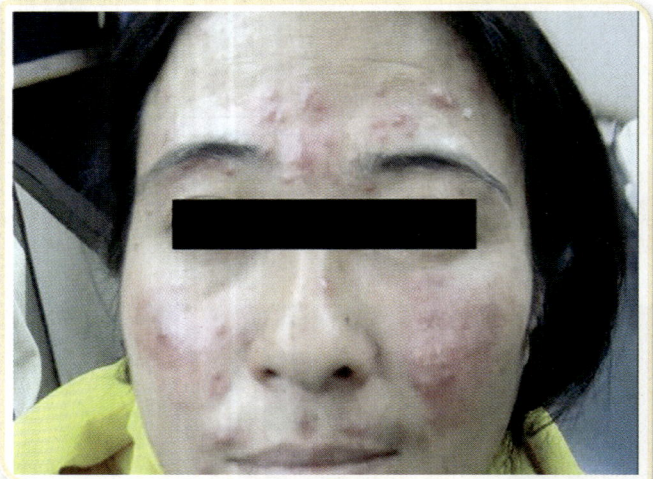

© MedEasy © Dr Ishad Aggarwal IPGIMER Kolkata

ACNE ROSACEA

The given image can lead to two main differentials; acne vulgaris and acne rosacea. However, the clinching points which favour the diagnosis of Acne rosacea are exacerbation on sweating, sun exposure and emotional disturbance

Acne Rosacea	
❑ Chronic inflammatory condition of facial pilosebaceous units with increased vascular hyperreactive ❑ Common in fair-skinned patients with peak in the third to fifth decade ❑ Presents with easy flushing and gradual reddening of complexion ❑ Exacerbating factors may include particular foods (especially spicy), alcoholic beverages, UV exposure, hot weather, warm beverages, and exercise. ❑ **Unlike Acne vulgaris, Acne rosacea are exacerbation on sweating, sun exposure and emotional disturbance etc.**	
Histology	Early lesions with dilated blood and lymphatic vessels; later lesions show lymphectasia, perivascular and perifollicular lymphohistiocytic infiltrate, ± poorly organized granulomas, dermal fibrosis, sebaceous gland hyperplasia, ± Demodex folliculorum mites within infundibula.
Type	**Predominant Feature**
Erythematotel-angiectatic	❑ Persistent centrofacial erythema ❑ Flushing ❑ Telangiectasias ❑ Skin sensitivity
Papulopustular	❑ Persistent centrofacial erythema ❑ Papules ❑ Pustules/papulopustules ❑ Overlap with other subtypes may occur

Contd...

Phymatous	Thickened, nodular skin ❑ Prominent pores ❑ Can affect nose (rhinophyma, most common), chin (gnathophyma), forehead (metophyma), ears (otophyma), eyelids (blepharophyma) ❑ May be associated with other features of rosacea or occur in isolation	
Ocular		❑ Dry, gritty sensation ❑ Blepharitis ❑ Conjunctivitis ❑ Chalazia and hordeola ❑ Keratitis, episcleritis, scleritis, iritis (rare)
Treatment	Skin care regimen	Sunscreen, moisturizer containing humectant, avoid cosmetics and toners and harsh exfoliation, avoid triggers
	Topical therapy	Metronidazole or azelaic acid best for inflammatory lesions, sodium sulfacetamide/sulfur
	Oral therapy	Tetracyclines, macrolides, isotretinoin
	Lasers	Pulsed-dye laser or intense pulsed light
	Surgical ablation	Phymatous lesions

DERMATOLOGY PLATE 35

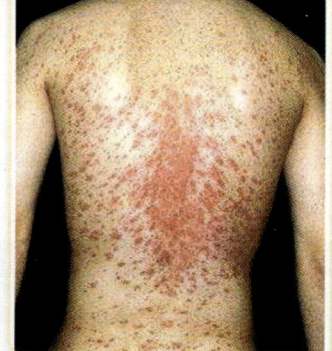

PITYRIASIS ROSEA

Pityriasis rosea is an acute, self-limiting disease, probably infective in origin, affecting mainly children and young adults, and characterized by a distinctive skin eruption and minimal constitutional symptoms
Etiology: The cause of Pityriasis rosea is not known, following agents are implicated: HHV-6, HHV-7, Pityriasis rosea is common, particularly during the winter,

Clinical Features

❑ It mainly affects children and young adults.
❑ Prodromal symptoms are usually absent.

- The first manifestation of the disease is usually the appearance of one plaque (the 'herald' or 'mother' plaque) before the others which is often mistaken for ringworm. It is larger and more conspicuous than the lesions of the later eruption and is usually situated on the **upper trunk (most commonly)**, thigh or upper arm, neck; rarely it may be on the face, scalp or the penis. It is a sharply defined, erythematous, round or oval plaque, soon covered by fine scale. It rapidly reaches its maximum size, usually 2–5 cm in diameter but occasionally much larger.
- After an interval, which is usually between 5 and 15 days, but may be as short as a few hours or as long as 2 months, the general eruption begins to appear in crops at 2 to 3-day intervals over a week or 10 days.
- In its classical form the eruption consists of discrete oval lesions, dull pink in colour and covered by fine, dry, silvery-grey scales. The centre tends to clear and assumes a wrinkled, atrophic appearance and a tawny colour, with a marginal **collarette of scale** attached peripherally, with the free edge of the scale internally. The long axes of the lesions characteristically follow the lines of cleavage parallel to the ribs in a **Fir tree of Christmas tree appearance** on the upper chest and back. The scaly lesions are commonly associated with pink macules of varying size and the eruption may be exclusively macular.
- When stretched across the long axis, the scales tend to fold across the line of stretch, the so called **Hanging curtain sign.**
- Usually the disease is self-limiting and no treatment is required.
- Secondary syphilis is common differential diagnosis and must be ruled out.

DERMATOLOGY PLATE 36

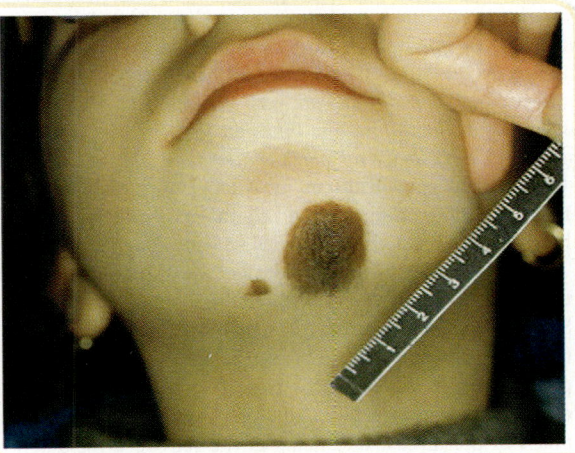

 KEY

CONGENITAL MELANOCYTIC NEVUS
This is classic congenital melanocytic nevus

Congenital Melanocytic Nevus	
Incidence	Congenital nevi are found in about 1% of newborn infants
Size	On the basis of the size, they are categorized as small CMN (diameter less than 1.5 cm), medium-sized CMN (between 1.5 and 19.9 cm) and large or giant CMN (20 cm or greater).

Contd...

Congenital Melanocytic Nevus	
Clinical features	They are usually solitary. The growth of a congenital nevus is very rapid and disproportionate to the growth of the particular body area in the first six months of age. In adults, the nevus remains static unless there is infection, trauma or development of malignancy. Small and medium nevi appear as hyperpigmented macules, solitary or multiple, at birth. Their growth is gradual and the **nevi darken, appear raised and develop coarse hair**, often in a spurt during puberty. Large CMN (also called giant, garment nevi or bathing trunk nevi) are commonly situated on the back and thighs, but may involve the arms or legs. Smaller satellite lesions are also found in the vicinity as well as at a distance from the main nevus. The nevi becomes larger, darker and more rugose as the child grows and develop a warty surface and nodules. The hairs become coarse like terminal hair and are often concentrated in the center.
Special forms	Cerebriform CMN in scalp, Neurocutaneous CMN associated with melanotic tumours of meninges
Malignant transformation	They can have potential of **malignant transformation.** High risk for giant congenital melanocytic nevus. Clinically, changes such as sudden appearance of nodules, very dark pigmentation (especially in fair-skinned individuals), itching, pain, bleeding or ulceration should arouse the suspicion of malignant melanoma
Histopathology	The classic histological features of congenital nevi after the neonatal period are: - Presence of nevus cells in the reticular dermis - Extension of nevus cells in the collagen bundles in a single row ('Indian file' appearance), sheets or combinations - Higher concentration of nevus cells around blood vessels, nerves and adnexal tissues

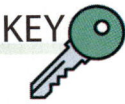

DERMATOLOGY PLATE 37

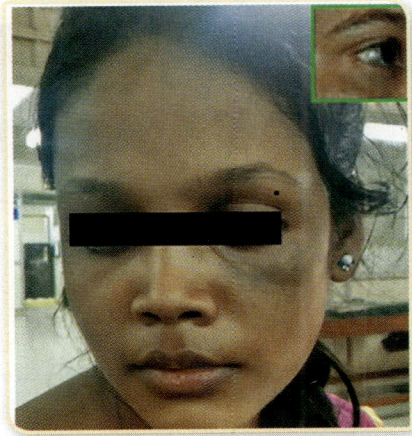

© MedEasy © Dr Ishad Aggarwal IPGIMER Kolkata

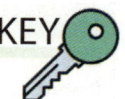

NEVUS OF OTA

A lady came with complaints of a bluish lesion over left side of forehead and left eye. An irregular bluish lesion is seen over the left superior conjunctiva. This is a clinical picture of Nevus of Ota.

- Nevus of Ota is a persistent, somewhat speckled, macular, slate brown or bluish hyperpigmentation in the distribution of the ophthalmic and maxillary division of the trigeminal nerve.
- It is commonly unilateral.
- It affects females more frequently than males and mostly presents at birth.
- Very rarely, the area supplied by the mandibular division of the trigeminal nerve may also be involved.
- Various shades of pigmentation (black, blue-back, slate blue, purple, purplish-brown or brown) have been observed.
- Hyperpigmentation of the sclera, cornea, iris, retina, fundus, optic nerve, extraocular muscles, retrobulbar fat, orbit, hard palate, pharynx, nasal mucosa, buccal mucosa, tympanic membrane of the affected side may also be present.
- The blue to blue–grey color in nevus of Ota is due to melanin-producing melanocytes in the dermis

DERMATOLOGY PLATE 38

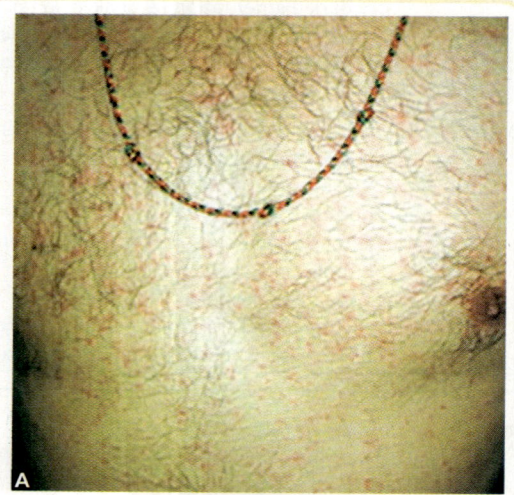

© Prashant S (Deccan College of Medical Sciences)

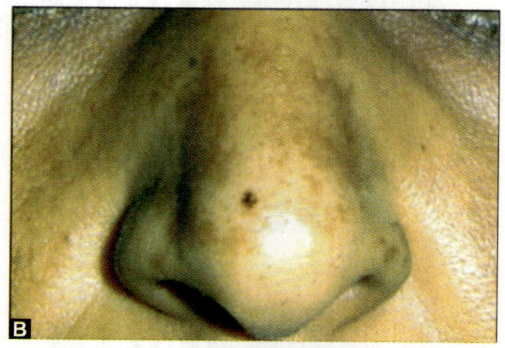

© Prashant S (Deccan College of Medical Sciences)

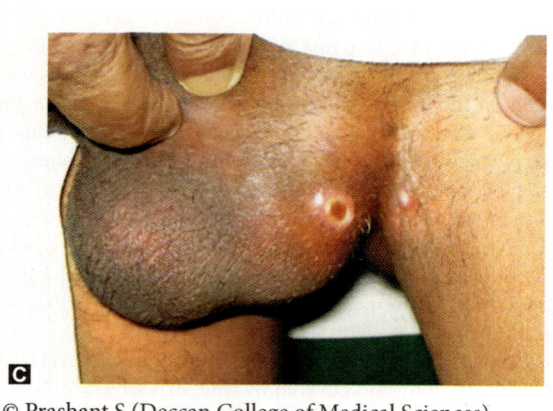

© Prashant S (Deccan College of Medical Sciences)

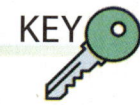

CUTANEOUS MANIFESTATIONS OF CHIKUNGUNYA FEVER

Chikungunya (CHK) is an acute onset, mosquito-borne viral disease characterized by high fever, predominant musculo-skeletal symptoms, and skin rash. The etiological agent is an RNA virus that belongs to the *alphavirus* genus of the family *Togaviridae*. The disease is transmitted to humans by the bite of infected **Aedes mosquito;** two species namely *Aedes aegypti* and *Aedes albopictus*. These mosquitoes generally bite throughout daylight hours with peaks of activity in the early morning and late afternoon. Approximately 4–7 days after the mosquito bite, patients display acute symptoms of painful polyarthralgia, high fever, myalgia, and headache. *Mucocutaneous involvement tends to be a prominent and significant finding in the acute phase of infection.* A host of mucocutaneous manifestations, occurring in 30–50% of all cases of Chikungunya infection, have been described. *Few of these are very characteristic and specific, and thus help in distinguishing the infection from its close differential of dengue fever and other viral febrile illnesses.*

A. **Generalized morbilliform maculopapular rash** with normal islands of intervening skin and characteristically sparing the face has been the most commonly (30–55%) reported manifestation. The rash develops within 3–4 days of the onset of fever and tends to subside in about a week without any sequel.
B. **Skin hyperpigmentation** is the next most commonly encountered finding. It occurs in the form of centrofacial pigmentation predominantly involving the nose (Chick sign). It is the most commonly described pigmentation developing during the acute phase of the disease and helps in the retrospective diagnosis of infection
C. Nonhealing ulcers and **genital ulcers** on the scrotum, vulva, and groins may occur.
  - Vascular response in the form of facial flushing, erythema, and edema of ear lobules resembling Milian's ear sign, erythema of striae in females have been described
  - Infants younger than 12 months tend to have different spectrum of skin lesions that include acrocyanosis and symmetrical superficial vesiculobullous lesions.
  - Subepidermal blisters and TEN like symptoms

DERMATOLOGY PLATE 39

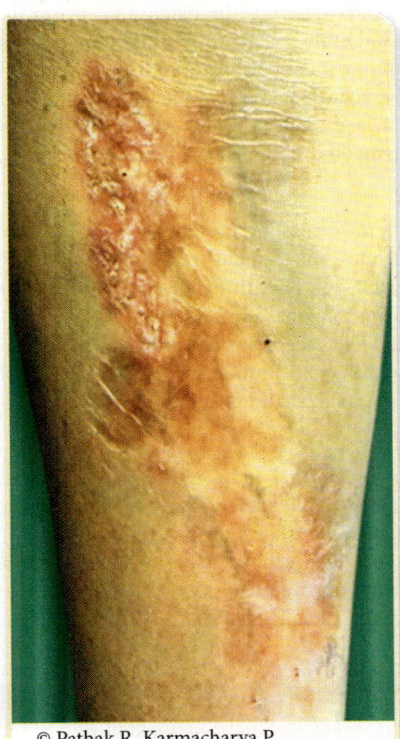
© Pathak R, Karmacharya P

NECROBIOSIS LIPOIDICA

Necrobiosis lipoidica (NL; also known as necrobiosis lipoidica diabeticorum) is a fairly distinct clinical entity that although not the most common, is the best recognized cutaneous marker of diabetes mellitus. It may be seen outside of the setting of diabetes mellitus, although up to three-quarters of patients with NL have or will have diabetes mellitus. Necrobiosis lipoidica is a chronic granulomatous dermatosis characterized by one or more yellow-brown, telangiectatic plaques with central atrophy and raised violaceous borders, typically in the pretibial regions.

Differential Diagnosis of Necrobiosis lipoidica

- **Diabetic dermopathy** is a constellation of well-demarcated, hyperpigmented, atrophic depressions, macules, or papules located on the anterior surface of the lower legs that is usually found in patients with DM. It is the most common cutaneous marker of DM. Other cutaneous markers of DM are loss of hair over the legs, acrochordons, pruritus, acanthosis nigricans, ichthyosis, cutaneous amyloidosis, syringoma, callosity, and brittle nails.
- **Hyperthyroidism:** Patients with hyperthyroidism have warm, moist, erythematous skin Many develop Onycholysis and scalp hair loss. In addition, patients with Grave's disease develops Pretibial myxedema and Acropachy. Myxedema can occur anywhere in the body but most commonly at pretibial location and is characterised by non pitting thickening and induration of the skin.
- **Sarcoidosis:** Cutaneous lesions of sarcoidosis are classified as specific (Non-caseating granulomas) and non-specific lesions (Erythema Nodosum). It is seen as localised lesion of scalp or as a manifestation of systemic disease. These lesions range from brownish red to violaceous papule and plaque that blanch on diascopy revealing "Apple jelly" colour. The lesions are most commonly seen in the head and neck region however the lesion may occur anywhere. There are case reports of Cutaneous Sarcoidosis mimicking Necrobiosis lipoidica-like skin lesions on both shins.

DERMATOLOGY PLATE 40

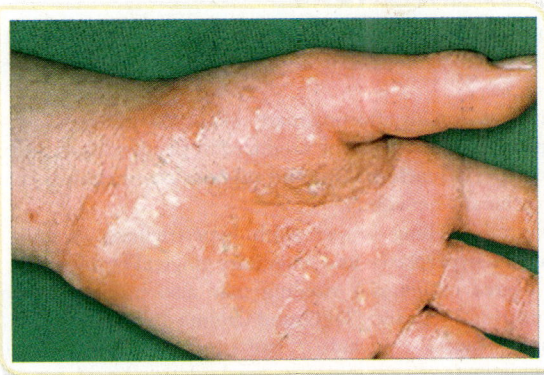

VESICULOBULLOUS HAND ECZEMA (POMPHOLYX, DYSHIDROSIS)

- Idiopathic acute vesicular hand dermatitis is not related to blockage of sweat ducts, although palmoplantar hyperhidrosis is common in these patients and control of hyperhidrosis improves the eczema.
- Acute pompholyx, also known as cheiropompholyx if it affects the hands, presents with severe, sudden outbreaks of intensely pruritic clear vesicles appear deeply seated and '**sago-grain** like:
- Primary lesions are macroscopic, deep-seated multilocular vesicles resembling tapioca on the sides of the fingers, palms, and soles.
- The eruption is symmetrical and pruritic, with pruritus often preceding the eruption. Coalescence of smaller lesions may lead to bulla formation severe enough to prevent ambulation.
- Individual outbreaks resolve spontaneously over several weeks. Bullous tinea or an id reaction from a dermatophyte should be excluded, and patch testing should be considered to rule out allergic contact dermatitis.

DERMATOLOGY PLATE 41

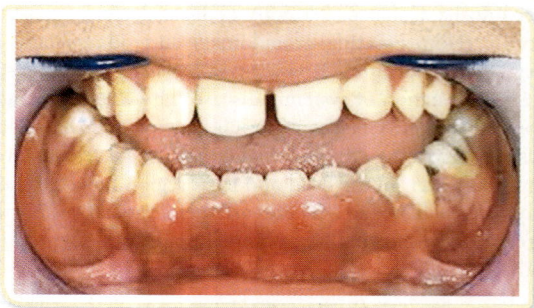

GINGIVAL HYPERPLASIA

- Localized gingival swellings (epulides) may be of local etiology or can be manifestations of pregnancy, a neoplasm or systemic disease.
- Gingival swelling affecting many areas is most commonly seen in chronic gingivitis, may be produced by drugs such as **phenytoin, ciclosporin (cyclosporin) and calcium channel blocker**s and is occasionally hereditary.
- Gingival swelling is seen with hypertrichosis in both drug-induced hyperplasias and hereditary gingival fibromatosis.
- A degree of gingival swelling may also be seen in herpetic stomatitis, pregnancy, OFG, and Crohn's disease.
- Rare causes include leukaemia, scurvy, Wegener's granulomatosis, sarcoidosis, amyloidosis, lipoid proteinosis, hypoplasminogenaemia, mucopolysaccharidoses and other disorders.

DERMATOLOGY PLATE 42

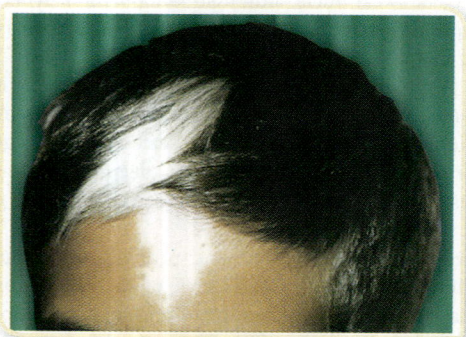

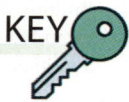

PIEBALDISM

- Piebaldism is a rare **autosomal dominant** condition characterized by stable areas of *vitiligo-like amelanotic skin associated with a white forelock*
- Piebaldism is an uncommon autosomal dominant disorder characterized by poliosis and congenital, stable, circumscribed areas of leukoderma due to an **absence of melanocytes** within involved sites.
- Patches of skin totally devoid of pigment are present at birth and usually remain unchanged throughout life.
- Most common is a *frontal median or paramedian patch*, associated with a mesh of white hair (**white forelock**); rarely, this may be the only lesion. Often, white patches occur on the upper chest, abdomen and limbs, bilaterally but not necessarily symmetrically.
- Piebaldism can easily be distinguished from vitiligo where the lesions are acquired later in life and their configuration and distribution are quite different Also the presence of islands of normal pigmented skin in the hypomelanotic areas is typical

Pathology

- Missense and frameshift mutations of the kit proto-oncogene, which encodes the cellular receptor tyrosine kinase for the mast cell/stem cell growth factor, are responsible for a range of phenotypes with piebaldism.
- Functioning KIT receptor is required for the normal development of melanocytes, both immediately before melanoblast migration from the neural crest and postnatally

Treatment

- Autografts of normal skin into amelanotic areas, including grafting of autologous melanocytes, are a therapeutic option, but this typically requires multiple procedures.
- Cosmetic products can be used to camouflage affected areas; protection against sunburn is also necessary.

DERMATOLOGY PLATE 43

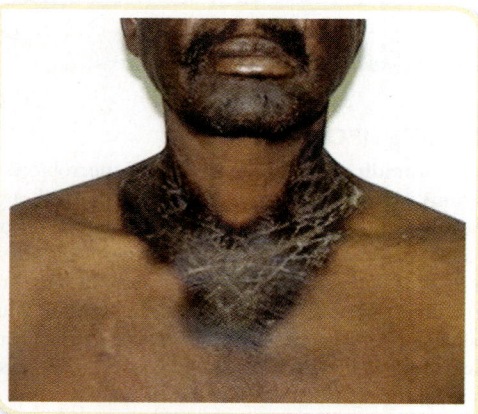

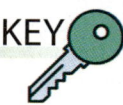

DERMATOLOGICAL MANIFESTATIONS OF PALLEGRA

- The name pellagra is derived from the Italian pelle agra, sharp [i.e., rough] skin. Pallegra was considered a public health problem in many maize consuming African and Asian countries throughout the 1960s and 1970s.
- Pellagra (vitamin B3/ niacin and/ or Tryptophan deficiency) is clinically manifested by the 4 D's: Photosensitive dermatitis, Diarrhea, Dementia and Death.
- The skin lesion starts with erythema resembling sunburn, which is symmetrically distributed on the parts of the body exposed to direct sunlight—the backs of the hands and forearms up to the rim of the sleeves (**"pellagra gloves"**), the forehead, and on the nose and cheeks in a butterfly distribution.
- The typical band of dermatitis encircling the neck has been referred to as **Casals collar or necklace** (dermatomes C3 and C4)

DERMATOLOGY PLATE 44

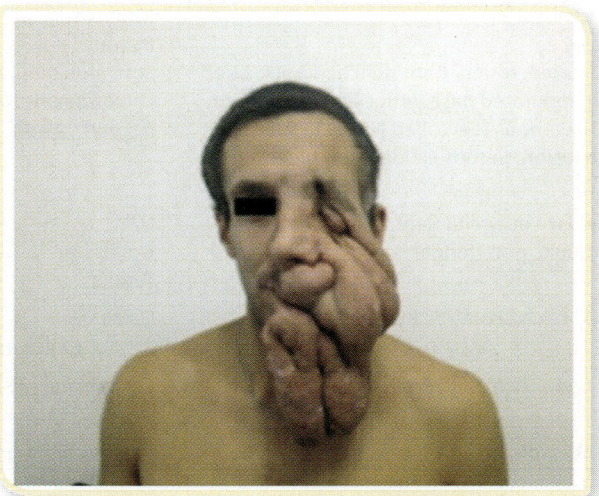

© Tchernev G et al

PLEXIFORM NEUROFIBROMA

Plexiform neurofibromatosis is a relatively common but potentially devastating manifestation of neurofibromatosis type 1 (NF1). Plexiform neurofibromas (PNF) are benign tumors that originate from nerve sheath cells or subcutaneous peripheral nerves, and can involve multiple fascicles. The image shows severe disfiguration of the left side of the face, due to overhanging folds of skin affecting the temporal, orbital, and cheek areas.

DERMATOLOGY PLATE 45

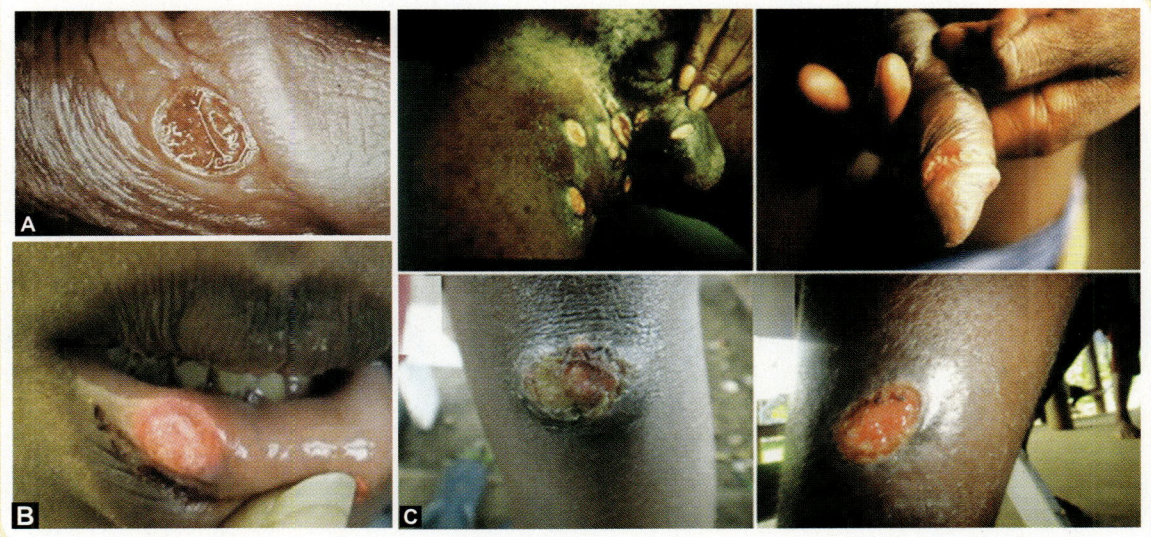

CHANCRE

A. **Penile hard chancre of syphilis:** Indurated, slightly elevated erosion with clean, smooth bases on the coronal sulcus
B. Mucosal chancre of syphilis
C. **Soft chancroid of *Hemophilus ducreyi*** in gernital and skin.[AIIMS PG]

STD	Syphilis (Hard chancre)	Chancroid (Soft chancre)
Etiology	Treponema pallidum	Haemophilus ducreyi
Incubation period	9-90 days	3-5 days
C/F, Mor	Single, Painless, Well demarcated, round, hard punched out/ raised edges, firm indurated base with clean granulation tissue, cartilagenous feel called **Nickel in funnel** or **Button like lesion**. Serous exudate, **no bleeding on touch**	Multiple Painful Soft/ non indurated base, Undermined, soft ragged edges. **Bleeds on touch.** **Mnemonic** = DUcreyi= **Do You Cry= Painful ulcer**
Inguinal Lymph Node	Generalized LN Pathy; Indolent bubo- rubbery, discrete, mobile, non- tender	U/L Unilocular Tender
Diagnosis	Dark ground microscopy, VDRL, TPi, FTAbs	Gram –ve **School of fish appearance**
Treatment	Benzathine penicillin	Ceftriaxone (250 mg IM stat) or Azithro (1 gm oral stat)
Treatment of Partner	Treat as early syphilis	Treat as if patient

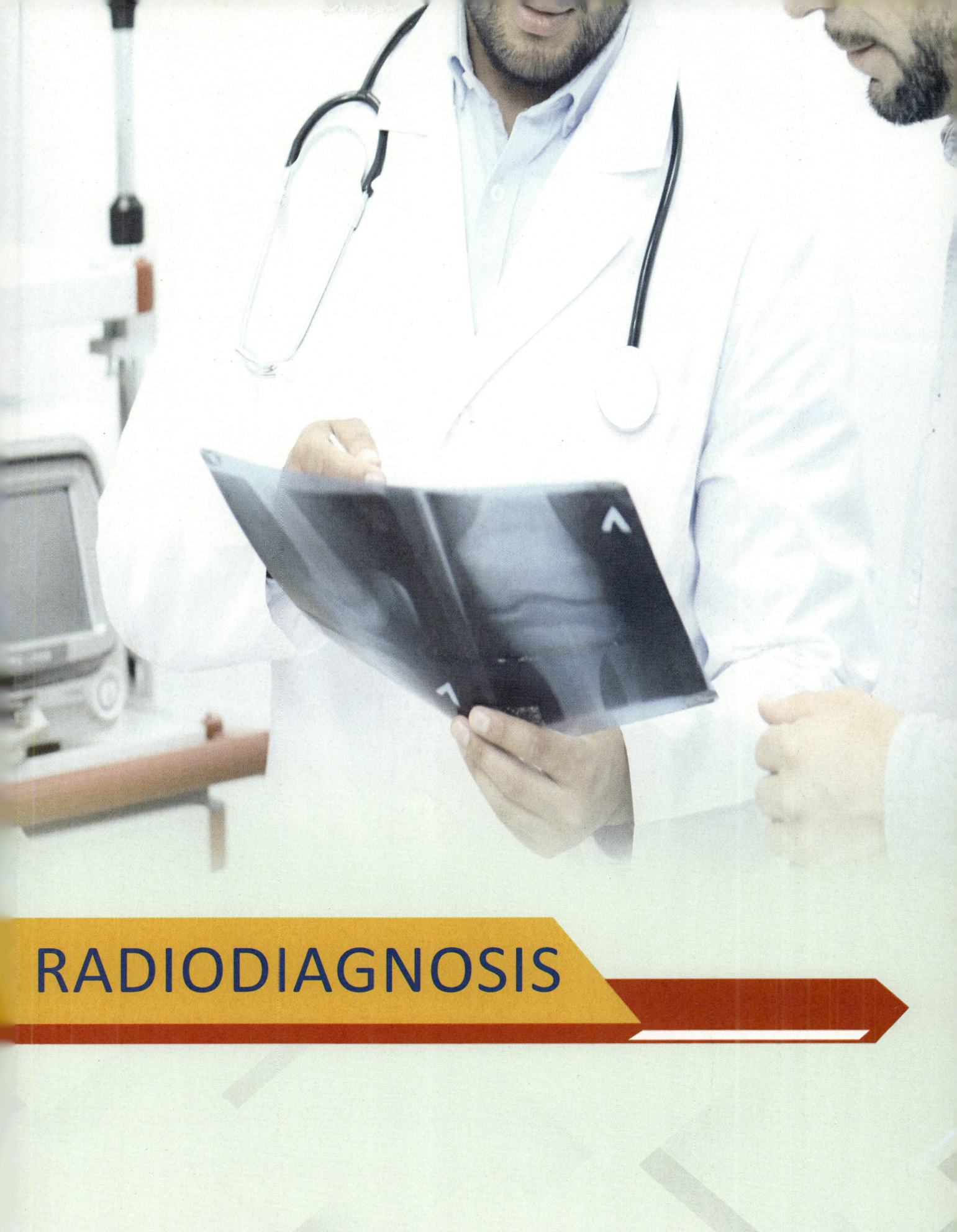

RADIODIAGNOSIS

RADIO PLATE 1

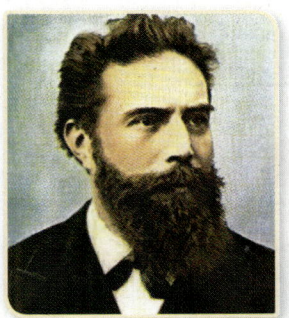

WILHELM CONRAD RONTGEN
Wilhelm Conrad Röntgen was born on **March 27, 1845**, at Lennep in the Lower Rhine Province of Germany. On 8 November 1895, he produced and detected electromagnetic radiation in a wavelength range today known as X-rays or Röntgen rays, an achievement that earned him the **first Nobel Prize in Physics in 1901**.

RADIO PLATE 2

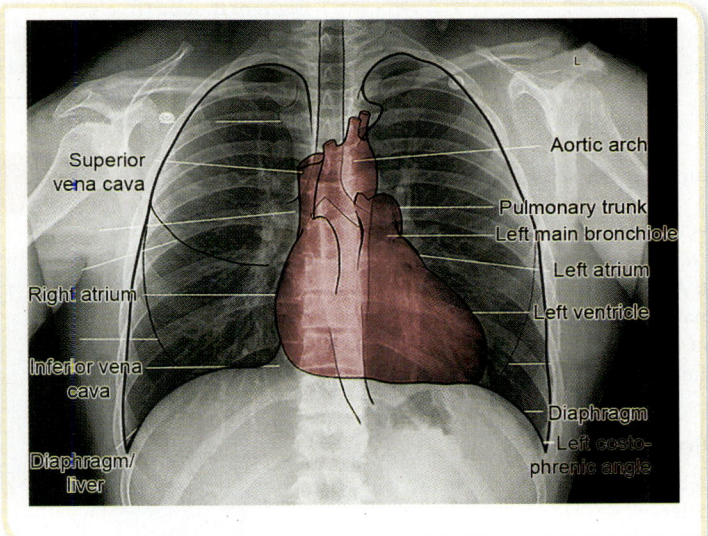

NORMAL CHEST X-RAY PA VIEW
Assessment of Heart Size
- The cardiothoracic ratio should be less than 0.5 in adults and 0.6 in infants.
- A cardiothoracic ratio of greater than 0.5 in adults and 0.6 in infants (in a good quality film) suggests cardiomegaly.

Assessment of Cardiomediastinal Contour
- Right heart border: Superior vena cava (SVC), Right Atrium
- Left heart border: Aortic Knuckle, Main pulmonary trunk, Left atrial appendage (when enlarged), Left ventricle
- Anterior aspect: Right ventricle
- Cardiac apex: Left ventricle

Assessment of Hilar Regions

- Both hilar should be concave. This results from the superior pulmonary vein crossing the lower lobe pulmonary artery. The point of intersection is known as the hilar point (HP).
- Both hilar should be of similar density.
- The left hilum is usually superior to the right by up to 1 cm.

RADIO PLATE 3

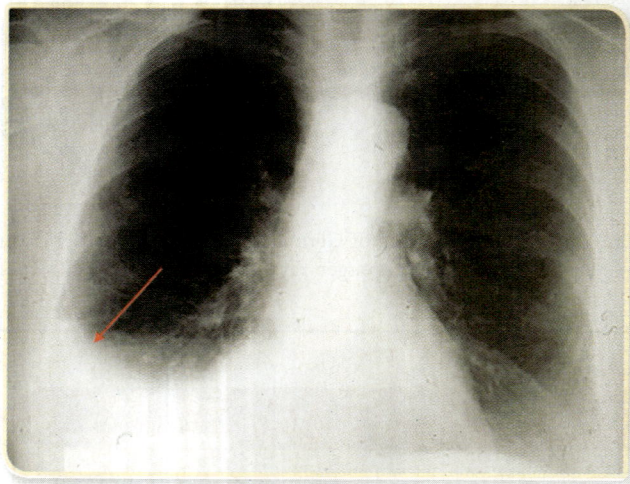

RIGHT PLEURAL EFFUSION

Note the meniscus-shaped upper surface of the right pleural effusion (Red arrow)

Pleural Effusion: Denotes a collection of fluid within the pleural space. On a routine erect chest x-ray as much as 300 ml of fluid is required before it becomes evident. **A lateral decubitus film is most sensitive**, able to identify even a small amount of fluid (detects about 50 ml of fluid). **Very small amount of fluid even 3-5ml is detected on ultrasound and CT**. Both PA and AP erect films are insensitive to small amounts of fluid.

Radiological Features of Pleural Effusion

- CXR (PA film) – effusions up to 300 ml may not be visible.
- Blunting of the costophrenic angles.
- Blunting of cardiophrenic angle
- Eventually a **meniscus** shaped upper surface will be seen, on frontal films seen laterally and gently sloping medially (if a hydropneumothorax is present, no such meniscus will be visible). They may be large extending up to the apex and causing mediastinal shift away from the effusion.
- Look for differential increased density projected beneath the diaphragm. Elevated apex of the diaphragm laterally, in keeping with a subpulmonic effusion.
- Fluid within the horizontal or oblique fissures
- With large volume effusions, mediastinal shift occurs away from the effusion (Note: if coexistent collapse dominates then mediastinal shift may occur towards the effusion).

RADIO PLATE 4

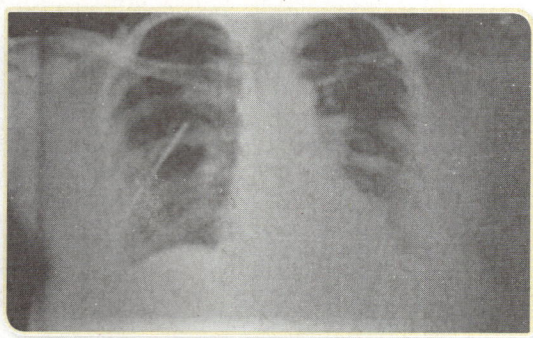

CHEST X-RAY SHOWING INTERCOSTAL TUBE PLACED FOR PLEURAL EFFUSION

Chest X-ray PA view showing **intercostal tube placed for pleural effusion.** The chest tube is in correct place draining the effusion fluid with expanded right lung. Mediastinal shift (tracheal shift) is not very clearly visible in this picture is however likely to be present. Always look for any additional findings like:

- Subcutaneous emphysema
- Signs of trauma (fracture)
- Signs of chest tube blockage (lack of expansion, kinking)
- Hydropneumothorax (Air fluid levels)

RADIO PLATE 5

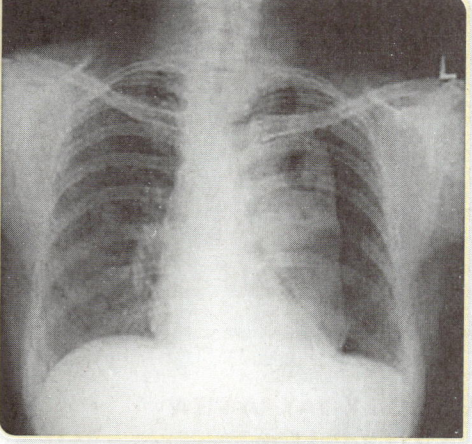

LEFT PNEUMOTHORAX

Pneumothorax refers to the presence of gas (air) in the **pleural space** and on chest X-ray.

Radiological Features

- **Simple pneumothorax:** Visceral pleural edge visible (thin sharp white line) with dark area lacking vascular markings laterally. Loss of volume on the affected side (e.g. raised hemidiaphragm). A small pneumothorax may not be visualized on a standard inspiratory film. An expiratory film may be of benefit.
- **Tension pneumothorax:** This is a clinical and not a radiological entity. Radiological signs are similar to Simple pneumothorax
- Associated mediastinal shift to the opposite side is seen.
- Pneumothorax may be difficult to visualize on frontal films, particularly on supine films. Look for increased lucency over the costophrenic recess (The **deep sulcus sign**).

RADIO PLATE 6

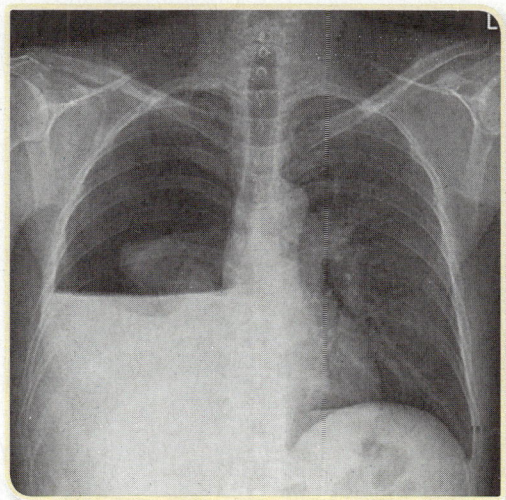

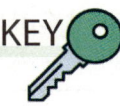 KEY

HYDROPNEUMOTHORAX

Hydropneumothorax is a term given to the concurrent presence of a **pneumothorax** as well as a **hydrothorax** (i.e. air and fluid) in the pleural space. On an erect chest radiograph, recognition of hydropneumothorax is classically shown as an air-fluid level. On the supine radiograph, this may be more challenging where a sharp pleural line is bordered by increased opacity lateral to it within the pleural space may sometimes suggest toward the diagnosis.

RADIO PLATE 7

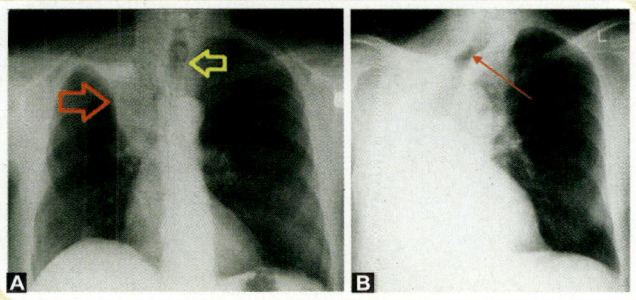

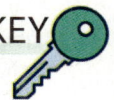 KEY

PLATE LEGENDS

A. **Right upper lobe collapse:** Red arrow–Well defined opacity of right upper lobe collapse, Yellow arrow–Tracheal shift towards the collapse
B. **Total Right lung collapse:** Red arrow–Tracheal shift to same side

Radiological Features of Lung Collapse

It is important to recognize the common lobar collapses on a frontal CXR.

- **Left upper lobe:** Veiled opacification throughout the left hemithorax with obscuration of the left heart border. Visible left margin of the aortic arch (Luftsichel sign). Horizontal orientation and splaying of the lower lobe bronchovascular markings. Almost all cases have a proximal tumor, which may only be visible on CT scans.
- **Left lower lobe:** Reduced lung volume. Small left hilum. Triangular density behind the heart with obscuration of the medial aspect of the left hemidiaphragm. Bronchial reorientation in a vertical direction.
- **Right upper lobe:** Reduced lung volume. Elevated right hilum. Triangular density abutting right medial mediastinum. A mass lesion at the right hilum may be present (Golden – S sign).
- **Right middle lobe:** Obscuration of the right heart border. A lateral CXR may be necessary to confirm the collapse.
- **Right lower lobe:** Reduced lung volume. Triangular density medially at the right base obscuring the medial aspect of the right hemi diaphragm. Bronchial reorientation in a vertical direction.
- **Total lung collapse:** Causes include misplaced endotracheal tube or large proximal tumor. Opacification of affected hemithorax with mediastinal shift to the collapsed lung.

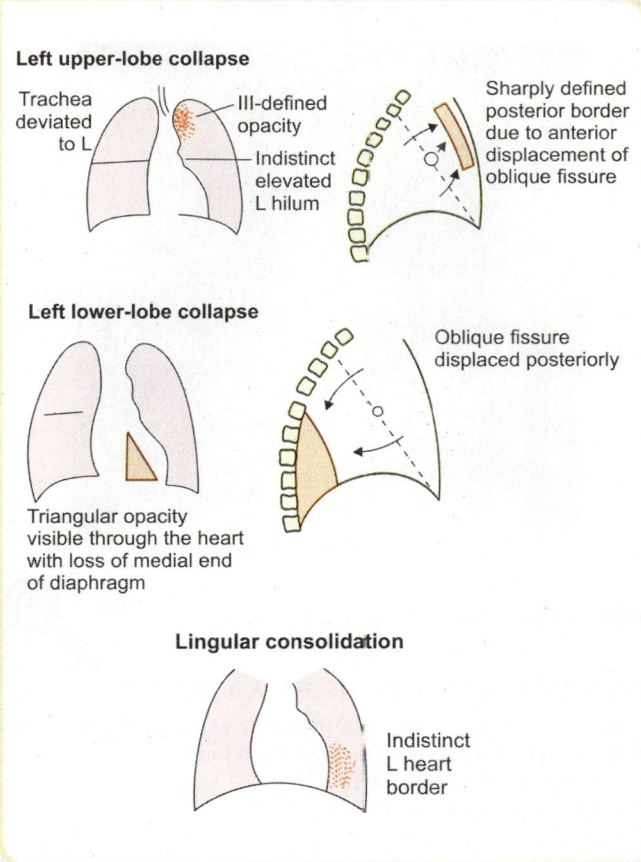

415

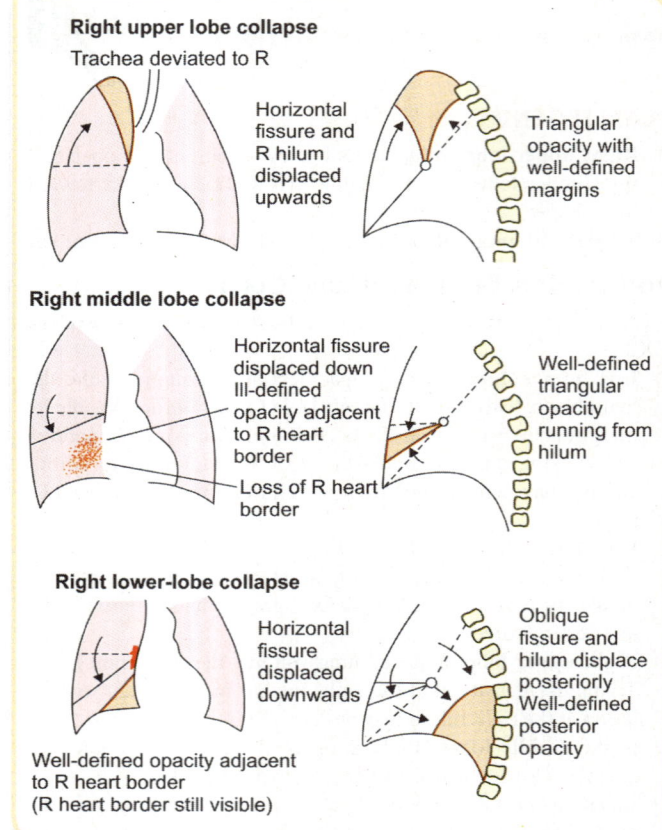

- Bronchial breath sounds
- Post primary TB: Ill-defined consolidation in the apical segments, which may cavitate.
- Right middle and lower lobe pneumonia: Loss of the outline of the right heart border and the right hemidiaphragm silhouette respectively.
- Lingular segment pneumonia: Loss of the outline of the left heart border.
- Left lower lobe consolidation: Typically obliterates an arc of left hemidiaphragm. Look 'through the heart' for loss of diaphragmatic outline.

RADIO PLATE 9

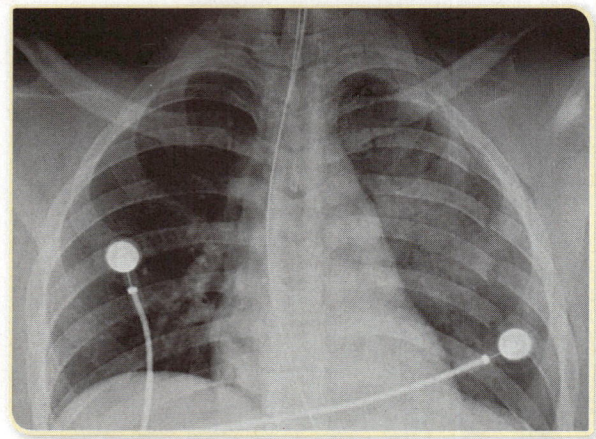

KEY

FLAIL CHEST
Two or more than two consecutive rib fracture from 2 places are seen.

RADIO PLATE 10

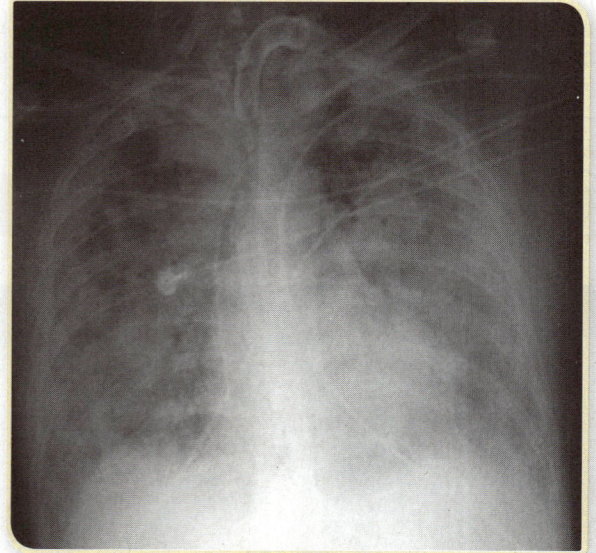

RADIO PLATE 8

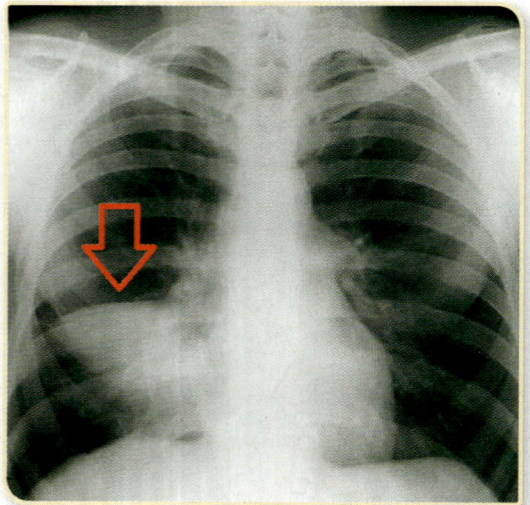

KEY

RIGHT MIDDLE LOBE CONSOLIDATION[AIIMSPG]

Dense opacification in the right mid zone (Arrow); this abuts the horizontal fissure and effaces the right heart border.
- No mediastinal/tracheal shift
- Air bronchograms may be present
- Increased vocal fremitus
- Dullness on percussion

ACUTE RESPIRATORY DISTRESS SYNDROME

Findings in this Chest X-ray are:
- Bilateral diffuse fluffy infiltrates
- Right subclavian central line seen
- Tracheostomy tube seen
- ECG leads can be seen.

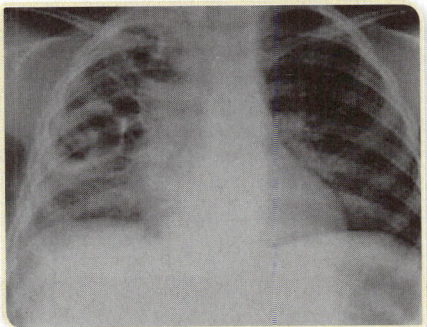

RADIO PLATE 11

PNEUMATOCELE

Chest X-ray shows right sided pneumonia with the presence of pulmonary infiltrates and characteristic multiple air filled spaces (**pneumatoceles**). Pneumatocoeles are intrapulmonary air-filled cystic spaces, which may contain air-fluid levels. **Staph aureus** is the most likely organism to present in this fashion.

Causes of Pneumatocoele

- **Pneumonia:** (*Staphylococcus aureus* (most common), *Streptococcus pneumoniae*, *Haemophilus influenzae*, *Escherichia coli*, Group A streptococci, *Klebsiella pneumoniae*, Adenovirus, Primary pulmonary tuberculosis).
- Trauma: Usually blunt trauma
- Positive pressure ventilation, especially in preterm neonates
- Hydrocarbon ingestion

RADIO PLATE 12

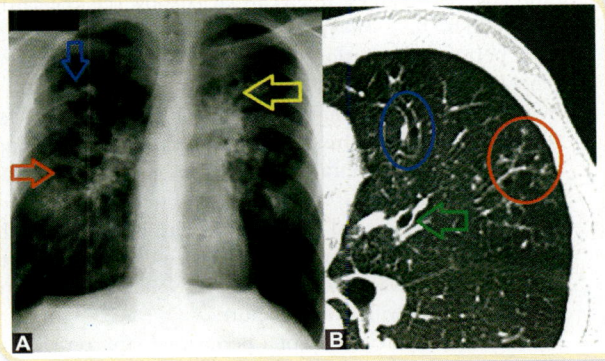

BRONCHIECTASIS AND/OR CYSTIC FIBROSIS

Bronchiectasis is a chronic condition characterized by local, irreversible dilatation of bronchi, usually associated with inflammation.

A. **Chest radiography:** Reveals abnormalities in the majority of cases.
   - Bilateral cystic-appearing lesion with air fluid levels
   - There is hyperinflation (**earliest sign**) with flattened diaphragm.
   - Areas of hyperlucency in the left upper lobe peripherally, mucus plugs (blue arrow), enlarged hilar shadows.
   - Clusters of **ring shadows** (red arrow), some containing air fluid levels, may be visible, together with evidence of air trapping, lobar or segmental collapse or consolidation may be visible.
   - Bronchial wall thickening and dilatation and scarring produces a characteristic parallel line opacity AKA- **Tram line shadow** pattern (Yellow arrow).
   - Pulmonary vessels may appear increased in size and may be indistinct because of adjacent peribronchial inflammation fibrosis.
   - This is consistent with chronic bronchiectasis and/or cystic fibrosis; the latter is more likely due its upper zone predominance. Cystic fibrosis has upper lobe predominance, whereas bronchiectasis associated with ABPA is central in location.

B. **Chest CT (HRCT) is more specific for bronchiectasis and is the imaging modality of choice for confirming the diagnosis.**
   - CT findings include airway dilation detected as parallel "**tram tracks**" (blue circle)
   - **Bronchial Dilatation:** the internal diameter of a bronchus is greater than the diameter of the adjacent pulmonary artery branch (i.e., the **broncho arterial ratio > 1**) giving the "**Signet-ring**" **sign.** (green arrow)
   - **Lack of Bronchial Tapering** (including the presence of tubular structures within 1 cm from the pleural surface), the diameter of the airway should remain unchanged for at least 2 cm distal to a branching point.
   - **Abnormal Bronchial Contours:** bronchiectasis may be classified as cylindrical, varicose, or cystic. Cylindrical bronchiectasis—"**tram-tracks**" Varicose bronchiectasis—"**string of pearls**" Cystic bronchiectasis—"**cluster of grapes**"
   - Bronchi visible within 1 cm of the costal pleural surfaces.
   - **Bronchial Wall Thickening**
   - Presence of mucus- or fluid-filled bronchi.
   - "**Tree-in-bud**" pattern; (red circle) centrilobular nodules (which are usually 2-4 mm in diameter and peripheral, within 5 mm of pleural surface) connected by opacified or thickened branching structures extending proximally (representing the dilated and opacified bronchioles.

> **Note**
> Other causes of Tree in bud appearance are endobronchial tuberculosis (mc cause), bronchiolitis, tumor emboli, sarcoidosis.

Bronchiectasis is often classified as cylindrical, varicose, saccular/cystic, or traction.

1. **Cylindrical or tubular bronchiectasis** is due to uniform fusiform dilation and is seen as "tram-track" lines on X-ray and CT.
2. **Varicose bronchiectasis** in which the bronchi have a bulbous/beaded appearance with alternating areas of bronchial dilatation and constriction.

417

3. **Saccular or cystic bronchiectasis** is manifested by marked bronchial dilation with peripheral ballooning of the cystic spaces and air-fluid levels and is often associated with bronchial stenosis with associated bronchial neovascularization and ulceration
4. **Traction bronchiectasis** is the result of fibrotic distortion of the lung caused by infection, radiation, or end-stage lung disease, and is seen most commonly in the lung periphery.

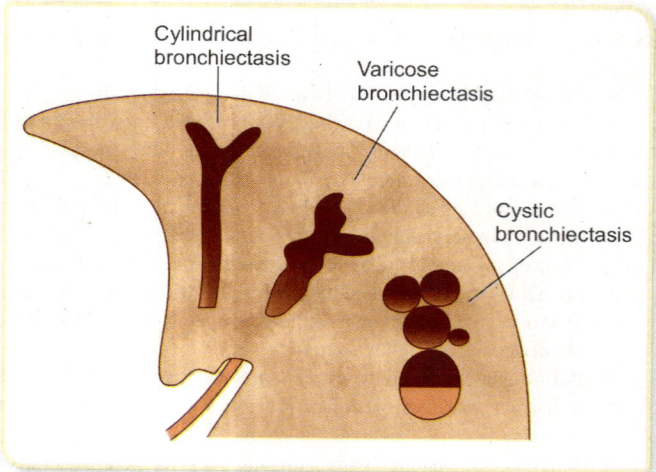

- Miliary Shadow: Pulmonary hemosiderosis seen as punctuate densities.
- **Cardiomegaly** (which is a 3 chamber phenomenon, excluding left ventricle)
- Alveolar Flooding Edema: PCWP> 25 mm Hg (Normal PCWP = 5-12 mm Hg)
- Lifting up of left bronchus.

Stages of Pulmonary Venous Hypertension

Stage	Radiological signs
Stage 1: Redistribution/Cephalization of the blood flow (pulmonary venous pressure ranges from **13-19 mm**)	▫ Constriction/blurring of lower lobe vessels ▫ Effacement of hilar angle ▫ Dilatation of upper lobe vessels
Stage 2: Interstitial Edema (venous pressure ranges from **20-24 mm**)	▫ Kerley lines ▫ Peribronchial cuffing ▫ Septal and interstitial edema ▫ Pleural effusion
Stage 3: Alveolar Edema (venous pressure of ≥ 25 mm)	Milking of edema fluid towards the hilum leads to "**Bat Wing appearance**"

RADIO PLATE 13

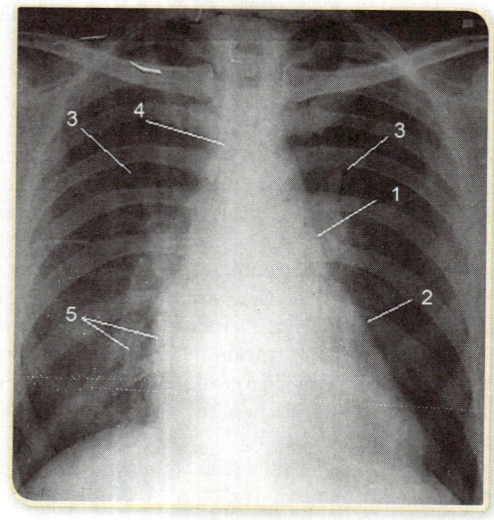

CHEST X-RAY SIGNS OF PULMONARY VENOUS HYPERTENSION:

Due to Mitral stenosis, Left ventricular heart failure etc.
- Loss of aortic window
- **Mitralization:** Straightening of left atrial border (Earliest sign)
- **Mouastache Sign/Batwing Sign/Cephalization:** Distention of upper lobe veins, Constriction of lower lobe veins, At PCWP > 13-19 mm hg (Stage 3 pulmonary venous hypertension)
- Posterior enlargement causing esophageal displacement
- **Double atrial shadow** (less dense left atrial shadow and more dense right atrial shadow)
- **Interstitial Edema/ Kerley B Lines:** Kerley B lines are caused by interstitial fluid and are defined as subpleural perpendicular lines 1-3 cm in length *(stage 2 of pulmonary venous hypertension)*.

RADIO PLATE 14

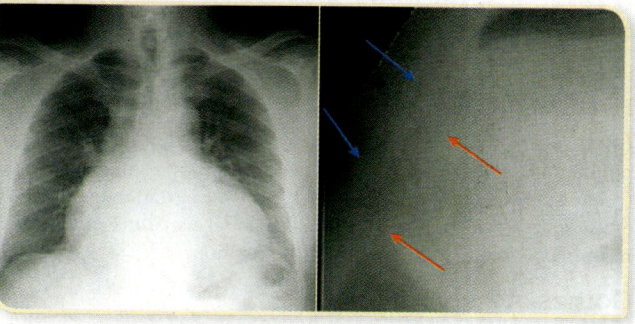

PERICARDIAL EFFUSION

- Pericardium is rarely distinctly definable on plain chest X-ray, however in two conditions it can be seen, effusion and constriction.
- Flask shaped heart, Pear shaped heart, Leather bottle heart, Money bog shaped heart: is seen in pericardial effusion.
- **On chest X-ray, how do I distinguish a pericardial effusion from cardiac enlargement?** Both cardiomegaly and pericardial effusion give rise to an enlarged cardiac shadow (i.e. the cardio-thoracic ratio is> 0.5). However:
  a. In a pericardial effusion, the heart enlargement must be generalized; in the former case it doesn't need to be.
  b. In a pericardial effusion, the lung fields should appear clear, whereas in cardiac failure, the lung fields should show changes, such as 'bat wing' infiltrates, upper lobe blood diversion and pleural effusions.
  c. Less reliably, pericardial effusions can bring forth two other changes. The cardiac shadow may cover both hila, and the superior vena cava may be enlarged. Neither of these two features are seen with cardiac failure.
  d. A lateral film and close up of a pericardial effusion showing the anterior mediastinal fat (blue arrows) and epicardial fat

(red arrows) separated by a soft tissue stripe reflecting the pericardial effusion seen edge-on. It is highly reliable and specific of pericardial effusion but is seen in later stages.

RADIO PLATE 15

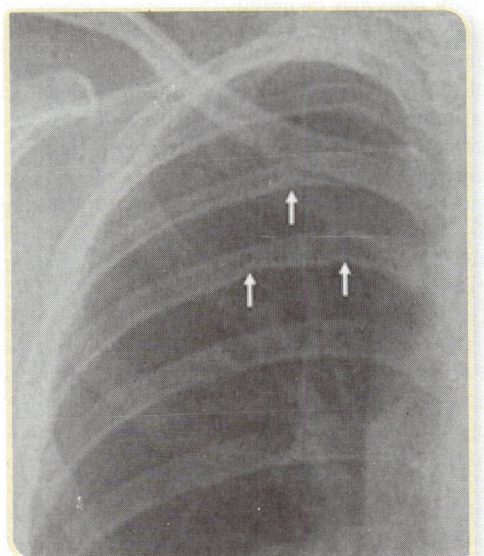

RIB NOTCHING

The image shows Inferior rib notching.

Rib Notching	
Inferior Rib notching	**Superior Rib notching**
Arterial	**Connective tissue diseases**
☐ Coarctation of the aorta – Affects 4th–8th ribs bilaterally, Unilateral and right-sided if the coarctation is proximal to the left subclavian artery.	☐ Rheumatoid arthritis*
	☐ Systemic lupus erythematosus
	☐ Scleroderma
	☐ Sjögren's syndrome
	Metabolic
	Hyperparathyroidism
☐ Aortic thrombosis – Usually the lower ribs bilaterally.	**Miscellaneous**
	☐ Neurofibromatosis
☐ Subclavian obstruction – most commonly after a Blalock operation, Unilateral rib notching of the upper three or four ribs on the operation side.	☐ Restrictive lung disease
	☐ Poliomyelitis
	☐ Marfan's syndrome
	☐ Osteogenesis imperfecta
	☐ Progeria
☐ Pulmonary oligaemia	
Venous	
Superior vena caval obstruction.	
Arteriovenous	
☐ Pulmonary arteriovenous malformation.	
☐ Chest wall arteriovenous malformation.	
Neurogenic	
Neurofibromatosis – 'ribbon ribs' may also be a feature.	

RADIO PLATE 16

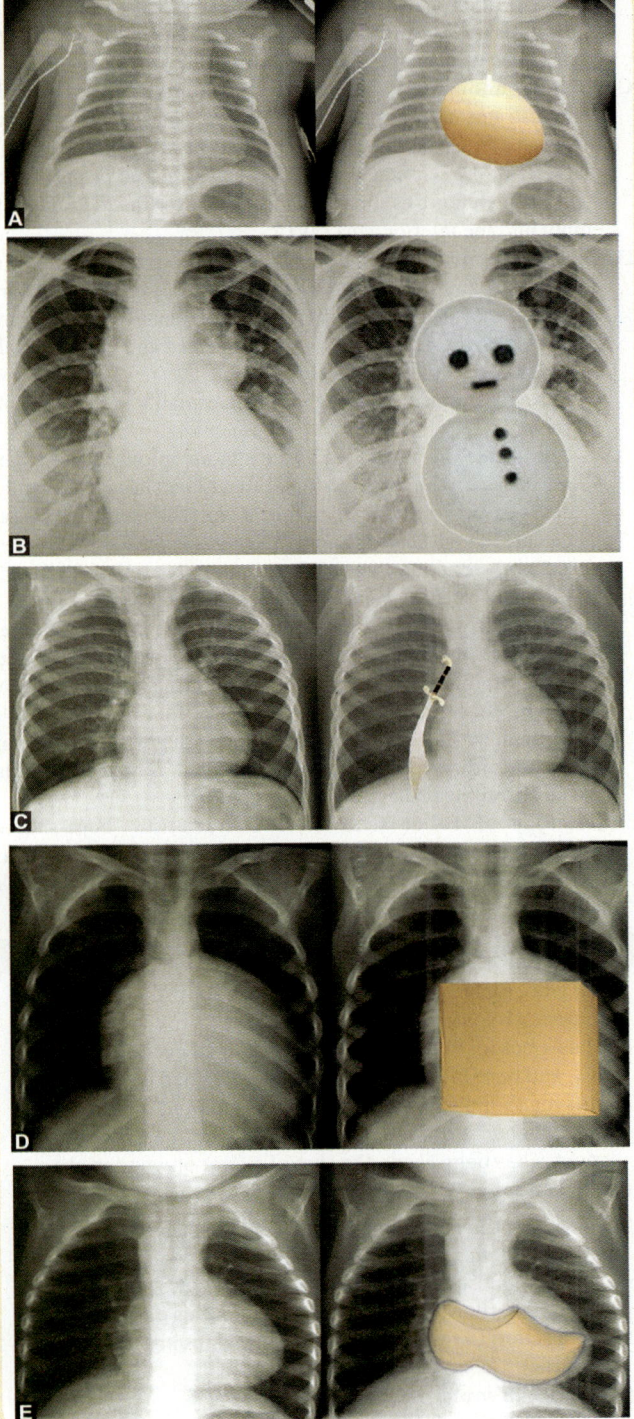

PLATE LEGENDS

A. **Transposition of the great arteries CXR:** Shows narrowing of the superior mediastinum, enlargement of the cardiac silhouette (**egg-on-a-string sign**) with abnormal convexity of the right atrial border, and increased vascular flow.

B. **TAPVR CXR:** Classic **Snowman sign or Figure of 8 sign** on X-ray is seen in Total Anomalous pulmonary venous connection **(TAPVC).** Since the pulmonary veins drain into right atrium in TAPVC, The right atrium and ventricle are dilated and hypertrophied, and the pulmonary artery segment is enlarged. The so-called "figure-of-8" or "snowman" heart is due to enlargement of the heart and the presence of a dilated right superior vena cava, innominate vein, and left vertical vein.

C. **Partial anomalous pulmonary venous return CXR:** Demonstrates a prominent curvilinear opacity that extends downward from the right hilum the **"scimitar sign".** The luminal diameter of the scimitar vein, which may drain all or part of the right lung, enlarges as the vein descends below the diaphragm to empty into the inferior vena cava

D. **Ebstein anomaly CXR:** Show massive cardiomegaly with decreased pulmonary flow best depicts the **box-shaped heart,** an appearance caused by enlargement of the right atrium and hypoplasia of the pulmonary trunk. Elongated and enlarged right atrium may result in an elevated apex.
   - Ebstein's anomaly is a congenital abnormality of the tricuspid valve.
   - The septal and mural leaflets are more apically placed than normal i.e. if the tricuspid septal attachment lies more than 1.5 cm "beneath" the apex than mitral septal attachment, this can be considered Ebstein anomaly (in adults, the measurement is 2 cm), resulting in a malfunctioning, regurgitant tricuspid valve and atrialization of the proximal right ventricle.
   - The consequence is gross right atrial enlargement and raised right atrial pressure. The anomaly is usually associated with an ASD and there is thus right-to-left shunting at the atrial level and subsequent cyanosis.
   - Ultimately, Ebstein's anomaly results in gross enlargement of the cardiac contour with a prominent curved right atrial border on the plain chest radiograph.

E. **Tetralogy of Fallot CXR**[NEETPG]: Characteristic **boot-shaped sign** produced by upturning of the cardiac apex because of right ventricular hypertrophy and by the concavity of the main pulmonary artery.

Tetralogy of Fallot

Roentgenographically, the typical configuration as seen in the anteroposterior view consists of a narrow base, concavity of the left heart border in the area usually occupied by the pulmonary artery, and normal heart size. The hypertrophied right ventricle causes the rounded apical shadow to be uptilted so that it is situated higher above the diaphragm than normal. The cardiac silhouette has been likened to that of a boot or wooden shoe **("coeur en sabot")**

TOF is one of the **conotruncal family** of heart lesions in which the primary defect is an anterior deviation of the infundibular septum (the muscular septum that separates the aortic and pulmonary outflows). The consequences of this deviation are:
- Obstruction to right ventricular outflow (pulmonary stenosis)
- Ventricular septal defect (VSD)
- Dextroposition of the aorta with override of the ventricular septum
- Right ventricular hypertrophy

The degree of pulmonary outflow obstruction varies, with the severity of the obstruction determining the degree of the patient's cyanosis.

Note: Fallot's pentalogy consists of Tetralogy of Fallot plus ASD.

Contd...

Tetralogy of Fallot

Associated anomalies with TOF:
- An associated PDA may be present, and defects in the atrial septum are occasionally seen.
- A right aortic arch occurs in ≈20% of patients with the tetralogy of Fallot, and other anomalies of the pulmonary arteries and aortic arch may also be seen.
- **Persistence of a left superior vena cava draining into the coronary sinus may be noted.**
- Multiple VSDs are occasionally present and must be diagnosed before corrective surgery.
- Tetralogy of Fallot may also occur with an atrioventricular septal defect, often associated with Down syndrome
- **Congenital absence of the pulmonary valve**
- **Absence of a branch pulmonary artery**
- As one of the conotruncal malformations, the tetralogy of Fallot can be associated with the spectrum of lesions known as **CATCH 22 (cardiac defects, abnormal faces, thymic hypoplasia, cleft palate, hypocalcemia).**
- CATCH 22 includes patients with clinical features of the **DiGeorge syndrome** (hypocalcemia, thymic hypoplasia, mild facial anomalies) or the **Shprintzen velocardiofacial syndrome** (abnormal facies, cleft palate).
- Cytogenetic analysis using fluorescence in situ hybridization demonstrates deletions of a large segment of chromosome 22q11 known as the DiGeorge critical region.
- Deletion or mutation of the gene encoding the transcription factor *Tbx1* has been implicated as a possible cause of DiGeorge syndrome.

RADIO PLATE 17

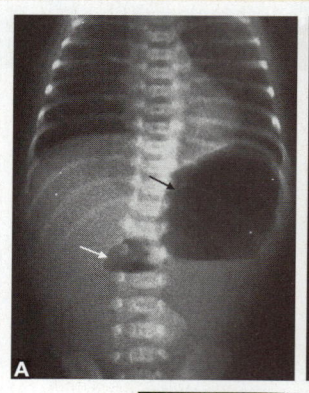
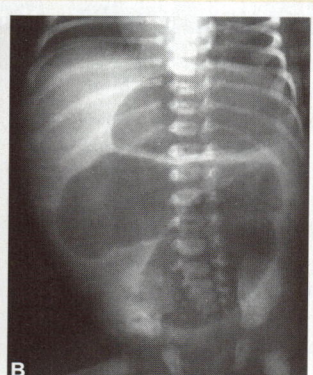
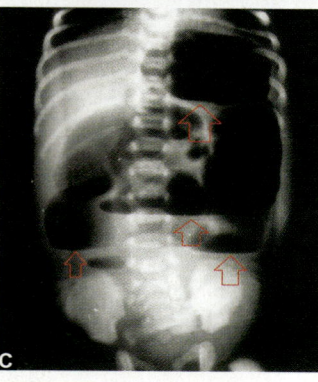

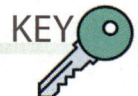 

INTESTINAL OBSTRUCTION

A. **Duodenal obstruction: Double bubble sign** consists of an air-distended stomach (black arrow) and proximal duodenum (white arrow) and is characteristic of duodenal obstruction which can be due to following reasons:
   - Ladd's bands, malrotation
   - Annular pancreas
   - Duodenal atresia, stenosis, web, duplication, obstruction

B. **Jejunal obstruction: Triple bubble sign** - Jejunal obstruction with air in stomach, duodenum, and proximal jejunum.

C. **Ileal atresia:** Upright radiograph shows **multiple air-fluid levels** occupying the entire abdominal cavity. Barium enema study shows numerous dilated, air-filled loops of bowel and a small, unused colon.

Signs of Small Bowel Obstruction

1. **Dilated small bowel:** (double headed arrow) Small bowel with a diameter greater than 30mm is considered to be dilated. Small bowel can dilate up to around 50mm. If the small bowel has a diameter of 70mm or greater it probably isn't small bowel.
2. **The 3,6,9 Rule:** The maximum diameter of the bowel is shown as follows:

	Maximum Normal Diameter
Small bowel	30mm
Large bowel	50-60mm
Caecum	90mm

3. **Step ladder pattern:** (Blue arrows) The appearance of multiple air-fluid levels on erect abdominal film is sometimes referred to as a step ladder sign. It has also been suggested that uneven levels in a bowel loop (i.e. more fluid on one side of the loop than the other) are diagnostic of SBO rather than ileus.
4. **Stretch/slit sign:** Slit sign is a result of small amounts of air caught in the valvulae of fluid-filled bowel.

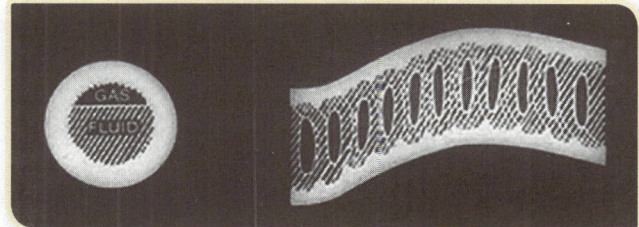

5. **String of pearls/beads sign:** (White arrow) The appearance is considered to be diagnostic of obstruction (as opposed to ileus) and is caused by small bubbles of air trapped in the valvulae of the small bowel. A similar appearance is sometimes seen in the large bowel but can usually be differentiated by the fact that the gas bubbles are larger
6. **Coiled spring sign:** (Red circle) The coiled spring appearance only occurs in the dilated air-filled small bowel. It also is most noticeable in the jejunum where the valvulae conniventes are closely spaced.

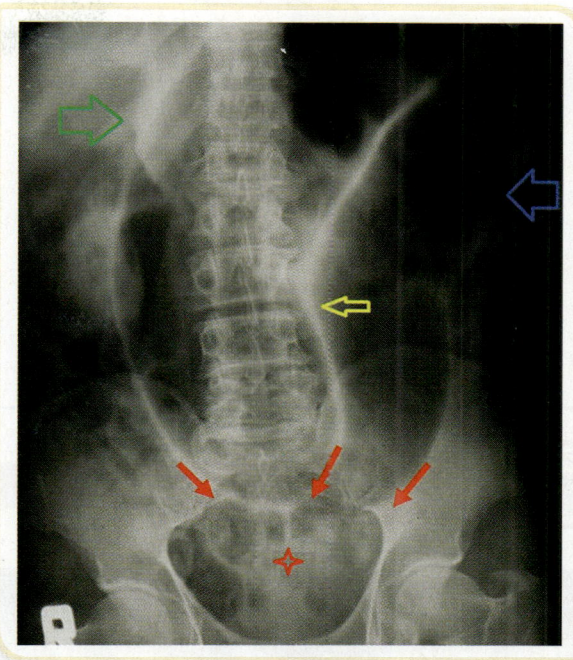

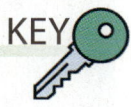

SIGMOID VOLVULUS PLAIN RADIOGRAPH

Most common volvulus (60-75 %).
Abdominal radiographs will demonstrate:
- Large dilated loop of colon
- Air fluid levels with air fluid ratio greater than 2:1
- Absent rectal gas (contrary to caecal volvulus)
- **Inverted U sign:** Dilated loop present as inverted U
- **Apex of the sigmoid volvulus:** usually lies very high in the abdomen above the level of T10, on the left side overlapping the transverse colon, under the left hemidiaphragm
- **Coffee bean sign** (yellow arrow)
- **Frimann Dahl's sign** - three dense lines converge towards site of obstruction (red arrow and star)
- The ahaustral margin can often be identified overlapping respectively the lower border of the liver shadow (the **liver overlap sign;** green arrow), the haustrated, dilated descending colon (the **left flank overlap sign**; blue arrow) and the left side of the pelvis (the pelvic overlap sign)
- **Loss of haustra:** The most important diagnostic point of a sigmoid volvulus rather than a large redundant distended loop of sigmoid colon is the absence of haustra.

Sigmoid Volvulus–Diagrammatic

1. Counterclockwise torsion at base of mesentery.
2. Adhesions at base of sigmoid mesocolon leading to formation of fixed omega loop that is susceptible to repeat torsion.

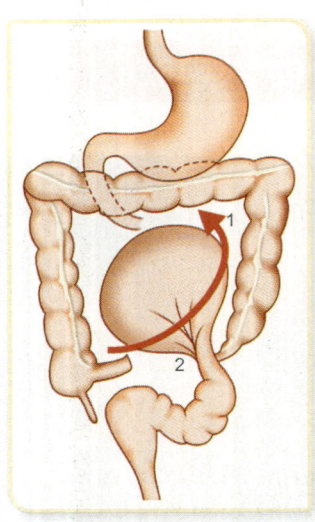

- Paucity of gas in the ascending colon
- Gas in the rectum (contrary to absence of gas in rectum in sigmoid volvulus)
- Embryo sign:

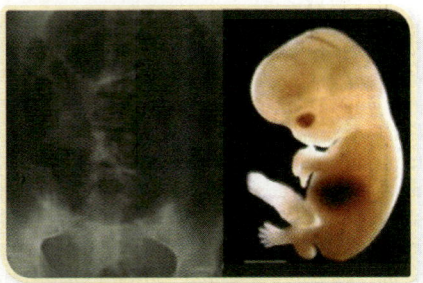

- One or two haustra can be seen
- Identification of attached gas filled appendix confirms the diagnosis
- Two types: In one half cecum twists and inverts so that the pole of caecum occupy the left upper quadrant (A), in other half caecum twists in axial plane without inversion occupying the right half or central part of abdomen (B)

Caecal Volvulus–Diagrammatic

1. Clockwise torsion of mesentery of cecum, ascending colon, and terminal ileum.
2. Absence of dorsal mesenteric attachments of cecum and proximal ascending colon, leading to lack of fixation to retroperitoneum.

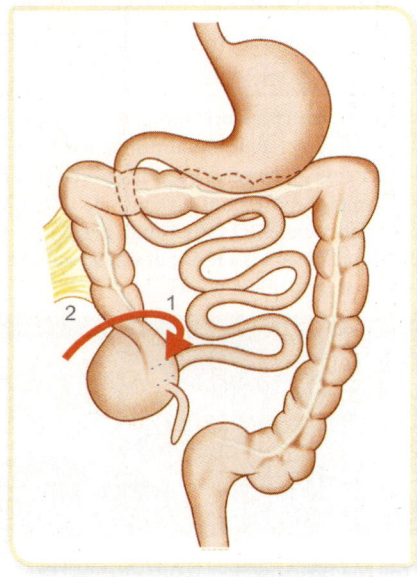

RADIO PLATE 19

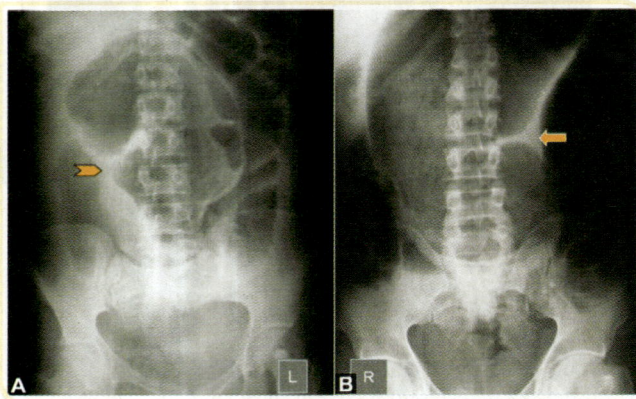

KEY

CAECAL VOLVULUS PLAIN RADIOGRAPH
- Distended upturned caecum with the configuration of a **reversed letter C**
- There is gas-filled small bowel.

RADIO PLATE 20

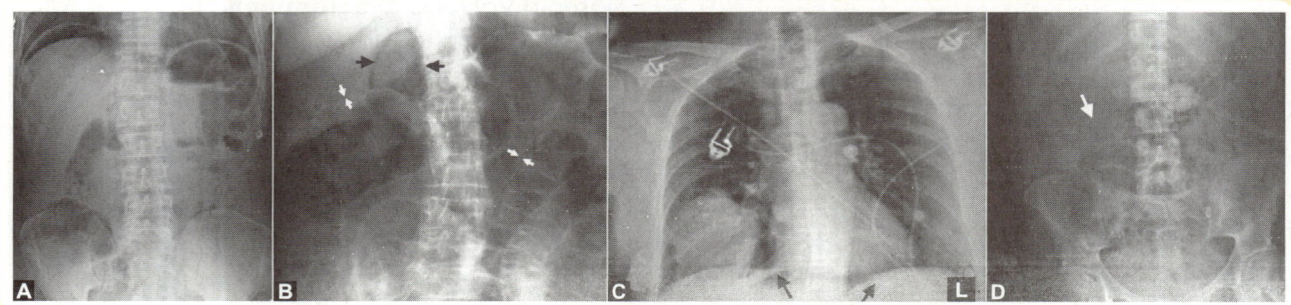

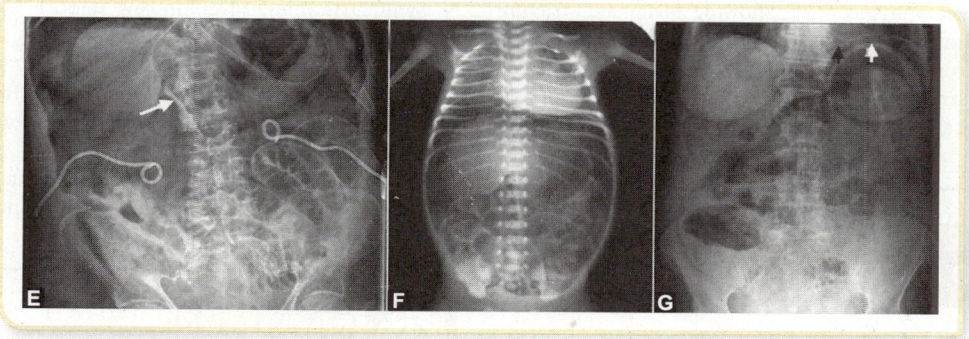

PNEUMOPERITONEUM

The most common cause is a perforation of the abdominal viscus—most commonly, a perforated ulcer, although a pneumoperitoneum may occur as a result of perforation of any part of the bowel; other causes include a benign ulcer, a tumor, or trauma.

X-ray signs of Pneumoperitoneum are:
A. **Gas under diaphragm:** The above X-ray abdomen (erect) shows presence of gas under the right dome of diaphragm suggestive of pneumoperitoneum. **The erect chest radiograph is superior to the erect abdominal view for the demonstration of free intra-abdominal gas since, in the erect abdominal view, the X-ray beam is passing through any free gas under the diaphragm at an oblique angle.** CT is superior to plain radiographs in detecting minute quantities of pneumoperitoneum
B. **Doges Cap sign** refers to free air in Morrison's pouch. Morrison's pouch is normally a potential space between the right kidney and the liver. This is a particularly difficult sign of pneumoperitoneum for several reasons. Firstly, it may be the only sign of pneumoperitoneum and may be very subtle. Secondly, it can be easily misinterpreted as gas in the duodenum. The Italian Doges wore this distinctively shaped cap. Gas in Morrison's pouch is only loosely shaped like a Doges cap and should not be taken too literally. Gas in Morrison's pouch on supine Radiographs may have the following features:
   - Triangular in shape
   - Concave medial border
   - Positioned inferior to the right 11th rib
   - Positioned superior to the right kidney.

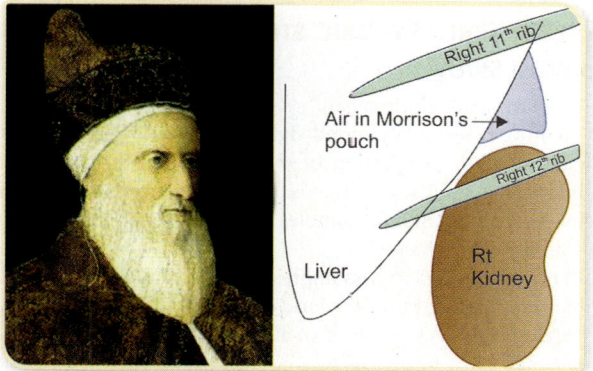

C. **Cupola sign:** Air accumulates underneath the central tendon of the diaphragm in the midline.
D. **Rigler's sign** (double wall sign) is seen when air is present on both sides of the intestine.
E. **Falciform ligament sign** in which falciform ligament is outlined with air in a supine patient with free abdominal gas.
F. **Football sign** is seen in massive pneumoperitoneum, where the abdominal cavity is outlined by gas from a perforated viscus.
G. **Double bubble sign** is an appearance of subdiaphragmatic gas under the left hemidiaphragm in which there are two collections of overlapping gas, one of these collections is subdiaphragmatic free gas and the other is normal gas within the fundus of the stomach.

RADIO PLATE 21

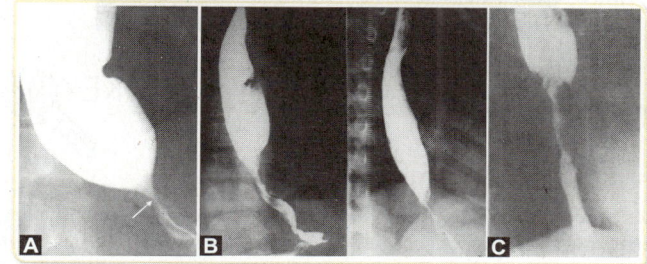

© Hedawoo JB et al

PLATE LEGENDS

A. **Rat–tail appearance of achalasia cardia:** Barium swallow with dilated esophagus with a tapering, **"bird's beak" or Rat–tail–like narrowing of the distal end**. There is usually an air-fluid level in the esophagus from the retained food and saliva on plain radiograph

   Sutton's radiology 7th ed vol 1 page 552 "In achalasia cardia barium swallow will show gastro esophageal junction failing to open fully and tapering to a rat tail or bird beak appearance"

   > **Note**
   > While going through the different text you will find both bird-beak beak appearance and Rat–tail appearance to be seen in both Achalsia cardia and Carcinoma esophagus.

   Duke Radiology Case Review: Imaging, Differential Diagnosis, and Discussion by James M. Provenzale, Rendon C. Nelson, Emily N. Vinson page 119 clears all doubts by quoting that **"Apart from Achalsia cardia Rat–tail appearance or bird-beak appearance is an important radiological sign of pseudoachalsia or secondary achalsia due to malignancy of gastric cardia or lower esophagus".**

B. **Rat tail appearance of Lower esophageal carcinoma:** See secondary achalasia producing rat tail appearance. It can be differentiated by mucosal irregularity and filling defect (malignant stricture) in comparison to smooth surface of primary achalasia.

C. **Carcinoma mid esophagus**[NEETPG]: Showing malignant stricture in the form of luminal narrowing with irregular mucosal surface with proximal contrast pooling. Also note shouldering of the proximal end (arrow) due to mass lesion. Note that upper and mid esophagus carcinoma will not produce secondary achalasia or Rat tailing.

RADIO PLATE 22

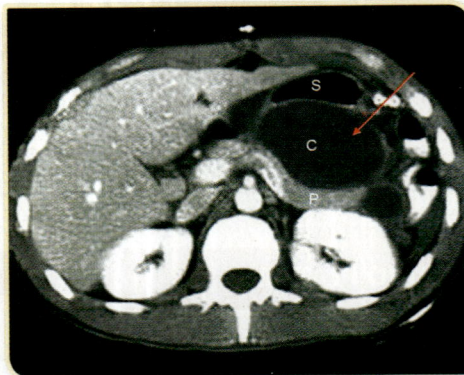

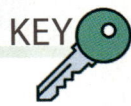

PSEUDOPANCREATIC CYST
If the level of CT is at the desired level then you will see three key structures: the hypodense well circumscribed cyst (C) posterior or around the gastric/stomach shadow (S) and a banana shaped pancreas (P).

RADIO PLATE 23

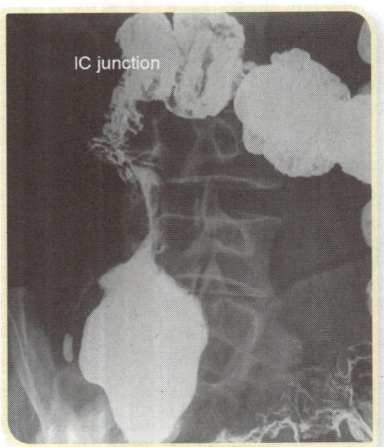

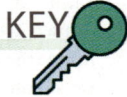

FINDINGS OF ILEOCAECAL (IC) TUBERCULOSIS ON BARIUM EXAMINATION
- Spasm and edema of Ileocecal valve
- Thickening of an incompetent IC valve with narrowing of terminal ileum (**Fleischner sign; inverted umbrella defect**)
- Symmetric annular **Napkin ring stenosis** with conical shrunken caecum
- Rapid emptying of fixed and narrowed terminal ileum into shortened, rigid obliterated caecum (**Stierlin's sign**)
- Obtuse/Widening of IC angle (normal IC angle is 90°)
- Contracted pulled up caecum
- Exuberant mucosal thickening (greater than Crohn's disease)
- Can cause **apple core** colonic stricture (indistinguishable from carcinoma).

RADIO PLATE 24

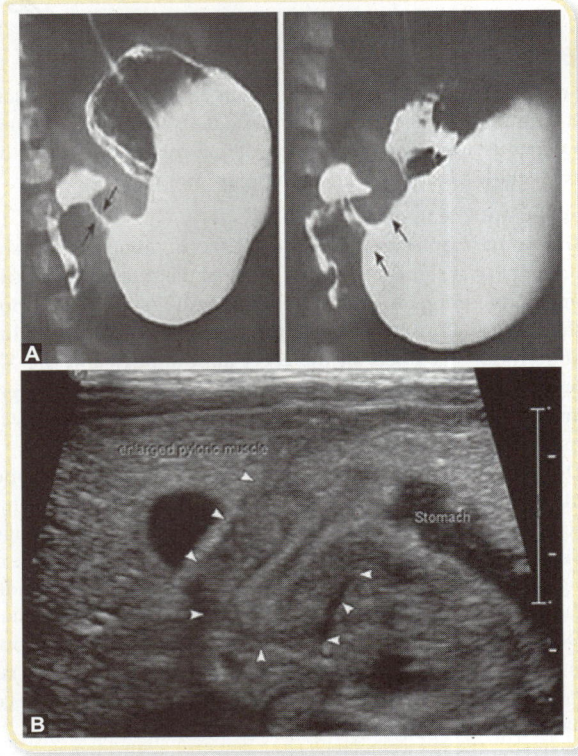

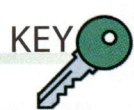

HYPERTROPHIC PYLORIC STENOSIS
Contrast Study
- Narrowing of pyloric canal
- **Twining recess** = "**diamond sign**" = transient triangular tentlike cleft/niche in midportion of pyloric canal with apex pointing inferiorly secondary to mucosal bulging between two separated hypertrophied muscle bundles on the greater curvature side within pyloric channel
- "**Antral beaking**" = mass impression upon antrum with streak of barium pointing toward pyloric channel
- "**String sign**" = passing of small barium streak through pyloric channel
- "**Double/triple track sign**" = crowding of mucosal folds in pyloric channel
- The enlarged muscle mass encroaches upon the lumen of the antrum proximally, resulting in the "**shoulder sign**"
- **Kirklin sign** = "**mushroom sign**" = indentation of base of bulb (in 50%)
- Gastric distension with fluid
- "**Caterpillar sign**" = gastric hyperperistaltic waves

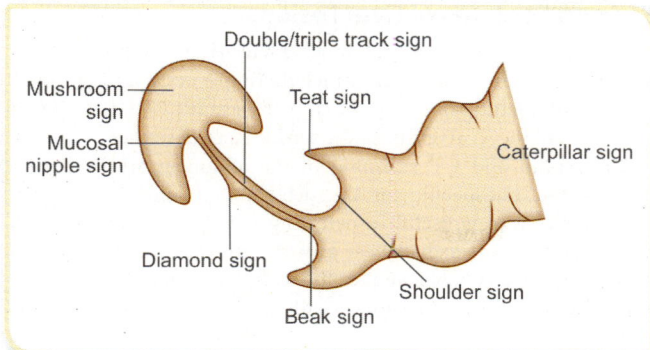

USG

- Palpation of the pyloric tumor (also called the olive) in the epigastrium or right upper quadrant by a skilled examiner is pathognomonic for the diagnosis of HPS. If the olive is palpated, no additional diagnostic testing is necessary.
- When the olive cannot be palpated, the diagnosis of HPS can be made with an ultrasound exam or fluoroscopic UGI series.
- USG has now replaced barium meal as **first line investigation** in infant with non bilious vomiting to whom HPS is suspected (Sutton 7th ed vol 1 page 854)
- "Target sign" = hypoechoic ring of hypertrophied pyloric muscle around echogenic mucosa centrally on cross-section
- Elongated pylorus with thickened muscle: Elongated **pyloric canal ≥ 15 mm in length, Pyloric muscle wall thickness ≥ 3 mm**
- Pyloric volume >1.4 cm^3
- "Cervix sign" = indentation of muscle mass on fluid-filled antrum on longitudinal section
- "Antral nipple sign" = redundant pyloric channel mucosa protruding into gastric antrum
- Exaggerated peristaltic waves
- Delayed gastric emptying of fluid into duodenum.

- Gastroesophageal junction (arrow) and the stomach slide to lie above the diaphragm
- Usually reducible in erect position.

RADIO PLATE 26

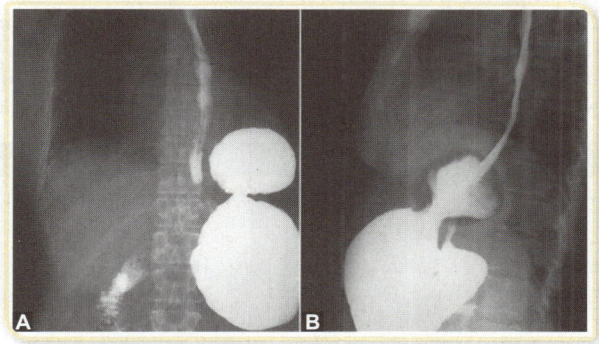

ROLLING/PARAESOPHAGEAL HIATUS HERNIA
(Contrast AP & Lateral view)

- Rare type of hiatus hernia
- Cardia remains below the diaphragm and fundus herniates through the hiatus and lies along the lower esophagus
- Gastro-esophageal junction lies in a normal position
- Mostly non reducible
- Can be mixed type (with sliding hiatus hernia).

RADIO PLATE 25

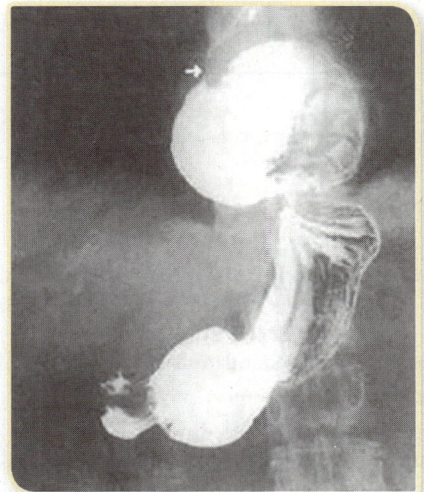

SLIDING HIATUS HERNIA

- Most common type of diaphragmatic hernia
- Wide hiatus measuring more than 3 cm
- Pouch of stomach protrudes more than 2 cm above the hiatus

RADIO PLATE 27

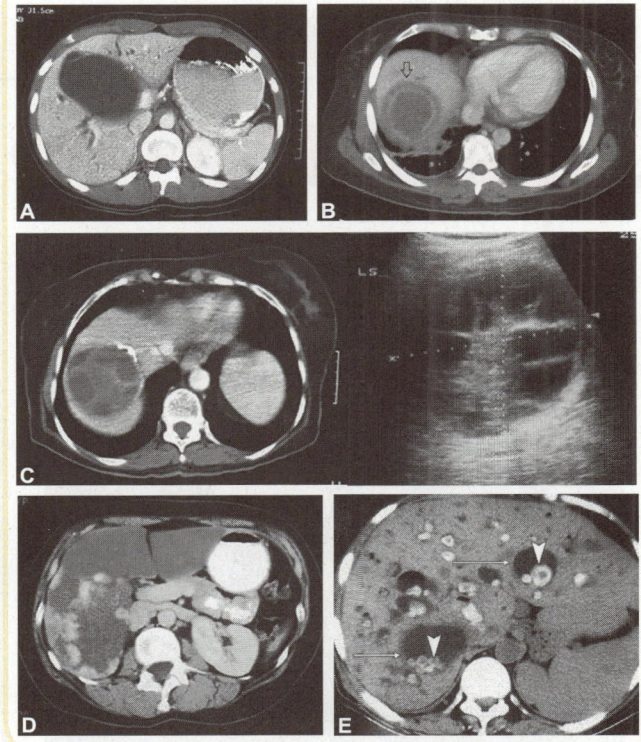

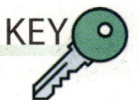

PLATE LEGENDS
A. **Simple liver cyst**
B. **Amoebic liver abscess**
C. **Hydatid cyst on CT and USG**
D. **Hemangioma of liver**
E. **Caroli disease:** Unenhanced CT scan shows multiple stones (arrowheads) within dilated bile ducts (arrows). Dilatation of intrahepatic bile ducts. Note the **"central" or "eccentric" dot** within many of the cystic structures, representing portal radicles.

CT Scan Features of Liver Lesions

Hepatic sonography is useful in characterizing many focal liver lesions. Cystic lesions of the liver include simple cysts, multiple cysts arising in the setting of polycystic liver disease (PCLD), parasitic or hydatid (echinococcal) cysts, cystic tumors, and abscesses.

Ultrasound and CT scanning of the abdomen are both very sensitive but nonspecific for the detection of amebic abscesses. CT scanning also is useful in detecting extrahepatic involvement. Amebic abscesses usually appear as well-defined low-density round lesions that have enhancement of the wall. They also usually appear somewhat ragged in appearance with a *peripheral zone of edema (Arrow).*

	Number	Echogenicity	Septa	Debries
Simple liver cyst	Solitary Multiple (1/3rd)	Anechoic (Echo Free)	No septa	No
Liver abscess	Solitary	Homogeneous Anechoic/ Hypoechoic (earlier, mostly) Hyperechoic (later)	No septa	Present
Hydatid cyst	Mostly solitary	Heterogeneous Hypoechoic (Type I &II- Anechoic)	Multiple cysts (septa) within parent cyst	Fine debris or hydatid sand
Hemangioma	Solitary or Multiple (10-30%)	Homogeneous, Hyperechoic. Certain large hemangiomas exhibit the **"chameleon phenomenon"**: when the patient assumes a different position, they change their echogenicity	No septa	No debris
Caroli's disease	Multiple dilated IHBD	Anechoic (Echo Free)	No septa	Intraductal Sludge and stones

Footnote:
- *Caroli's disease* is a rare disorder characterized by congenital, segmental, saccular dilatations of the intrahepatic bile ducts without other hepatic histological abnormalities
- Differentiation between an amoebic and pyogenic abscess is not possible with sonography.
- The presence of nodules or septae in liver cyst may indicate infection or neoplasm.

Signs of Hydatid Cyst on USG: (Echinococcus)
- Meniscus/crescent/double arch sign:
- Floating membrane sign:
- Spoke wheel/Cart wheel appearance
- Cumbo sign
- **Water lily sign:** Camalote sign: A cyst with an undulating membrane. Detachment of the germinal layer from the cyst wall in Hydatid cyst typically forms "water lily sign" in ultrasound
- Serpent sign

 RADIO PLATE 28

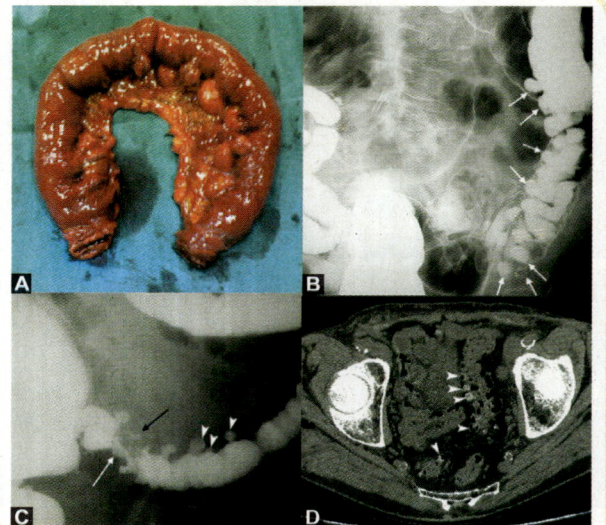

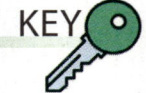

DIVERTICULAR DISEASE
Diverticulosis & Diverticulitis
Diverticulosis: Mucosal herniation through vascular entry sites into the pericolic fat often between the mesenteric and antimesenteric taeniae.
Diverticulitis: Superimposed inflammation on diverticulosis

Diverticulosis
Commonest cause of lower GI bleeding.
A. **Diverticulosis specimen:** A section of colon reveals numerous diverticula, which protrude from the edge of the Taenia coli US: Abnormal wall thickening of more than 4 mm involving a segment 5 cm or longer at the point of maximal tenderness.
B. **Barium enema:** Lower GI showing Diverticula as flask like rounded out pouching (arrow). Distribution and severity is best demonstrated on barium enema. They produce **ring shadow** when seen en face. Differentiation from polyps is done on the basis of projection beyond the bowel wall and presence of air fluid level. Muscular changes results in **Concertina like or Serrated appearance.**

C. **Diverticulitis with Abscess:** Diverticulitis is a condition that occurs when diverticula become infected and inflamed. Complications of diverticulitis are Abscess, Bleeding, Fistula, Obstruction and Perforation. **White arrow:** Diverticula, **White arrow:** Narrowed lumen, **Black arrow:** Perforation with intramural abscess

D. **CT scan:** Arrowheads point to multiple diverticula arising from the recto sigmoid. CT is the imaging procedure of choice to evaluate diverticular disease, as it can show many aspects of disease that are not recognizable by other studies. CT scan can assess complications better. For inflammation or abscess, helical CT with colonic contrast has a sensitivity and specificity of 97 and 100%.

CT Based Classification of Diverticulitis	
Stage 0	Mural thickening
Stage 1	Abscess/phlegmon <3 cm in diameter
Stage 2	Abscess 5-15 cm in diameter
Stage 3	Abscess beyond confines of pelvis
Stage 4	Fecal peritonitis

RADIO PLATE 29

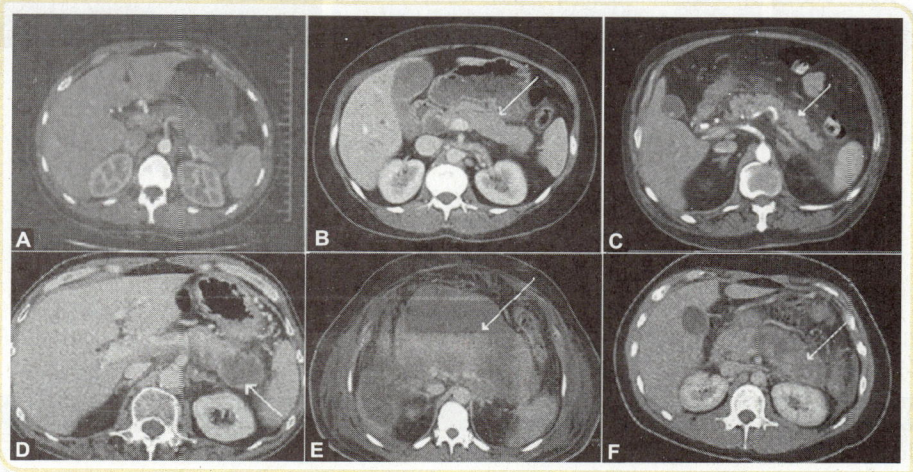

PLATE LEGENDS

A. **Normal CT Abdomen:** Balthazar Grade A
B. **Balthazar Grade B:** Focal/diffuse enlargement of pancreas (arrow)
C. **Balthazar Grade C:** Peripancreatic inflammation (arrow)
D. **Balthazar Grade D:** Fluid collection at single location (arrow)
E. **Balthazar Grade E:** Gas bubbles (arrow)
F. Pancreatic necrosis >50%, 6 points.

Computed Tomography Severity Score (CTSI)

CT scanning with bolus IV contrast has become the gold standard for detecting and assessing the severity of pancreatitis. Currently, IV (bolus) contrast-enhanced CT scanning is routinely performed on patients who are suspected of harboring severe pancreatitis, regardless of their Ranson's or APACHE scores. **Maximum score 10 (>6 indicates severe pancreatitis).** The numerical CTSI has a maximum of ten points, and is the sum of the Balthazar grade points and pancreatic necrosis grade points:

Computed Tomography Severity Score (CTSI)		
Balthazar Grade	**Appearance on CT**	**CT Grade Points**
Grade A	Normal CT	0 points
Grade B	Focal or diffuse enlargement of the pancreas	1 point
Grade C	Pancreatic gland abnormalities and peripancreatic inflammation	2 points
Grade D	Fluid collection in a single location	3 points
Grade E	Two or more fluid collections and/ or gas bubbles in or adjacent to pancreas	4 points
Necrosis score		
Necrosis score		**Points**
No necrosis		0 points
0 to 30% necrosis		2 points
30 to 50% necrosis		4 points
Over 50% necrosis		6 points

RADIO PLATE 30

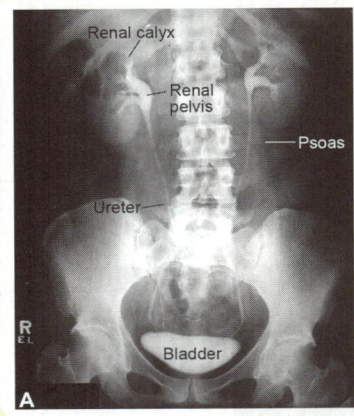
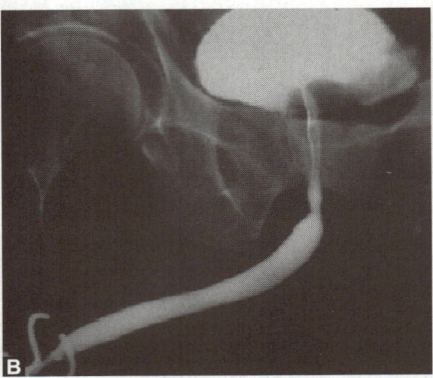
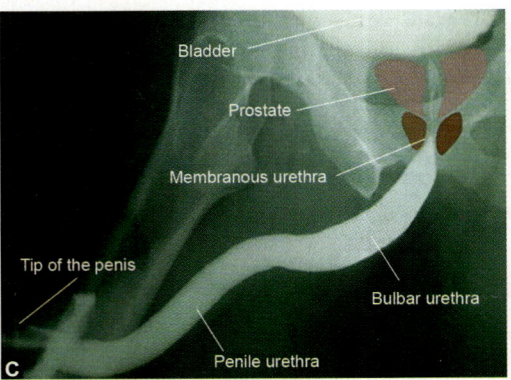

PLATE LEGENDS

A. **Normal IVP**
B. **Normal MCU**
C. **Normal RUG:** This is an X-ray obtained in a patient with a normal urethra. This test is called a retrograde urethrogram (RUG). X-ray contrast is instilled through the tip of the penis towards the bladder. As the contrast is injected, a film is obtained. The contrast is clear and looks like water, but is white on an X-ray

	IVP	MCU	RGU
Full form	Intravenous pyelography	Micturating cystourethrogram	Retrograde urethrography
Other names	Excretory urography	Voiding cystourethrogram/ Descending urography	Ascending urography
Definition	Invasive radiological imaging technique in diagnosis of urinary tract disease which requires the use of X-rays after the injection of contrast.	**MCU** remains essential and a primary tool for the diagnosis and evaluation of infants and young children with many genitourinary disorder.	**Retrograde urethrography** involves the use of x-ray pictures to provide visualization of structural problems or injuries to the urethra.
Indications	▫ Hematuria ▫ Renal colic ▫ Renal trauma ▫ Persistent pyuria ▫ Prior to per-cutaneous uro-procedures to define renal anatomy. ▫ Prior to surgery involving risk of ureteric injury ▫ Work-up of live donor in renal transplant ▫ After surgery (ureteric surgery) ▫ Renal artery stenosis ▫ PUJ obstruction ▫ Ectopic Kidney	▫ Vesicoureteric reflux in children - in recurrent UTI ▫ Stress incontinence ▫ Urethral stricture ▫ Bladder dysfunctions ▫ Anomalies of bladder neck and urethra ▫ Suspected bladder trauma	▫ Congenital abnormalities ▫ Fistulas or false passages ▫ Lacerations ▫ Strictures ▫ Valves, known as "posterior urethral valves" ▫ Tumors ▫ Post operative
Contraindications	▫ Previous serious reaction ▫ Pregnancy ▫ DM in renal insufficiency ▫ Myeloma ▫ Sickle- cell disease	▫ Current - urinary tract infection ▫ Contrast media allergies	▫ Pregnancy ▫ Recent urethral instrumentation ▫ Current UTI ▫ Recent surethral surgery
Contrast	Intravenous	Through the catheter, contrast is instilled. Patient is asked to micturate & films are taken while micturition	Contrast is instilled through the external urethral meatus.

Contd...

	IVP	MCU	RGU
Structures seen	Kidneys, ureter and bladder	Bladder and posterior urethra (prostatic and membranous urethra)	Anterior urethra (penile and bulbar urethra)
Complications	☐ Spontaneous rupture of collecting system ☐ Contrast medium induced nephropathy ☐ Adverse reactions to cont. media ☐ Infection and septicemia	☐ Temporary Dysuria ☐ Transient Haematuria from catheterization. ☐ Cystitis	☐ Urethral trauma and bleeding per urethra ☐ Intravasation of contrast medium (predisposing factors: excessive injection pressure in the presence of stricture, recent urethral instrumentation, active urethral inflammation) ☐ Urinary tract infection

RADIO PLATE 31

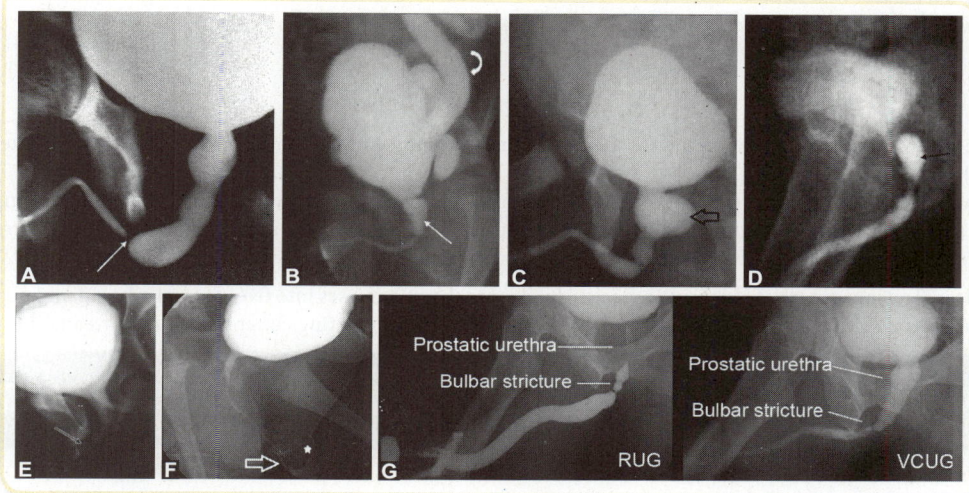

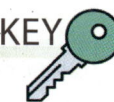 KEY

PLATE LEGENDS

A. **Anterior urethral valve:** VCUG image shows urethral dilatation proximal to an anterior urethral valve (arrow) and narrowing distal to it. Note the abrupt change in the caliber of the urethra below the valve. **Note: Voiding cystourethrography (VCUG)** Voiding cystourethrography (VCUG, synonym being **micturating cystourethrogram** or MCUG) refers to a fluoroscopic technique complemented by radiographic imaging performed as an examination of lower urinary tract, by introducing contrast media into the bladder via a catheter. VCUG examination is performed combining fluoroscopic and radiographic imaging that starts with abdominal radiography prior to the aseptic catheterization of the bladder, followed by application of nonionic iodinated contrast media via a catheter. Fluoroscopic screening and radiographic images are obtained within ALARA principle (As Low As Reasonably Achievable) during contrast application, when the bladder is filled (frontal view with full bladder, left and right oblique), during voiding (oblique in male patients) and following micturition. If the contrast moves into the ureters and back into the kidneys, the radiologist makes the diagnosis of vesicoureteral reflux, and gives the degree of severity a score. The volume of contrast material depends on estimated bladder capacity, which can be calculated as follows: for children less than 1 year old V (mL) = Weight (kg) X 7, for children older than 1 year V (mL) = [Age (years) + 2] X 30.

B. **Posterior urethral valve** in a male child. An oblique MCU image shows a dilated posterior urethra (arrow) with an abrupt transition to a normal-caliber anterior urethra. Note the bladder neck hypertrophy, the irregular trabeculated bladder wall, and the left-sided vesicoureteric reflux (curved arrow) leading to recurrent UTI. Posterior urethral valves (PUV) are the most common obstructive anomaly in male children. Voiding cystourethrography is the only procedure that confirms PUV, showing a filling defect followed by reduced caliber of urethra between disproportionately dilated posterior urethra and a narrow anterior urethra, associated with secondary changes- bladder neck hypertrophy, and trabeculation or sacculation of the bladder, with or without vesicoureteral reflux.

C. Large **posterior urethral diverticulum** in a male child presenting with recurrent urinary tract infection. An oblique MCU image reveals a large wide-neck diverticulum (arrow) arising from the prostatic urethra.

D. **Prostatic utricle**. Oblique RGU image reveals a blind-ending outpouching, filled with the contrast, arising from the prostatic urethra (arrow). The anterior urethra appears normal.

E. An oblique VCUG image of a young male shows a short **epispadiac urethra** opening on the dorsal surface of the penile shaft (arrow)

F. An oblique VCUG image of a young male shows a short **Hypospadias** urethra opening on the ventral surface of the penile shaft (arrow) and short malformed penis (star) Imaging in patients with hypospadias is usually accomplished by retrograde urethrography (RUG) and less commonly by voiding cystourethrography (VCUG).

G. **Stricture of bulbar urethra**[NEETPG] in RUG with proximal narrowing of the lumen. Stricture of bulbar urethra in same patient on VCUG/MCU with distal narrowing of lumen.

RADIO PLATE 32

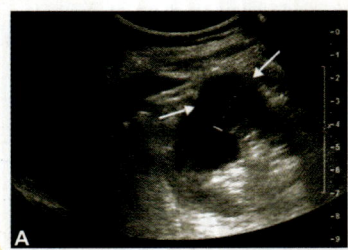
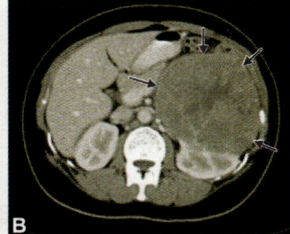
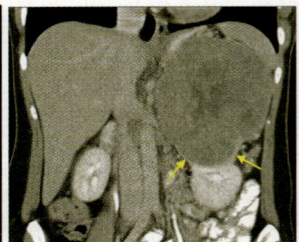
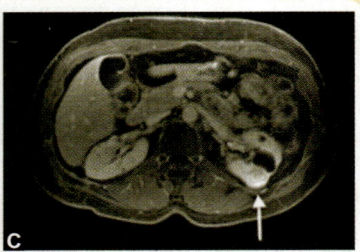

PLATE LEGENDS

A. **USG kidney:** The renal cell carcinoma is identified as a rounded mass extending off the posterior kidney (arrows). Note the dark area next to the mass, which represents a renal cyst.
B. **Transverse and coronal CT.** This patient presented with a huge left upper pole mass (arrows). One of the helpful imaging signs is called the **'claw sign'**, where a small claw-like parenchyma from the organ extends around the tumor, as indicated by the yellow arrows on the coronal CT. This allowed us to correctly predict that the tumor was arising from the left kidney.

The **Bosniak classification system** of renal cystic masses divides renal cystic masses into five categories based on imaging characteristics on contrast-enhanced CT. It is helpful in predicting a risk of malignancy and suggesting either follow up or treatment.

Bosniak Renal Cyst Classification System							
Category	Description	Cyst wall	Septa	Calcification	Contrast enhancement	Malignant %	Management
I	A simple cyst of water density (0-20 HU)	Hairline thin and smooth	No	No	Non enhancing	0%	No follow up
II	**Minimally complicated benign cysts.** Uniformly high-attenuation lesions **<3 cm** (so-called high-density cysts) that are well marginated and do not enhance are included in this group.	Hairline thin and smooth	& or 1 or 2 hairline thin septa (<1 mm in thickness). However no enhancement	&/ or Fine calcification (not measurable) may be present in the wall or septa	Perceived enhancement may be present (10-15 HU)	0%	No follow up
IIF ("F" for follow-up)	**Moderately complex cyst.** Totally intrarenal, non enhancing, high-attenuation renal lesions **>3 cm** are also included in this category.	Minimal thickening with Perceived but not measurable enhancement	Multiple **hairline septa** with minimal thickening and with Perceived but not measurable enhancement	Their wall or septa may contain calcification that may be thick and nodular	Perceived enhancement of their septa or wall may be present. (10-15 HU)	5%	Follow up to demonstrate stability
III	**"Indeterminate complex cyst"** masses	Thick wall with or without wall Nodularity with measurable contrast enhancement	More numerous or irregularly thickened septae (>1 mm) with measurable enhancement	Their wall or septa may contain calcification that may be thick and nodular	Measurable enhancement is present (>15 HU)	55%	Surgery in most cases or Strict follow up

Contd...

Bosniak Renal Cyst Classification System							
Category	Description	Cyst wall	Septa	Calcification	Contrast enhancement	Malignant %	Management
IV	**Complex cystic masses** with inhomogenous solid components. These lesions include cystic carcinomas and require surgical removal.	Thick wall with or without wall Nodularity with measurable contrast enhancement	Thickened irregular or smooth walls or septa with measurable enhancement	Their wall or septa may contain calcification that may be thick and nodular	Measurable enhancement is present (>15 HU). Plus Enhancing soft tissue components adjacent to, but independent of, the wall or septa	100%	Surgery

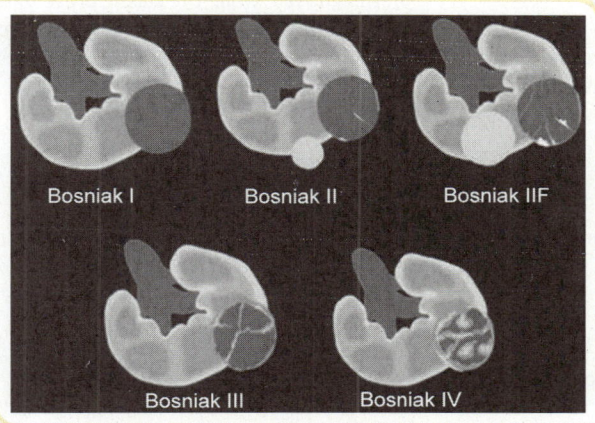

C. **Contrast-enhanced MRI:** The renal cell carcinoma is identified as an avidly enhancing rounded mass along the posterior left kidney (arrow).

 **RADIO PLATE 33**

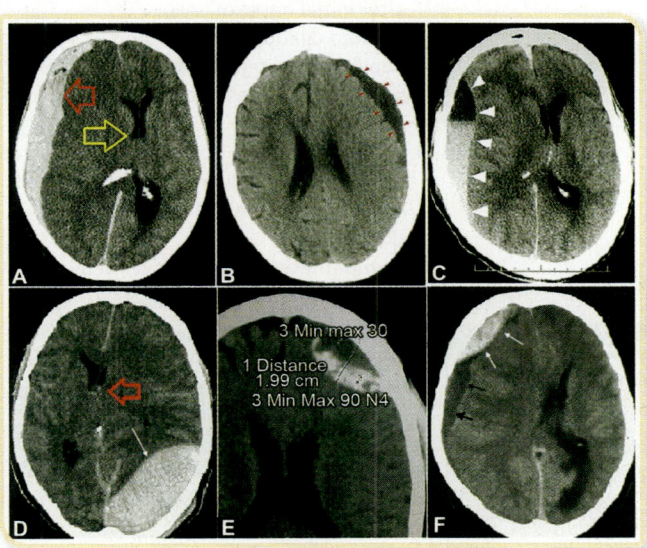

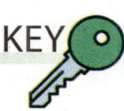 **KEY**

PLATE LEGENDS

A. **Acute Subdural hemorrhage:** On head CT scan, the clot is bright white (hyperdense) or mixed-density, **Crescent/ Lunate-shaped** (Red arrow) with a concave surface away from the skull, may have a less distinct border, and does not cross the midline due to the presence of the falx. A midline shift is also noted if the hemorrhage is large (Yellow arrow). While MRI is superior for demonstrating the size of an acute subdural hematoma (SDH) and its effect on the brain, noncontrast head CT is the primary means of making a diagnosis and suffice for immediate management purposes

B. **Chronic subdural hematoma:** Acute hematomas are bright white (hyperdense) on CT scan for approximately 3 days, after which they fade to isodensity with brain (subacute), and then to hypodensity after 2 to 3 weeks (Chronic). A true chronic SDH will be as dark as CSF on CT (Red arrowhead).

C. **Acute-on-chronic subdural hematoma:** *Arrowheads* outline the hematoma. The acute component is slightly denser and is seen as the hyperdense area in the dependent portion. (White arrowhead)

D. **Acute Extradural hemorrhage:** On head CT the clot is bright white (hyperdense), **biconvex/lentiform (while arrow),** and has a well-defined border that usually respects cranial suture lines. Epidural hematoma (EDH) forms an extra axial, smoothly marginated, lenticular, or biconvex homogenous density. A midline shift is also noted if the hemorrhage is large (red arrow).

 Note

EDH is mostly associated with fractures whereas SDH is rarely associated.

E. **Chronic Extradural hemorrhage with ossification:** Hypodense extradural hematoma with margins of the hematoma which increased in thickness and density (Hyperdense), HU comparable to bone density.

F. **Chronic subdural hematoma with Acute Extradural hematoma:** CT-scan showed right frontal extra-axial collections suggesting an acute extradural hematoma (white arrows) associated to chronic subdural hematoma (black arrows). The **swirl sign** refers to the non-contrast CT appearance of acute extravasation of blood into a hematoma, for example an extra dural hematoma. It represents un-clotted fresh blood which is of lower attenuation than clotted blood which surrounds it.

Traumatic Intracranial Hematomas

	Extradural hemorrhage	Subdural hemorrhage	Subarachnoid hemorrhage
Cause	Lower-energy trauma with less resultant primary brain injury causing rupture of middle meningeal artery, usually traumatic coup injury (rapid because it is usually from arteries) 10% of epidural bleeds may be venous, 70-80% of epidural hematomas (EDHs) are located in the temporoparietal region	High energy impacts with rupture of bridging veins (superior cerebral vein) slower onset than those of epidural hemorrhages because the lower pressure veins bleed more slowly than arteries, most often around the tops and sides of the frontal and parietal lobes, A subdural hematoma (SDH) is the most common type of intracranial mass lesion	Head trauma (MC) > Rupture of berry's aneurysm (2nd MC) Intracerebral hematomas and subarachnoid hemorrhages can also result from strokes.
Peak Age	Younger than 20 years	Bimodal age 60 and older,	50 years
History	Following injury, the patient may or may not lose consciousness	Subdural hematomas are divided into acute, subacute, and chronic, depending on the speed of their onset. **Risk factors:** ☐ Shaken baby syndrome ☐ Blood thinners (anticoagulants) ☐ Long-term alcohol abuse ☐ Dementia ☐ Elderly ☐ Alcoholics	Subarachnoid hemorrhage (SAH) range from subtle prodromal events to the classic presentation. Prodromal events often are misdiagnosed, while the classic presentation is one of the most pathognomonic pictures in all of clinical medicine.
Signs and Symptoms	☐ Hypertension ☐ Bradycardia ☐ Bradypnea ☐ Severe headache ☐ Vomiting ☐ Seizures EDH has a classic three-stage clinical presentation that is probably seen in only 20% of cases. The patient is initially unconscious from the concussive aspect of the head trauma. The patient then awakens and has a <u>lucid interval</u> while the hematoma sub clinically expands. As the volume of the hematoma grows, the decompensated region of the pressure-volume curve is reached, ICP increases, and the patient becomes lethargic and herniates. **Uncal herniation from an EDH classically causes ipsilateral third nerve palsy and contralateral hemiparesis.**	☐ Loss of consciousness ☐ Irritability ☐ Seizures ☐ Disorientation ☐ Ataxia ☐ Altered breathing pattern ☐ Blurred vision ☐ Persistent headache, ☐ Fluctuating drowsiness, ☐ Confusion ☐ Memory changes ☐ Paralysis on the side of the body opposite the hematoma ☐ Speech or language impairment	☐ Severe headache with a rapid onset ("thunderclap headache") ☐ Confusion or a lowered level of consciousness ☐ Seizures ☐ Photophobia ☐ Focal neurologic deficit (hemiparesis, aphasia, hemineglect, cranial nerve palsies memory loss) ☐ Motor neurologic deficits ☐ Sub hyaloid retinal hemorrhage & papilledema ☐ ↑Temperature (secondary to chemical meningitis) ☐ ↑Blood pressure ☐ Neck stiffness usually presents six hours after initial onset of SAH, ☐ Isolated dilation of a pupil and loss of the pupillary light reflex may reflect brain herniation as a result of rising intracranial pressure ☐ Oculomotor nerve abnormalities (affected eye looking downward and outward and inability to lift the eyelid on the same side) or palsy, ☐ **"sympathetic surge"** i.e. over-activation of the sympathetic system
Grading	Nil	**Bender grading system** | Group 1	Normal mental function, no focal signs | | Group 2 | Lethargic, focal neurologic signs | | Group 3 | Stuporous, marked focal neurologic signs | | Group 4 | Coma, sign of hibernation (pupillary dilation, decerebrate or decorticate posturing, respiratory arrest). |	**World Federation of Neurosurgeons (WFNS) classification:** | Grade | GCS | Focal neurological deficit | |---|---|---| | 1 | 15 | Absent | | 2 | 13–14 | Absent | | 3 | 13–14 | Present | | 4 | 7–12 | Present or absent | | 5 | <7 | Present or absent |

Contd...

	Traumatic Intracranial Hematomas		
	Extradural hemorrhage	**Subdural hemorrhage**	**Subarachnoid hemorrhage**
		Markwalder grading system	**Fischer scale (CT scan appearance)**
		Group 0 – No neurologic signs Group 1 – Headache, reflex asymmetry Group 2 – Altered mental status, hemiparesis Group 3 – Stupor but responsive, hemiplegia Group 4 – Coma, decerebrate or decorticate posturing	Grade 1 – None evident Grade 2 – Less than 1 mm thick Grade 3 – More than 1 mm thick Grade 4 – Diffuse or none with intraventricular hemorrhage or parenchymal extension
CT Scan	See PLATE	See PLATE	See PLATE
Treatment	Patients who meet all of the following criteria may be managed conservatively: clot volume <30 cm³, maximum thickness <1.5 cm, and GCS score >8. Open craniotomy for evacuation of the congealed clot and hemostasis is indicated for EDH which are not managed conservatively	Open craniotomy for evacuation of acute SDH is indicated for any of the following: thickness >1 cm, midline shift >5 mm, or GCS drop by two or more points from the time of injury to hospitalization. Nonoperatively managed hematomas may stabilize and eventually reabsorb, or evolve into chronic SDHs	Medical management by **"Triple H therapy"**; Hypervolemia, Hypertension & Hemodilution. Prompt neurosurgery or radiologicaly guided interventions with medications & other treatments to help prevent recurrence of the bleeding and complications. Many aneurysms are treated by a less invasive procedure called "coiling", which is carried out by instrumentation through large blood vessels.
Mortality	15 and 20%	30% overall, 60 to 80% in acute SDH	Up to half of all cases of SAH are fatal and 10–15% of casualties die before reaching a hospital
Poor prognosis	☐ Advanced age ☐ Intradural lesions ☐ Temporal location ☐ Increased hematoma volume ☐ Rapid clinical progression ☐ Pupillary abnormalities ☐ Increased intracranial pressure ☐ Lower Glasgow coma scale (GCS) ☐ No lucid interval	☐ Acute subdural hematomas ☐ Glasgow coma scale <7 ☐ Age >80 ☐ Acute duration ☐ hypodensity of SDH on CT scan	

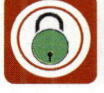 **RADIO PLATE 34**

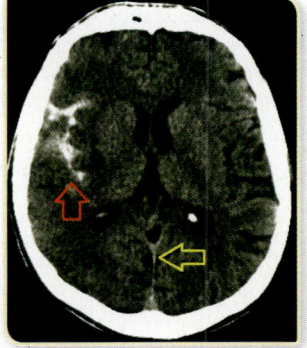

indicates rupture of a saccular aneurysm. Sensitivity of 98% within the first 12 hours & 93% within 24 hours.

 **RADIO PLATE 35**

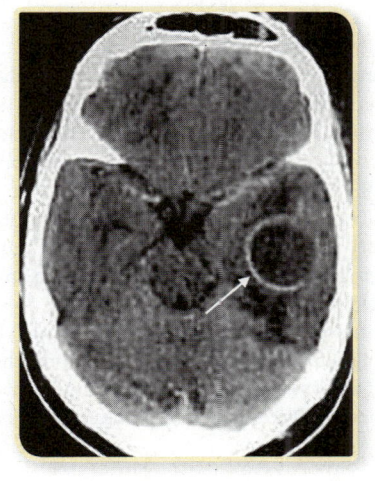

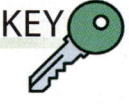 KEY

SUBARACHNOID HEMORRHAGE
In general, blood localized to the basal cisterns, the sylvian fissure (Red arrow), or the intra-hemispheric fissure (Yellow arrow)

CT SCAN SHOWING CEREBRAL ABSCESS

- Ring of iso/hyperdense tissue, typically of uniform thickness
- Central low attenuation (fluid/pus)
- Surrounding low density (vasogenic edema)
- Ventriculitis may be present, seen as enhancement of the ependyma
- Obstructive hydrocephalus will be seen when intraventricular spread has occurred

RADIO PLATE 36

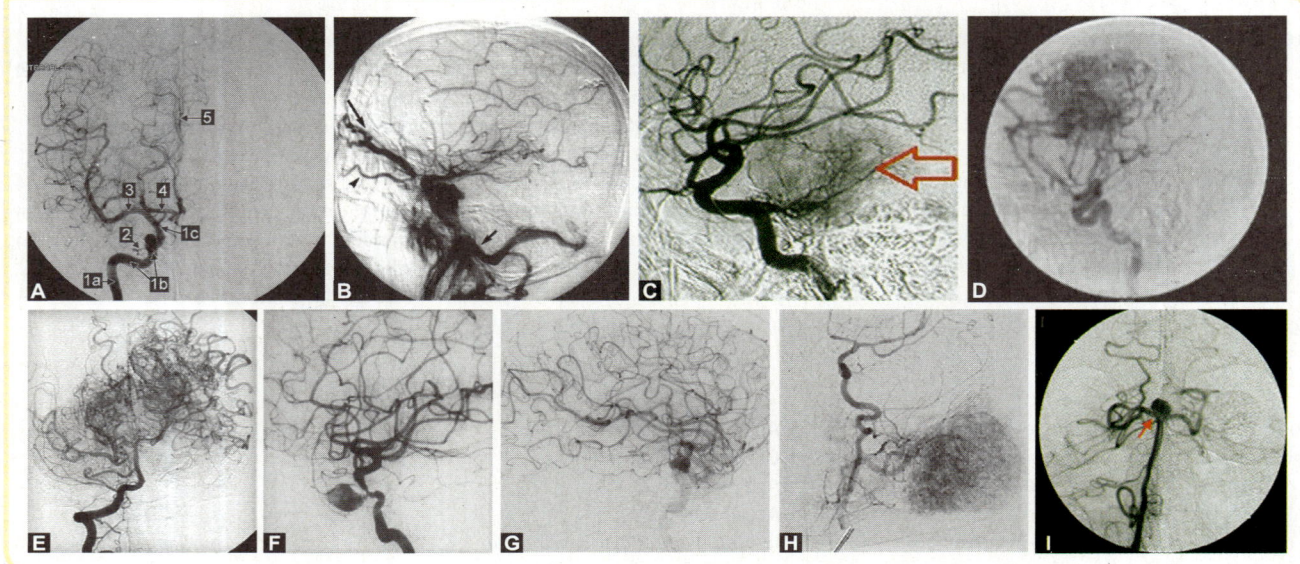

PLATE LEGENDS

A. **Normal Cerebral arteriogram-AP arterial phase**
   1. Internal carotid artery (ICA)
   1a. Cervical ICA
   1b. ICA in carotid canal and cavernous sinus
   1c. Carotid siphon
   2. Ophthalmic artery
   3. Middle cerebral artery
   4. Anterior cerebral artery
   5. Pericallosal artery

B. **Cerebral angiography carotid cavernous fistula** - Left internal carotid artery angiogram in lateral projection, showing direct CCF with drainage into sigmoid sinus (short arrow), superior ophthalmic vein (long arrow) and inferior ophthalmic vein (arrowhead). DSA is a required for definitive diagnosis and treatment. The findings are typical. Rapid shunting of Internal carotid artery into cavernous sinus. There are enlarged draining vessels. Retrograde flow from cavernous sinus, most commonly into ophthalmic veins.

C. **Cerebral angiography hypervascular tumor blush**, due to angiofibroma supplied predominantly by branches of the right meningohypophyseal trunk from the right internal carotid artery (ICA). Tumor blush is enhancement of tumor after administration of contrast

D. **Cerebral angiography- cerebral proliferative angiopathy (CPA)**- left internal carotid artery injection showing diffuse proliferative angiogenesis with feeders supplied from branches of left anterior cerebral artery and left middle cerebral artery.

E. **Cerebral angiography Moyamoya disease:** Moya Moya is Japanese for **'puff of smoke'**, it is a progressive **idiopathic arteriopathy** non-atherosclerotic, non-inflammatory narrowing of distal internal carotid arteries and proximal circle of Willis with collateral formation and the net like vessels give the characteristic **puff of smoke appearance.** Mainly seen in Japan and the Pacific Rim. *A Moya Moya-like pattern may be found in other conditions such as sickle cell disease, Down's syndrome, previous radiotherapy or tuberculous meningitis and Type 1 neurofibromatosis.*

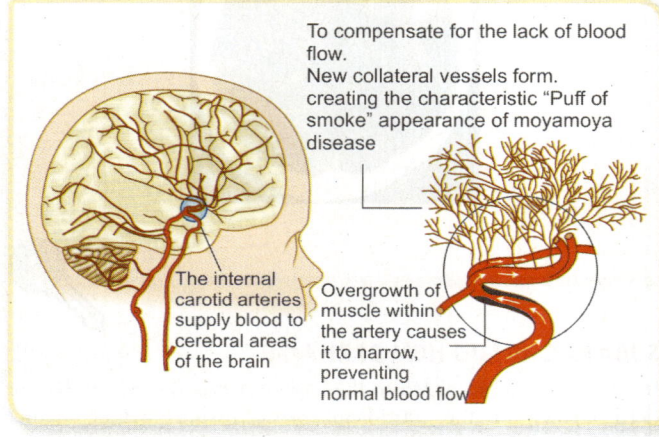

F & G Cerebral angiography ICA Pseudoaneurysm: Irregular pseudo-aneurysm at the cavernous part of the internal carotid artery. A patent pseudoaneurysm sac has the appearance of a focal outpouching from the artery of origin. On CTA a thrombosed pseudoaneurysm or thrombosed false lumen appears as an eccentric and usually smooth filling defect in or adjacent to the true lumen.

Distinguishing between true aneurysms and pseudoaneurysms on imaging is often difficult, even with cerebral angiography, because the difference between them is essentially histopathologic. In true intracranial aneurysms, the intima and adventitia are intact, whereas in intracranial pseudoaneurysms the artery is perforated and the "dome" of the pseudoaneurysm is contained within extraluminal clot.

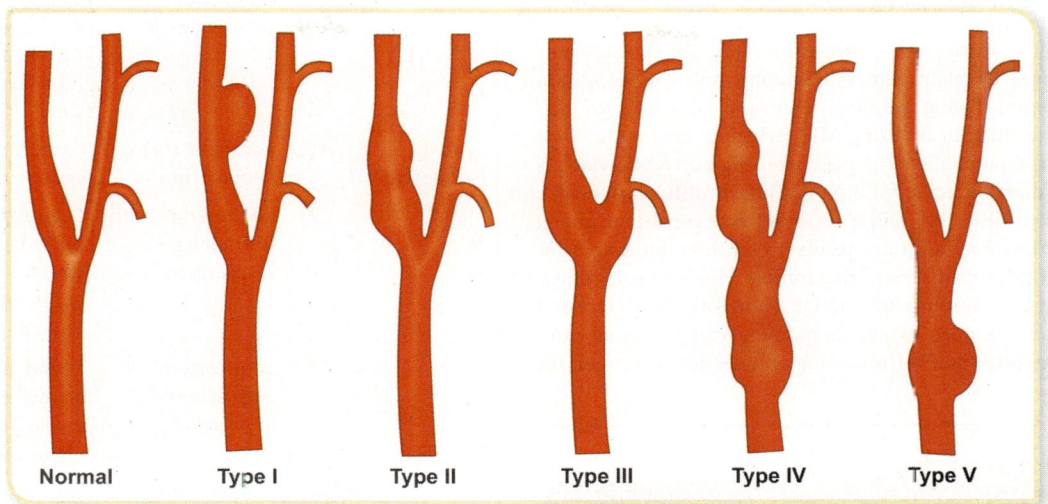

Morphological classification of the extracranial carotid artery aneurysm or Pseudoaneurysm:
- Type I: Aneurysm of the internal carotid artery above the carotid bulb
- Type II: Aneurysm of the internal carotid artery
- Type III: Aneurysm of the carotid bifurcation
- Type IV: Aneurysm of the internal carotid artery and the common carotid artery
- Type V: Aneurysm of the common carotid artery

H. DSA of hemangioma would show pooling of contrast, tumor blush and flow voids

I. **Basilar artery aneurysm:** Basilar artery aneurysms are less common than anterior circulation aneurysms, and rupture less frequently.

DIGITAL SUBSTRACTION ANGIOGRAPHY

Digital subtraction angiography (DSA) was introduced in the 1980s as a method for intravenous injection of contrast for imaging the arterial system, as the contrast in the arterial system following intravenous injection was too dilute to be imaged with standard X-rays.

DSA is based upon fluoroscopy. **Fluoroscopy** is an imaging technique that uses X-rays to obtain real-time moving images of the interior of an object. In traditional angiography, images are acquired by exposing an area of interest with time-controlled X-rays while injecting contrast medium into the blood vessels. The image obtained includes the blood vessels and all overlying and underlying structures. DSA is a modality in which these background structures are substracted from the image to allow better visualization of the vessels. In order to remove these distracting structures to see the vessels better, first a mask image is acquired. The mask image is simply an image of the same area before the contrast is administered. The radiological equipment used to capture this is usually an X-ray image intensifier, which then keeps producing images of the same area at a set rate (1 to 7.5 frames per second). Each subsequent image gets the original "mask" image subtracted out.

Contrast Agents

Nonionic contrast agents are safer and less allergenic than ionic preparations.

Iohexol (Omnipaque), a low osmolality, nonionic contrast agent, is relatively inexpensive and probably the most commonly used agent in cerebral angiography.
1. Diagnostic angiogram: Omnipaque, 300 mg I/mL
2. Neurointerventional procedure: Omnipaque, 240 mg I/mL
3. Patients with normal renal function can tolerate as much as 400–800 mL of Omnipaque, 300 mg I/mL without adverse effects.

 **RADIO PLATE 37**

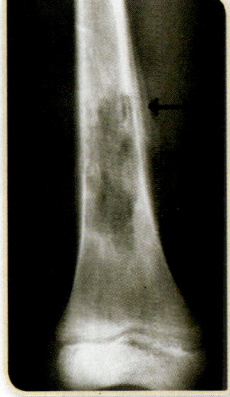

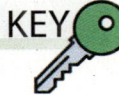

ACUTE OSTEOMYELITIS X-RAY

Acute osteomyelitis showing widespread destruction of the cortical and medullary portions of the metaphysis and diaphysis of the distal femur, together with periosteal new bone formation and a large subperiosteal abscess is evident.

Anteroposterior radiograph demonstrates a lesion in the medullary portion of the distal femoral diaphysis (Metaphysis is most common) with a moth-eaten type of bone destruction, associated with a lamellated periosteal reaction and a small soft-tissue prominence (Black arrow).

The most common radiographic appearance is permeative moth-eaten osteolytic lesion with partial cortical destruction, a cortical sclerotic rim surrounding the zone, and osteolysis with pathological fracture. All lesions may mimic malignant bone tumors especially Ewing's sarcoma, thus making diagnosis more difficult based on radiographic findings alone. The absence of a definite soft-tissue mass and the short symptomatic period, however, point to the correct diagnosis of osteomyelitis

It is difficult to distinguish between osteomyelitis of the femur and bone tumors by plain film radiography, and this condition commonly mimics Ewing sarcoma. Accurate diagnosis of this condition is also difficult by using MRI, which is believed to be a sensitive and useful modality. The **penumbra sign** on MRI, which is reported to be highly specific for osteomyelitis, is difficult to detect. However, elevated CRP levels and ESRs found to be consistent among the cases with this condition are relatively sensitive indicators for distinguishing osteomyelitis from bone tumors. However sometimes, Ewing sarcoma can present with similar laboratory data. Hence, it is recommended that open biopsy should be performed in all cases for accurate diagnosis and for obtaining an adequate specimen for culture.

Jones Classification of Chronic Hematogenous Osteomyelitis in Children

Class		Explanation	Example X-ray
Type A		Brodie abscess[NEETPG] (Subacute osteomyelitis)	Solitary circumscribed oval cavity surrounded by a zone of sclerosis A1 = Upper end of tibia A2 = Femur AP view A3 = Femur frog leg view
Type B (sequestrum involucrum)	B1	Localized cortical sequestrum	Localized cortical sequestrum of tibia
	B2	Sequestrum with normal structural involucrum	Sequestrum (black arrow) with normal structural involucrum (white arrow) of proximal humerus
	B3	Sequestrum with sclerotic involucrum	Sequestrum (white arrow) with sclerotic involucrum (black arrow head) of radius
	B4	Sequestrum without/ Inadequate structural Involucrum	Sequestrum without/ inadequate structural involucrum of tibia
Type C		Sclerotic	Sclerotic tibia

RADIO PLATE 38

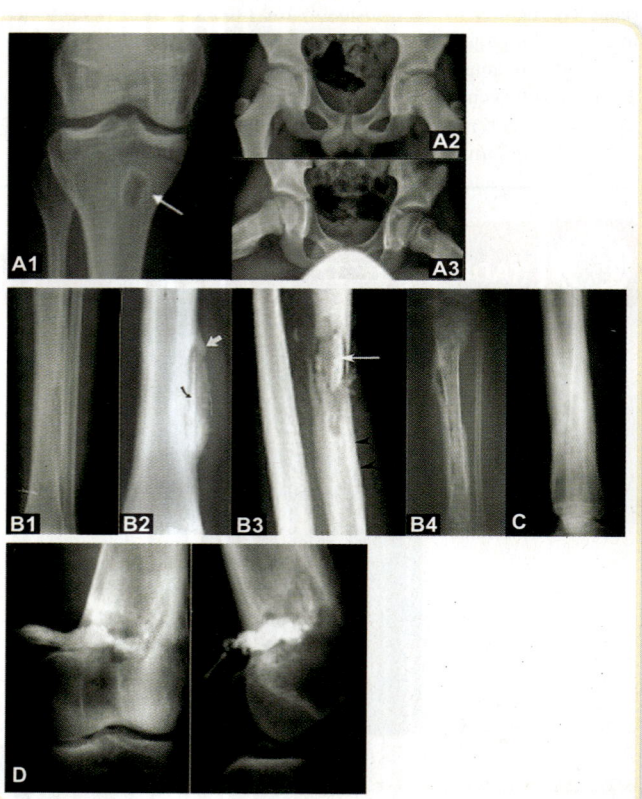

D. Sinogram in Chronic osteomyelitis: AP and Lateral roentgenograms of a sinogram in with chronic osteomyelitis that tracks into the intramedullary cavity.

RADIO PLATE 39

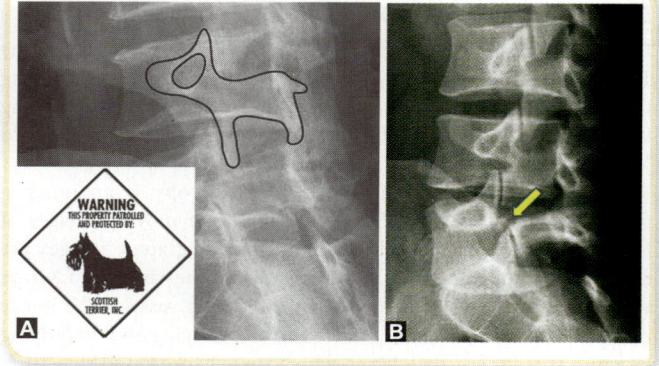

CHRONIC OSTEOMYELITIS X-RAY

Jones et al. described a classification of chronic hematogenous osteomyelitis in children in which three main types are identified based on radiographic appearance:

PLATE LEGENDS

A. Normal vertebra with **Scottish dog sign** (without collor and without beheading). The Scotty dog sign refers to the normal appearance of the lumbar spine when seen on oblique radiograph. It is important to remember the body parts of the dog corresponding to the parts of vertebra as shown in the following figure.

- The **transverse process** being the nose
- The **pedicle** forming the eye
- The **inferior articular facet** being the front leg
- The **superior articular facet** representing the ear
- The **pars interarticularis** (the portion of the lamina that lies between the facets) equivalent to the neck of the dog.

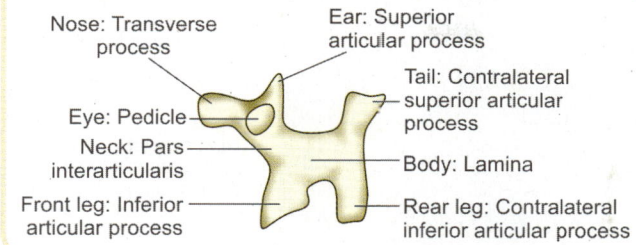

B. **Spondylolysis** is seen as a broken neck or a collar on the 'Scotty dog' (arrow). Oblique X-ray views of the lumbar spine showing the 'Scotty dog' figure, the ear of which is the superior articular process, the eye is the pedicle, the nose is the transverse process, the neck is the pars interarticularis and the front limb is the inferior articular process. If spondylolysis is present, the pars interarticularis, or the neck of the dog, will have a defect or break. It often looks as if the dog has a collar around the neck. Spondylolysis is a defect in the **pars interarticularis** of the neural arch, the portion of the neural arch that connects the superior and inferior articular facets. It is commonly known as pars interarticularis defect or more simply as pars defect.

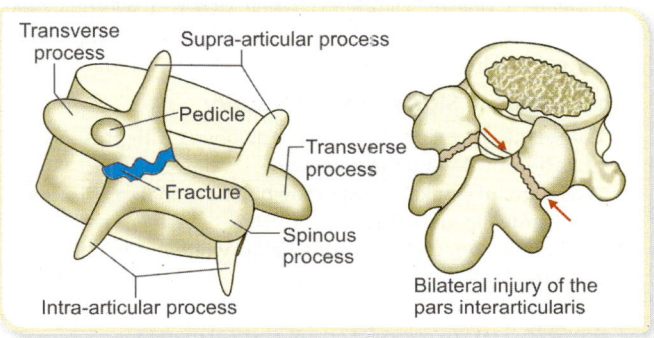

A. In spondylolisthesis the defect in pars interarticularis is seen as if the Scotty dog is beheaded in the oblique view, it is also known as Terrier sign.
B. **Inverted napoleon hat sign** is seen on anterior posterior radiograph indicating spondylolisthesis of L5 over S1.

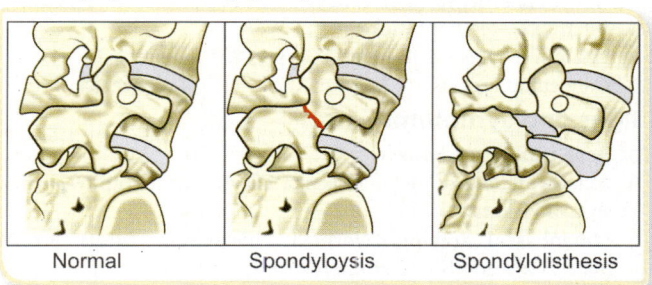

Spondylolisthesis Grades	
Grade 1	0- 25% of vertebral body has slipped forward
Grade 2	20- 50%
Grade 3	50- 75%
Grade 4	75- 100%
Grade 5	100%, Vertebral body completely fallen off (i.e., spondyloptosis)

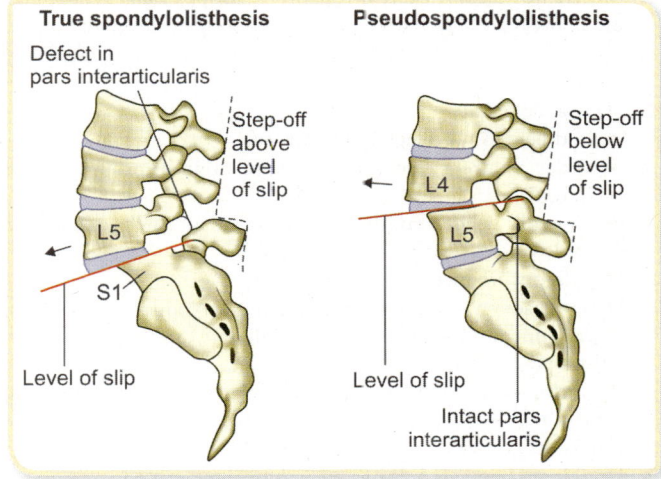

RADIO PLATE 40

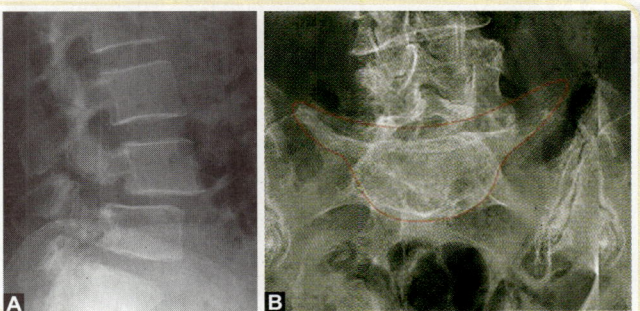

PLATE LEGENDS

Spondylolisthesis[NEETPG] is the forward displacement of a vertebra, especially the fifth lumbar vertebra, most commonly occurring after a fracture.

RADIO PLATE 41

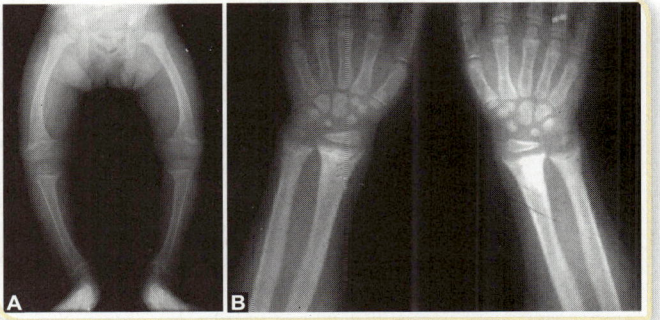

PLATE LEGENDS

A. Rickets of Lower limbs
B. Rickets of Upper limbs

Rickets is a softening of bones in children due to deficiency or impaired metabolism of vitamin D, magnesium, phosphorus or calcium, potentially leading to fractures and deformity.

Types
- Nutritional Rickets
- Vitamin D Resistant Rickets
- Vitamin D Dependent Rickets (Type I & Type II)
- Congenital Rickets

Signs and Symptoms
- Bone pain or tenderness
- Axial widening of metaphysis aka **Fraying of metaphysis (first sign of rickets)**
- **Metaphyseal fraying:** Normally metaphysis meets growth plate as a smooth line of sclerosis known as zone of provisional calcification. Serrated metaphyseal ends seen in rickets is known as fraying.
- **Metaphyseal cupping** refers to the inward bulging of the metaphysis.
- During infancy and early childhood, the long bones show the greatest deformity, both at the cartilage-shaft junctions and in the diaphyses resulting in characteristic bowing deformities of the arms and legs.
- Dental problems
- Muscle weakness (rickety myopathy or **"floppy baby syndrome"** or "slinky baby" (such that the baby is floppy or slinky-like)
- Increased tendency for fractures (easily broken bones), especially greenstick fractures
- Skeletal deformity
    - Toddlers: **Bowed legs (genu varum)**
    - Older children: **Knock-knees (genu valgum)** or "windswept knees"
    - Cranial, pelvic, and spinal deformities (such as lumbar lordosis)
- Growth disturbance
- Hypocalcaemia (low level of calcium in the blood)
- Tetany (uncontrolled muscle spasms all over the body)
- **Craniotabes** (soft skull)
- Costochondral swelling (aka "rickety rosary" or **"rachitic rosary"**)
- Harrison's groove
- **Double malleoli sign** due to metaphyseal hyperplasia
- Widening of wrist raises early suspicion, it is due to metaphyseal cartilage hyperplasia.

Diagnosis
- Blood tests: Serum calcium may show **low levels of calcium, serum phosphorus may be low, and serum alkaline phosphatase may be high.**
- Arterial blood gases may reveal metabolic acidosis
- An X-ray or radiograph of an advanced sufferer from rickets tends to present in a classic way: **bow legs or Genu Varum** (outward curve of long bone of the legs) and a deformed chest. Changes in the skull also occur causing a distinctive **"square headed" appearance.** These deformities persist into adult life if not treated. Long-term consequences include permanent bends or disfiguration of the long bones, and a curved back.
- **Reappearance of the zone of provisional calcification is the most important sign of healing rickets.**

RADIO PLATE 42

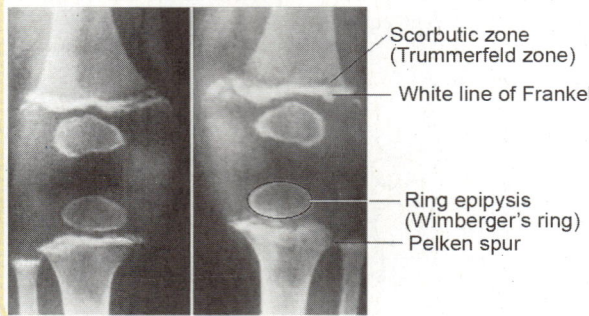

KEY

SCURVY

"Two radiological eponyms carry the name of Wimberger. Wimberger sign refers to bilateral metaphyseal destruction in the medial proximal tibias seen in congenital syphilis. Wimberger's ring or Wimberger's ring sign is a sclerotic ring around the ring shaped epiphysis indicating loss of epiphyseal density in children with scurvy".

Radiological Signs Seen in Scurvy
- **Wimberger ring sign:** Ring shaped epiphysis with presence of a sclerotic rim around epiphysis
- **White line of frankel:** Dense zone of provisional calcification at the growing metaphysis
- **Trumerfeld zone:** A lucent zone below white line due to lack of mineralization
- **Pelkan spur:** Also known as metaphyseal spurs, as the area is prone to fractures manifesting at cortical margin
- Osteoporosis
- Subperiosteal hemorrhage

RADIO PLATE 43

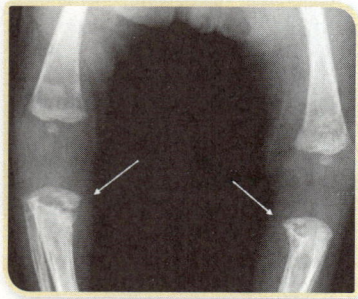

CONGENITAL SYPHILIS

Bilateral focal destruction of the medial aspect of proximal tibial epiphysis (Arrow) is pathognomic of congenital syphilis (**Wimberger's sign**).

RADIO PLATE 44

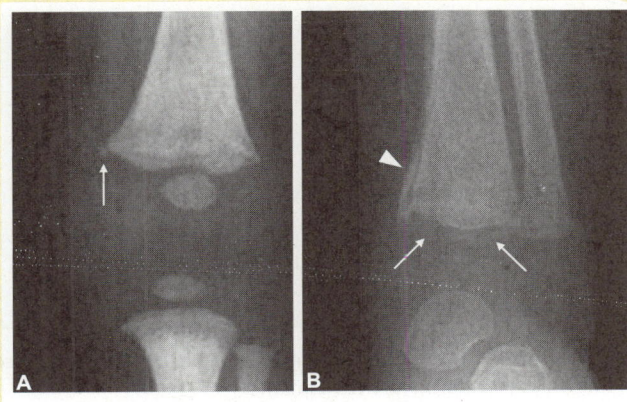
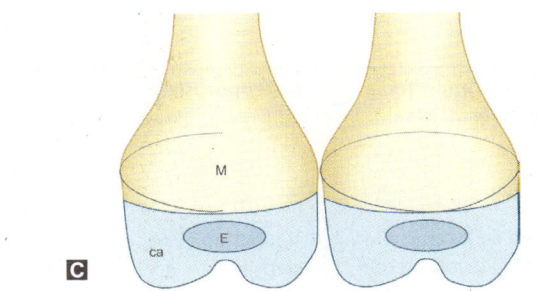

PLATE LEGENDS

A. Anteroposterior radiograph of the knees in a child having undergone NAI reveals **"corner" fracture** (arrows) on the medial aspect of the distal femur.

B. Anteroposterior radiograph of the ankle in a child having undergone NAI evidences a **"bucket-handle" fracture** (arrows) of the distal tibia. Since the lesion is extensive, an associated periosteal reaction is seen (arrowhead).

C. Diagram of a **classic metaphyseal lesion** depicts a "corner" incomplete fracture (left) and a "bucket-handle" complete fracture (right). M = metaphysis; E = osseous portion of the epiphysis; ca = cartilaginous portion of the epiphysis. The black line corresponds to the fracture line.

Radiology of Nonaccidental Injury

The spectrum of injuries encompassed by the terms nonaccidental injury (NAI) or child abuse range from the well-documented physical and sexual abuse to the less frequently publicized emotional abuse, neglect, deprivation and abandonment. The radiologist's role is to provide an objective assessment of the radiology and this is best carried out in the absence of any contact with the patient or his/her family.

Metaphyseal Fractures

Also known as corner or bucket handle fractures, metaphyseal fractures are highly characteristic of and specific for NAI with an incidence of between 11% and 28%. They are most commonly seen in nonmobile abused infants under 18 months of age, and are most frequent around the knees and ankles but also occur at the shoulder, elbow, wrists and hips. They may be bilateral. Metaphyseal fractures do not usually occur in children over 2 years of age.

Diaphyseal fractures are the most common fracture in child abuse and are said to occur four times more frequently in NAI than metaphyseal fractures. The femur, humerus and tibia are the most frequently injured bones. No one pattern or type of diaphyseal fracture is specific to NAI.

RADIO PLATE 45

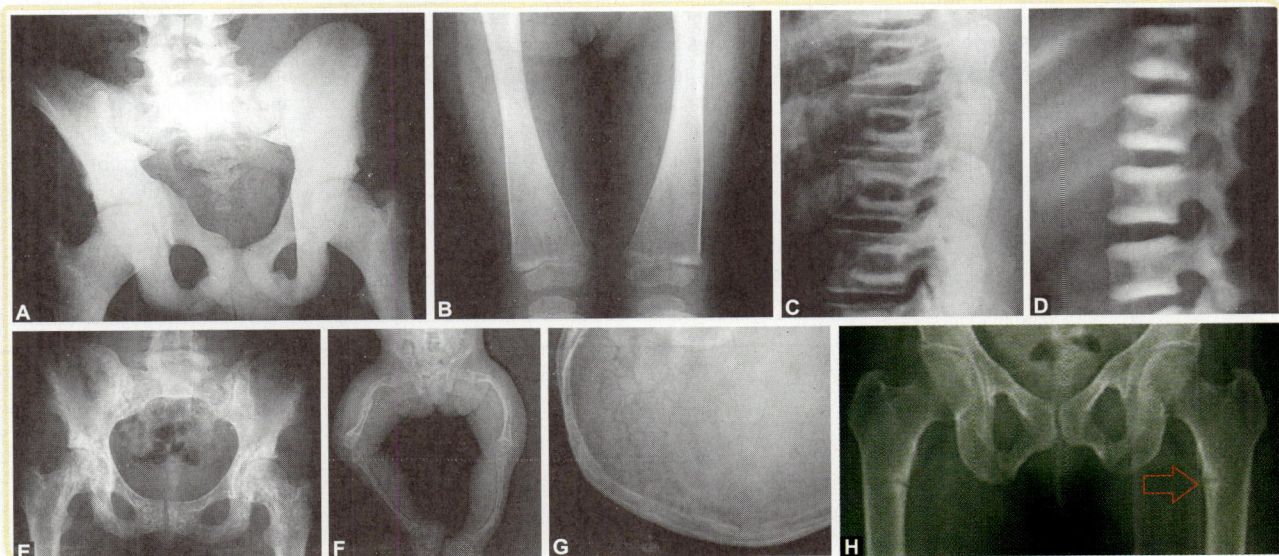

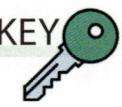

PLATE LEGENDS

A. Osteopetrosis: Diffuse osteosclerosis (increased bone density), Cortical thickening with medullary cavity being replaced.

B. Erlenmeyer flask deformity: An Erlenmeyer flask deformity is characterized by the flaring at the metaphysis/ ends of the bones (Femur in the given picture) and is named for its resemblance to an Erlenmeyer flask, a type of beaker used in chemistry labs.

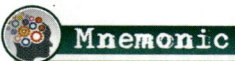

This deformity is seen in = **CHONG**= Craniodiaphyseal dysplasia, Hemoglobinopathies (Thalassemia, sickle cell anemia), Osteopetrosis, Niemann Pick disease, Gaucher's disease)

C. Bone within bone appearance: Appearance of tiny bone (vertebrae in the given picture) within larger bone. Seen in Normal (in the spine of infants), Thorotrast (thorium dioxide) administration, Osteopetrosis, Paget disease, Sickle cell disease or thalassemia, Lead poisoning, Acromegaly, Congenital syphilis, Hypervitaminosis D, Complex Regional Pain Syndrome

D. Sandwich vertebrae: dense bands of sclerosis along superior and inferior end plates, much more dense and sharply defined than Rugger Jersey spine. Alternating sclerotic + radiolucent transverse metaphyseal lines (phalanges, iliac bones) indicate fluctuating course of disease

E. Osteopoikilocytosis: Multiple punctate sclerotic **bone islands** or foci of compact bone located in cancellous bone around the joint.

F. Osteogenesis Imperfecta: Severe osteopenia is seen throughout the skeleton with multiple bone fractures and deformities of the ribs and long bones severe osteopenia is seen throughout the skeleton with multiple bone fractures and deformities of the ribs and long bones **severe osteopenia is seen throughout the skeleton with multiple bone fractures and deformities of the ribs and long bones**

G. Wormian bone in Osteogensis imperfecta: Wormian bone is accessory bones within a suture of the skull, most often the lambdoid suture. Usually a normal variant. Pathological only when greater than 10 in number or large that lend a **"mosaic" or "paving"** appearance to the cranial vault.

Mnemonic

PORK CHOP Down
P - Pyknodysostosis
O - Osteogenesis imperfecta
R - Rickets
K - Kinky hair syndrome
C - Cleidocranial dysostosis
H - Hypothyroidism/Hypophosphatasia
O - otopalatodigital syndrome
P - primary acroosteolysis (Hajdu-Cheney)/pachydermoperiostosis/progeria
Down = Down's syndrome

H. Osteoporosis: Decreased bone density with Looser's zone also known as Pseudofracture (Red arrow).

	Osteopetrosis (Albers Schonberg disease/osteosclerosis/ Marble bones/chalk bones)	Osteopoikilosis or Osteopoikilocytosis	Osteogensis imperfecta (Brittle bone disease)	Osteoporosis
Pathology	Defective osteoclasts, i.e., osteoclasts fail to resorb bone. Bones become thick & dense	Benign, autosomal dominant sclerosing dysplasia of bone	Defective collagen I production involving the connective tissue & bones	Reduction in bone mineral density
X-ray	Diffuse osteosclerosis Cortical thickening with medullary involvement. **Erlenmeyer flask deformity, Bone within bone appearance, Sandwich vertebrae**	Multiple punctate sclerotic **bone islands** or foci of compact bone located in cancellous bone around the joint. Particularly in the pelvis, metaphysis and epiptysis of long bones, tarsals, and carpals. Long axis of lesion is along the long axis of bone. May be mistaken for sclerotic metastases but Osteopoikilosis is **symmetrical, periarticular** and the lesions are uniform in size	Severe osteoporosis. MC affect appendicular skeleton, especially lower limbs, but upper limbs and skull may be involved. Excessive bone malleability and plasticity. Deformed (overtubulated) bones. Cortical thinning. Hyperplastic callus. **Wormian bones. Codfish vertebrae.**	More than 30-50% bone loss is required to appreciate decreased bone density and **Looser's zone (Pseudofracture)** Vertebral osteoporosis manifests as: penciling of vertebrae, loss of cortical bone (**picture frame vertebra**) and trabecular bone (**ghost vertebra**), compression fractures and vertebra plana Loss of trabeculae in proximal femur

RADIO PLATE 46

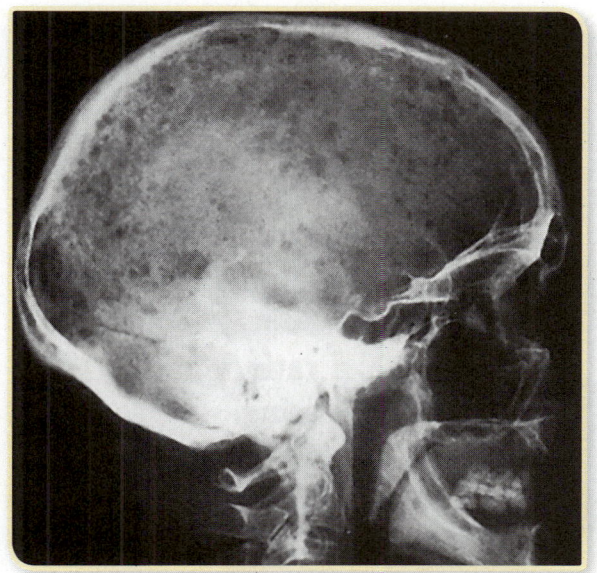

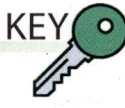

MULTIPLE MYELOMA
The classical appearance of **Multiple Myeloma (MM)** consists of well-defined **'punched-out' lesions** throughout the skeleton, *most characteristic in the skull*. The only common differential diagnosis in this age group is metastatic disease. The presence of multiple small (up to 20 mm), well-defined, round or oval lesions is more suggestive of MM.

RADIO PLATE 47

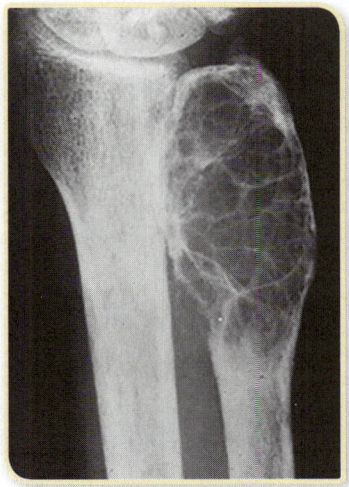

BROWN TUMOR OF HYPERPARATHYROIDISM
When this lesion involves the metaphyseal-epiphyseal region, as it does in this case, it may mimic exactly a giant cell tumor. The pathological differentiation can also be difficult without appropriate blood studies showing the elevated calcium and low phosphorus.

Radiological Signs of Hyperparathyroidism
With the increased number of patients with primary hyperparathyroidism being diagnosed with asymptomatic hypercalcemia, the majority (95%) of patients will have no radiological abnormalities. The radiologic features of secondary hyperparathyroidism are similar to those of the primary form of the disease. Hyperparathyroid 'brown tumors' should be considered in the differential diagnosis of atypical cyst-like lesions of long bones.

- **Brown tumor** (osteitis fibrosa cystica): The common sites of brown tumors is Mandible followed by long bones, pelvic girdle, clavicle, ribs. Brown tumors have a slightly greater frequency in primary than in secondary hyperparathyroidism (3% versus 2% solitary finding). However, secondary hyperparathyroidism is much more common than primary hyperparathyroidism, therefore most of brown tumors that are seen are associated with secondary hyperparathyroidism. These cysts are less commonly seen now
- **Subperiosteal erosions:** Hallmark/ classical/ pathognomonic – feature, which should always be sought, is sub-periosteal cortical resorption of cortical bone, particularly radial side of the middle phalanges of the 2nd and 3rd (index and middle) fingers. Other sites may be involved including the distal phalanges (acro-osteolysis), the outer ends of the clavicle, the symphysis pubis, the sacroiliac joints, the proximal medial cortex of the tibia, the proximal humeral shaft, ribs and femur. However, if no subperiosteal erosions are identified in the phalanges, they are unlikely to be identified radiographically elsewhere in the skeleton. Subperiosteal erosions in sites other than the phalanges indicate more severe and long-standing hyperparathyroidism, such as found in secondary to chronic renal impairment.
- **Chondrocalcinosis:** The deposition of calcium pyrophosphate dihydrate (CPPD) causes articular cartilage and fibrocartilage to become visible on radiographs. This is most likely to be identified on radiographs of the hand (triangular ligament), the knees (articular cartilage and menisci) and symphysis pubis. Other joints less commonly involved are the shoulder and the hip. Clinically the patients may present with acute pain resembling gout, but on joint aspiration pyrophosphate crystals, rather than urate crystals, are found. *Affected joints may however be asymptomatic, and chondrocalcinosis noted radiographically might bring the diagnosis of hyperparathyroidism to light in an asymptomatic patient.* The combination of chondrocalcinosis in the symphysis pubis and nephrocalcinosis on an abdominal radiograph is diagnostic of hyperparathyroidism. *Chondrocalcinosis is a feature of primary disease, rather than that secondary to chronic renal impairment.*
- **Salt and pepper skull/pepper pot skull**
- **Basket work appearance:** Of cortex with loss of corticomedullary junction.

RADIO PLATE 48

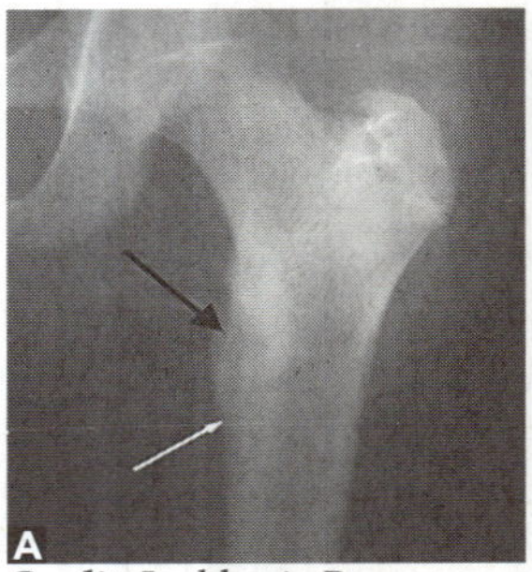

Credit: Jankharia B

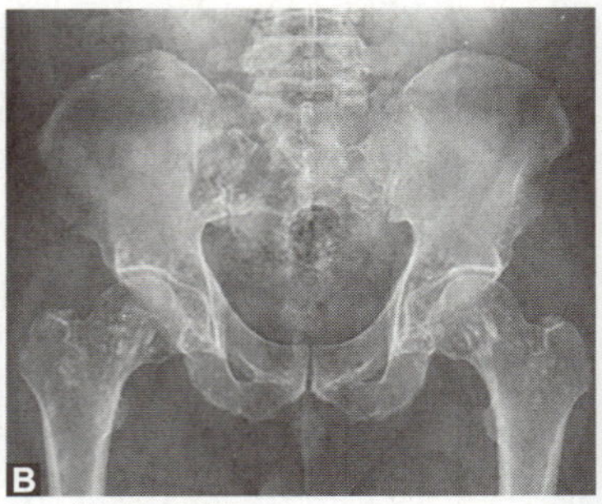

Credit: Tsai SY

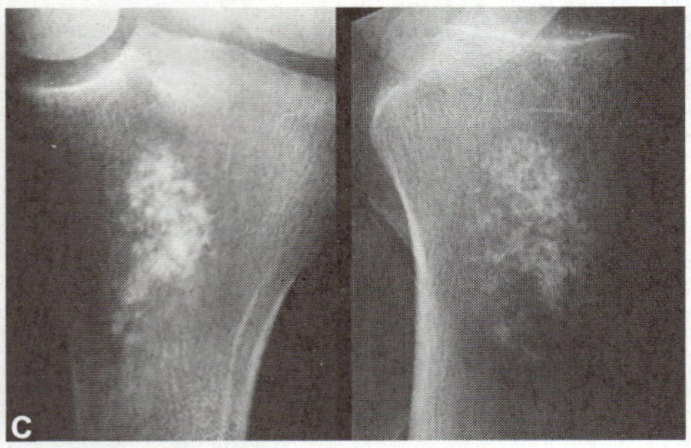

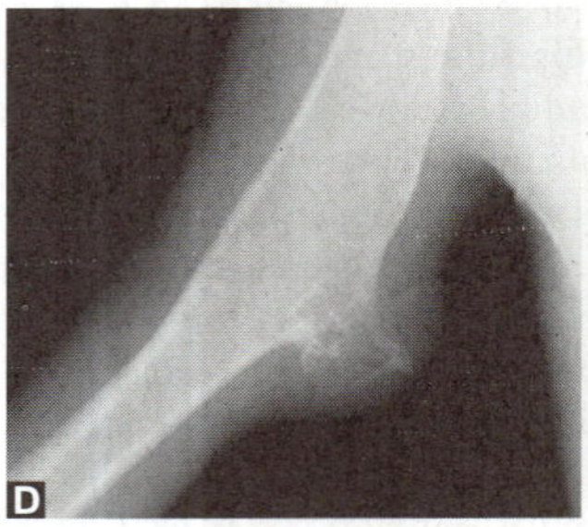

Credit: Maras Ozdemır Z

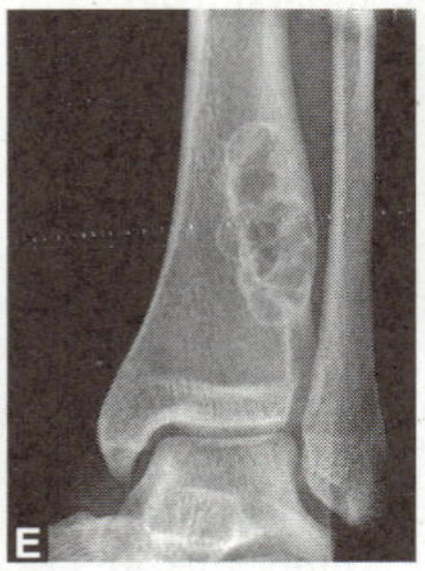

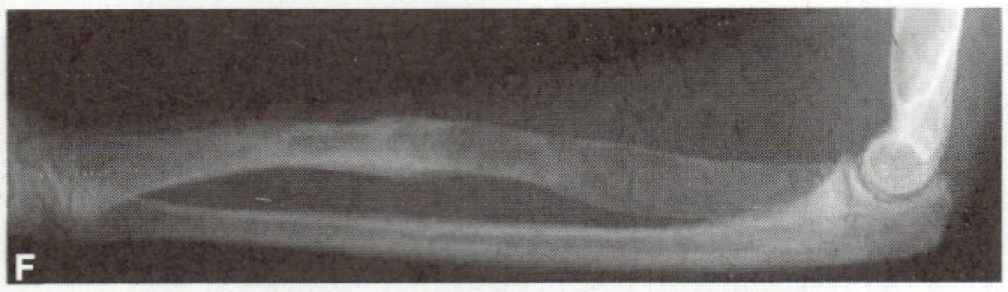

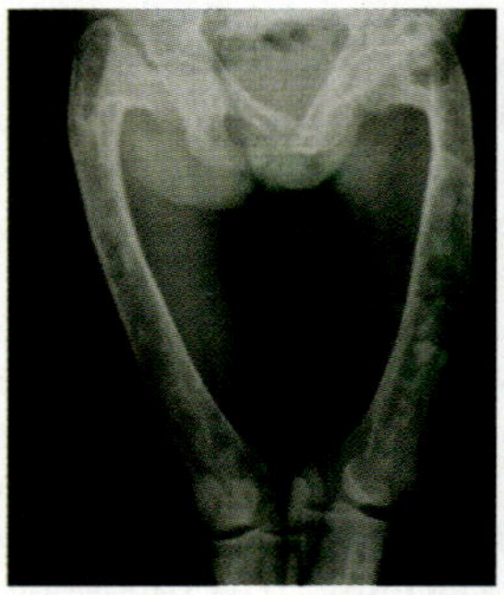

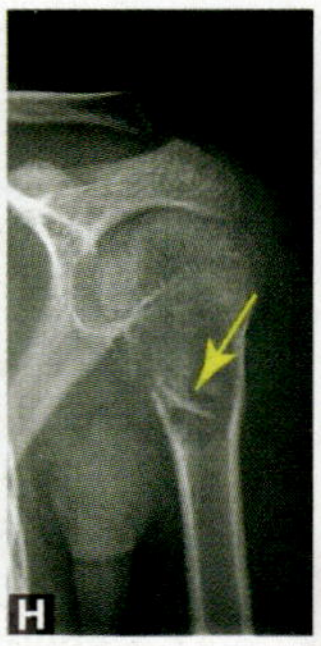

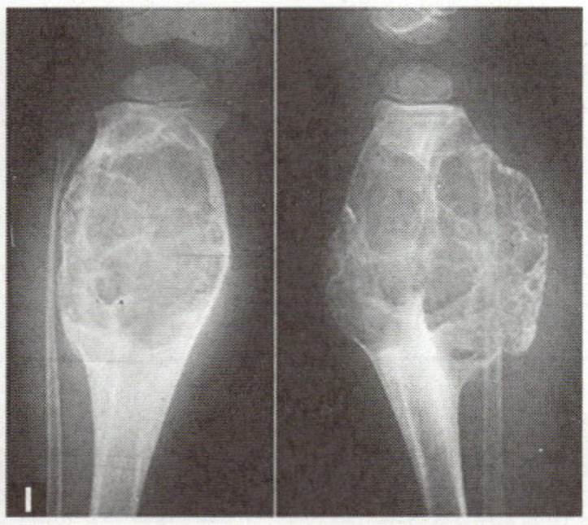

KEY

BENIGN TUMORS OF BONE

A. **Osteoid osteoma:** Plain radiograph shows a typical metadiaphyseal cortical osteoid osteoma involving the upper end of the femur. The **nidus** is well seen (black arrow) along with the surrounding cortical thickening (white arrow).

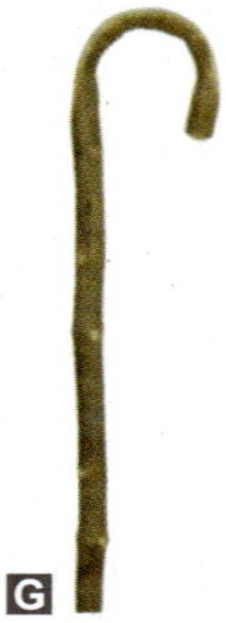

B. **Enostosis (Bone island):** Radiograph of pelvis showed multiple bone islands symmetrically distributed at the skeleton, primarily on pelvic bone, sacrum, and bilateral proximal femur. The lesion appears as an ovoid, round, or oblong focus, homogeneously dense and sclerotic, in the cancellous bone. It is commonly oriented with the long axis of the bone parallel to the cortex. Characteristic of this lesion are radiating bony streaks, referred to as *"thorny radiation" or "pseudopodia". Osteopoikilosis results in multiple enostoses.*

C. **Enchondromas,** also known as chondromas, are relatively common intramedullary cartilage neoplasms with benign imaging features. Characterized by intralesional *punctate/popcorn calcification.* It is the most common primary benign bone tumor of hand/wrist

D. **Osteochondroma:** Oblique radiograph of the right humerus shows soft tissue swelling overlying a broad-based osteochondroma.

E. **Non-ossifying fibroma:** The oblique radiograph of the ankle shows an expansile lytic lesion centered in the cortex of the distal diaphysis/metaphysis of the tibia. The lesion has a narrow zone of transition and a sclerotic rim. It does not abut the growth plate and does not cause any periosteal reaction.

F. **Fibrous dysplasia** of radius with radiolucency as ground glass appearance. Cortex is thinned out but no periosteal reaction. The **rind sign** is seen when a lesion is surrounded by a layer of thick, sclerotic reactive bone and is suggestive of fibrous dysplasia.

G. **Shephard's crook deformity**^{Q} of femur in fibrous dysplasia

H. **Simple/Unicameral bone cyst**^{Q}**:** Centrally located, purely radiolucent lesion, Concentrically expands cortex. Thinned cortical fragment falls into base of lesion, pathognomic **"fallen fragment sign**

I. **Aneurysmal bone cyst (ABC)**^{AIIMSPG} is benign expansile lytic lesion that elevates the periosteum but remain inside the thin cortical bone. Eccentrically located in the metaphysis with well-defined margins. The term is a misnomer, as the lesion is neither an aneurysm nor a cyst. Managed by curettage and autograft^{AIIMSPG}

	Demography	Site	Presentation	Imaging	Histology	Treatment	Comments
Benign Tumors of Bone & Other Non Neoplastic Conditions							
Bone forming							
Osteoid osteoma	2nd–3rd Decades, M:F - 3:1	Lower limb long bones Posterior elements spine Diaphyseal	Pain; worse at night, responds to NSAIDs	Cortical radiolucent **nidus** <1.5 cm with marked cortical thickening	Trabeculae surrounded by loose fibrovascular tissue	NSAIDs Burr down technique Radiofrequency ablation	High levels of cyclooxygenases & prostaglandins in the lesion
Enostosis (Bone island)	Adults, M= F	Pelvis, Femur	Usually Asymptomatic	Small round area of increased density in cancellous bone with radiating spicules at periphery	Mature bone with thickened trabeculae that merge with normal bone at the periphery	Observation	Osteopoikilosis—multiple bone Islands
Cartilage lesions							
Enchondroma	Adults, M= F	MC tumor of Hand. Proximal humerus Distal femur Proximal tibia	Usually Asymptomatic	Intralesional **punctate/ popcorn calcification** Minimal cortical erosion (except in hand)	Benign-appearing hyaline cartilage	Observation Curettage if symptomatic	**Ollier disease**—multiple enchondromas (malignant transformation common) **Maffucci syndrome**—Multiple enchondromas with soft tissue Hemangiomas (malignant transformation common)
Osteochondroma	2nd–3rd Decades, M> F	Metaphysis of long bones	Mass; may be painful secondary to irritation of soft tissue structures, fracture, or overlying bursa	Pedunculated or sessile bone lesion that communicates with intramedullary canal of host bone Lesion has overlying cartilage cap	Similar to epiphysis that undergoes endochondral ossification	Observation if asymptomatic Resection if symptomatic; cartilage cap must be removed entirely	Malignant transformation to chondrosarcoma is rare Multiple hereditary exostoses (MHE) is autosomal dominant with incomplete penetrance MHE—mutation of EXT1 or EXT2
Nonossifying fibroma (NOF)	1st–2nd Decades, M=F	Metaphysis of long bones	Asymptomatic; usually discovered incidentally on plain radiographs unless pathological fracture	Geographic, eccentric lesion located in metaphysis of long bones Multilobulated appearance with well defined sclerotic margins	Bland-appearing spindle cells arranged in a storiform pattern in a collagenous matrix	Observation Curettage if large Fractures usually treated nonoperatively	**Jaffe-Campanacci Syndrome:** multiple Non ossifying fibromas with café-au-lait spots

Contd...

Benign Tumors of Bone & Other Non Neoplastic Conditions

	Demography	Site	Presentation	Imaging	Histology	Treatment	Comments
Fibrous dysplasia	1st–3rd Decades, M=F	Femur Tibia epiphysis, metaphysis, or diaphysis.	Pain Deformity Cutaneous pigmentation Endocrine abnormalities	**Ground glass appearance** with well defined sclerotic rim. Severe **"shepherd's crook"** deformity of the proximal femur, usual in polyostotic form.	Irregular woven bone spicules with a fibrous stroma	Prophylactic fixation of impending fractures Correction of deformity Bisphosphonates for severe cases	**McCune-Albright Syndrome:** polyostotic fibrous dysplasia, cutaneous pigmentation, endocrine abnormalities **Mazabraud syndrome:** polyostotic fibrous dysplasia, intramuscular myxomas
Osteofibrous dysplasia	1st–2nd Decades, M=F	Tibia & fibula (diaphyseal, may encroach metaphysis)	Asymptomatic unless pathological fracture Anterior bowing	Multicentric radiolucent lesions in the cortex of the tibia	Irregular trabeculae with prominent osteoblastic rimming Loose fibrous stroma	Observation Fractures usually treated nonoperatively Surgery for correction of deformity	(ossifying fibroma of long bones, also known as **Campanacci disease**)
				Cystic lesions			
Unicameral bone cyst	1st–2nd Decades, M:F 2:1	Proximal humerus Proximal femur	**Asymptomatic** unless Pathological fracture (2/3 rd patients)	Centrally located, purely radiolucent lesion Concentrically expands cortex. Thinned cortical fragment falls into base of lesion, pathognomic **"fallen fragment sign"**	Cyst filled with **straw-colored fluid** Thin fibrovascular Lining	Observation Aspiration/ injection (steroids, bone marrow, bone graft substitute, sclerosant) Curettage	
Aneurysmal bone cyst	1st–2nd Decades, F>M	Proximal humerus Distal femur Proximal tibia Spine (posterior elements)	Pain	Eccentric expansile radiolucent lesion Thin cortical shell Fluid/fluid levels on MRI	Hemorrhagic cavernous spaces Septae of fibroblasts, histiocytes, hemosiderin-laden macrophages, and giant cells	Extended curettage Consider preoperative embolization for pelvic lesions	

RADIO PLATE 49

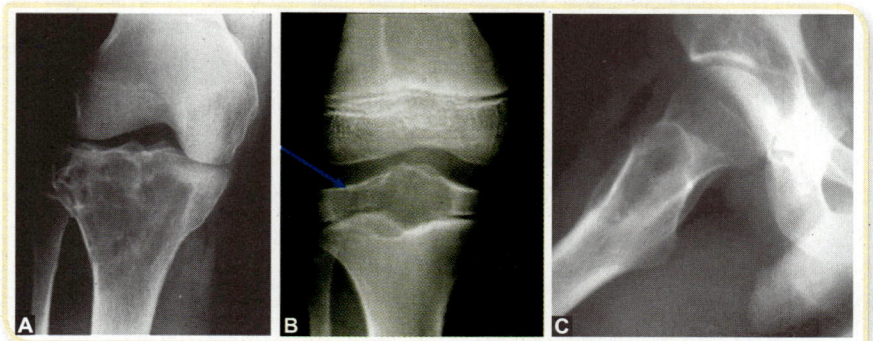

A B C

BENIGN AGGRESSIVE BONE TUMORS

A. **Giant cell tumor**[NEET PG]: Radiograph of proximal tibia with characteristic Soap bubble appearance. Well-defined, Eccentric tumor of epiphysis with non-sclerotic margins. No matrix calcification or mineralization
B. **Chondroblastoma** is a benign cartilaginous neoplasm of the epiphysis. It is eccentrically placed. Well-defined. Eccentric tumor of epiphysis with sclerotic margins. 50% show calcification.
C. **Osteoblastoma:** lytic or mixed lytic-blastic lesion with radiolucent nidus > 2cm reactive sclerotic bone

	Demography	Site	Presentation	Imaging	Histology	Treatment	Comments
Giant cell tumor	20–40 yrs F> M	Eccentrically located in epiphysis, Distal femur Proximal tibia Distal radius	Pain Pathological fracture (10%–30%)	Purely radiolucent (no matrix formation) Usually no rim of reactive bone Abuts subchondral Bone may exhibit cortical destruction with soft tissue extension Metaphyseal in skeletally immature patients	Multinucleated **giant cells** in sea of mononuclear cells Nuclei of mononuclear cells identical to nuclei of giant cells	Extended curettage Resection if residual bone stock inadequate Consider radiation for spinal/sacral tumors Resection of pulmonary metastases	3% incidence of **benign pulmonary metastases**
Chondroblastoma	10–25 yrs M: F -2 : 1	Epiphysis, Distal femur Proximal tibia Proximal Humerus	Pain Symptoms can mimic chronic synovitis	Well circumscribed lesion in epiphysis or apophysis May cross an open physis Frequently with rim of bone, 30%–50% with matrix calcification	Sheets of chondroblasts **(polygonal cells** with distinct cytoplasmic outlines) **"chicken wire" calcification Multinucleated giant Cells**	Extended curettage Resection of pulmonary metastases	1% incidence of **benign pulmonary metastases** Secondary aneurysmal bone cyst in 20%
Chondromyxoid fibroma	10–30 yrs M> F	Proximal Tibia	Pain Can present with painless mass in hands and feet	Well-circumscribed bubbly lesion Thin rim of reactive bone (appearance similar to nonossifying fibroma)	Lobules of hypocellular myxoid cartilaginous tissue Lobules separated by cellular fibrous tissue	Extended curettage	Important to distinguish from chondrosarcoma
Osteoblastoma	10–30 yrs M: F- 3 : 1	Posterior elements of spine Any bone	Pain Painful scoliosis Neurological symptoms	Bone forming lesion in posterior elements of spine. Variable/nonspecific radiographic appearance outside of spine	Fibrovascular stroma Osteoid/woven bone Osteoblastic rimming Histologic appearance similar to osteoid osteoma	Extended curettage or resection Might require spinal stabilization	Important to distinguish from low-grade Osteosarcoma

Contd...

Benign Aggressive Tumors of Bone

	Demography	Site	Presentation	Imaging	Histology	Treatment	Comments
Langerhans cell histiocytosis	< 20 yrs M: F- 2 : 1	Vertebral bodies Flat bones Diaphysis of long bones	Bone lesions may be painful or asymptomatic Can mimic osteomyelitis (pain, fever, local signs)	Vertebra plana "hole within a hole" appearance in flat bones Aggressive, permeative appearance with periosteal reaction in long bones Radiographic appearance varies from very benign to very aggressive. Can be multifocal Bone scan sometimes falsely negative	Large histiocytic cells with indented Nucleus & abundant cytoplasm **S-100 positive** Clusters of eosinophils **Birbeck granule** seen on electron microscopy	Observation of asymptomatic lesions (usually resolve) Steroid injection for symptomatic lesions Curettage/ grafting for impending fractures Chemotherapy for systemic disease	**Hand-Schüller-Christian disease** triad of skull lesions, exophthalmos, & diabetes insipidus **Letterer-Siwe disease**—fever, lymphadenopathy, Hepatosplenomegaly & multiple bone Lesions

 RADIO PLATE 50

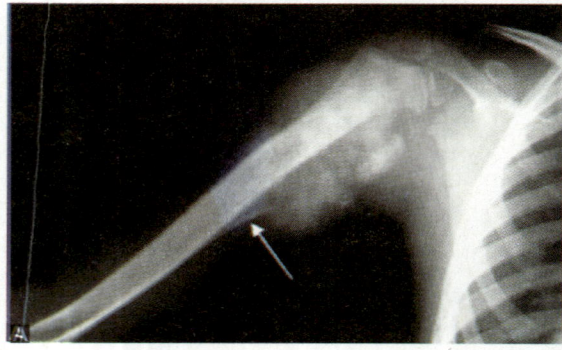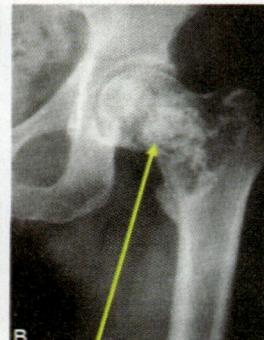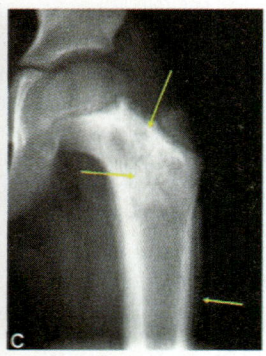

 KEY

MALIGNANT TUMORS OF BONE

A. **Osteosarcoma:** Lytic, sclerotic or mixed metaphyseal lesion with **Permeative margins** (borders of the lesion cannot be clearly delineated) with wide zone of transition from lytic/sclerotic areas of tumor to normal bone. Periosteal elevation in the form of **Codman's triangle** (arrow) and **Sunburst appearance** of the tumor.

B. **Chondrosarcoma:** Rings and arcs calcification (arrow) is characteristic of chondrosarcomas. It is due to enchondral mineralization of multiple hyaline cartilage. No sclerotic rim. Low grade Osteosarcoma presents with thin but intact cortex. High-grade chondrosarcoma presents with cortical destruction and soft tissue mass.

C. **Ewing sarcoma:** Femur is most common location. Involves Diaphysis. Top arrow indicates reactive sclerosis, Middle arrow indicates **Permeative reaction** (Most common pattern- borders of the lesion cannot be clearly delineated), Lower arrow indicates Onion skin periosteal reaction. Permeative pattern is poorly demarcated with multiple small irregular holes suggestive aggressive process. Acute osteomyelitis mimics Ewing's sarcoma both clinically and radiologically

Malignant Tumors of Bone

Tumor	Demography	Site	Presentation	Imaging	Histology	Treatment	Comments
Osteosarcoma	2nd decade M> F	Metaphyseal Distal femur Proximal tibia Proximal humerus	Progressive Pain	Mixed lytic and blastic appearance Cortical destruction Periosteal reaction (Codman triangle or hair-on-end) Soft tissue mass	Osteoproduction from malignant spindle cells Marked nuclear pleomorphism Abundant mitotic figures	Chemotherapy and wide resection	Rarely associated with hereditary form of retinoblastoma, Rothmund-Thomson syndrome, or Li-Fraumeni syndrome
Chondrosarcoma	5th–7th Decades, M> F	Pelvis Proximal femur Proximal humerus	Progressive Pain	Punctate calcification, **Rings and arc calcification.** Cortical erosion Soft tissue mass	Cartilaginous matrix Binucleate cells Grade related to degree of hypercellularity Entrapment of bony trabeculae	Wide resection (extended curettage for low-grade intramedullary tumors) No role for chemotherapy or radiation	Important to correlate symptoms, radiographic findings, and histology
Ewing sarcoma	1st–3rd Decades. M> F	Flat bones Metadiaphysis of long bones	Pain and swelling May have systemic Complaints, **Mimics osteomyelitis**	Permeative bone destruction Large soft tissue mass "Onion skin" periosteal reaction	Small round blue cells **CD99/MIC-2 positive**	Chemotherapy Surgery and/or radiation for local control	t(11,22)
Chordoma	5th–7th Decades, M: F 3 : 1	Sacrum Base of skull	Pain Neurological signs/ symptoms	Midline lesion Soft tissue mass anterior to sacrum	Cells arranged in long strands or "cords" Mucinous background Vacuolated cytoplasm physaliferous cells	Wide resection	
Adamantinoma	2nd–3rd Decades. M=F	Tibial diaphysis	Pain of long duration	Sharply demarcated radiolucent lesions in tibial diaphysis based in anterior cortex	Islands of epithelial cells in a fibrous stroma	Wide resection	
Malignant fibrous histiocytoma (MFH) / Fibrosarcoma	After 1st Decade. M=F	Distal femur Proximal tibia	Pain 20% with pathological fracture	Purely lytic Destructive	Pleomorphic spindle cells MFH—**storiform pattern** Fibrosarcoma— **Herring bone pattern**	Chemotherapy and wide resection	25% are secondary to Pre existing condition such as Paget disease, radiation, giant cell tumor, or bone infarct

Contd...

Malignant Tumors of Bone

Tumor	Demography	Site	Presentation	Imaging	Histology	Treatment	Comments
Plasmacytoma/ multiple myeloma	6th–7th Decades. M:F- 2:1	Axial location Proximal femur Proximal humerus	MC= Bone pain. Plus Systemic Complaints. Pathological facture; spine> Rib > pelvis	**Bone scan negative.** X-ray; Multiple purely lytic sharply demarcated **"punched out" lesions**	Sheets of plasma Cells with clock face nuclei and perinuclear halo. Abundant Amyloid	Chemotherapy Irradiation for symptomatic bone lesions Surgery for impending or actual pathological fractures	Diagnosis often made by serum or urine protein electrophoresis, which demonstrates a monoclonal gammopathy
Metastatic carcinoma	5th–8th Decades. M=F	Axial location Proximal femur Proximal humerus	Pain Symptoms referable to the primary lesion	**Blastic:** breast, prostate **Lytic:** kidney, thyroid mixed, lung	Histology usually similar to the primary tumor	Systemic treatment for the primary tumor Irradiation for symptomatic bone lesions Surgery for pathological fractures	Breast & prostate most common. Kidney & lung most common if patient presents with bone metastases & no known primary tumor

RADIO PLATE 51

RADIO PLATE 52

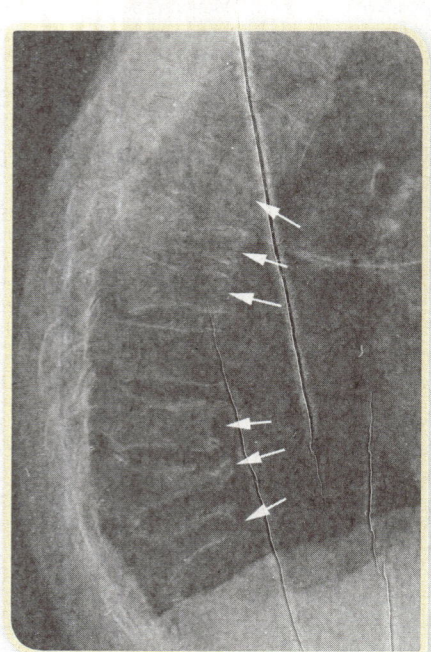

 KEY

WEDGE COMPRESSION FRACTURE
Dorsal spine lateral radiograph showing multiple vertebral wedge compression fracture in osteoporotic bones most commonly in post menopausal female.

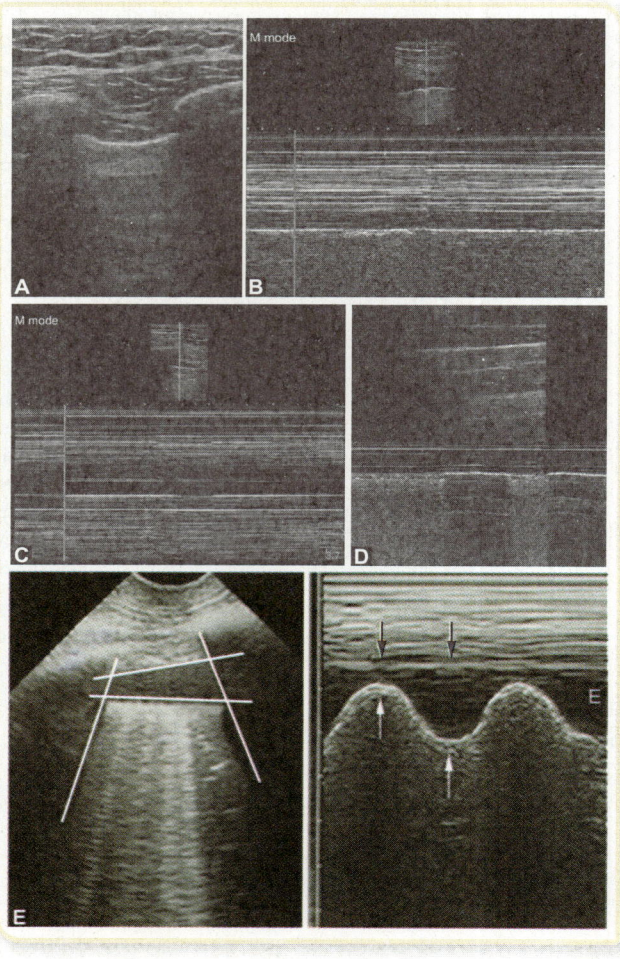

LUNG ULTRASOUND SIGNS

A. **Bat sign:** Normal USG thorax/ lung in B mode obtained with a linear probe showing two convex hyperechoic lines (blue lines) representing ribs, with posterior acoustic shadowing and the concave line, between them, (green line) corresponds to the pleural line. The superficial hyperechoic ribs represent the bat's wings and the body is made up of the pleural line underneath and between the wings

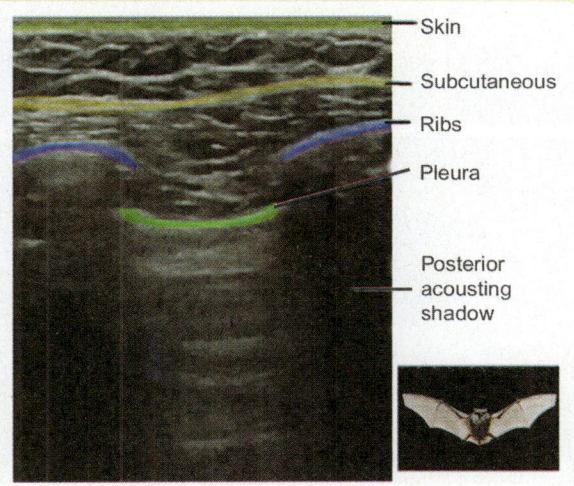

B. **Seashore sign:** M-mode image of the normal lungs with seashore sign. Above the pleura, the scan reveals wave-like lines, generated by the movement of muscles (waves) and the skin (sky). Underneath the pleura, the image shows a grainy pattern resembling the sand. Sliding of pleura results in comet tail artifact which produces granular pattern of sand.

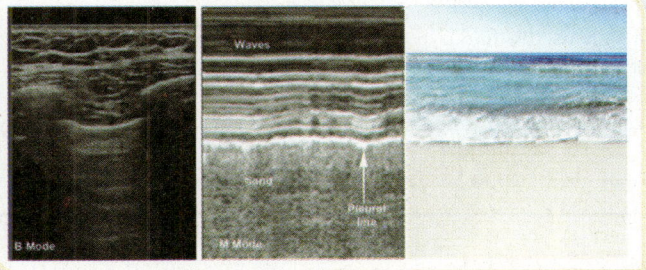

Fig: Seashore sign M mode in middle image compared with B mode image and the real seashore

C. **Stratosphere or Barcode sign**[AIIMSPG]: M-mode showing the "stratosphere" or "barcode" sign in pneumothorax where there is no pleural sliding.

D. **Lung point sign:** It is the point of transition of normal lung and pneumothorax. Hence a transition of Seashore sign and stratosphere sign is seen on M mode.

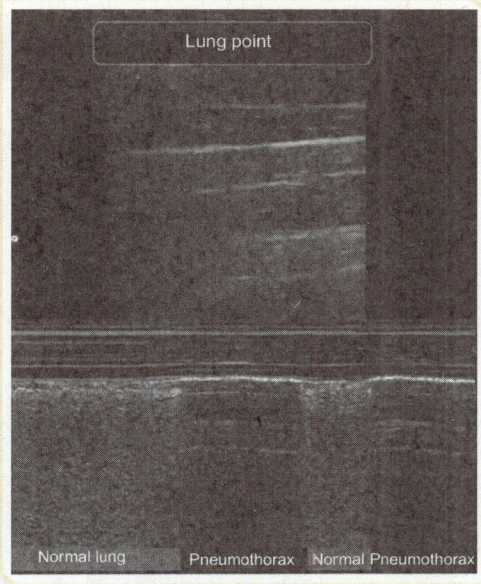

Fig: Lung point sign with seashore (representing normal lung) and stratosphere (representing pneumothorax) both on M mode.

E. **The quad sign and the sinusoid sign of pleural effusion on USG thorax.** The quad sign and sinusoid sign are universal, as opposed to the anechoic pattern of the effusion, which is applicable only to uncomplicated effusions. They are highly sensitive and specific.

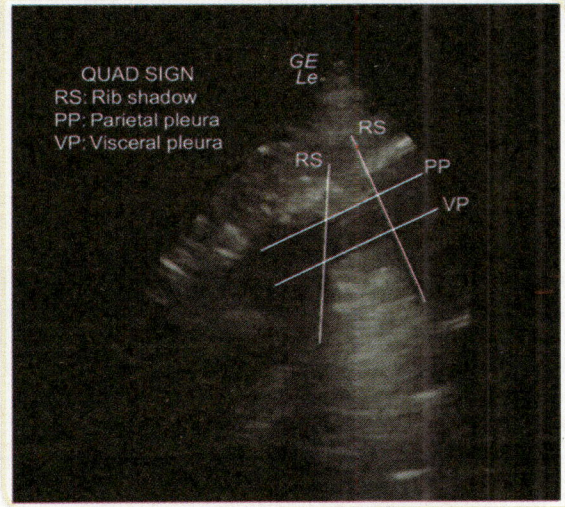

Fig: Quad sign for Pleural effusion shown in USG thorax B mode curvilinear probe.

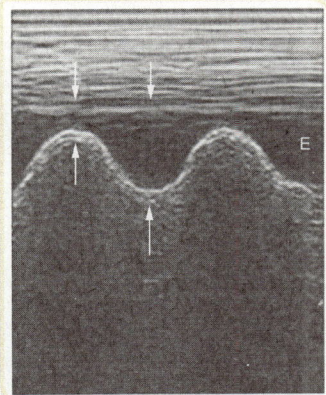

Fig: Sinusoid sign for pleural effusion on M mode linear probe with E, representing pleural effusion (white arrow = Visceral pleura, black arrow = Parietal pleura)

RADIO PLATE 53

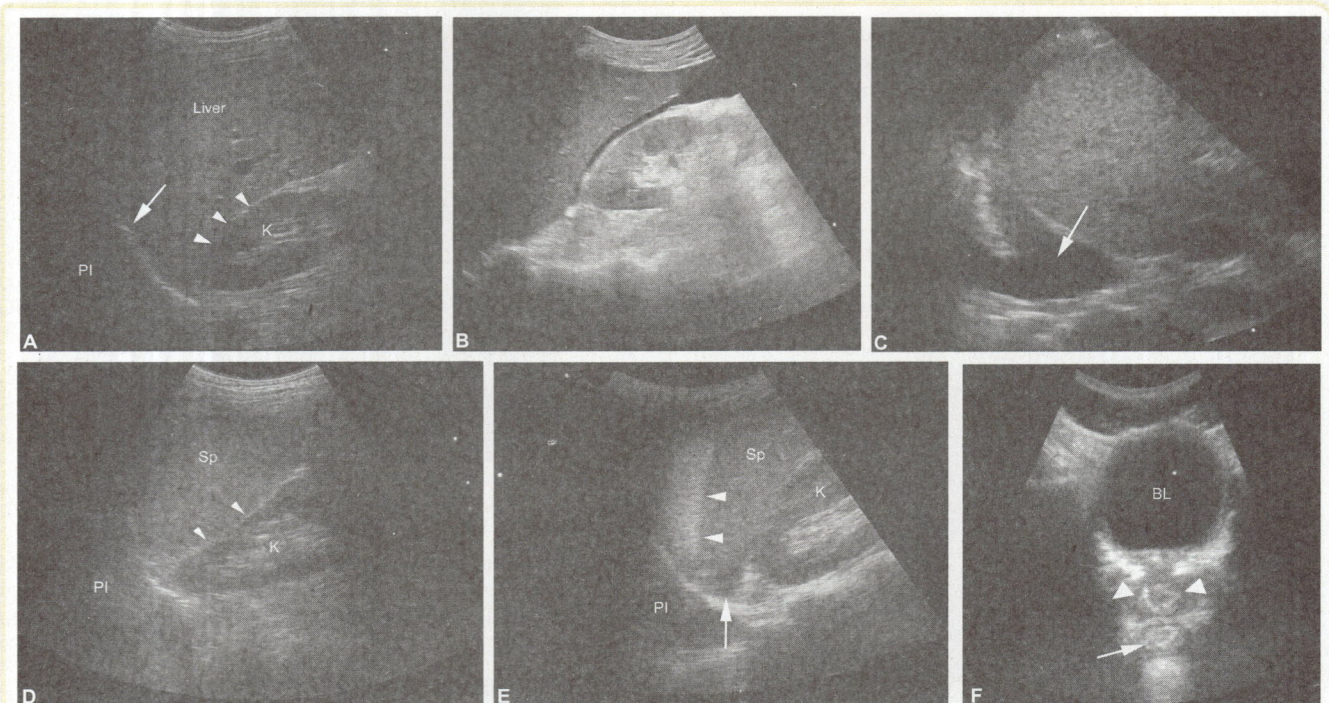

USG FAST IMAGES

A. **Normal Right upper quadrant:** Showing liver, Kidney (K), Pleural space (Pl), Diaphragm (long arrow) and hepatorenal pouch/ Morrison's pouch (arrow heads)
B. **Fluid in Morrison's pouch in right upper quadrant**[AIIMSPG]: In trauma patients, the fluid is likely to be Hemoperitoneum
C. **Fluid in Right pleural space (arrow):** Pleural effusion or hemothorax
D. **Normal left upper quadrant:** showing spleen, left kidney, pleural space (PL) and Lenorenal interface (arrowhead)
E. **Fluid in Left upper quadrant** (arrow) with clots (arrowhead) most likely due to splenic injury. In the setting of clots the free fluid is likely to be blood.
F. **Normal suprapubic/ pelvic scan:** Showing urinary bladder (BL), prostate gland (arrow heads) and rectum (Long arrow)

RADIO PLATE 54

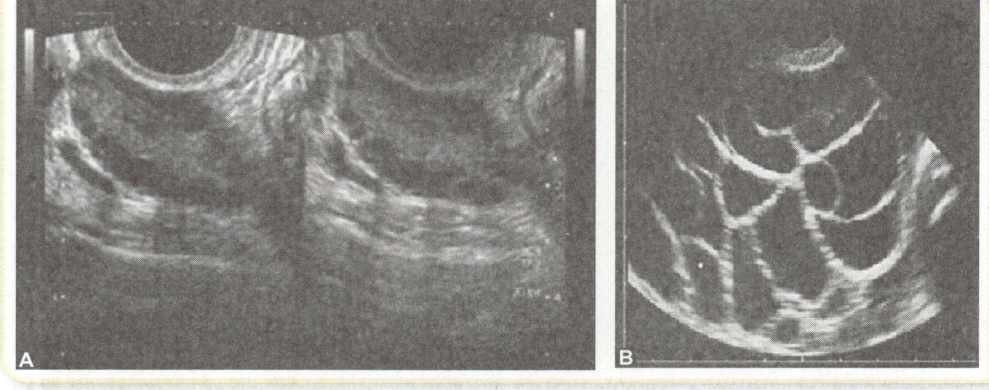

KEY

A. **Necklace sign of PCOD:** Bulky ovaries with multiple small follicles arranged like a string of pearls or necklace around the ovarian rim with echogenic stroma
B. **Ovarian Hyperstimulation Syndrome (OHSS):**[NEETPG] Grossly enlarged ovaries with large cysts (2-4 cm) arranged in cart wheel pattern. Preexisting PCOD and gonadotrophins treatment for infertility are two risk factors. Once OHSS is suspected, the diagnosis of OHSS is aided by ultrasound findings including presence and volume of abdominal ascites, degree of ovarian enlargement, presence or absence of pleural effusions, and Doppler studies showing venous thromboembolism.

RADIO PLATE 56

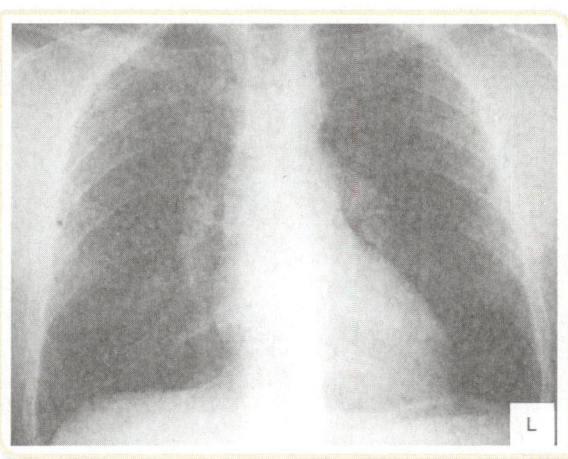

COARCTATION OF THE AORTA

Coarctation of the Aorta[NEETPG] is a congenital heart anomaly involving constriction of an aortic segment. Aortic coarctation is rare, most commonly affecting the aortic isthmus (95% of cases) and rarely the more distal thoracic and abdominal aorta. There may be a '3' sign due to enlargement of the left subclavian artery above the coarctation.

Rib notching usually takes several years to develop. It is caused by pressure erosion of the inferior aspects of the upper adjacent ribs by enlarged and tortuous intercostal arteries. It is usually bilateral but asymmetric, and most often spares the first two ribs where intercostal arteries arise from the costocervical trunk proximal to the usual site of coarctation and do not form part of the collateral circulation.

RADIO PLATE 55

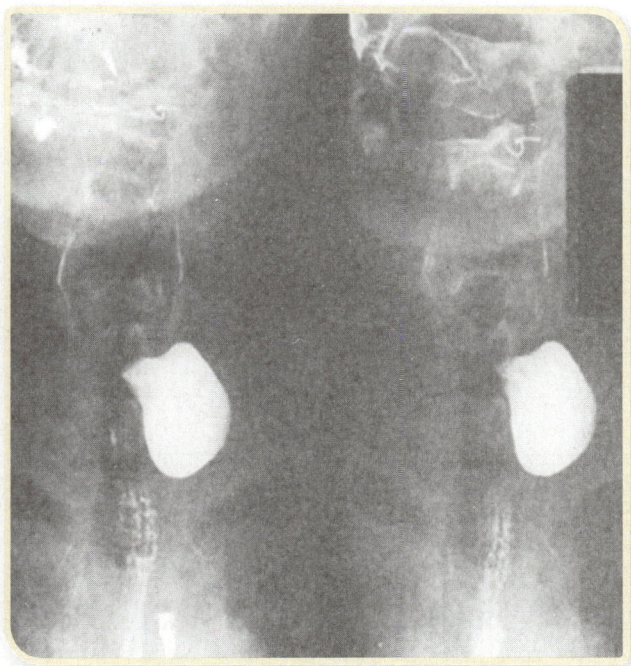

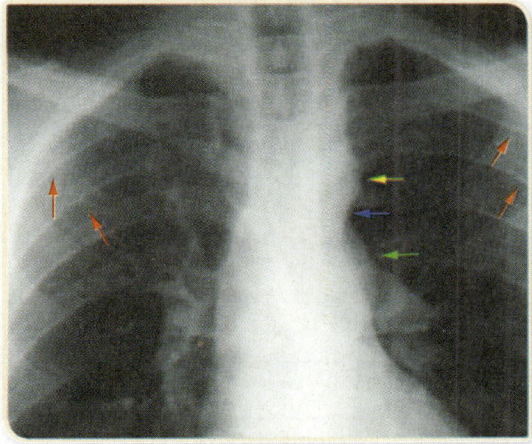

Fig: Chest radiograph in a patient with coarctation of aorta. There is rib notching (red arrow) and enlargement of the left subclavian artery causing a '3' sign. Yellow arrow Ao arch; blue – coarctation; red-thinned rib areas – collateral network; green – the post-stenotic area.

ZENKER'S DIVERTICULUM[NEETPG]

It Arises in the hypopharynx proximal to the upper oesophageal sphincter. Located in the posterior midline at the plane between the circular and oblique fibers of the cricopharyngeus – Killian Dehiscence. Barium pools in an outpouching lying posterolateral to the hypopharyngeal esophagus at the level of the cervicothoracic junction. These are classic appearances of a pharyngeal pouch, also known as a **Zenker diverticulum**. Typically present with dysphagia, halitosis or regurgitation.

NOTES

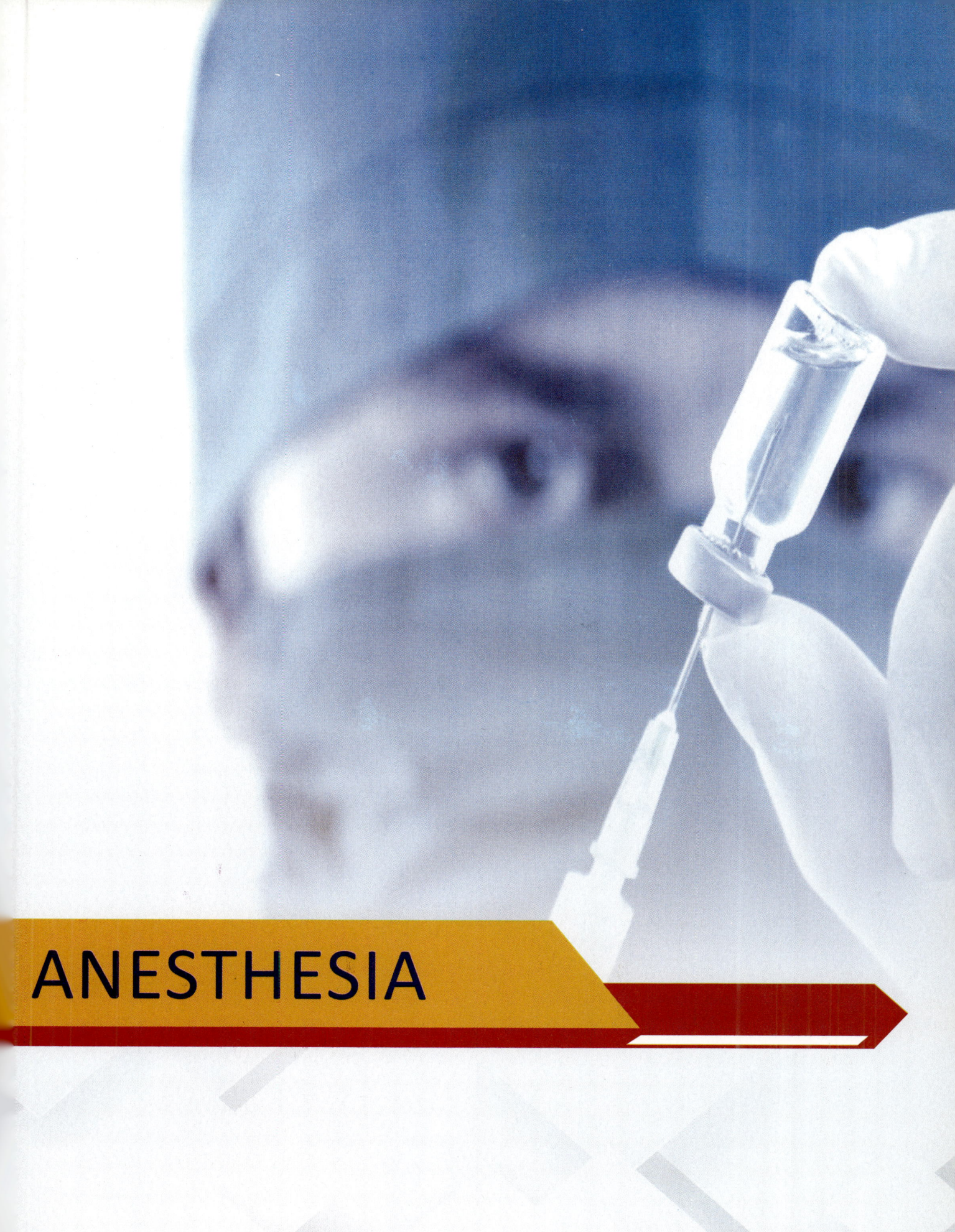

ANESTHESIA

ANESTHESIA PLATE 1

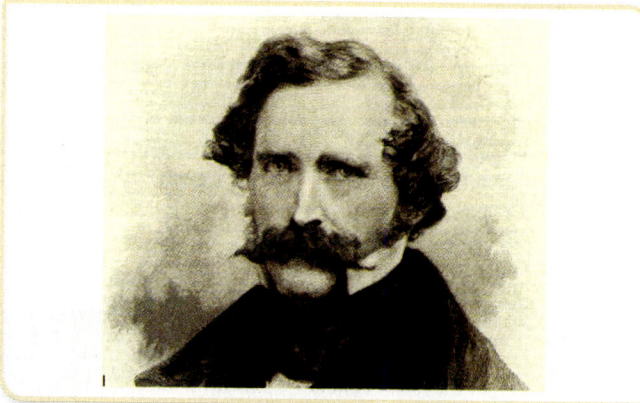

KEY

WILLIAM T. G. MORTON

William T. G. Morton was born in 1819 on a farm near Charlton, Massachusetts. During the summer of 1844, Morton, on the advice of Charles T. Jackson, used sulfuric **ether** for painless tooth extractions, and study of this agent eventually led to his successful demonstration of ether anesthesia at Massachusetts General Hospital on October 16, 1846. The remainder of Morton's life was spent in efforts to patent and receive monetary recognition for the discovery of ether anesthesia. Broken and despondent, he died of a cerebral hemorrhage in New York City in July 1868.

"Ether dome" is an amphitheater in the Bulfinch Building at Massachusetts General Hospital in Boston. It served as the hospital's operating room from its opening in 1821 until 1867. It was the site of the first public demonstration of the use of inhaled ether as a surgical anesthetic on 16 October 1846 ("Ether day"/now considered as World Anesthesia Day), and now commemorates the beginning of modern anesthesia.

ANESTHESIA PLATE 2

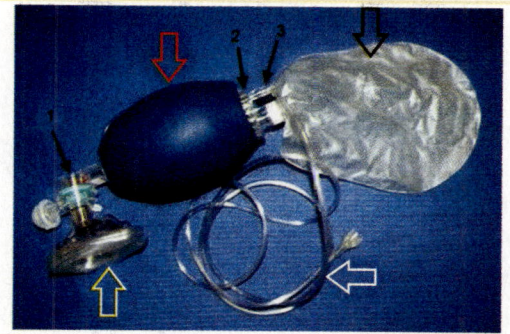

KEY

BAG MASK VENTILATION/AMBU BAG

- The bag-valve mask concept was developed in 1953 by the German engineer, **Dr. HolgerHesse,** and his partner, Danish anesthetist **Henning Ruben**
- Ventilation in the prehospital setting is most commonly achieved by **bag-mask-valve ventilation.**
- It is a hand-held device commonly used to provide **positive pressure ventilation** to patients who are not breathing or not breathing adequately.
- Resuscitation bags (AMBU bags or bag-mask units) are commonly **used for emergency ventilation** because of their simplicity, portability, and ability to deliver almost 100% oxygen *Black arrow: Reservoir bag, Red arrow: Ventilation bag, White arrow: Tube to oxygen inlet, 1= non rebreathing Patient valve, 2= intake valve, 3= Reservoir valve*
- Contains 3 valves:
  1. The **patient valve** opens during controlled or spontaneous inspiration to allow gas flow from the ventilation bag to the patient. Rebreathing is prevented by venting exhaled gas to the atmosphere through exhalation ports in this valve.
  2. The compressible, self-refilling ventilation bag also contains an **intake valve.** This valve closes during bag compression, permitting positive-pressure ventilation. The bag is refilled by flow through the fresh gas inlet and across the intake valve. Connecting the reservoir to the intake valve helps prevent the entrainment of room air.
  3. The **reservoir valve** assembly is really two unidirectional valves: the inlet valve and the outlet valve. The inlet valve allows ambient air to enter the ventilation bag if fresh gas flow is inadequate to maintain reservoir filling. Positive pressure in the reservoir bag opens the outlet valve, which vents oxygen if fresh gas flow is excessive.
- Bag and valve combinations can also be attached to an alternate airway adjunct, instead of to the mask. For example, it can be attached to an endotracheal tube or laryngeal mask airway.
- A bag-valve mask can be used without being attached to an oxygen tank to provide "room air" (21% oxygen) to the patient, however manual resuscitator devices also can be connected to a separate bag reservoir which can be filled with pure oxygen from a compressed oxygen source – this can increase the amount of oxygen delivered to the patient to nearly 100%.
- Bag-valve masks come in different sizes to fit infants, children, and adults. The face mask size may be independent of the bag size

Sizes of AMBU bag		
Size	Ventilation bag capacity	Reservoir bag capacity
Adult size (>30kg)	1600 ml	2600 ml
Child size (7-30 kg)	500 ml	2600 ml
Infant size (<7kg)	240 ml	600 ml

ANESTHESIA PLATE 3

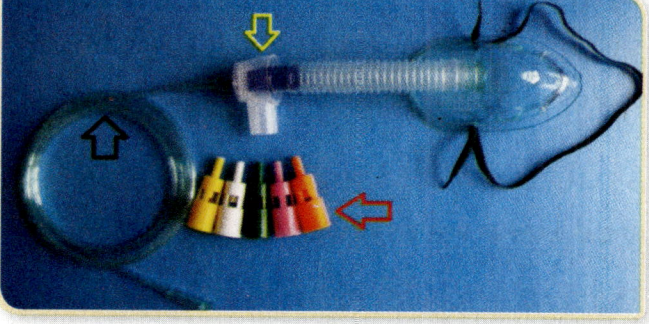

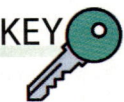

VENTURI MASK

- The mask was invented by **Moran Campbell** as a replacement for intermittent oxygen treatment
- The gas delivery approach with **air-entrainment masks** is somewhat different than with an oxygen reservoir. The goal is to create an **open system with high flow** about the nose and mouth, with a **fixed FIO$_2$**. Masks are known as **"Venturi"** or **"Venti-" masks,** or **high-airflow with oxygen-entrainment (HAFOE) systems.**
- A Venturi mask **mixes oxygen with room air**, creating high-flow enriched oxygen of a settable concentration.
- This is because venturi masks are able to provide total inspiratory flow at a specified FIO$_2$ to patient's therapy. The kits usually include multiple jets in order to set the desired FIO$_2$ which are usually color-coded.
- The mechanism of action depends on the **venturi effect**
- The Venturi effect is the reduction in fluid pressure that results when a fluid flows through a constricted section of pipe.
- The air-entrainment masks are a logical choice for patients whose hypoxemia cannot be controlled on lower FIO$_2$ devices such as the cannula.

Black arrow: Oxygen supply tube, Yellow arrow: Removable adapter, Red arrow: Oxygen diluter

Venturi mask diluter color code		
Diluter color	**Oxygen %**	**Oxygen flow**
Blue	24%	3 Lit/min
Yellow	28%	6 Lit/min
White	31%	8 Lit/min
Green	35%	12 Lit/min
Pink	40%	15 Lit/min
Orange	50%	15 Lit/min

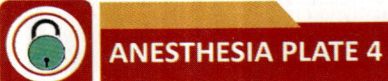

ANESTHESIA PLATE 4

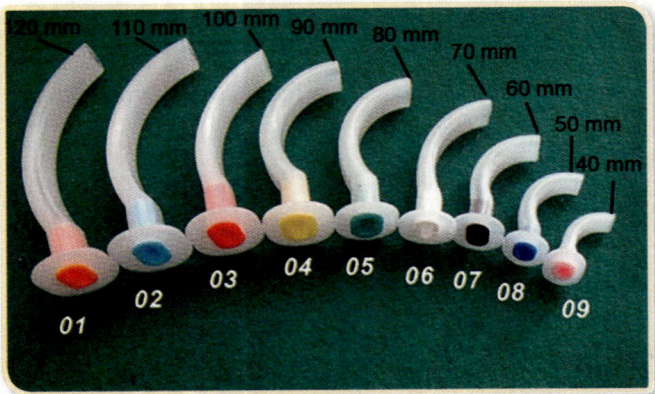

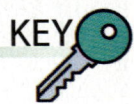

GUEDEL'S AIRWAY

- It is an oropharyngeal airway.
- Colored broad end is called the flange, while the other end is the pharyngeal end
- The purpose of the airway is to lift the tongue & epiglottis away from the posterior pharyngeal wall, & prevent them from obstructing the space above the larynx in anesthetized patient and in unconscious patient to secure airway
- The appropriate size of Guedel's airway is determined approximately. It should approximately be measured as that extends from the **incisor teeth to the tip reaching angle of mandible.** Too large an airway causes the tip to press the epiglottis against the posterior pharyngeal wall or larynx, obstructing both the device and the patient's physiologic airway. Too small an airway causes pushing the tongue against the posterior pharyngeal wall, and thereby causing obstruction.

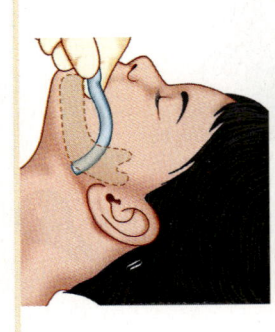 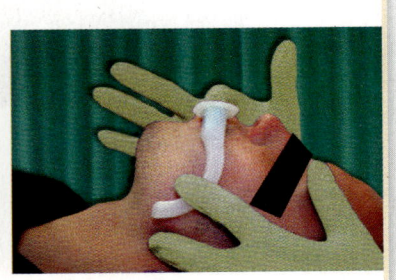

ANESTHESIA PLATE 5

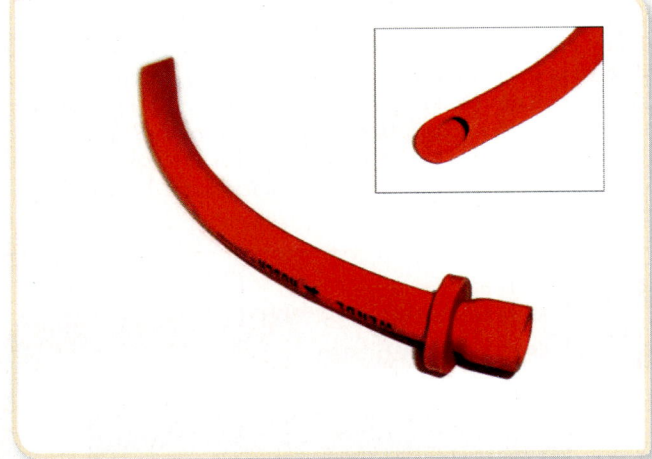

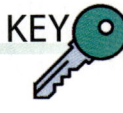

NASOPHARYNGEAL AIRWAY

Material: Made of soft plastic, polyurethane or latex rubber.

Description

- **Proximal end:** either a fixed or adjustable flange which limits insertion of an excessive length so that the device lies just above the epiglottis.
- The tube is curved to fit the curvature of the nasopharynx.
- **Distal end:** Beveled → makes its passage through the nose less traumatic.
- Sometimes there may be a hole cut into the wall opposite the bevel which ensures airway patency even if the bevel becomes blocked with mucus during insertion.

Advantages

Better tolerated in a semi-awake patient than an oral airway. Less likely to be accidentally displaced or removed. Can be used in patients with limited mouth opening, awkward or fragile dentition, trauma or pathology of oral cavity, or where oral airway is frequently displaced by marked overlapping bite.

Contraindications

- CSF rhinorrhea
- Bleeding diathesis
- Trauma or pathology inside nasal cavity

ANESTHESIA PLATE 6

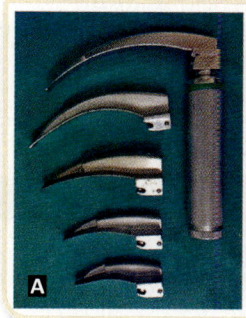
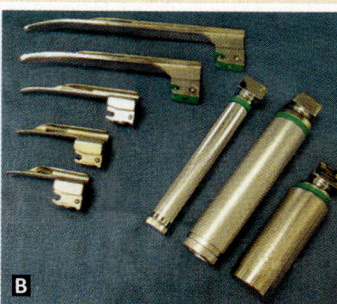
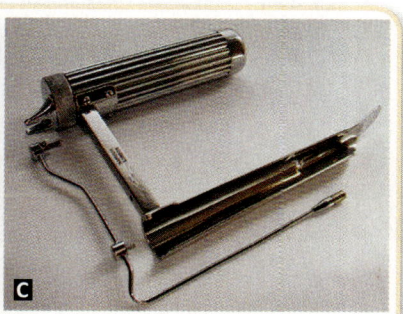

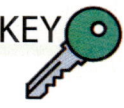
KEY

LARYNGOSCOPE

A. Laryngoscope handle with an assortment of **Macintosh blades** *(Most commonly used)* (large adult, small adult, pediatric, infant, and neonate). Curved blades
B. Laryngoscope handles with an assortment of **Miller blades** (large adult, small adult, pediatric, infant, and neonate). Straight blades
C. **Magill laryngoscope** with the light carrier detached. **Magill's blades** (minimum or no blind area) are used in infants. Straight blades

 Note

- Upper incisors are commonly injured during Laryngoscopy
- Laryngoscope blades are available in 0 to 5 sizes, Size 0 is used in Infants while Size 5 is used in Large adults. Miller blade is also available in 00, 0, 1, 2, 3, 4
- Straight blades are often preferred in infants as the epiglottis is larger, soft and floppy as cartilaginous framework is not yet developed. The epiglottis is inclined at 45° to the glottis. The larynx in more anterior and high up in the neck opposite to C3 C4 vertebral body. In this case the straight blades are places behind or posterior to the epiglottis, where it is lifted out of the way of vocal cords (epiglottis is "included").

Direct laryngoscopy	
Technique	- Direct laryngoscope is **held in non-dominant hand** so as to keep dominant hand free for instrumentation or surgery
- **Neck position in laryngoscopy:** Extension of atlanto-occipital joint, flexion of the cervical spine "SNIFFING THE MORNING AIR" position.
- Mouth opening using the **scissors technique**. This is accomplished by placing the thumb on the lower teeth and the index finger on the upper teeth.
- Initial blade insertion is from the left side as the mouth is scissored open, and the blade is then directed initially from left to right to position the blade flange ultimately toward the left side of the patient's mouth on complete insertion of the blade
- The blade is advanced carefully and directed in a midline approach until the epiglottis is visualized. After the soft palate tissue and tongue are lifted in a direction along the axis of the laryngoscope handle and the glottic opening is exposed, a tracheal tube can be inserted using the right hand and advanced from the right corner of the patient's mouth and through the vocal cords
- The laryngoscope should never be hinged at the incisors while lifting.

Contd...

Direct laryngoscopy	
Diagnostic indications in ENT	▫ When indirect laryngoscopy is not possible as in infants and young children, and the symptomatology points to larynx and/or hypopharynx, e.g. hoarseness, dyspnea, stridor and dysphagia. ▫ When indirect laryngoscopy has not been successful, e.g. due to excessive gag reflex or overhanging epiglottis obscuring a part of a complete view of the larynx. ▫ To examine hidden areas of: *Hypopharynx:* Base of tongue, vallecula and lower part of pyriform fossa. *Larynx:* Infrahyoid epiglottis, anterior commissure, ventricles and subglottic region. ▫ To find the extent of growth and take a biopsy.
Therapeutic indications in ENT	▫ Removal of benign lesions of larynx, e.g. papilloma, fibroma, vocal nodules, polyps or cysts. ▫ Removal of foreign bodies from larynx and hypopharynx. ▫ Dilatation of the laryngeal structures.
Contraindications	▫ Diseases or injuries of the cervical spine. (Video laryngoscope may be used) ▫ Limited mouth opening where the laryngoscope cannot be introduced
Caution	▫ Highly stimulates the sympathetic system hence to be carefully used in patients with heart disease, raised Intracranial pressure etc. If essential, a quick laryngoscopy (15 seconds) may be done or adjuvants which lower BP or heart rate can be used during laryngoscopy e.g., esmolol ▫ Loose teeth

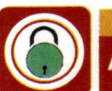

ANESTHESIA PLATE 7

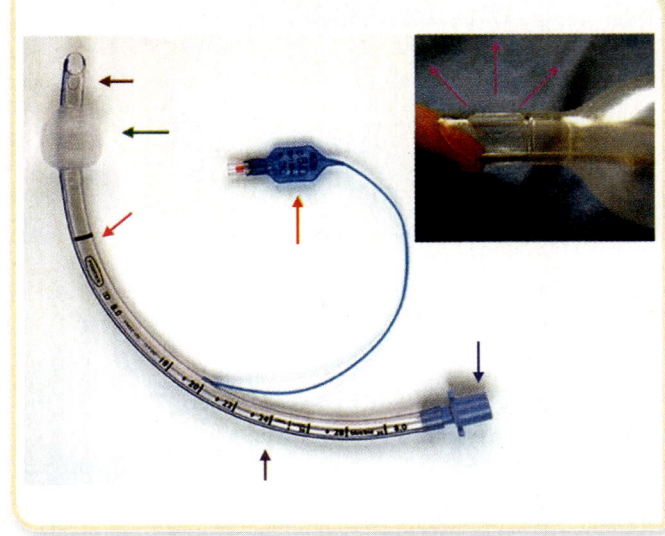

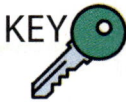

KEY

ENDOTRACHEAL TUBE

▫ The brown arrow indicates Murphy's eye
▫ **The Murphy's eye is situated just above the tip of the tube. It serves to ventilate the lungs in case the tip of the endotracheal tube is blocked.**
▫ Green arrow shows the **cuff**. It protects the airway against aspiration, and also holds the tube in its place.
▫ Pink arrow shows the **black line** which should be placed at the level of vocal cords, to ensure that the cuff does not damage the vocal cords on inflation.
▫ The purple arrow shows **markings which indicate the level at which the tube is fixed at the angle of mouth.**
▫ The blue arrow denotes the **connector (Universal size is 15 mm)**
▫ The red arrow shows the pilot balloon, which indicates the degree of inflation of the cuff.
▫ **Sizes:** The size of the tube is its internal diameter in mm. the commonly used sizes range 2.5 (in premature) to about 8- 8.5 in adult males. Generally, the larynx of females being smaller, an endotracheal tube of size 7- 7.5 usually suffices.
▫ **Uses:** Prevents against aspiration (cuffed tubes), Useful for positive pressure ventilation, Useful for long duration surgeries and postoperative ventilation.

ANESTHESIA PLATE 8

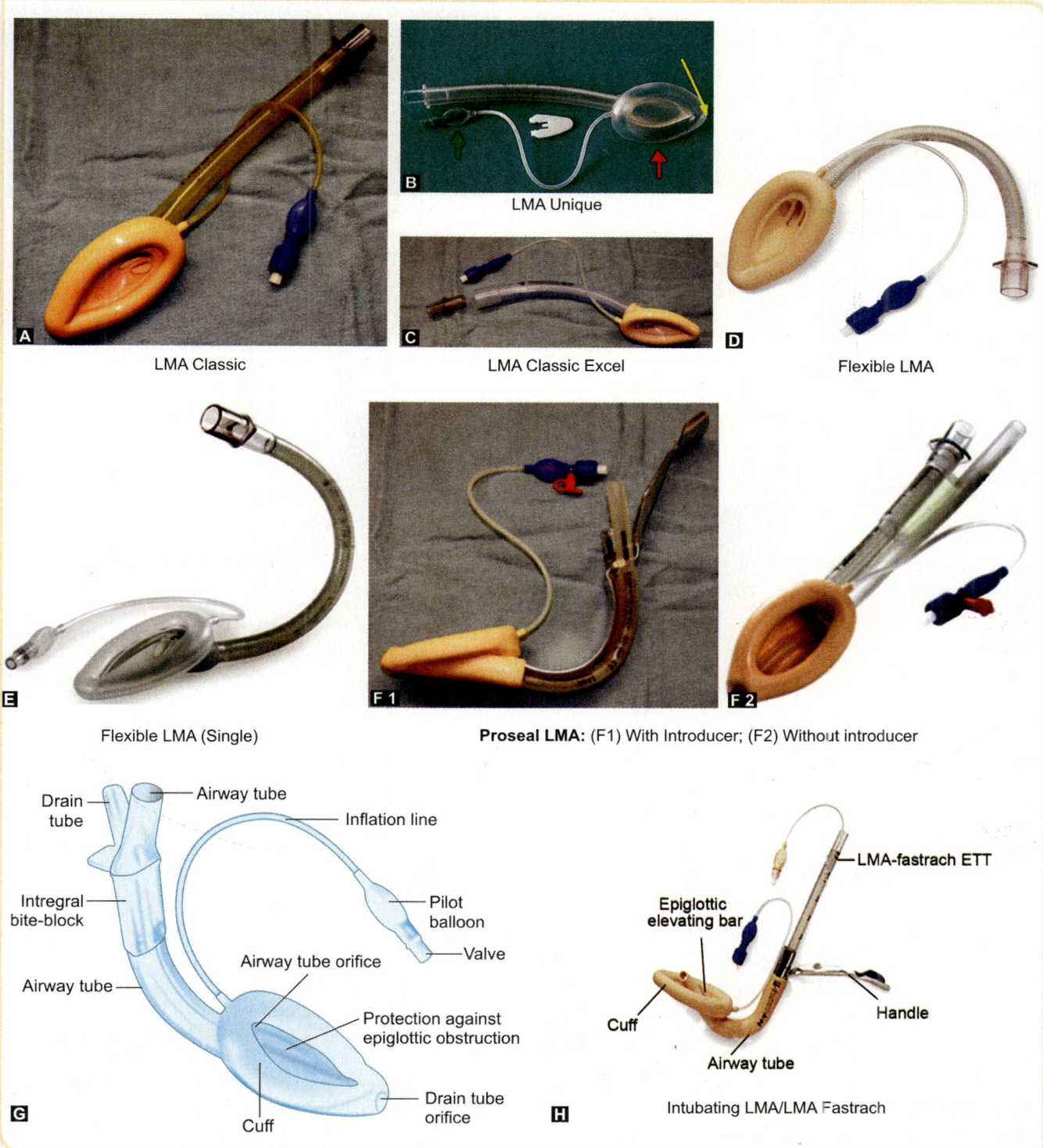

Fig: Parts of LMA Supreme

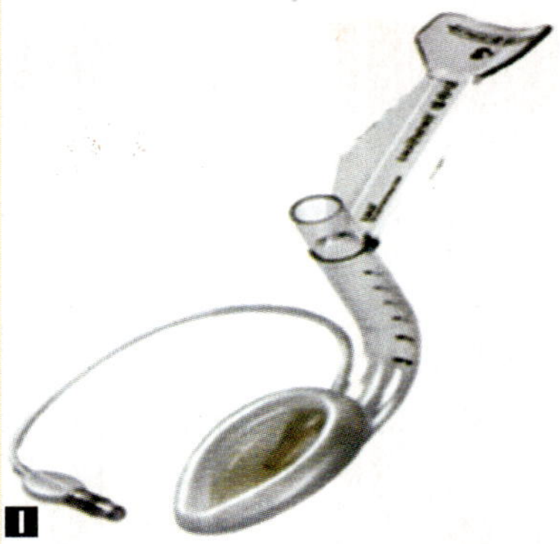

PICTURE MEDEASY

I — Single use LMA Fastrach/Intubating LMA

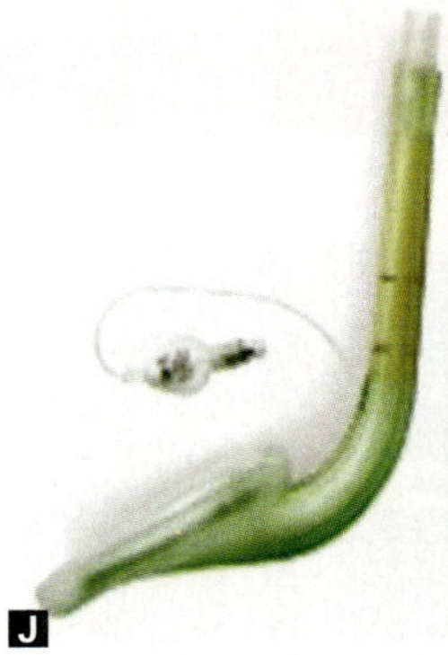

J — AMBU LMA

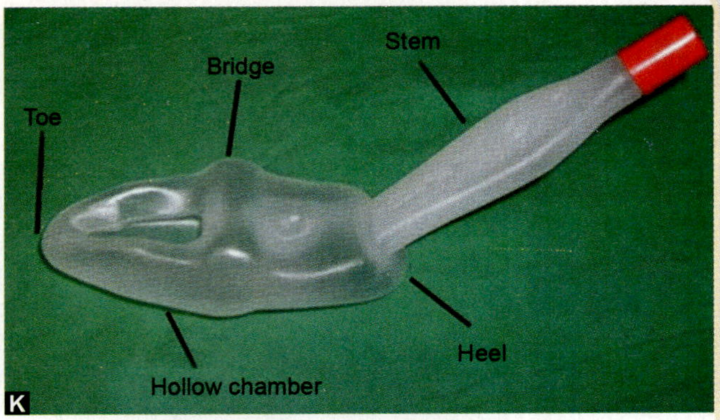

K — SLIPA- Streamlined Liner of Pharyngeal Airway 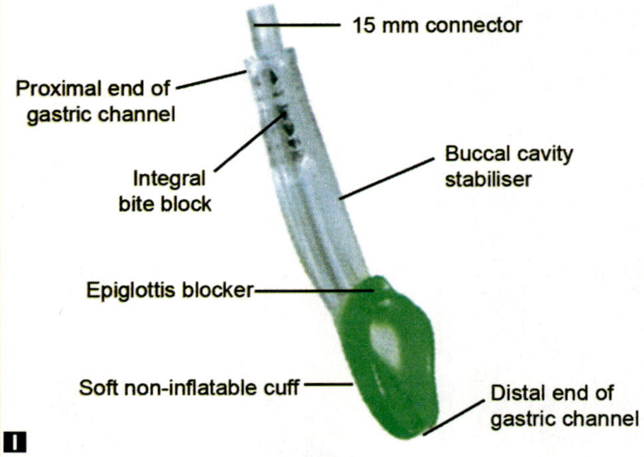
(Toe, Bridge, Stem, Hollow chamber, Heel)

L — IGel
(15 mm connector, Proximal end of gastric channel, Integral bite block, Buccal cavity stabiliser, Epiglottis blocker, Soft non-inflatable cuff, Distal end of gastric channel)

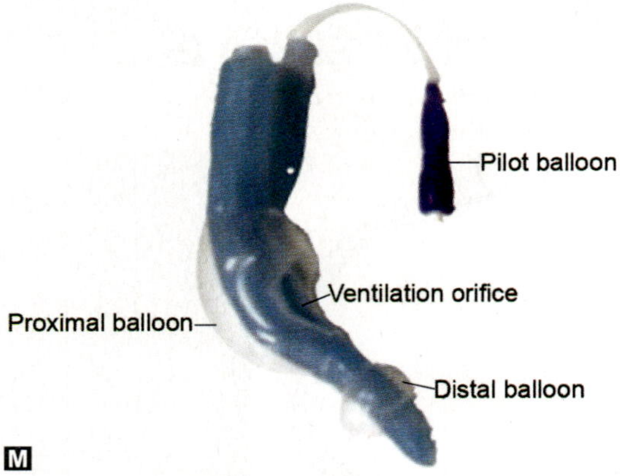

M — Elisha airway device
(Pilot balloon, Ventilation orifice, Proximal balloon, Distal balloon)

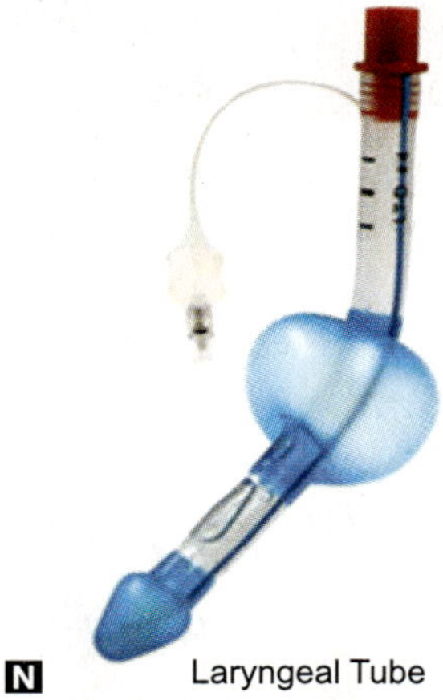

N — Laryngeal Tube

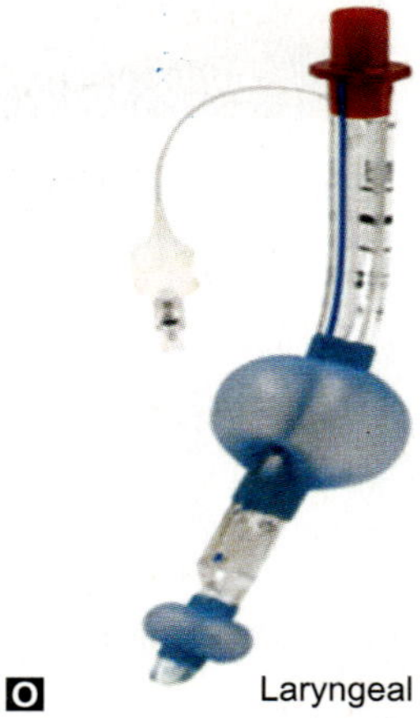

O — Laryngeal Tube S

KEY

TYPES OF LMA

A. **Classic LMA:** Prototype. Can be autoclaved and reused 40 times
B. **LMA Unique:** Single use version of Classic LMA
C. **LMA Classic excel:** Is adapted for intubation through LMA. **Clue for identification:** *The connector is detachable so as to facilitate intubation*
E. **Flexible LMA:** Has a wire reinforced tube to avoid kinking on flexion
E. **Single use flexible LMA**
F. **ProSeal LMA:** F1, with introducer; F2 without introducer. The device shown in the picture is Proseal LMA which has internal drainage (gastric) tube which is *lateral* to the airway tube and ends at the tip of the mask for aspiration of gastric contents in the event of passive regurgitation, and hence the tip is placed just above the esophageal opening It is not performed and requires an introducer for insertion.
G. **LMA Supreme (Parts of LMA Supreme):** Preformed 2nd generation LMA with gastric port *above* the airway tube.
H. **LMA Fastrach:** Especially designed for intubation through LMA with a special Endotracheal tube that comes as a part of the kit. It has a metal handle attached to the LMA to help maneuver the tube.
I. **Single use LMA Fastrach/Intubating LMA**
J. **Ambu LMA:**
Clue for identification: *Looks like classic LMA in a Preformed form and is green color*
K. **SLIPA (Streamlined Liner of Pharyngeal Airway):** Cuffless device. Slipper shaped. Size determined by distance between thyroid cornuae

L. **I gel:** Cuffless. Made of thermoplastic elastomer. Contorts to the airway anatomy
M. **Elisha Airway device:** Has 3 separate channels for gastric tube, ventilation and fiberoptic intubation. Endotracheal tube can be inserted through fiberoptic intubation.
N. **Laryngeal tube**
O. **Laryngeal tube Suction:** note the difference in tips of the tubes

Laryngeal Mask Airway (LMA) (AKA: Supraglottic Airway Device)

- **Invented by Archie Brain**
- Red arrow indicates the cuff, while green arrow shows the pilot balloon. Yellow arrow indicates the tip
- It is a supraglottic airway device. It is commonly inserted by a **blind technique** (without the aid of a laryngoscope) & is useful for short procedures, and can be a backup when one is not able to ventilate or intubate, since it is a blind technique.
- Also, it does not require a lot of skill. However, it is easily displaced & there is some risk of aspiration.
- The LMA was designed by British anesthesiologist **Archie Brain** and is also known as Brain's airway.
- "The LMA is usually suitable for minor oral surgeries only like tooth extractions but not for other oral and pharyngeal surgeries"
- Generally, a size of 3 is suitable for small adults, 4 for medium adults, and 5 for large adults. Most commonly, 3 is used for Indian females while 4 is used for Indian males.
- The size of the LMA to be inserted depends upon the weight. *Note that this rule applies to most LMA's but there are exceptions where the appropriate LMA size is not determined by the weight of the patient. e.g: size of SLIPA is determined by the distance between thyroid cornuae*

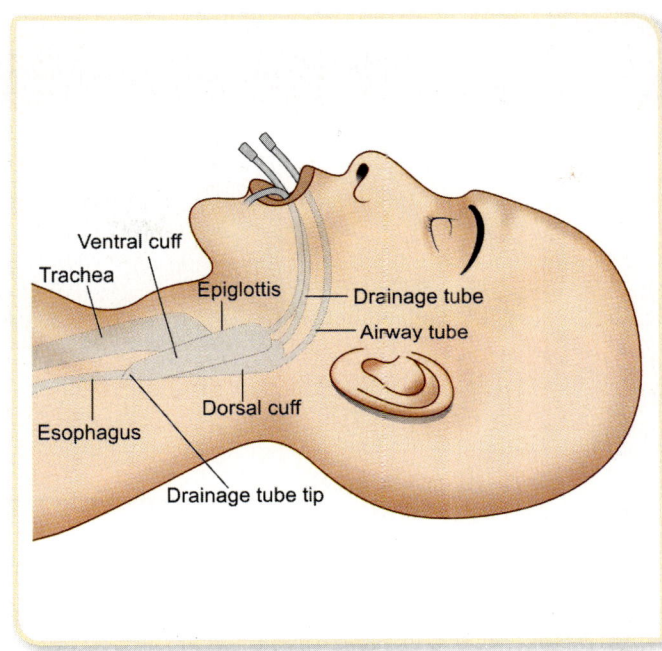

Fig: Placement of LMA

LMA Sizes	Weight of patient	Length of LMA	Volume of cuff up to (ml)	Largest size of tracheal tube that fits into LMA
1	Neonates/infants up to 5 kg	8	4	3.5
1.5	Infants between 5 and 10 kg	10	7	4
2	Infants/children between 10 and 20 kg	11	10	4.5
2.5	Children between 20 and 30 kg	12.5	14	5
3	Children 30 to 50 kg	16	20	6
4	Adults 50 to 70 kg	16	30	6
5	Adults 70 to 100 kg	18	40	7
6	Adults over 100 kg	18	50	

Advantages of LMA	Disadvantages of LMA
- Easy to insert - Doesn't require muscle relaxant and laryngoscope, can be inserted blindly - Can be inserted without interrupting CPR - Leaves the anesthetist's hands free to manage other aspects of the anesthesia procedure - They do not cause much sympathetic stimulation during insertion as endotracheal tubes and will not traumatize the larynx - Doesn't require any specific position of cervical spine so can be used in cervical spine injuries - Can be used by paramedics and does not require special training	- Doesn't prevent aspiration completely, so not used for full stomach patients - LMA does not replace the ETT (especially in longer cases and when protection from aspiration is important) - They do not protect the airway from aspiration reliably, may become dislodged intraoperatively, and may cause as much sore throat as an endotracheal tube. - Although they do not damage the larynx, the distension of the pharynx can (rarely) lead to temporary vocal cord palsy.

Miller's Classification of Supraglottic Airway Devices				
Cuffed				**Cuffless preshaped sealers**
Cuffed perilaryngeal sealers		**Cuffed pharyngeal sealers**		
Without directional sealing	With directional sealing	Without esophageal sealing cuff	With esophageal sealing cuff	SLIPA
Classic LMA	Proseal LMA	COBRA	Laryngeal Tube	
Intubating LMA			Laryngeal Tube suction	IGEL
Soft Seal LM			Combitube	Baska mask
AMBU LM			Easytube	

ANESTHESIA PLATE 9

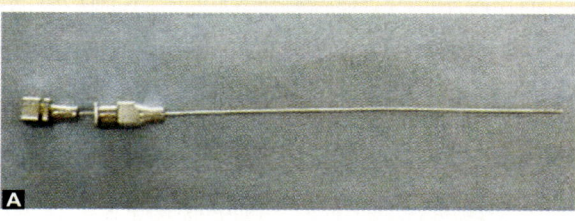

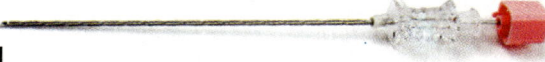

LUMBAR PUNCTURE NEEDLE
A. Metal; reusable
B. Disposable; single use
Points of Identification: Thin slender, steel needle with stillate, having gauge No: 22-24

Lumbar Puncture	
Indications: □ For the diagnosis of various types of Meningitis. □ CSF pressure study □ Spinal anesthesia □ Myelography □ Intrathecal administration of the drugs □ Subarachnoid hemorrhage □ CNS Malignancy □ Demyelinating diseases □ Guillain-Barré syndrome □ Unexplained Coma	**Precaution:** Patients with an altered level of consciousness, focal neurologic deficit, new-onset seizures, papilledema, or an immunocompromised state are at increased risk for potentially fatal cerebellar or tentorial herniation following LP. Neuroimaging should be obtained in these patients prior to LP to exclude a focal mass lesion or diffuse swelling
Contraindications: **Absolute contraindications:** Patient refusal, patient's inability to maintain stillness during the needle puncture and raised intracranial pressure, which may theoretically predispose to brainstem herniation. **Relative contraindications** intrinsic and idiopathic coagulopathy, skin or soft tissue infection at the proposed site of needle insertion, severe hypovolemia; and lack of anesthesiologist experience. **Legal contraindication:** The often-cited relative contraindication of preexisting neurologic disease (e.g., lower extremity peripheral neuropathy) is not usually based on medical criteria but rather on legal considerations	**Complications:** □ CSF leakage □ Infections □ Injury to spinal cord, paralysis □ Patients with coagulation defects including thrombocytopenia are at increased risk of post-LP spinal subdural or epidural hematomas, either of which can produce permanent nerve injury and/or paralysis.
Patient positioning: □ **The lateral decubitus** position is the most commonly used because it allows easier administration, less dependent on assistant and allow a more accurate measurement of the opening pressure. □ **The sitting position** when low lumbar and sacral levels of sensory anesthesia are adequate for the surgical procedure (perineal and urologic operations), or when obesity or scoliosis makes identification of midline anatomy difficult in the lateral position □ **The prone position** should be chosen when the patient is to be maintained in that position during the surgical procedure (rectal, perineal, or lumbar procedures) The procedure should be performed on a firm surface; if the procedure is to be performed at the bedside, the patient should be positioned at the edge of the bed and not in the middle. The patient is asked to lie on his or her side, facing away from the examiner, and to "roll up into a ball." The neck is gently anteflexed and the thighs pulled up toward the abdomen; the shoulders and pelvis should be vertically aligned without forward or backward tilt.	**Site of puncture:** The spinal cord terminates at approximately the L1 in adults and L3 in infants. Although the spinal cord ends at the lower border of L1 in adults, the subarachnoid space continues to S2. LP is therefore performed at or below the **L3–L4 interspace.** A useful anatomic guide is a line drawn between the posterior superior iliac crests, which corresponds closely to the level of the L3–L4 interspace. The interspace is chosen following gentle palpation to identify the spinous processes at each lumbar level. A line joining both iliac crests **(Tuffier's line)** passes across the spine of L4 and is a reliable landmark for locating the L3 / 4 interspace, which is usually easily defined and is the one most often used. or sometimes the L4-5 space. **Note:** The incidence of post dural puncture headache is less when the **needle bevel is placed in the long axis of the neuraxis, parallel to dural fibres**- i.e, bevel faces laterally in sitting position, while it faces upwards in lateral position.

Contd...

Lumbar Puncture

Procedure: Sterilize the skin over the lumbar spine and raise a skin wheal with lidocaine 1% over the appropriate interspace. Inject 2–3 ml more lidocaine into the subcutaneous tissue. Insert the needle or introducer in the midline in slightly cephalad angle (15 degrees) Feedback from the needle tip will monitor the progress of the needle through the supraspinous and interspinous ligaments, ligamentum flavum and sometimes the dura mater. If bone is contacted, withdraw the needle to the subcutaneous tissue and redirect slightly cephalad in the first instance. Puncture of the dura is usually obvious, and when the stylet is removed CSF should flow freely. **The first snap or giveaway or loss of resistance is seen after puncture of ligamentum flavum.** This first loss of resistance is used for identifying the epidural space. When trying to put an epidural catheter, we do not go any further in. The second loss of resistance is due to puncture of the dura and is used for identifying the subarachnoid space. Once we feel the second giveaway, we withdraw the stylet and look for CSF.

During lumbar puncture the needle passes through the following structures in that sequence
- Skin
- Subcutaneous tissue
- Supraspinatous ligament
- Interspinous ligament
- Ligamentum flavum (First snap/loss of resistance)
- Dura mater
- Arachnoid mater
- Subarachnoid space (Target)

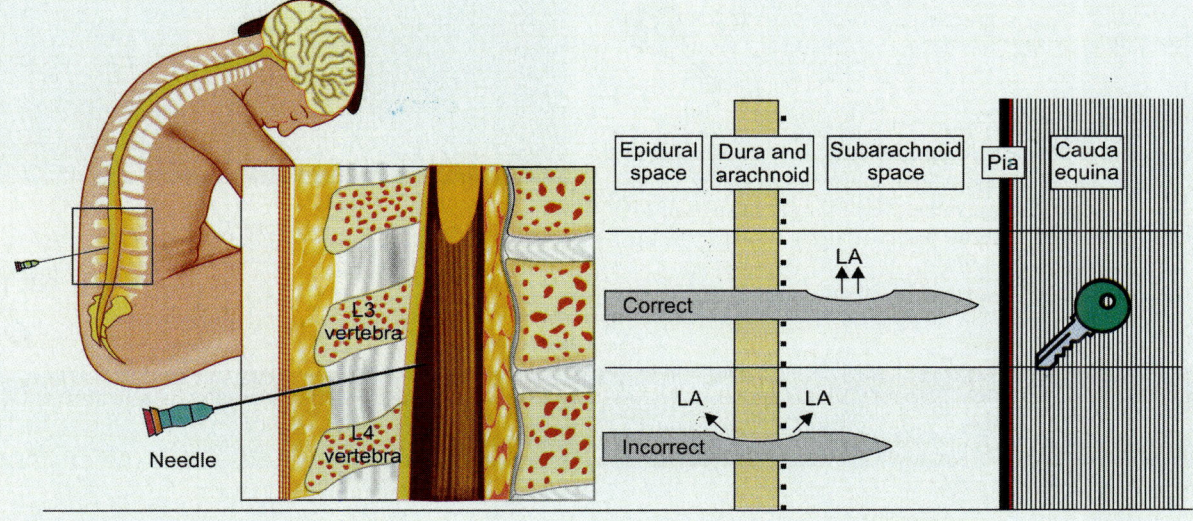

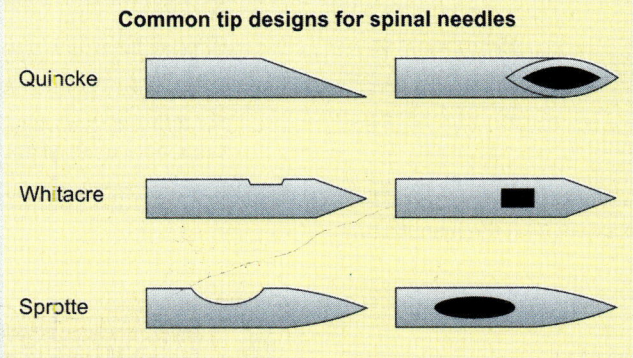

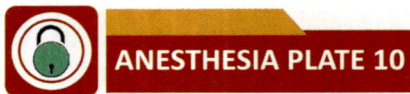
ANESTHESIA PLATE 10

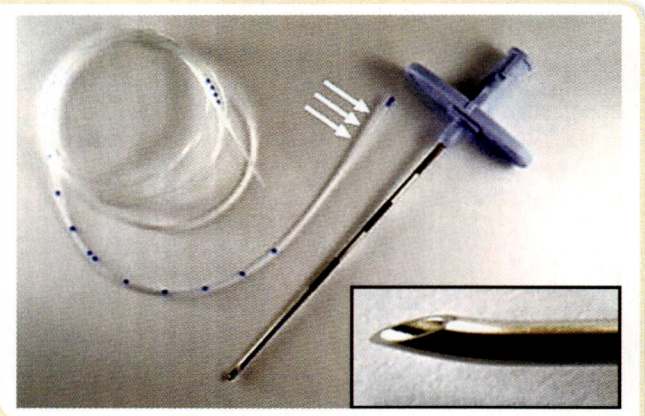

on the shaft (As marked by arrow). Standard Tuohy needle is 11 cm in length with 8 cm shaft and 3 cm hub assembly. Diameter is most commonly 16-18 G for adults and 19 G for pediatrics. Spinal needle is about 20mm longer than the Tuohy needle

ANESTHESIA PLATE 11

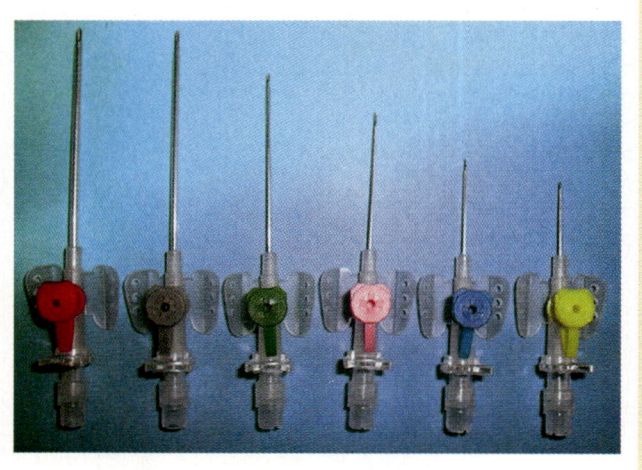

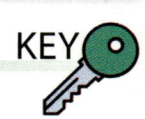 KEY

TUOHY NEEDLE

The Tuohy needle is a hollow hypodermic needle, very slightly curved at the end, suitable for inserting epidural catheters. The Tuohy needle with a Huber tip and an epidural catheter emerging at an angle of 20° to the shaft. The epidural catheter has openings just below the tip,

 KEY

Cannula Sizes and Color Codes					
Color code	Gauge (G)	External Dia (mm)	Length (mm)	Flow Rate (ml/min)	Uses
Red	14	2.2	32	325	For emergency use (e.g., shock)
Grey	16	1.7	50	196	For use in large blood transfusions and emergency use (Shock)
Green	18	1.3	45	96	Suitable for IV fluids and smaller blood transfusions
Pink	20	1.1	33	61	Suitable for the majority of patients that require IV fluids.
Blue	22	0.9	25	36	For difficult hand veins - elderly patients with fragile veins. May be used in slightly older children
Yellow	24	0.7	19	22	Used commonly in pediatric patients

\# Size and flow data may vary to some extent with the manufacturer

 Mnemonic

To remember the color codes of IV cannula in increasing order of calibre - **Rahul Gandhi Grows Pink Before Yelling (for Red, Grey, Green, Pink, Blue, Yellow)**

 Note

- These values may differ amongst different manufacturers.
- The larger the gauge size, the smaller the diameter. This is because the gauge size denotes how many cannulas of that size will fit into a tube of fixed diameter. E.g., 22 cannulas of 22 G will fit into the tube of fixed diameter

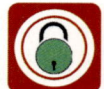
ANESTHESIA PLATE 12

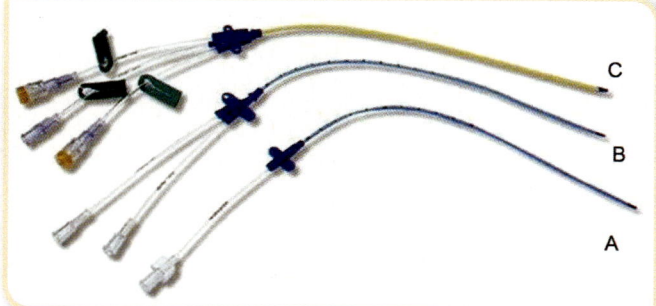

CENTRAL VENOUS CATHETERS
A. Single lumen central venous catheter
B. Double lumen central venous catheter
C. Triple lumen central venous catheter

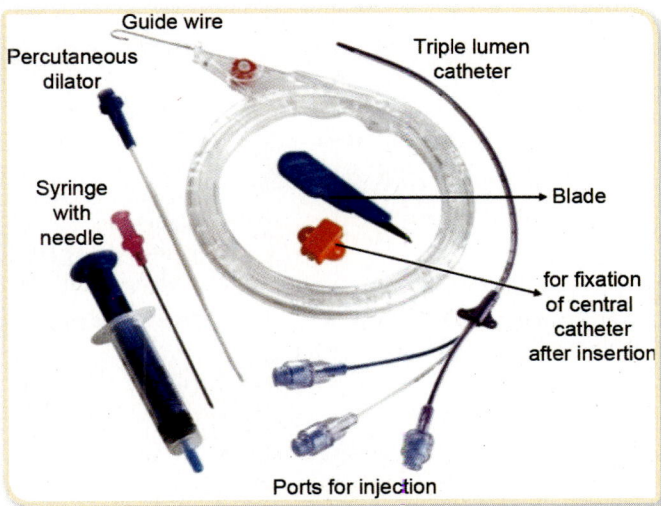

Fig: Central venous catheter kit (labelled)

Scan QR Code to See Full Video Demonstration of Central Line Insertion

http://opn.to/a/S9fHb

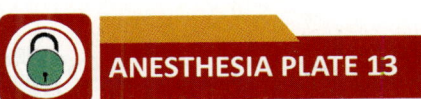

ANESTHESIA PLATE 13

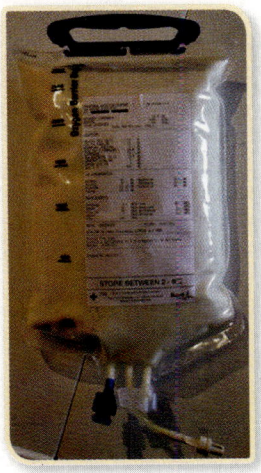

TOTAL PARENTERAL NUTRITION

TPN, also referred to as *central parenteral nutrition*, requires access to a large-diameter vein to deliver the entire nutritional requirements of the individual. Dextrose content of the solution is high (15 to 25%), and all other macronutrients and micronutrients are deliverable by this route.

Access: TPN solutions must be administered through a central venous catheter. A dedicated single-lumen catheter or a multilumen catheter can be used. Catheters should be replaced for unexplained fever or bacteremia.

TPN solutions: TPN solutions generally are administered as a 3-in-1 admixture of protein, as amino acids (10%; 4 kcal/g); carbohydrate, as dextrose (70%; 3.4 kcal/g); and fat, as a lipid emulsion of soybean or safflower oil (20%; 9 kcal/g). Alternatively, the lipid emulsion can be administered as a separate intravenous "piggyback" infusion. Standard preparations are used for most patients. Special solutions that contain low, intermediate, or high nitrogen concentrations as well as varying amounts of fat and carbohydrate are available for patients with diabetes, renal or pulmonary failure, or hepatic dysfunction.

Complications Associated with TPN

☐ **Catheter associated complications:** Catheter thrombosis and catheter-related sepsis are the most important complications of indwelling catheters. Patients with indwelling central vein catheters in whom fever develops without an apparent source should have their lines changed over a wire or removed immediately, the tip quantitatively cultured, and antibiotics begun empirically. Quantitative tip cultures and blood cultures will help guide further antibiotic therapy. Catheter-related sepsis occurs in 2–3% of patients even if maximal efforts are made to prevent infection.

Metabolic Complications of Parenteral Nutritional Supports		
Complication	**Common causes**	**Possible solutions**
Hyperglycemia	Too rapid infusion of dextrose, "stress," corticosteroids	Decrease glucose infusion; insulin; replacement of dextrose with fat
Hyperosmolar nonketotic dehydration	Severe, undetected hyperglycemia	Insulin, hydration, potassium
Hyperchloremic metabolic acidosis	High chloride administration	Decrease chloride
Azotemia	Excessive protein administration	Decrease amino acid concentration
Hyperphosphatemia, hypokalemia, hypomagnesemia	Extracellular to intracellular shifting with refeeding	Increase solution concentration

Selected Metabolic Disturbances and their Corrections

Disturbance	Cause	Corrective action with PN
Hyperglycemia	Too rapid infusion of dextrose, "stress," corticosteroids	Decrease glucose infusion; insulin; replacement of dextrose with fat
Hyperosmolar nonketotic dehydration	Severe, undetected hyperglycemia	Insulin, hydration, potassium
Hyperchloremic metabolic acidosis	High chloride administration	Decrease chloride
Hyponatremia	Increased total body water or decreased total body sodium	Decrease free water or increase sodium
Hypernatremia	Occurs commonly with excessive isotonic or hypertonic fluid followed by diuretic administration with free water clearance; can also occur with dehydration and normal total body sodium	Increase free water to produce net positive fluid balance maintaining sodium and chloride balance
Hypokalemia	Inadequate intake relative to need	Use supplements
	Excessive diuresis, tubular dysfunction	Use supplements
	Magnesium deficiency	Increase magnesium
	Metabolic alkalosis	Correct alkalosis
	Hyperinsulinemia	Maintain constant PN, increase potassium
Hyperkalemia	Excessive provision	Reduce supplements
	Metabolic acidosis	Evaluate acidosis, treat with PN acetate salt and decrease potassium
	Renal deterioration	Evaluate patient and adjust PN as indicated
Hypocalcemia	Reciprocal response to phosphorus repletion	Increase calcium
	Critical illness effect	Increase calcium
	Severe malabsorption	Supplement calcium
Hypercalcemia	Excessive administration or pathologic (cancer, hyperparathyroidism)	Reduce or eliminate calcium
Hypomagnesemia	Increased requirements due to diuretic use, alcoholism, malabsorption, malnutrition	Supplement magnesium
	Critical illness	Supplement magnesium

Contd...

Selected Metabolic Disturbances and their Corrections

Disturbance	Cause	Corrective action with PN
Hypophosphatemia	Inadequate intake relative to needs related to malnutrition, alcohol use	Supplement phosphorus
	Increased calcium intake	Use supplements
Hyperphosphatemia	Excessive administration or worsening renal function	Reduce phosphorus
Azotemia	Excessive amino acid infusion or worsening renal function	Reduce amino acid level but consider renal replacement therapy if cannot provide 1 g protein per kg for prolonged periods
Liver enzyme abnormalities	Lipid trapping in hepatocytes, fatty liver	Decrease dextrose
Acalculous cholecystitis	Biliary stasis	Oral fat
Zinc deficiency	Diarrhea, small bowel fistulas	Increase concentration
Copper deficiency	Biliary fistulas	Increase concentration

ANESTHESIA PLATE 14

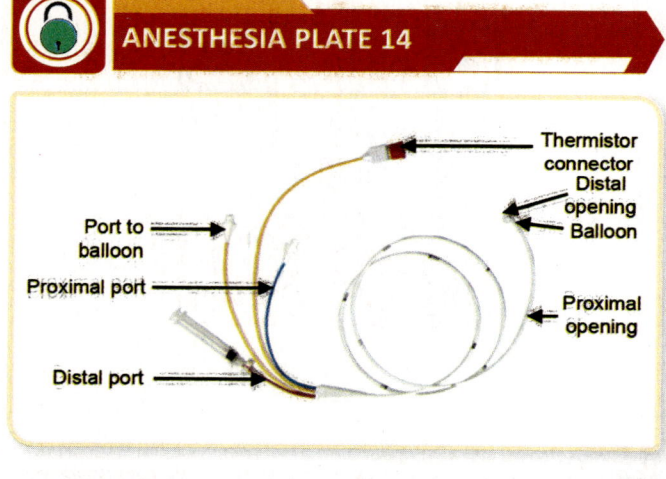

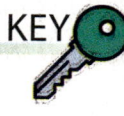

KEY

SWAN GANZ CATHETER

A Swan-Ganz catheterization is a type of pulmonary artery catheterization procedure. The procedure itself is sometimes called right heart catheterization. This is because it can measure the pressure of your blood as it flows through the right side of your heart. The pulmonary artery catheter (PAC) is a balloon tipped thermo dilution **catheter 110 cms long,** that is inserted via a large vein and floated into the pulmonary artery. It is used to obtain hemodynamic measurements.

It measures the pressure at three different places:
1. Right atrium
2. Pulmonary artery
3. Pulmonary capillaries

Indications	Contraindications
A pulmonary artery catheter is indicated for assessment of: Shock states Cardiovascular function Pulmonary function Hemodynamic function peri, intra and post cardiac surgery Fluid requirements and the effectiveness of therapy Multiorgan failure	Coagulation defects Tricuspid or pulmonary valve replacements Right heart mass/thrombus/tumor Tricuspid or pulmonary valve endocarditis High risk of dysrhythmias Caution with LBBB (5% risk of complete heart block)

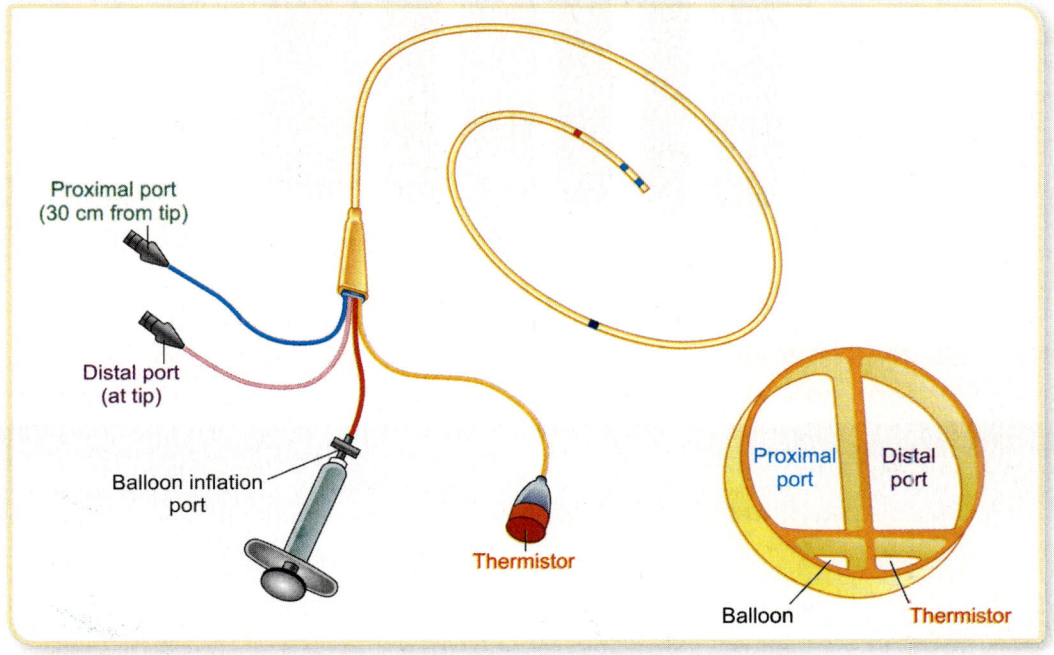

Fig: Diagrammatic representation of Swan Ganz catheter

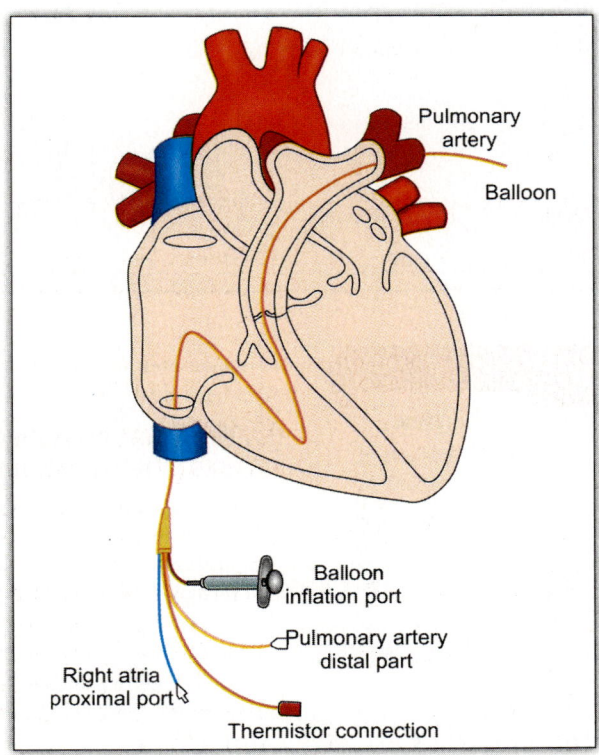

Fig: Diagrammatic representation of Swan Ganz catheter insertion

The distance from tip is marked on the catheter according to the following code

I	II	III	IIII	▪	▪I	▪II	▪III	▪IIII	▪▪
10	20	30	40	50	60	70	80	90	100

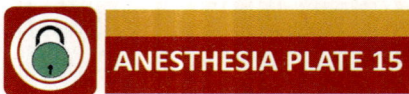

ANESTHESIA PLATE 15

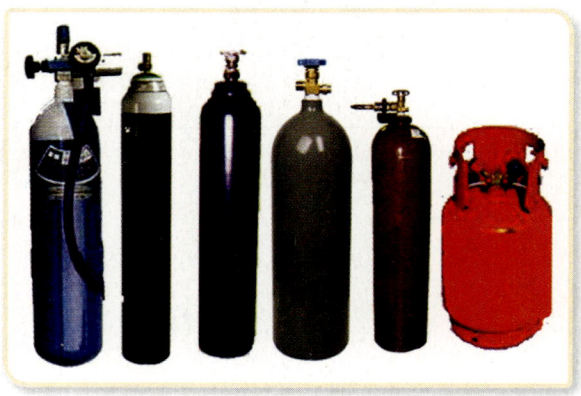

GAS CYLINDERS USED IN ANESTHESIA

From left to right: Entonox cylinder, oxygen cylinder, N_2O cylinder, CO_2 cylinder (pure), Helium cylinder, Cyclopropane cylinder

Gas cylinders used in anesthesia							
Substance	State	Color coding			Pin Index	Pressure (PSIG)	Critical Temp.
		Body	Shoulder	Central supply			
Oxygen	Gas	Black	White	Green	2,5	1900	-1180C
AIR	Gas	Black	White/black	Yellow (U.S)	1,5	1900	
Nitrous Oxide	Gas + Liquid (below 980F)	Blue	Blue	Blue	3,5	745	36.50C
Entonox N2O/ O2	Gas & Vapor	Blue	White/Blue	NA	7		
O2-CO2 (Cylinder with only CO2 is fully grey)		Black	White/ Grey	NA	2,6 (CO2 <7.5%) 1,6 (CO2 >7.5%)		310C (for CO2)
Helium	Gas	Black	White/ Brown	NA		1600	
Cyclopropane		Orange	Orange	NA	3,6		

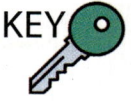

ANESTHESIA PLATE 16

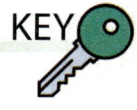

TEMPERATURE MEASUREMENT PROBES (THERMOMETERS)

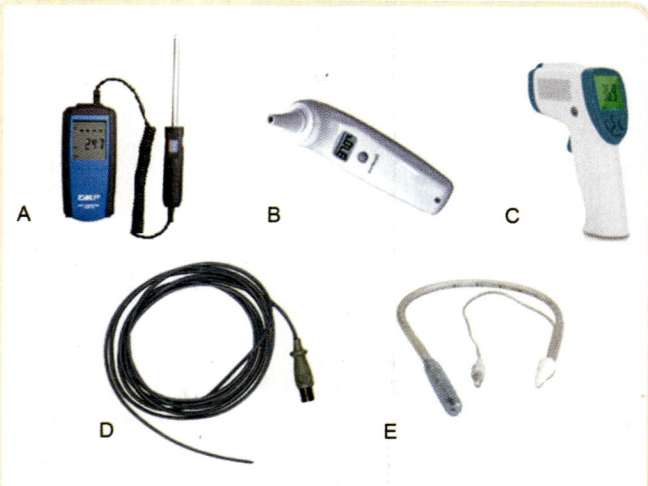

A. **Electronic thermometer:** For oral, axillary and rectal temperature measurement. Most widely used method. Measures body temperature in brief time between 4–20 seconds.

B. **Tympanic W temperature probe:** Placed in auditory canal. Detects body temperature radiated from the body. Used in children less than 6 years of age and for uncooperative patients. Determination time less than 2 seconds.

C. **Forehead/ Temporal artery temperature probe:** They are placed on the temporal artery (forehead or just behind the ear) and reads the infrared heat. Can be used in all age groups. Results are similar to rectal temperature measurement.

D. **Esophageal temperature probe:** Placed at the lower third of esophagus behind the heart where the heart sound is loudest.

E. **Esophageal stethoscope cum temperature probe:** Esophageal temperature probes are often combined with esophageal.